754

EDW

Genital Dermatology Atlas

SECOND EDITION

Genital Dermatology Atlas

Libby Edwards, MD

Chief of Dermatology
Carolinas Medical Center
Charlotte, North Carolina

Peter J. Lynch, MD

Frederick G. Novy Jr. Professor of Dermatology
Department of Dermatology
University of California, Davis
Sacramento, California

With contributions from

Sallie M. Neill, MD, FRCP

Consultant Dermatologist
St. Johns Institute of Dermatology
Guy's and St. Thomas' NHS Trust,
London, United Kingdom

Wolters Kluwer | Lippincott Williams & Wilkins
Health

Philadelphia • Baltimore • New York • London
Buenos Aires • Hong Kong • Sydney • Tokyo

Acquisitions Editor: Sonya Seigafuse
Product Manager: Kerry Barrett
Production Manager: Bridgett Dougherty
Senior Manufacturing Manager: Benjamin Rivera
Marketing Manager: Kim Schonberger
Design Coordinator: Stephen Druding
Production Service: MPS Limited, A Macmillan Company

530 Walnut Street
Philadelphia, PA 19106 USA
LWW.com

Printed in China

Library of Congress Cataloging-in-Publication Data

Genital dermatology atlas/edited by Libby Edwards, Peter J. Lynch; with contributions from Sallie M. Neill.—2nd ed.
      p. ; cm.
   Includes bibliographical references and index.
   ISBN 978-1-60831-079-1
   1. Genitourinary organs—Diseases—Atlases. 2. Skin—Diseases—Atlases. I. Edwards, Libby. II. Lynch, Peter J., 1936- III. Neill, Sarah M.
   [DNLM: 1. Genitalia—pathology—Atlases. 2. Skin Diseases—diagnosis—Atlases. 3. Genital Diseases, Female—diagnosis—Atlases. 4. Genital Diseases, Male—diagnosis—Atlases. WR 17 G331 2011]
   RC872.G46 2011
   616.5—dc22

                                                                     2010006910

To purchase additional copies of this book, call our customer service department at (800) 638-3030 or fax orders to (301) 223-2320. International customers should call (301) 223-2300.

Visit Lippincott Williams & Wilkins on the Internet: at LWW.com. Lippincott Williams & Wilkins customer service representatives are available from 8:30 AM to 6 PM, EST.

10 9 8 7 6 5 4 3 2

To my Aunt Sara, who brings me joy and comfort

and

To Marrise Phillips, who, for her whole life, has brought joy and comfort to her patients, family, and friends

Libby Edwards

To Barbara, my best friend and wife for nearly 50 years, to Deborah and Timothy, our wonderful children together with their families: your love and support are a glorious gift that gives my life meaning and happiness.

Peter Lynch

CONTENTS

Patients with disorders of the external genitalia are cared for by individuals with many different educational backgrounds: dermatologists, gynecologists, urologists, primary care physicians, nurse practioners, and physician assistants. Unfortunately, the training programs for each of these areas rarely provide the necessary educational preparation needed to offer the level of care that patients with genital disease want and deserve. This textbook, which is based on the authors' 70 years of combined experience, is designed to offer additional comprehensive, practical information that is needed to supplement whatever baseline knowledge is being brought to the clinic.

Making the correct diagnosis represents both the first and most important step in caring for these patients. Most disorders of the external genitalia are in the broadest sense dermatologic in nature. Those trained in areas other than dermatology are likely to have appreciable difficulty in recognizing any but the most common of these conditions. Moreover, because these diseases often have an atypical appearance due to their location in the warm, moist environment of the genital area, even dermatologists often experience diagnostic difficulty. For this reason, one of the key features of this book is the arrangement of information in a manner that provides immediate diagnostic help.

Conventional textbooks almost always present information organized by etiology or pathophysiology. In these books, diseases are arranged in sections such as "infectious diseases," "neoplastic diseases," etc. To use such a book, the clinician must a priori know what the diagnosis is before he or she can look up other relevant information such as laboratory evaluation and treatment options. In contradistinction, the information in our book is organized on the basis of clinical morphology. Once the appearance of the condition is determined, use of the diagnostic algorithm found in Chapter 2 quickly directs one to the chapter containing those disorders that constitute the differential diagnoses for the unrecognized disease. At that point, a short review of the photos and the narrative clinical information generally allows for identification of the single most likely diagnosis. Using this approach, it is even possible to correctly recognize a disease that one has never previously encountered!

Many genital diseases present with a variety of clinical appearances. To allow for correct diagnosis of these variants, such disorders are listed in multiple chapters with the main coverage being located in the chapter representing the most common presentation. The very large number of photos included in this book is also helpful in this regard, as this allows for visual depiction of the many clinical variants of these diseases. We have also included additional helpful material regarding normal anatomy (including common variants), symptoms (itching and pain), special considerations (immunosuppressive, psychologic, pediatric, and geriatric issues), basic diagnostic and therapeutic procedures, and patient handout material.

Libby Edwards, MD
Peter J. Lynch, MD

CHAPTER 1

Genital Anatomy

LIBBY EDWARDS

Dermatoses on genital skin often present differently than when occurring on extragenital dry, keratinized skin surfaces. Scaling is inapparent in damp skin folds, and some diseases, such as lichen sclerosus, preferentially affect modified mucous membrane skin rather than true mucous membrane. A knowledge of anatomy helps with the recognition of both normal structures and pathologic findings, as well as choices of therapy.

FEMALE GENITALIA

Vulva

The vulva consists of the mucocutaneous structures that compose the external female genitalia (Fig. 1-1 and Table 1-1). The vulva extends from the mons pubis anteriorly to the perineum posteriorly and from the crural folds laterally to the hymen and hymeneal ring medially.

The labia majora (singular = labium majus) are two fatty folds of skin that are derived from ectodermal tissues. The labia minora (singular = labium minus), medial to the labia majora, are much thinner folds of connective tissue and squamous epithelium. The vestibule, or introitus, is mucous membrane that extends from the medial origin of the labia minora to the hymeneal ring. The mons and labia majora cover and protect more delicate structures such as the clitoris, the clitoral hood, the labia minora, the vestibule, and the posterior fourchette, which is the posterior vestibule, extending to the perineal body.

The vulva exhibits several different types of epithelium. The lateral aspect of the labia majora is covered with dry, keratinized, conspicuously hair-bearing skin. Each hair follicle is part of a pilosebaceous unit comprising the follicle itself, its hair shaft, sebaceous gland, and the erector pili apparatus—a smooth muscle that contracts to form gooseflesh.

Although the medial aspect of the labia majora and the entire labia minora are generally considered to exhibit hairless mucous membrane epithelium, these areas actually are covered with partially keratinized skin that contains several structures, including subtle hair follicles. Numerous apocrine sweat glands lie on the modified mucous membranes of the labia minora, and ectopic sebaceous glands are often prominent, especially on the medial aspect of these skin folds. Sebaceous glands appear as small, yellow to white, lobular papules that occasionally enlarge to become nearly confluent (Figs. 1-2 and 1-3). A variably distinct line of demarcation (the Hart line) is evident at the base of the medial aspect of each labium minus, separating modified mucous membrane from the mucous membrane skin of the vestibule. The medial aspect of the labia majora and the entire labia minora display moist, partially keratinized modified mucous membrane. Mucosa, unkeratinized, non–hair-bearing epithelium with mucus-secreting glands, extends from the Hart line to and including the vagina and the external surface of the cervix. Mucosa is defined as ectodermal tissue that lines tubular structures and comprises the epithelium, basement membrane, lamina propria mucosa, and lamina muscularis mucosa. Mucous membrane skin also differs from keratinized squamous epithelium by the absence of a granular layer. In general, mucous membrane skin is non–hair-bearing epithelium that contains mucus-secreting glands. Both the vagina and the vestibule are mucosae, with surfaces that are variably wet (depending on estrogen status) as a result of mucous produced by associated glands and the cervix.

The vestibule, the innermost portion of the vulva, extends from the Hart line to the hymen. Variable numbers of mucus-secreting vestibular glands open onto the mucous membrane of this area. These glands are shallow pits lined with secretory cells; these primarily open circumferentially around the external aspect of the hymeneal ring and between the hymen and urethra (Fig. 1-4). They supplement lubrication in young, postpubertal women. Bartholin glands are paired glands that lie under the posterior portion of the vestibule, with duct openings just outside the hymen at the 5 and 7 o'clock positions. Skene glands exit into the distal urethra.

The vulva undergoes marked change from birth until puberty (see Chapter 14). The skin of the mons and the lateral labia majora is characterized by fine vellus hair at birth, but with puberty, coarse terminal hair appears. In addition, the labia minora are almost absent until puberty, and they enlarge at puberty. Apocrine glands become better developed with sexual maturity.

Normal Variants

Similar to the mucous membrane epithelia of the mouth and conjunctivae, mild erythema of the vulva and

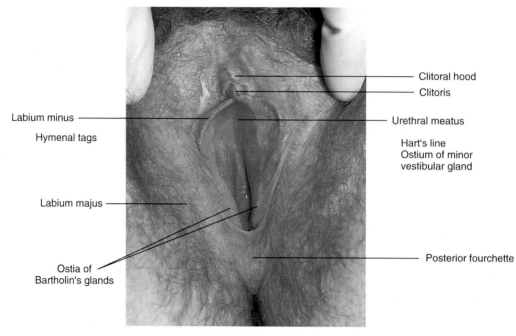

Clitoral hood
Clitoris
Urethral meatus
Hart's line
Ostium of minor
vestibular gland
Posterior fourchette
Labium minus
Hymenal tags
Labium majus
Ostia of
Bartholin's glands

FIG. 1-1. Normal vulva.

vagina is normal and varies from patient to patient. In one reported series of premenopausal women, 43% showed erythema (Fig. 1-5) (1). This redness is more evident in patients of light complexion, especially those with a naturally ruddy complexion. This finding is often misinterpreted by patients and their physicians as indicative of inflammation because the asymptomatic vulva is rarely examined critically. In addition, more than half of the women with vestibular erythema report no dyspareunia, but experience pain when the area is touched with a cotton-tipped applicator (the Q-tip test). This indicates that redness and a positive Q-tip test are normal findings and do not, alone and in the absence of real-life symptoms, constitute vulvodynia/vestibulodynia/vulvar vestibulitis syndrome.

Vulvar papillae (see Chapter 12) are also common normal variants, occurring in about one third of premenopausal women (Figs. 1-6 through 1-10). When these occur in the vestibule, they are called vestibular papillae. These variants are often mistaken for signs of disease, usually condylomata acuminata. Initial descriptions of vulvar papillomatosis reported biopsies consistent with human papillomavirus (HPV) infection as the cause. However, biopsies of even normal vulvar skin generally show large, clear keratinocytes that mimic koilocytes of HPV infection. More recent studies have evaluated for the

TABLE 1.1	Genital comparative anatomy
Female anatomy	**Male anatomy**
Glans of the clitoris	Dorsal aspect of the penis
Labia minora	Urethral folds
Labia majora	Scrotum
Urethra	Prostatic urethra
Paraurethral glands of Skene	Prostate gland
Bartholin glands	Bulbourethral glands of Cowper
Vestibular glands	Bulb of the penis
Minor vestibular glands	Glands of Littré

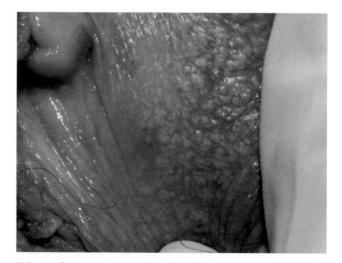

FIG. 1-2. Fordyce spots, which are enlarged sebaceous glands, occur on modified mucous membranes, particularly the medial aspect of the labia minora. These appear as multilobular, yellow-white papules.

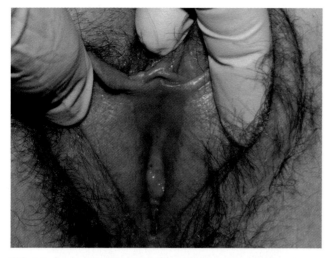

FIG. 1-3. Occasionally, sebaceous glands can be small and coalesce, forming almost sheetlike white plaques. This vulva also is a clear demonstration of Hart line, and the normal redness of the mucous membranes of the vulva.

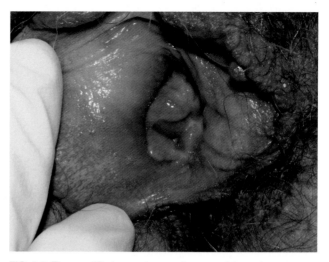

FIG. 1-5. The modified mucous membranes of the vulva are normally pink, in varying degrees. Patients with very light complexion, particularly red-headed women, tend to exhibit much deeper redness normally. Women, in general, do not examine the vulva except when symptoms occur, so they perceive this redness as indicative of inflammation in the setting of symptoms.

actual presence of the virus. The current consensus is that vestibular papillomatosis is a variant of normal, and this morphology is distinct from HPV infection (2,3). These small, filiform, soft, monomorphous, tubular projections are located symmetrically within the vestibule, whereas papillae of other areas of the vulva are more likely to be dome-shaped and less filiform. Vulvar papillae differ from condylomata acuminata by their rounded rather than acuminate tips, symmetric pattern, and discrete rather than fused base of adjacent lesions. Moreover,

genital warts are often keratinized and appear white in this moist area. Occasionally, similar dome-shaped, smooth papules that coalesce into a cobblestone texture to the inner labia minora occur in some women. Sometimes, these lesions form papules on the edge of the labia minora. These changes are also often mistaken for warts. Although vulvar papillae were once believed to produce itching or pain, they are now known to be asymptomatic.

The whitening of vulvar skin following the application of 5% acetic acid has been believed to be pathognomonic of HPV infection. However, this is a nonspecific finding occurring with any condition that produces hyperkeratosis or thickening of the skin. Some investigators have

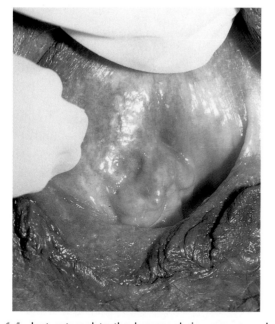

FIG. 1-4. Just external to the hymeneal ring are several pits *(arrows)* that represent openings to the vestibular glands. Occasionally, these can be found in other areas of the vestibule.

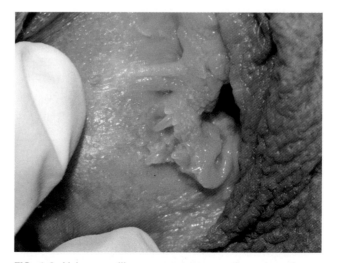

FIG. 1-6. Vulvar papillae are common on the vulva of premenopausal women and are found most often within the vestibule.

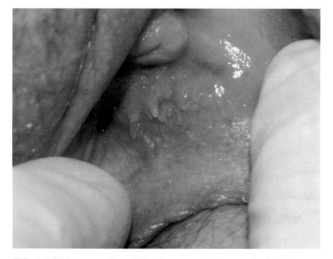

FIG. 1-7. Vulvar papillae differ from genital warts in their dome-shaped tips, symmetric distribution, and the discreteness of individual papillae, rather than being fused at the base, as occurs with genital warts.

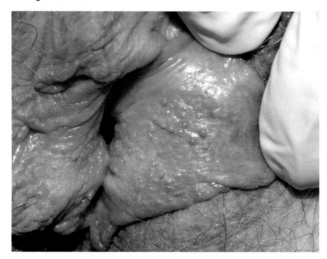

FIG. 1-8. Occasionally, vulvar papillae occur outside the vestibule, and they can occur in small patches of one or two lesions, rather than larger patches or lines.

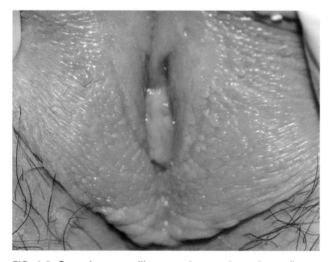

FIG. 1-9. Sometimes, papillae are short and nearly confluent, producing a cobblestone texture to the skin.

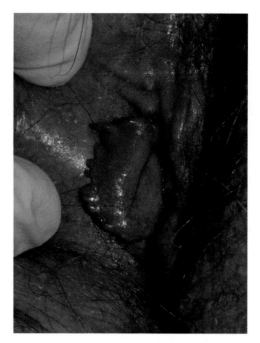

FIG. 1-10. Although vulvar papillae are found most often in the vestibule, they can occur on the labia minora, as seen here.

found that 5% acetic acid predictably produces acetowhitening of all vulvar skin (1).

Labia minora exhibit wide morphologic variability. These folds of skin can be large and pendulous, so small as to be nearly absent, or very asymmetric (Figs. 1-11 through 1-15). The anterior origin of the labia minora is the frenulum of the clitoris, but often the anterior origin is bifid, with a contribution from the skin lateral to the clitoral hood

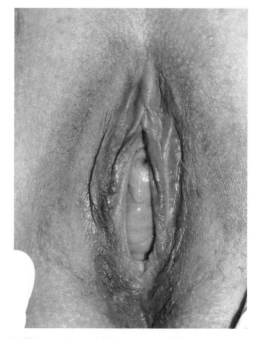

FIG. 1-11. This patient exhibits very small but symmetrical labia minora.

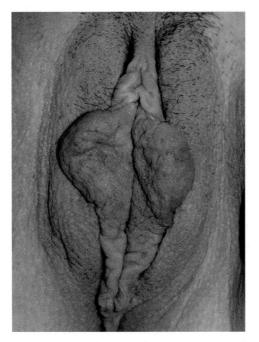

FIG. 1-12. This teenager has very large labia minora that protrude beyond the labia majora.

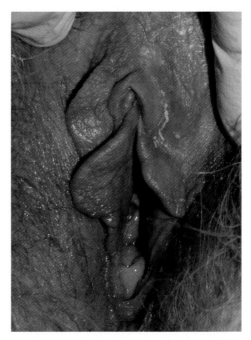

FIG. 1-14. Often, the labia minora originate with the frenulum of the clitoral hood. Sometimes, the labia minora attach at other areas of the vulva.

(Fig. 1-14). In addition, there is variability of the clitoral hood and the clitoris. In some, the clitoral hood is thick and redundant, and in other, the clitoral hood is thin, with the clitoris partially exposed. Adhesions of the clitoris to the clitoral hood are sometimes a sign of a previous scarring dermatosis; however, this is a normal finding in as many as one in four young women, with the youngest women most likely to be affected (4).

Physiologic hyperpigmentation of the vulva is common, especially in women with a darker natural complexion, patients who are pregnant, and women with systemic hormone exposure (Figs. 1-13 and 1-16). This discoloration is generally poorly demarcated and is located symmetrically on the lateral edges of the labia minora, on the perianal skin, and sometimes on the hair-bearing portion of the labia majora.

Although sebaceous glands on the modified mucous membrane skin of the vulva are regularly present in premenopausal women, some women exhibit unusually large or numerous sebaceous glands, called Fordyce spots (see Chapter 8). This finding is an asymptomatic normal variant that is occasionally mistaken for genital warts. However, the distribution, yellowish color, and lobular, monomorphous pattern are diagnostic for sebaceous glands.

Often, because very small hair follicles are present on the labia minora, firm, white, or yellowish epidermal cysts and comedones are relatively common (Fig. 1-17). These are unimportant unless they become secondarily inflamed.

Small, purple or red papules called angiokeratomas (see also Chapter 7) represent common, medically unimportant benign blood vessel tumors that occur on the labia majora (Figs. 1-18 and 1-19).

Vagina

The vagina is a tube that connects the introitus to the cervix. This structure is covered by squamous mucous membrane skin, and it is a potential space that is flattened with the anterior and posterior walls in contact. The

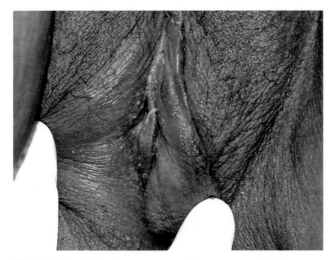

FIG. 1-13. The labia minora are very often asymmetric. They may be asymmetric in shape or in size, as seen here, with the left labium minus much larger than the right.

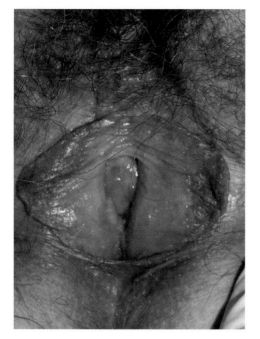

FIG. 1-15. The labia minora can also fuse posteriorly.

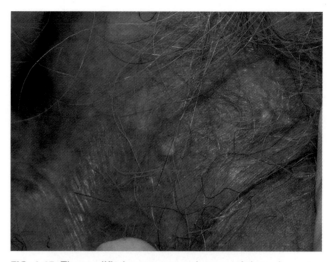

FIG. 1-17. The modified mucous membranes of the vulva actually contain vestigial hair follicles that sometimes become blocked with desquamated epithelium (comedone), resulting in the underlying distention of the underlying follicle, which enlarges to form epidermal cysts. There are three white epidermal cysts on this labium minus.

vaginal epithelium of estrogen-deficient prepubertal girls and many postmenopausal women is pale, smooth, dry, and fragile, whereas well-estrogenized women normally exhibit pink, wet, resilient vaginal skin that forms folds, or rugae. Postmenopausal women who are sexually active often have skin that does not appear estrogen deficient.

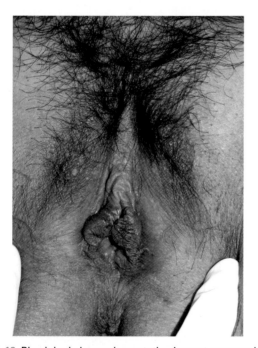

FIG. 1-16. Physiologic hyperpigmentation is most common in patients who have naturally dark complexion or who have recently experienced hormonal changes by virtue of pregnancy or therapy. The labia minora and, sometimes, the posterior fourchette are the most commonly involved areas.

The cervix normally lies in the proximal anterior wall of the vagina, and the small pouch between the posterior cervix and the apex of the vagina is called the cul de sac.

The vagina is rich with colonizing organisms. Predominant organisms in the well-estrogenized vagina are *Lactobacillus* and *Corynebacterium* species. Because of the lactic acid produced by lactobacilli, vaginal secretions are normally acidic, showing a pH of 3.5 to 5. Other organisms include *Streptococcus*, *Bacteroides*, *Staphylococcus*, and *Peptostreptococcus*. A recent study showed that 21% of asymptomatic women were found to harbor *Candida albicans* as well, and after antibiotic use, this number increased to 37% (5).

A nonspecific reaction to inflammation in the vagina is monomorphous red 1 to 2 mm macules, analogous to the "strawberry cervix" characteristic of trichomonas.

Normal Variants

The vaginal mucosa, like the vulva, exhibits varying degrees of normal erythema, which can be difficult to use as a measure of inflammation. One method for evaluating subtle vaginal abnormalities is by a microscopic examination of vaginal secretions (see Chapter 15). More than one white blood cell per epithelial cells suggests the presence of inflammation.

The vaginal walls vary from one patient to another. Rugae can be subtle, or very folded. Occasionally, papillomatosis can occur in the vagina. Although vaginal HPV infection should be investigated, diffuse disease can also be a normal finding with negative HPV probes, and requires no therapy.

A major tool for the evaluation of the vagina is a microscopic examination of vaginal secretions. Secretions

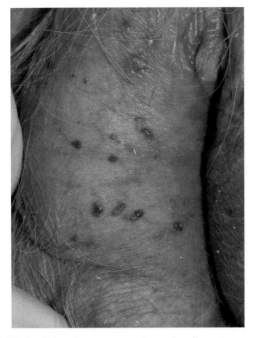

FIG. 1-18. Angiokeratomas are red-purple, discrete, asymptomatic papules that are common on the vulva.

result from mucus, desquamated epithelial cells, and bacteria. Normal estrogenized vaginal secretions microscopically reveal large, mature, flattened, epithelial cells with small nuclei, multiple rods representing lactobacilli, and one or fewer leukocytes per epithelial cell. The borders of the epithelial cells should be crisp and sharp, without the

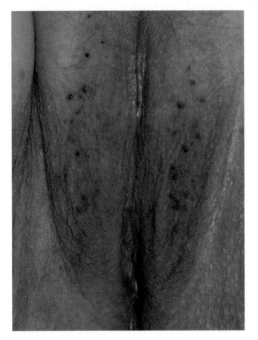

FIG. 1-19. The hair-bearing portion of the labia majora is the most common location for angiokeratomas, and these sometimes are so dark as to appear black.

ragged, granular appearance of a clue cell indicative of bacterial vaginosis. Fungal elements and *Trichomonas* should be absent. The pH of vaginal secretions should be lower than 5.

MALE GENITALIA

Genital disease of males occurs differently in circumcised men as compared to uncircumcised men, and the appearance of normal skin and normal structures is different as well. Skin disease is far less common in the uncircumcised man, with circumcision being curative for several diseases such as lichen sclerosus and balanitis plasmacellularis (the Zoon balanitis).

The male genitalia encompass the pubis anteriorly, the perineum posteriorly, the scrotum posterolaterally, and the penis medially.

Penis

The male and female genitalia exhibit analogous structures (see Table 1-1). In contrast to the female external genitalia, in which the urethra and the vagina are independent, the penis is a shaft that contains the urethra, the common outlet for urine and semen (Fig. 1-20). The penis is composed of ectodermal, mesodermal, and endodermal structures. Three major cylindric erectile structures are enclosed by a dense white fibrous capsule, the tunica albuginea. These three structures are the paired dorsal bodies, called the corpora cavernosa, and the ventral, midline corpus spongiosum. The urethra runs through the root and body of the penis. At the distal aspect of the penis is the glans penis, and the border of the glans is called the corona, separating the glans from the shaft. The shaft of the penis is covered by keratinized epithelium, and modified mucous membrane skin is found on the glans. The slitlike opening at the distal tip of the glans is the external urethral meatus.

At the distal aspect of the penis, the overlying mucosa is infolded to form the prepuce (foreskin); the prepuce, in turn, covers the glans. Circumcision is the surgical removal of the prepuce. There have been heated debates for years regarding the benefits and risks of circumcision. Pain and possible infection in newborn boys have been weighed against the risk of squamous cell carcinoma in uncircumcised men (slight, but much higher than the risk in circumcised men) and the difficulty of hygiene. More recently, dermatoses such as psoriasis, erosive lichen planus, and lichen sclerosus have been shown to occur almost exclusively on the uncircumcised penis, and circumcision protects against both sexually transmitted diseases and candidiasis (6). On the ventral aspect of the glans is the median fold or raphe, which extends from inferior to the opening of

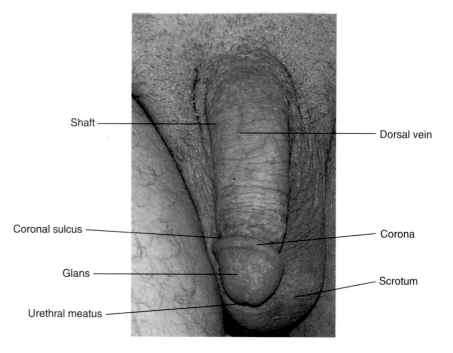

Shaft —

Coronal sulcus —

Glans —

Urethral meatus —

— Dorsal vein

— Corona

— Scrotum

FIG. 1-20. Normal penis with landmarks indicated.

the urethra to the base of the glans and represents the area of fusion.

At birth, the mons pubis, the fatty pad of tissue anterior to penis and scrotum, is characterized by fine, vellus hair. As puberty approaches, terminal hair develops. In addition, apocrine glands become better developed at this time. The modified mucosa of the penis contains both apocrine and eccrine sweat glands, but only rarely are pilosebaceous structures evident.

Normal Variants

Ectopic sebaceous glands (Tyson glands) are found commonly on the shaft of the penis (Fig. 1-21). These lobular, skin-colored papules are sometimes mistaken for

genital warts or mollusca contagiosa (7). In addition, pearly penile papules are found in up to 34% of uncircumcised men (Figs. 1-22 and 1-23) (8). These are small (1- to 2-mm) soft, monomorphous, flesh-colored papules that occur in rows around the edge of the corona (see Chapter 12). Sometimes, there are several parallel rows. These papules are sometimes elongated into papillae with

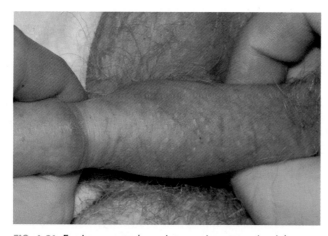

FIG. 1-21. Fordyce spots (prominent sebaceous glands) occur on the penile shaft at times and can resemble genital warts, except for their monomorphous appearance. (Courtesy of Errol Craig, MD.)

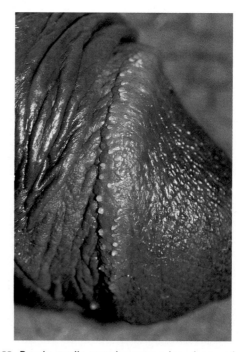

FIG. 1-22. Pearly penile papules occur in a large minority of uncircumcised men and are sometimes confused with genital warts.

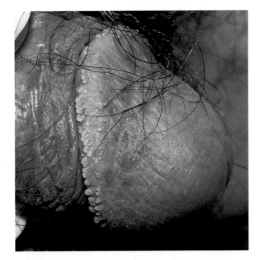

FIG. 1-23. Pearly penile papules can be differentiated from genital warts by the monomorphous, symmetric appearance and by the finding that each is discrete. These papules are most often located on the corona in circumferential, parallel rows.

rounded tips. Rarely, pearly penile papules can occur on the glans or shaft of the penis, where the diagnosis is less obvious. Like vestibular papillomatosis, pearly penile papules have been mistaken for HPV infection, but these monomorphous papules in a characteristic distribution have been found to have no association with this viral infection. For those men wanting treatment of these lesions for cosmetic reasons, CO_2 laser has been reported beneficial (9) as has been cryotherapy (10).

At times, hair follicles on the shaft are prominent, making differentiation from warts, Tyson glands, and pearly penile papules of the shaft difficult.

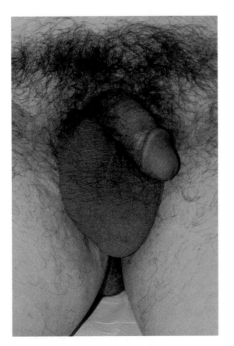

FIG. 1-24. Physiologic hyperpigmentation is most common on the scrotum. (Courtesy of Errol Craig, MD.)

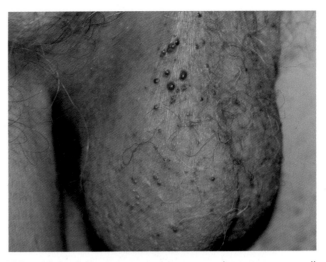

FIG. 1-25. Angiokeratomas are common on the scrotum as well as on the vulva, and they are asymptomatic in both locations.

Scrotum

The scrotum consists of two sacs that are separated by a septum and covered with keratinized squamous epithelium. The testicles rest within the sacs, attached by the vas deferens. The scrotum, from the outside in, consists of an outer skin layer, the dartos (smooth) muscle, the external spermatic fascia with the cremasteric (skeletal) muscle, the internal spermatic fascia, and the tunica vaginalis.

Normal Variants

Ridges or folds of skin called rugae are common on the scrotum, although some men exhibit smooth scrotal skin. The scrotum is variably red, with many showing skin-colored epithelium, others exhibiting erythema, and still others being hyperpigmented (Fig. 1-24). As occurs in women, redness may not be appreciated until the patient

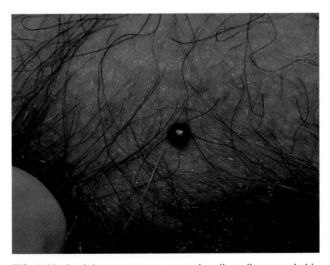

FIG. 1-26. Angiokeratomas are occasionally solitary, and this plus a very dark color suggests an erroneous diagnosis of a nevus or nodular melanoma in this man.

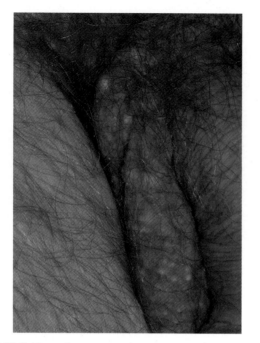

FIG. 1-27. Epidermal cysts sometimes occur on the scrotum as a normal finding, manifested as small, firm white nodules.

experiences symptoms, and both the patient and health care provider misinterpret this redness as a pathologic sign of inflammation.

Red-purple angiokeratomas, 1 to 5 mm in diameter, are also common and innocuous (Figs. 1-25 and 1-26), and some men exhibit skin-colored or white, firm nodules of inconsequential scrotal epidermal cysts (Fig. 1-27).

REFERENCES

1. van Beurden M, van der Vange N, de Craen AJ, et al. Normal findings in vulvar examination and vulvoscopy. *Br J Obstet Gynaecol.* 1997;104:320–324.
2. Micheletti L, Preti M, Bogliatto F, et al. Vestibular papillomatosis. *Miverva Ginecol.* 2000;52(suppl. 1):87–91.
3. Beznos G, Coates V, Focchi J, et al. Biomolecular study of the correlation between papillomatosis of the vulvar vestibule in adolescents and human papillomavirus. *Scientific World Journal.* 2006;12:6:628–636.
4. Wiesmeier E, Masongsong EV, Wiley DJ. The prevalence of examiner-diagnosed clitoral hood adhesions in a population of college-aged women. *J Low Genit Tract Dis.* 2008;12:307–310.
5. Pirotta MV, Garland SM. Genital *Candida* species detected in samples from women in Melbourne, Australia, before and after treatment with antibiotics. *J Clin Microbiol.* 2006;44: 3213–3217.
6. Morris BJ. Why circumcision is a biomedical imperative for the 21(st) century. *Bioessays.* 2007;29:1147–1158.
7. Ena P, Origa D, Massarelli G. Sebaceous gland hyperplasia of the foreskin. *Clin Exp Dermatol.* 2009;34:372–374.
8. Hogewoning CJ, Bleeker MC, van den Brule AJ, et al. Pearly penile papules: still no reason for uneasiness. *J Am Acad Dermatol.* 2003;49:50–54.
9. Lane JE, Peterson CM, Ratz JL. Treatment of pearly penile papules with CO_2 laser. *Dermatol Surg.* 2002;28:617–618.
10. Porter WM, Bunker CB. Treatment of pearly penile papules with cryotherapy. *Br J Dermatol.* 2000;142:847–848.

SUGGESTED READING

Agrawal SK, Bhattacharya SN, Singh N. Pearly penile papules: a review. *Int J Dermatol.* 2004;43:199–201.

CHAPTER 2

Principles of Genital Diagnosis and Therapy

PETER J. LYNCH

GENERAL PRINCIPLES OF DIAGNOSIS

Correct diagnosis is the sine qua non for the care of any patient with any disorder. If you don't know the diagnosis you can't establish the cause, provide the prognosis, or institute appropriate therapy. For patients with mucocutaneous disease a working diagnosis is almost always first established on the basis of clinical symptoms and signs. If necessary, this clinical diagnosis can subsequently be confirmed through procedures such as biopsy, cytology, and microbial culture (see Chapter 3).

There are two major approaches to using clinical symptoms and signs to establish a working diagnosis: the use of visual memory and the use of a morphologically determined diagnostic algorithm. Dermatologists by virtue of repeated exposure to patients with both common and uncommon diseases almost always depend on visual memory. And, because it works for them, they consistently use that same approach when teaching medical students and other clinicians. Thus, in the classroom or at continuing medical education courses, they bombard their audience with clinical photo after clinical photo, leaving the participants with a jumbled mass of impossible to remember images of skin disease.

The use of visual memory works for the dermatologist because of sufficient, repetitive exposure to these diseases. But other clinicians, encountering fewer patients with mucocutaneous disorders, lack the opportunity for sufficient visual reinforcement to dependably recognize uncommon and rare diseases. By analogy, they are put in the position of someone attending a large gathering where they know few of the guests. In spite of many introductions, the names of those they have met quickly disappear from memory. At best, on subsequent encounter, one might remember the face as vaguely familiar but find it impossible to identify the person by name. The same problem occurs for the nondermatologist in a clinical setting. In this situation, when faced with an unrecognized mucocutaneous disorder, one might futilely turn to a standard dermatology textbook but find that the diseases in it are organized on the basis of etiology or pathophysiology. This is, of course, of no help, as one must know the diagnosis first before it is possible to make use of the material contained in such a book. As a last resort one might then end up paging through an atlas hoping to stumble on a disease that matches what was just found on examination of the patient. At best this offers a hit or miss approach and even when it is helpful, it is an inefficient and mostly inaccurate approach to diagnosis.

A better diagnostic approach for the nondermatologist is the use of a diagnostic algorithm in which the diseases are organized on the basis of clinical morphology. This type of diagnostic algorithm directs the clinician to a cluster of diseases that share similarities in appearance. Once having arrived at the correct group of diseases, reading a small amount of text describing the characteristic diagnostic features together with perusal of the associated clinical photos for each disease within that group allows one to arrive at a likely diagnosis that then can be confirmed by a biopsy or other diagnostic test. Importantly, this approach even allows a clinician to make a correct diagnosis of a disorder that he or she has never previously encountered.

Of course, to use a morphologic approach like this, one must be able to describe in dermatologic terms the features that one has seen on examination. This is not very difficult because, as is true for most "foreign" languages, a relatively small number of words can serve one's basic needs. The dermatologic words that are required for this approach together with the diagnostic algorithm that uses them (Table 2-1) are contained below.

As is true in all fields of medicine, history and physical examination represent the first two steps in diagnosis; they are covered in this chapter. A third step, that of utilizing diagnostic procedures to confirm a clinical diagnosis, is covered in the next chapter.

Initial Approach to the Patient: History and Physical Examination

There are at least two good approaches that can be used in obtaining the initial history. Some clinicians prefer using a questionnaire that can be completed by the patient either at home or in the office prior to first contact with the clinician. One of us (LE) utilizes this approach and she has made her questionnaire available at her online site, www.libbyedwardsmd.com. This may be downloaded, modified, and subsequently used by any clinician. This approach allows the patient to express what he or she feels is important and minimizes any discomfort a patient may have about beginning a discussion

TABLE 2.1	Algorithm for the diagnosis of genital disorders

Are there visible changes?

No, only symptoms are present
   1) Pruritus   See Chapter 4
   2) Pain   See Chapter 5

Yes, visible changes are present

   Nearly all of the lesional epithelium is lifted
      (blistered) or missing
      3) Pustules   See Chapter 8
      4) Blisters and/or erosions   See Chapter 9
      5) Ulcers   See Chapter 10
   Lesions are red, with or without erosions or
      excoriations
      6) Red patches and plaques   See Chapters 4
                                          and 6
      7) Red papules and nodules   See Chapter 7
   Lesions are some color other than red
      8) Skin-colored lesions   See Chapter 12
      9) White lesions   See Chapter 11
      10) Brown, blue, and
             black lesions   See Chapter 13

about genital and/or sexual problems. Alternatively, one of us (PJL) takes the initial history after the patient is placed in the examination room but, importantly, before the patient is asked to disrobe. With either alternative a more directed history is then taken during or after the examination.

The two key points in examination of patients with genital problems are exposure and illumination. First, in a misguided attempt to protect patient modesty, some clinicians erroneously allow the patient to determine the extent of clothing to be removed. This leads patients to believe that they can simply pull underwear partially down or to one side whereas, in fact, all clothing covering the anogenital area must be completely removed.

Second, nearly all examinations should take place with the patient lying supine on the examination table. Women can then be examined either in a "frog leg" position or with their feet in stirrups. The latter is preferred as it allows for good visualization of the anal area. Men are usually examined the "frog leg" position as they fairly strenuously resist being placed in stirrups. For men, the anal area can be examined either with the patient rolled to his side or with him standing but bending forward over the examination table. It cannot be emphasized strongly enough: the genital area in men cannot be adequately examined with the patient seated or standing.

Good lighting is required for all examinations. This requires use of a light separate from a fixed ceiling light: one that is adequately bright and that is flexible enough so that it can be moved to illuminate every aspect of the anogenital region. Needless to say, except in extraordinary circumstances examination of a patient of the sex opposite to that of the clinician should be carried out in the presence of a chaperone.

Definition of Dermatologic Terms

The definitions included here are very similar, though not necessarily identical, to those found in standard dermatology textbooks. The differences, where they occur, will not significantly interfere with the use of the diagnostic algorithm that follows.

Macule. A macule is a small (1.5 cm or less), nonelevated, nonpalpable area of color change. The surface of macules is usually smooth, though a small amount of powdery scale may be present.

Patch. A patch is a larger (greater than 1.5 cm), nonelevated, nonpalpable area of color change. It may be considered as a two-dimensional (length and width) increase in the size of a macule. Again, the surface is usually smooth but sometimes a small amount of powdery scale may be present.

Papule. A papule is a small (1.5 cm or less) palpable lesion. Usually, but not always, a papule is visibly elevated above the surface of the surrounding tissue. A palpable lesion contained within the skin is a papule whether or not it is visibly elevated. A papule may be considered as a one-dimensional (lesional thickness) increase in the size of a macule. Papules may be either smooth or rough surfaced. Roughness on the surface of a papule is due to the presence of either scale or crust.

Plaque. A plaque is a large (greater than 1.5 cm) flat-topped, palpable lesion. It may be considered as a two-dimensional (length and width) increase in the size of a papule. Plaques are usually, but not always, elevated above the surface of the surrounding tissue. As for papules, intracutaneous lesions that are palpable are termed plaques whether or not they are elevated. Likewise, plaques may be smooth or rough surfaced. Roughness on the surface of a plaque is due to the presence of scale or crust.

Nodule. A nodule is a large (greater than 1.5 cm) dome-shaped, palpable lesion. It may be considered as a three-dimensional (length, width, and depth) increase in the size of a papule. Nodules are usually smooth surfaced.

Vesicle. A vesicle is a small (1.0 cm or less) fluid-filled blister. It may be considered as a fluid-filled papule in which the fluid is loculated. Fluid-filled papules in which the fluid is nonloculated are known as *wheals*. Vesicles and wheals are differentiated clinically by the observation that when the surface of a blister is pierced, the fluid runs out and the blister collapses. When a wheal is pierced, a drop of fluid may appear on the surface but the papule remains as it was before the piercing. When the surface of a vesicle has been removed or has disintegrated, an erosion is left.

Pustule. A pustule is a vesicle that contains visibly purulent (pus-filled) fluid. That is, the lesion appears opaquely white, yellow, or yellow-white. This color occurs as a result of the presence of packed neutrophils and other white blood cells. Note that a vesicle may turn cloudy as it ages. This change does not make it a pustule. To be a pustule, a blister must have been purulent from the time of its inception.

Bulla (plural: bullae). A bulla is a large (greater than 1.0 cm) vesicle. Here too, the fluid is loculated. Usually the fluid is found in a single compartment occupying the whole of the lesion but, uncommonly, coalescence of closely set vesicles occurs to form a multiloculated bulla.

Erosion. An erosion is a shallow defect in the surface of the skin. In this context "shallow" means the epidermis is missing but the defect does not extend more deeply into the dermal component of the skin. The base of an erosion may be red and moist or the base may be covered with crust. In an erosion any crust that is present is yellow in color and is crumbly and easily removed. Erosions occur as the result of two mechanisms. They can develop subsequent to trauma, most often as a result of scratching. Erosions due to trauma are usually linear or angular in appearance. Alternatively, erosions may occur when the roof of a blister is removed or disintegrates. Such erosions are usually round and generally have a thin peripheral rim of scale. This is called "collarette" scale and it occurs as a result of fragments of the peripheral blister roof that remain intact at the edge of a previous blister.

Fissure. A fissure is a subtype of an erosion in which a thin (less than 1 mm wide), linear crack occurs into or through the epithelium. A fissure appears clinically as a thin red line and possibly may not be recognized as a true defect in the surface of the skin unless a magnifying lens is used. Fissures generally arise in the setting of an epithelial surface that is too dry. They are analogous to the cracked surface present in the bed of a dried pond or stream.

Ulcer. An ulcer is a deep defect in the surface of the skin. The defect is deeper than that of an erosion and extends into, or even through, the dermal connective tissue. Such a defect involves significant blood vessel damage and, as a result, the base of an ulcer may contain crust that includes heme pigment as well as plasma proteins. Such crust may be red, blue, or black. When considerable fibrin is present as well, the crust is very adherent to the base of the ulcer; such crust is known as "eschar."

Scale and crust. Scale is due to excess keratin on the surface of a lesion. It generally occurs as a result of epithelial hyperproliferation. The presence of scale indicates that the epithelial surface is intact. Scale is usually visible as gray, white, or silver "flakes" on the surface of a lesion. However, sometimes, especially on moist surfaces, scale is not visible at all and is only recognized as being present when a slight sense of roughness is palpable on the surface of a lesion. Crust is due to the presence of plasma proteins left after the water component of plasma has evaporated. It occurs as a result of an epithelial defect (erosion or ulcer). Crust is always visible and is usually yellow but may be red, blue, or black if heme pigment is present.

Margination. Margination refers to the zone of transition between normal and lesional tissue as would be visualized in a cross-sectional view of the lesion. This transition can be very distinct (sharply marginated) or somewhat indistinct (poorly, or diffusely marginated). Margination can be helpful in distinguishing the papulosquamous diseases such as psoriasis from the eczematous diseases such as atopic dermatitis.

Configuration. Configuration refers to the shape of the lesions when viewed from above. Most often, this shape is round or slightly oval. Gyrate (serpiginous) margination occurs in urticaria whereas linear and angular shapes suggest a traumatic etiology, especially that due to scratching.

Eczema. In this book, "eczema" is used synonymously with "dermatitis." Both refer to a pattern of disease characterized by the presence of red, scaling, poorly marginated papules and plaques displaying evidence of epithelial disruption. Epithelial disruption is identified by the presence of visible excoriations, fissures, weeping, crusting, and/or yellow-colored scale (see Chapter 4). Note, although we disagree with this usage, some clinicians use the term "eczema" as a synonym for "atopic dermatitis."

Lichenification. Lichenification refers to the presence of thickened, rough surfaced (scaling) skin with prominent skin markings. It occurs as a callus-like response due to chronic rubbing. Lichenification is characteristically seen in the two related conditions of atopic dermatitis and lichen simplex chronicus (see Chapter 4).

The Diagnostic Algorithm

In order to use the diagnostic algorithm, the clinician must accurately describe the lesion that was found on clinical examination. If more than one lesion was present, the description should be of the most prototypical lesion. This description needs to be in "standard dermatologic language" using the terms discussed in the section "Definition of Dermatologic Terms." In carrying out this description, it is helpful to start with whatever noun (macule, patch, papule, plaque, etc.) is most appropriate. Once the noun (primary lesion) is determined, one can then insert the necessary adjectives describing color, margination, surface characteristics, configuration, and degree of firmness on palpation. It is helpful to actually write down the description so that salient points are not overlooked or forgotten.

When the description is completed, it is easy to place the unidentified disease into one of the 10 categories (groups) listed in the diagnostic algorithm (Table 2-1).

Once that is done one simply refers to the chapter related to that category. A quick perusal of the disease discussed in that chapter allows the clinician to then put together a short list of differential diagnoses. Additional reading about each of the diseases on this short list almost always allows for identification of the single most likely diagnosis. The algorithm presented here is a simplified one designed for identification of genital diseases by nondermatologists. An earlier algorithm for genital disorders (1) and a more detailed algorithmic approach to the diagnosis of the 100 most common and important general dermatologic diseases can be found elsewhere (2,3).

GENERAL PRINCIPLES OF THERAPY

This section deals only with general therapeutic principles; the specifics of individual therapeutic agents and their use for a particular disorder are contained with the discussion of the diseases as they occur throughout this book.

One of the guiding principles of medical therapy is the recognition that a disease is occurring in an individual rather than existing as a separate, localized problem. This is particularly true for patients with genital disease where there are immense psychological, social, and sexual repercussions associated with every problem occurring in this region of the body. For instance, patients are highly likely to have a perception that negligence on their part regarding something they were responsible for, such as sexual activity or hygiene, led to the development of their problem. This, of course, may or may not be actually true. Therefore, look for the presence of anxiety, depression, guilt, or other aspects of psychological dysfunction in all patients with anogenital disorders. Offer support and counseling to include assistance in obtaining help by others where the magnitude of the problem warrants it. Failure to recognize the patient as a person is very likely to compromise the therapeutic outcome even when the disease itself is identified and treated correctly.

GENERAL CONSIDERATIONS

Environmental Factors

The anogenital area represents a very hostile environment for normal function of the mucocutaneous epithelial cells that make up the barrier between us and the outside world. Some of the detrimental factors that are involved include heat, sweat, vaginal secretion, urine, feces, clothing, friction, and excessive hygiene. These factors can cause disease, worsen minor problems, and retard normal healing.

Epithelial cells can generally withstand rather high temperatures but, unfortunately, with heat comes sweating. And sweat can be remarkably irritating as exemplified by the discomfort experienced when sweat gets in our eyes during exercise. The retention of sweat leads to maceration and this in turn leads to damage and possibly death of epithelial cells. This damage to the epithelial barrier allows the exposure of cutaneous nerve endings and results in symptoms of pruritus and/or pain. The presence of this warmth and moisture also fosters the overgrowth, and sometimes infections due to bacteria and *Candida* sp. Obesity, tight clothing, and prolonged sitting (especially on vinyl or plastic seats) are often responsible for such maceration. Improvement can be obtained with modification of these factors but at the practical level, this is difficult to achieve.

In women, vaginal discharge (whether physiologic or pathologic) and/or urinary incontinence cause irritation with subsequent inflammation and damage to epithelial cells. The end result is similar to that described for sweat retention. To make matters worse, women with urinary incontinence or vaginal discharge often turn to the use of panty liners on a continual basis. The cause of such vaginal secretions (see Chapter 15) should be determined and treated appropriately. Incontinence may require urologic consultation. In both sexes, fecal soiling can lead to irritation. More careful cleaning after defecation is desirable so that sweat does not liquefy and spread fecal material. Usually, careful use of ordinary toilet paper is sufficient but if that causes too much irritation, Cetaphil cleanser, mineral oil, or vegetable oil can be used for anal cleansing.

In terms of clothing, a change from tight pants (especially jeans) to looser fitting clothing can be helpful as is the use of cotton or cotton blend underwear. In spite of the frequent admonition to use only white undergarments, color of the underwear has not been demonstrated to be of any particular importance. Hair dryers, even at their lowest settings, should not be used for purposes of drying. It is our opinion that changes in laundering practices, such as double rinsing and avoidance of antistatic products, are not helpful.

Excessive hygiene, especially in women, is frequently overlooked as an environmental irritant. Hygienic practices are rarely volunteered by patients and are infrequently asked about by clinicians. More than twice daily cleansing of the anogenital area is unnecessary and is usually detrimental. Soap and water applied with the hands or with a washcloth suffices; scrubbing is never warranted. A hand-held showerhead can be used by those who are too obese to otherwise reach the anogenital area.

Additional information on environmental irritation can be found in the section "Irritant Contact Dermatitis" in Chapter 4.

Soaks

Soaks serve several purposes. First, they can offer symptomatic relief for symptoms such as pruritus and pain. Second, they offer a gentle approach to the debridement of any crust that is present. This removal of crust decreases bacterial and yeast overgrowth and removes a mechanical impediment to wound healing. Third, soaks temporarily restore a physiologic, moist environment that enhances epithelial healing. Fourth, soaks are one of the few approaches to therapy that can safely, appropriately, and usefully be suggested by telephone before one has the opportunity to examine the patient.

Dermatologists historically have made somewhat of a fetish out of ordering esoteric and complicated solutions for soaks. But in reality soaks can be accomplished very simply by filling a bathtub with ordinary tap water. The water temperature should be comfortably warm rather than very hot or very cold. Nothing further needs to be added to the water and in fact many of the products sold for such purpose make the floor of the bathtub dangerously slippery. Soaking should occur for a period of 15 or 20 minutes, following which the skin should be patted, rather than rubbed, dry. The soothing effect of a soak is lost within about 30 minutes as the water evaporates from the outer layers of the skin, but this can be delayed by the prompt application of a lubricant (see below). Soaks may be repeated several times per day if the severity of the patient's pain or itching requires it.

Soaks should be considered as "first aid" and not as something to be continued indefinitely. After several days of soaks, weeping and crusting should be markedly diminished, and there will usually be no further improvement in pain or pruritus. Moreover, prolonged use may lead to a detrimental excess drying effect on the epithelium. A perceived need for longer use of soaks generally suggests that the therapeutic plan may require revision.

General Aspects of Topical Therapy

Vehicles. Most products are available as creams or ointments. In the genital area, ointments are generally preferred because they are rarely accompanied by irritation and burning as often happens with creams. It is rarely appropriate to use gels, lotions, or solutions because of their irritating propensity.

Amount to be applied. Most patients have no idea how much of a topical product should be used for any one application. It is reasonable to suggest use of an amount about the size of a lead pencil eraser (~0.2 g). That amount, spread appropriately thinly, will cover all of the external genitalia. Nearly all products are most appropriately applied twice daily.

Site of application. Patients are often uncertain as to just where the product should be applied. Instructions in this regard should be given not only verbally but also by demonstration, using a patient-held mirror if the site is not otherwise visible to the patient.

Amount to be dispensed. Since an amount about the size of a lead pencil eraser (0.2 g), or even smaller, is applied each time, a 30-g tube would theoretically last 2 months

for most anogenital disorders. In practical terms, given waste and overapplication, a 30 g tube lasts about 1 month. Most products are available in larger sizes (60 to 80 g), and it may be economical to dispense these larger sizes if the patient is educated as to how long such an amount should last.

Lubrication

Epithelial cells are very sensitive to the amount of moisture in and around them. In the section above, we indicated that too much moisture leads to maceration and cell death. Epithelial cells are also very sensitive to too little moisture. When evaporative loss occurs faster than it is replaced by the underlying interstitial fluid, epithelial cells shrink in size and pull apart. This causes disruption of the barrier layer located in the outer portion of the epithelium. Such disruption allows for exposure and triggering of sensory nerve endings, resulting in pain and/or pruritus. Lubricants are used to retard evaporative loss and thus allow for a more physiologic environment and faster subsequent repair of the barrier layer.

There are two common circumstances in which the barrier layer becomes disrupted because of excess dryness. The first circumstance occurs as the result of excessive washing, utilization of harsh solvents, and various types of scrubbing. The use of soap and water on the genitalia more than twice a day removes the naturally present lipids and leads to excess water loss from the epithelial cells. The second circumstance occurs in the presence of disease-related thickening of the stratum corneum. In this situation, moisture from underneath cannot adequately diffuse into the outermost cells. This dry surface layer then tends to fissure, allowing even more water loss from the epithelial cells. In both of these situations, lubrication, by way of retarding evaporative water loss, restores a more physiologic environment for the epithelial cells and is very helpful in alleviating symptoms of itching and/or pain.

Many types of lubricants are available. Those that are petrolatum based (e.g., Vaseline) do the best job of preventing evaporative water loss but are messy, sticky and, if thickly applied, may be counterproductive by way of trapping sweat. Products such as these are best used in infants and young children, though some adults find them surprisingly acceptable. At the other end of the spectrum are lotions that can be poured or pumped out of a container. Although these are cosmetically very pleasing, they contain little in the way of lipids and therefore do a poor job of lubricating. Moreover, most contain alcohols and other chemicals that can cause stinging on application. This is particularly noticeable when applied to the tender skin of the anogenital region, especially in children. A reasonable compromise is the use of any one of the standard creams (hand cream) available for hand lubrication.

Anti-inflammatory Therapy

Anti-inflammatory therapy is the most important and most often used treatment in dermatology. Given the prime role for such therapy, it is discouraging to find that it is so often misused. Attention must be given to the route for use (topical, intralesional, or systemic), the dosage, the amount to be dispensed, and the duration for which the product is to be used.

Topical Steroid Therapy

Topical steroid therapy represents the mainstay of anti-inflammatory therapy. The number of topical steroid products available is unmanageably large. For our purposes, a clinician only needs to be familiar with four of these. All four are available either by brand or generically. Thus they can be found on essentially all formulary lists or can be purchased at reasonable prices if the patient lacks insurance coverage for medications.

Hydrocortisone is a low-potency steroid. It is available in 1.0% product (nonprescription strength) or 2.5% (prescription strength). Either of these is suitable as initial therapy for eczematous genital disorders in infants and children. Safety, even with long-term use is excellent but their level of effectiveness is correspondingly low. *Triamcinolone* is a mid-potency steroid. It is available in several strengths but only the 0.1% strength needs to be considered. Triamcinolone is appropriate for second-line therapy of eczematous disease in children and initial therapy of adults. Safety, even with long-term use is excellent. *Fluocinonide* is a high-potency steroid. It is available in several strengths but only the 0.05% strength needs to be considered. It is suitable for second-line therapy of eczematous disease in adults (first line for lichen simplex chronicus) and initial therapy of noneczematous disease. *Clobetasol* is a super potent steroid. It is suitable for second-line therapy of lichen simplex chronicus and for first-line therapy of noneczematous disorders such as lichen sclerosus, lichen planus, and psoriasis.

From a standpoint of *systemic* adverse effects, all of the products described above are reasonably safe even for long-term use. When the high and super potent products are restricted to use on the modified mucous membranes of the vulvar vestibule and the glans penis, safety in terms of *cutaneous* side effects is also excellent. However, when clobetasol is used (or is allowed to spread due to heat and sweat) extragenitally, especially on the upper inner thighs, there is a fairly high risk for the development of skin atrophy, telangiectasia, and striae. It is not clear whether this can happen with the use of fluocinonide, but caution is warranted.

Intralesional Steroid Therapy

Triamcinolone (Kenalog) is generally the only steroid used for intralesional injection. This route of administration is used when there has been failure (due to either inadequate penetration or noncompliance) of topically applied steroids. The commercial preparation is a 10 mg/mL multiuse vial. This product can be used at this strength or, to avoid the possibility of local atrophy, may be diluted to 5 mg/mL with equal parts of normal saline or lidocaine. An injection of 0.1 mL will spread to encompass about 1 cm^2; therefore, the number of injections can be planned according to the size of the involved area. As might be expected, these injections are rather painful due to the penetration of the needle and the tissue distension as the medication is injected.

Several practical points should be considered in using triamcinolone intralesionally. First, the stock preparation is a suspension and must be shaken before the medication is withdrawn from the vial. Likewise, the syringe should be shaken just prior to performing the injections. The size of the particles makes for difficulty in withdrawing and injecting the product through a 30-gauge needle. We prefer withdrawing the triamcinolone with a 27-gauge needle and often use that size needle for injection as well. It is preferable to use a 1-mL syringe ("tuberculin" or "diabetic" syringe) to improve accuracy while injecting.

Systemic Steroid Therapy

It is rarely necessary to use systemic therapy for disorders localized to the anogenital area, though this is occasionally necessary for patients with erosive lichen planus, aphthosis major, Behcet disease, Crohn disease, hidradenitis suppurativa, and lichen simplex chronicus. Systemic steroids (and other systemic immunomodulating agents) are regularly required in immunobullous disease, but such treatment lies outside the scope of this chapter.

Systemic steroid therapy can be administered orally. Prednisone is the product most often used. Generally a dose of 40 to 60 mg is given daily in the early morning. In most situations, this is given as a "burst," without taper, for 7 to 10 days. When therapy needs to be continued longer than that, the dose should be tapered both to reduce the likelihood of rebound and to allow for recovery of any hypothalamic–pituitary–adrenal suppression that has occurred.

When prednisone is used, there is obviously concern about blood sugar elevation, increased blood pressure, psychological problems (especially insomnia and agitation), and dangerous worsening of any underlying systemic infection. Adverse effects occurring with long-term use (osteoporosis, cataract formation, etc.) are not of concern if therapy is limited to less than a month.

Systemic steroids can also be administered intramuscularly. The product used is triamcinolone (Kenalog), which is available in a 40 mg/mL concentration. The usual dose of 60 to 80 mg (1.5 to 2.0 mL) is injected into the upper, outer quadrant of the buttock. A 1.5-inch needle should be used as injection with a shorter needle leads to superficial deposition with less effectiveness and greater risk of local atrophy. As with the intralesional preparation, this is a suspension and both the vial and the syringe must be shaken before use. There are several advantages related to the use of intramuscular triamcinolone: there is no concern regarding patient compliance, there is a built-in tapering of dose due to the depot effect, and fewer milligrams of steroid can be used for a given level of anti-inflammatory effect.

Topical Nonsteroidal Anti-inflammatory Therapy: Topical Calcineurin Inhibitors

There are concerns about both systemic absorption and cutaneous side effects with prolonged use of topical steroids. About a decade ago, topical calcineurin inhibitors were approved by the FDA. Two of these, tacrolimus 0.03% and 0.1% ointment (Protopic) and pimecrolimus 1% cream (Elidel) are currently being marketed. These calcineurin inhibitors lessen inflammation by reducing T-cell elaboration of inflammatory cytokines.

These two products, unlike topically applied potent steroids, do not cause cutaneous telangiectasia and atrophy. For this reason, they have been widely used for facial and intertriginous eruptions. Tacrolimus 0.1% appears to be slightly more effective than pimecrolimus 1%. Both are less effective than high and super potent topical steroids, though there have been instances of improvement in patients where these calcineurin inhibitors were used following failure with topical steroids. Both products are associated with an appreciable degree of stinging and burning on application.

Controversy exists about the use of these agents for genital disease. In 2006, the FDA required that a "black box" warning be included in the package information. This notice warns that long-term safety of these agents has not been proven due to rare reports of skin cancer and lymphoma. Most dermatologists believe that any relationship between their use and the development of malignancy is coincidental rather than causal, but it is easy to appreciate the potential for legal risk when these agents are used on certain mucocutaneous disorders (such as lichen sclerosus and lichen planus) that inherently have an increased risk for the development of squamous cell carcinoma. Indeed, a few such case reports have been published. These were reviewed in 2008 by Starritt and Lee (4).

Oral Nonsteroidal Anti-inflammatory Therapy

Multiple medications are regularly used by dermatologists as nonsteroidal anti-inflammatory agents. These include hydroxychloroquine, cyclosporine, tumor necrosis factor alpha inhibitors, mycophenolate mofetil, and a variety of other immunomodulating and cytotoxic agents. These are uncommonly indicated for the treatment of genital disease and therefore will be discussed only in the situations where they are most likely to be used rather than in this chapter.

Antipruritic Therapy

Itching is an extremely distressing symptom and may be even more troublesome than mild-to-moderate pain. It represents a major reason why patients with genital disorders seek medical attention.

General Measures

It stands to reason that if a specific underlying disease can be identified, treating it as effectively as possible will reduce the itching. But note that although treatment of such a disease is necessary it often is not sufficient, especially if the "itch–scratch" cycle is present. Other general approaches, as discussed previously, include improving the local environment and using soaks and lubrication as "first aid" measures.

Decreasing Inflammation

Inflammation occurring as a component of any genital disorder is often associated with itching. Using any of the anti-inflammatory approaches, especially the application of topical steroids, described in the section "Anti-inflammatory Therapy," almost always has a beneficial effect on pruritus.

Oral Antihistamines

The administration of oral antihistamines for pruritus has a time honored place in the dermatologic armamentarium. Traditionally, the agent most often used is hydroxyzine (Atarax, Vistaril). Because of its sedative side effect, it is best administered in the evening. However, if it is given just before going to bed, the patient may scratch while waiting for it to take effect and may wake up in the morning feeling drowsy. Therefore, it is best to suggest taking it approximately 2 hours before the patient's expected bedtime. Allowing the patient to subsequently experiment with the length of this interval increases both compliance and efficacy. The usual starting dose is 25 mg, but for a patient who is very "sensitive" to medications it may be appropriate to start with 10 mg. The dose is then increased weekly by 25 mg until there is no more nighttime scratching, or until side effects prevent further increase, or until a dose of 100 mg is reached. The entire dose is taken all at the same time. A rare patient can tolerate, and benefit, by taking 25 mg four times per day rather than just at night, but such patients must be warned about the hazards of driving and operating machinery.

Other antihistamines such as diphenhydramine (Benadryl) can be used instead of hydroxyzine, but most dermatologists feel that it is somewhat less effective than hydroxyzine. The dosing is the same as for hydroxyzine. Many clinicians use the "low-sedating" antihistamine cetirizine (Zyrtec) or the nonsedating antihistamines loratadine (Claritin), desloratadine (Clarinex), or fexofenadine (Allegra) for daytime treatment of itching. However, in our opinion, these agents are almost totally ineffective for the treatment of nonurticarial pruritus.

Tricyclic Medications

Use of the tricyclic agents can be remarkably effective in the treatment of both pruritus and pain. Although these drugs are approved and marketed primarily for the treatment of depression and anxiety, they are remarkable good antihistamines as well. In fact, for most clinicians they represent the second line of therapy for pruritus in situations where hydroxyzine has failed. When tricyclics are used, it is not clear whether it is the psychotropic, the antihistaminic, or the sedative component that is responsible for their beneficial effect. There is, however, some consensus that those with the greatest sedative effect work better than those that are less sedative. Doxepin (Sinequan) is the agent most often used for the treatment of itching, though amitriptyline (Elavil) works equally well.

The starting dose for either of these is usually 25 mg taken in the evening. An initial dose of 10 mg can be used in the elderly and for those with a history of being very "sensitive" to other medications. It is preferable to have the patient take the medication about 2 hours before bedtime so as to lessen drowsiness in the morning. The dose is then increased weekly by 25 mg until there is no more nighttime scratching, or until side effects prevent further increase, or until a dose of 100 mg is reached. The entire dose is taken all at the same time. In addition to drowsiness, there are a number of other possible adverse effects. These include dryness of the mouth and eyes, blurred vision, arrhythmias, and many drug–drug interactions. Lest these adverse effects lead to wariness about the use of the tricyclics, it should be emphasized that they occur almost only at doses above 75 mg/day.

Selective Serotonin Reuptake Inhibitors

Selective serotonin reuptake inhibitors (SSRIs) can be used quite effectively for daytime treatment of pruritus. These agents and their use are discussed in Chapter 4.

Topical Nonsteroidal Antipruritic Agents

Several topical products are available for the local treatment of itching. Some of the more commonly used agents include pramoxine (usually mixed with hydrocortisone), doxepin (Zonalon), benzocaine (in multiple products, notably Vagisil Cream), and lidocaine (Xylocaine and other products). In our opinion, none of these works well and several can cause allergic contact dermatitis.

Analgesic Therapy

Analgesics can be used both for idiopathic pain (vulvodynia, penodynia, scrotodynia, and anodynia) and for pain associated with any one of multiple dermatologic disorders (herpes zoster, erosive lichen planus, etc.). Note that opiate analgesics are rarely, if ever, used in the

treatment of genital pain and for that reason are not discussed here.

Oral Analgesics

The tricyclic antidepressants have historically been the mainstay of systemic therapy for genital pain of all types. These agents are used in the same doses and in the same schedules as are contained in the section "Antipruritic Therapy."

Other antidepressants such as duloxetine (Cymbalta) and venlafaxine (Effexor XL) are also used in the treatment of genital pain. Both agents are serotonin and norepinephrine reuptake inhibitors; venlafaxine additionally inhibits the uptake of dopamine. Specifically, duloxetine, but not venlafaxine, has been approved by FDA for the treatment of diabetic neuropathy and fibromyalgia. Duloxetine is given in a dose of 60 mg once daily. Venlafaxine is started in a dose of 37.5 mg/ day; this may be increased to 75 mg/day in a week. The total daily dose can eventually, and slowly, be increased to 225 mg/day. Both of these agents have drug–drug interactions and may have adverse central nervous system effects. Patients taking venlafaxine should have their blood pressure monitored regularly. These medications should be tapered when they are to be discontinued.

The antidepressants from the group known as the SSRIs have also been used off-label in the treatment of genital pain, but most clinicians believe they are less effective than duloxetine and venlafaxine. The use of SSRIs is discussed in Chapter 4 where they have an efficacious role for daytime treatment of pruritus.

The anticonvulsants carbamazepine (Tegretol), gabapentin (Neurontin), and pregabalin (Lyrica) are used in the treatment of idiopathic genital pain on the basis of their approval by FDA for treatment of trigeminal neuralgia (carbamazepine), postherpetic neuralgia (gabapentin), and neuropathic pain and fibromyalgia (pregabalin). Gabapentin and the related product, pregabalin, reduce calcium influx into nerve terminals. Gabapentin has few serious adverse effects and is the product most often used. It is started in a dose of 300 mg/day and is increased weekly by 300 mg increments until relief is obtained or a total daily dose of 600 mg t.i.d. is reached. Even higher dosing (up to 3600 mg/day) is possible, but little additional analgesic effect is obtained at doses above 1800 mg/day. The initial dose of pregabalin is 75 mg b.i.d.; this may be increased weekly to a total dose of no more than 300 mg b.i.d. Carbamazepine has several serious potential adverse effects and is the agent least often used. It is started at a dose of 100 mg b.i.d. This dose can be increased in steps to 400 mg b.i.d.

Topical Analgesics

The most commonly recommended topical medication for genital pain is 2% or 5% lidocaine (Xylocaine). The 5% ointment is the preferred product. A small amount (the size of a lead pencil eraser) can be applied four or five times per day. Lidocaine can be absorbed from the skin and mucous membranes. For this reason, no more than 15 g should be applied in the course of a day. The 5% lidocaine ointment is available by prescription only. Strengths up to 2.5% are available over the counter but are perceived to be less effective. Many topical analgesic products, including the widely used Vagisil Feminine Cream, contain benzocaine. Benzocaine is based on the PABA molecule and is chemically unrelated to lidocaine. Unfortunately, benzocaine causes allergic contact dermatitis with considerable frequency and for that reason we advise against its use on the genitalia.

Antibacterial Therapy

The two most common bacterial infections of the genital and perigenital skin are those due to *Staphylococcus aureus* and *Streptococcus pyogenes*. For this reason, the antibacterial therapy discussed here will apply only to these two agents. Therapy for other less commonly encountered infections, including those used for vaginitis and sexually transmitted disorders, will be discussed as these topics are covered elsewhere in this book.

Oral Antibiotics

The penicillins are bactericidal antibiotics that act by inhibiting the synthesis of bacterial cell walls. They are effective for streptococcal infections and non-methicillin-resistant staphylococcal infections. The most commonly used agent is dicloxacillin given in a dose of 250 to 500 mg q.i.d. Other frequently used drugs include penicillin V potassium in a dose of 250 to 500 mg q.i.d. and amoxicillin plus clavulanate (Augmentin) in a dose of 500 mg b.i.d. or t.i.d. Allergic reactions to the penicillins are fairly common and must be inquired about before these antibiotics are prescribed.

The cephalosporins are comparable in efficacy to the penicillins for streptococcal and non-methicillin-resistant staphylococcal infections. Cephalexin (Keflex) in a dose of 250 to 500 mg q.i.d. is the drug most commonly used. Allergic reactions to cephalosporins do occur, but they are less common than with the penicillins. There is a 2% or 3% crossover of allergic reactions between these two groups of antibiotics.

Other antibiotics have to be considered due to the rapid rise in the frequency of community-associated methicillin-resistant *S. aureus* (MRSA) infections. At least four generic oral antibiotics are generally effective for MRSA infections. These include trimethoprim-sulfa (1 or 2 double strength tablets b.i.d.), doxycycline (100 mg b.i.d.), minocycline (100 mg b.i.d.), and rifampin (600 mg/day). Linezolid (Zyvox) in an oral dose of 600 mg b.i.d. is very effective but is also extremely expensive. Vancomycin, given in an intravenous dose of 1 g every 12 hours, is used only for the most serious, life-threatening MRSA infections. The agent chosen from among these antibiotics should be based on drug resistance data for the clinician's local community.

Topical Antibiotics

There are several nonprescription products available for the topical treatment of staphylococcal and streptococcal infections. The two most commonly used preparations are neomycin and bacitracin applied t.i.d. or q.i.d. They are inexpensive, present in almost every home and have the sole drawback of causing allergic contact dermatitis with some degree of frequency. These agents are also available in mixtures with polymyxin B (Polysporin, Neosporin), but this combination offers no real therapeutic advantage for typical skin infections.

Mupirocin (Bactroban) is available only by prescription in a 2% ointment or cream. It is as effective as neomycin and bacitracin. It is more expensive but has the advantage of rarely, if ever, causing allergic contact dermatitis. A new prescription-only topical antibiotic, retapamulin (Altabax) ointment, was recently approved by the FDA. Its role in the treatment of staphylococcal and streptococcal genital infections has not yet been established. Both of these agents currently appear to be at least somewhat effective in the treatment of MRSA infections.

Antifungal and Anticandidal Therapy

The "azole" medications are very effective in the therapy of both dermatophyte fungal infections and most yeast infections due to *Candida* sp. They work by interfering with the synthesis and function of microbial cell walls. For practical purposes, the azoles have supplanted a variety of drugs whose usefulness was restricted to either fungal infections or yeast infections.

Topical Therapy

There are about 20 different azole and non-azole products available for the topical treatment of vaginal yeast infections and superficial genital fungal and yeast infections. Topically applied azoles are effective for both types of infection and in most instances these agents represent the first line of treatment. The most frequently used products are clotrimazole, ketoconazole, and miconazole creams and vaginal suppositories. Several of these topical azoles are available over the counter. All of them are essentially equal in efficacy. Nystatin, once the most widely used topical agent for candidiasis, is somewhat less effective than the azoles and is less often used. Therapeutic problems associated with vaginal non-albicans *Candida* sp. are discussed in Chapter 15.

Oral Therapy

Clinicians are gradually switching from topical to oral administration of the azoles for all forms of candidiasis in adults. This has occurred because of troublesome irritation from topical azoles, better patient compliance, and a decreasing cost of the oral preparations. The major products available for oral use include ketoconazole, itraconazole, and fluconazole. Fluconazole (Diflucan) is the product most frequently used. For simple problems related to infections with *Candida albicans* infections, a single oral dose of 150 or 200 mg is usually sufficient to resolve the problem. For more complicated situations, fluconazole can be administered in 150 or 200 mg once weekly doses as long as it is necessary. It has a very good safety record in terms of few adverse effects but because of its inhibition of cytochrome P450 enzymes, there are many potential drug–drug interactions.

Terbinafine, a member of the allylamine family, rather than the azole, is the drug most often used when oral administration is desired for dermatophyte fungal infections. Unfortunately, it is relatively ineffective for yeast infections. In adults, terbinafine is administered in a dose of 250 mg/day. Numerous adverse effects, including some severe cutaneous reactions, have been reported with the use of terbinafine. It, too, inhibits cytochrome P450 enzymes and for that reason it also is associated with many potential drug–drug interactions. All of the orally administered azoles mentioned above for candidiasis are also effective for dermatophyte fungal infections.

Antiviral Agents

Several drugs are available for the treatment of infections due to herpes simplex virus (HSV) and varicella zoster virus (VZV). Only those available for oral administration are included here as the topical agents are too ineffective for routine use. Three products are widely available: acyclovir (Zovirax), valacyclovir (Valtrex), and famciclovir (Famvir). All three are nucleoside analogues and have a similar mechanism of action whereby they are phosphorylated by viral thymidine kinase into very potent inhibitors of viral DNA polymerase. All three are equally safe and, in appropriate dosage, are equally effective. The recommended doses vary with the use of each of these and on clinician preference. For this reason, dosage is discussed in the chapter 9 covering HSV and VZV infection rather than in this section.

There are no effective topical or systemic medications for other genital viral infections such as molluscum contagiosum and HPV-related warts and malignancies. However, immunomodulating therapy with the topically applied product imiquimod (Aldara) 5% cream can be effective in both of these viral infections. It is most commonly used every other day three times per week until the problem resolves or 16 weeks elapse. However, many other regimens are also in clinical use. Imiquimod stimulates both the innate and the acquired types of immune response through multiple mechanisms. Its applicability is hampered by the development of intense, painful inflammatory reaction and by the long period over which it must be used. Needless to say, these problems lead to poor patient satisfaction and low levels of compliance.

REFERENCES

1. Lynch PJ, Edwards L. *Genital Dermatology*. New York: Churchill Livingstone Inc; 1994:7–10.
2. Lynch PJ. *Dermatology*. 3rd ed. Baltimore: Lippincott Williams & Wilkins; 1994:89–105.
3. Lynch PJ. Problem-oriented diagnosis. In: Sams WM Jr, Lynch PJ, eds. *Principles and Practice of Dermatology*. 2nd ed. New York: Churchill Livingstone; 1996:33–44.
4. Starritt E, Lee S. Erythroplasia of Queyrat of the glans penis on a background of Zoon's plasma cell balanitis. *Australas J Dermatol*. 2008;49:103–105.

Diagnostic and Therapeutic Procedures

LIBBY EDWARDS

The evaluation and diagnosis of anogenital diseases are a process that generally requires only a limited history, careful observation, and minor office procedures. Although there are several diagnostic procedures useful for the diagnosis of anogential procedures, the crucial aspects of evaluation are a careful visual examination, microscopy of vaginal fluid and some scaling skin conditions, and, at times, skin biopsy. The careful inspection of the skin requires a good light and, sometimes, simple magnification. The degree of magnification afforded by a colposcope is not required (1).

At times, the diagnosis of skin disease on the genitalia is obvious, with classic signs. However, the typical morphology of skin disease often is modified in the folds of genital skin, where the skin is often normally somewhat red, and where moisture, heat, and friction obscure scale and change the appearance of dermatoses. For those diseases that display objective abnormalities, the cause is nearly always infection, tumor, or noninfectious inflammation that is often immune mediated. Even when the exact diagnosis cannot be ascertained by examination or biopsy, infection and tumor can be ruled out by cultures and biopsies (Table 3-1). Those remaining diseases are categorized by the histologic description (see Appendix 1), and correlated with physical findings to generate a differential diagnosis. Most visible skin disease that is not tumor or infection is corticosteroid responsive. Sometimes a definitive diagnosis cannot be made, and when easily diagnosed and dangerous conditions have ruled out, presumptive therapy is reasonable and often beneficial.

Treatment of skin diseases is often time-consuming, because careful and sensitive patient education generally is required, and attention to multifactorial processes such as secondary infection and irritant contact dermatitis is important. Except for radiation therapy and the surgical removal of growths, the therapy of most genital disorders is medical, consisting of self-administered oral and topical medications. There are several office procedures, however, including intralesional therapy, cryotherapy, and the application of topical chemotherapy such as trichloroacetic or bichloroacetic acid, phodophyllum resin, or cantharidin.

DIAGNOSTIC PROCEDURES

In genital dermatology, most diagnostic procedures are performed in an outpatient setting or at the bedside. Required are only a microscope, glass slides and coverslips, 10% to 20% potassium hydroxide (KOH), and normal saline. Although these procedures are easy to perform, the interpretation of the microscopic findings requires extensive experience. Unexpected results or poor response to therapy should be followed by cultures or biopsies to corroborate the microscopic findings. Clinicians who care for patients with vulvar dermatoses or vulvar pain should invest in a narrow, straight Pederson speculum, which produces far less distention of the introitus and less pain on insertion than does the standard Graves speculum with its bulbous tip. However, visualization of the cervix is much more difficult with the Pederson speculum. The use of a speculum allows for visualization of the vaginal walls and sampling of vaginal fluid for microscopic examination and culture. Occasionally, biopsy specimens are obtained and sent to the laboratory for histologic evaluation. When biopsies are performed, the most likely diagnoses should be indicated on the pathology requisition, to provide the pathologist with information and to narrow the clinically possible diagnoses. Often, the "diagnosis" on the final laboratory report is a microscopic description (see Appendix 1) rather than a specific disease name, so that correlation of this description with the appearance of the skin is required to formulate the most likely diagnosis. Sometimes, one firm diagnosis is not possible, but possibilities can be narrowed to allow for initiation of therapy.

Cytologic Smears

Fungal Preparations

Fungal preparations are essential to the diagnosis of anogenital disease. Men generally interpret all anogenital itching as produced by "jock itch," or tinea infection, whereas women assume all vulvovaginal itching to result from candidiasis. The confirmation or elimination of these conditions is vital.

TABLE **3.1**	Diagnosis of unknown skin disease

Categorize by color, and other visible changes (i.e., red patch, white diseases, pustules) and see appropriate chapters in this book for differential diagnosis. If no diagnosis;

Perform indicated microscopy and/or cultures. If no diagnosis;

Biopsy. If no specific diagnosis;

    Classify according to Appendix 1 (lichenoid, spongiotic, etc.)

    Correlate with physical findings to generate differential diagnosis, and either formulate additional investigation or treat presumptively

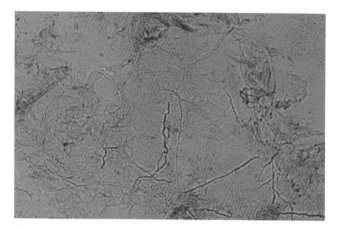

FIG. 3-1. Dermatophytosis of tinea cruris shows hyphae similar to candidiasis, but there are no budding yeast; the hyphae are long, branching, and cross cell membranes.

KOH 10% to 20% solution is a basic agent that dissolves the keratin of epithelial cells, allowing spores and fungal hyphae and pseudohyphae to be seen more clearly. The reliability of this test depends on the choice of the lesion to be sampled, adequate dissolution of cells so fungal elements are best visualized, and the experience of the examiner in distinguishing fungal elements from artifacts such as hair, fabric fibers, cell membranes, and fractures in crusts.

The specimens most likely to yield fungi include the peripheral scale from plaques of possible dermatophyte infection, pustule roofs, and white, cheesy material produced by suspected yeast. These elements are removed by scraping with the rounded surface of a number 15 scalpel blade. In the damp areas of the genitalia, the sample usually adheres to the scalpel blade and can be wiped onto the glass slide. Dry, hairbearing skin can be moistened with water so that the moistened specimen sticks to the blade until it is smeared onto the slide. Vaginal secretions are collected with a cotton-tipped applicator from secretions remaining on the blade of the withdrawn speculum, from a pool of secretions within the vagina (avoiding the cervical os) or by gently rolling the cotton tip along the vaginal walls.

Once the specimen is applied to the glass slide, a drop of KOH is placed on the material to dissolve the keratin from cells and to enhance the visibility of fungal elements. A coverslip is applied, and firm pressure to the coverslip with the back of a fingernail or a pencil eraser (to avoid distracting fingerprints on the coverslip) flattens and augments the dissolution of keratin. Although the unkeratinized epithelial cells in vaginal smears deteriorate quickly after exposure to KOH, the scale of keratinized skin requires further attention to dissolve so that fungi and yeasts can be easily detected. The examiner can use KOH mixed with dimethylsulfoxide to enhance dissolution or can simply allow 10 to 15 minutes for the KOH to disintegrate the cells. In addition, gentle warming of

the specimen over an alcohol flame dissolves cells from keratinized skin more quickly.

Fungal elements are best visualized by lowering the condenser and decreasing the light to increase the contrast between fungi elements and epithelial cells. Spores, buds, and hyphal elements appear refractile and sometimes very slightly green, and these are much smaller than common artifacts, such as hair and fibers. Dermatophytes appear as branching, septate hyphae that cross over cell membranes (Fig. 3-1). *Candida* appears as budding yeasts with or without hyphae or nonseptate, branching pseudohyphae (Fig. 3-2). At times, cell membranes in the process of dissolving resemble hyphae or pseudohyphae (Fig. 3-3). Pressure on the cover slip generally disrupts the cells and these partially dissolved membranes. The specific dermatophyte species cannot be recognized from the smear, and *Candida* species can be divided only into those characterized by hyphae or pseudohyphae (*C. albicans* or *C. tropicalis*) or yeast forms

FIG. 3-2. The hyphae and pseudohyphae of dermatophytosis and candidiasis are nearly indistinguishable, but on this higher power, budding yeast often can be seen in candidiasis.

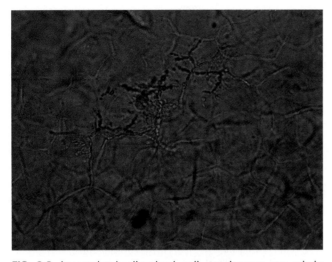

FIG. 3-3. Incompletely dissolved cell membranes can mimic fungal hyphae and yeast buds at times, as has occurred here.

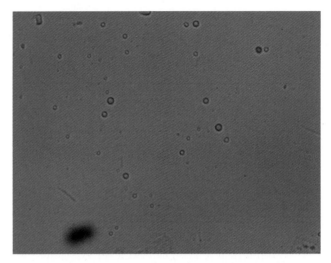

FIG. 3-5. Although these small, round structures resemble yeast buds, the variable sizes, lack of budding, and the very round rather than oval shape show that these are artifactual. In this case, these were air bubbles.

that exhibit budding yeast only (e.g., *C. glabrata* or *C. parapsilosis*) (Fig. 3-4). A culture is required to confirm the species if needed. Oil droplets and air bubbles can be confused with yeast buds at times, but the variability in size and very round shape distinguish these from yeast buds (Fig. 3-5). "Tinea" versicolor (which occurs uncommonly in the genital area) is a misnomer because it is a yeast rather than a dermatophyte or "tinea." It exhibits short, curved hyphae and spores/buds ("spaghetti and meatballs") microscopically.

Saline "Wet Drop" Preparation (see also Chapter 15)

A microscopic evaluation of vaginal secretions using normal saline under a coverslip permits an evaluation of

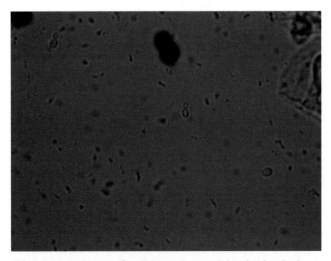

FIG. 3-4. Non*albicans Candida* can be much harder for the inexperienced provider to identify. There are no hyphae or pseudohyphae, but only tiny budding yeast as seen here; however, some of these yeast buds are generally seen in every high power field.

the morphology of cells, a screen for inflammation and estrogen effect, and a crude survey of colonizing and infecting organisms. Information from an examination of vaginal secretions is sometimes extremely important in the evaluation of the vulva and vagina (Table 3-2). Secretions are collected as described above for evaluation for *Candida* spp. However, the secretions are transferred from the cotton tipped applicator by touching (if abundant) or gently rolling (if scant) onto the glass slide. Care should be taken to avoid the thick application of secretions, which interferes with visualization.

In order to evaluate vaginal secretions for abnormalities, the examiner should be aware of the ranges of normal (Fig. 3-6). Mature epithelial cells shed from a well-estrogenized vaginal epithelium appear as large, often folded, polygonal cells with abundant cytoplasm and a small, condensed nucleus. A crude maturation index can be performed, in which the degree of maturation of epithelial cells is estimated. Immature epithelial cells, or parabasal cells, are much smaller and rounder than mature cells, with proportionately larger nuclei (Fig. 3-7). These less mature cells are seen in several settings and serve as a marker for atrophic, estrogen-deficient vaginal epithelium, erosions within the epithelium, and rapidly proliferative inflamed skin. Epithelial cells also appear abnormal in the setting of bacterial vaginosis and are pathognomonic for that condition. These clue cells occur when non *Lactobacillus* bacteria adhere to epithelial cells and obscure the sharp borders of the cells so that the edge appears ragged and the cytoplasm appears granular (Fig. 3-8).

Although many different organisms are normal vaginal inhabitants, lactobacilli are the most common bacteria seen on a saline preparation of normal vaginal secretions of a well-estrogenized woman. These appear as rods of variable lengths. Occasionally, lactobacilli attach

TABLE 3.2	Evaluation sheet for vaginal secretion microscopy			
Finding	None or normal	Few	Moderate	Many
Parabasal (immature epithelial) cells				
White blood cells				
Budding yeast				
Hyphae/pseudohyphae				
Clue cells				
Lactobacilli/rods				

to each other from end to end, to form very long filaments, formerly believed to represent Leptothrix (Fig. 3-9). These strands are sometimes confused with the hyphae of *C. albicans*. However, these filaments of lactobacilli are more delicate and smaller in caliber than yeast, and these are nonbranching, when compared to the hyphae and pseudohyphae of *C. albicans*.

Other parameters evaluable from a saline preparation are the numbers and types of white blood cells. Leukocytes are regularly present, normally at a ratio of 1:1 with epithelial cells. Inflammation, which can be produced by *Trichomonas* infection, an irritated or superinfected atrophic vagina, erosive vaginal dermatoses, or desquamative inflammatory vaginitis, is characterized by an increase in white blood cells (Fig. 3-10). Some clinicians believe that bacterial infections (excluding bacterial vaginosis) are more likely to be characterized by a dense neutrophilic infiltrate, whereas noninfected, inflamed dermatoses, such as lichen planus, are more likely to result in an influx of lymphocytes. This author

has noted most vaginal inflammation is characterized by neutrophils, but both neutrophils and lymphocytes can be seen with either infectious or noninfectious causes of inflammation.

Tzanck Preparation

When performed by experienced examiners, Tzanck smears can confirm the presence of a herpetic blister, but these cannot distinguish between herpes simplex virus and varicella-zoster virus (herpes zoster and chicken pox). Some very practiced clinicians can tentatively detect abnormalities consistent with pemphigus vulgaris with this test. The base of an erosion left by an unroofed blister is scraped with a number 15 scalpel blade, and the material on the blade transferred to a glass slide. Giemsa or Papanicolaou stain is applied to reveal nuclear characteristics of cells. A Tzanck preparation of a herpes blister base shows extremely large, multinucleated epithelial cells and intracytoplasmic inclusions. However, the correct interpretation of Tzanck

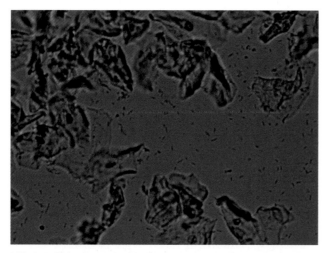

FIG. 3-6. This photograph illustrates the normal vaginal secretions of a premenopausal woman. The epithelial cells are flattened, folded, and mature. There are fewer than one white blood cell per epithelial cell, and lactobacilli are present.

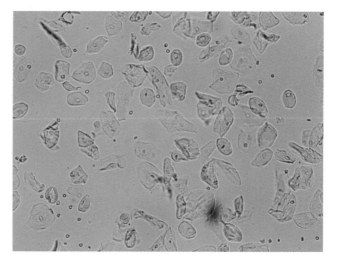

FIG. 3-7. The vaginal secretions of this patient illustrate the presence of immature epithelial cells (parabasal cells) as well as mature squamous epithelial cells. The immature cells are smaller and round.

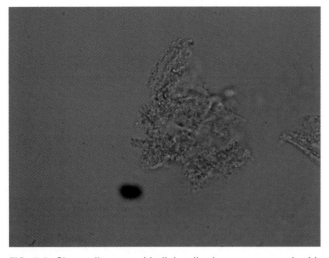

FIG. 3-8. Clue cells are epithelial cells that are covered with granular-appearing bacteria so that the borders of the cells are obscured and appear ragged rather than crisp.

smears requires experience, and results from even confident dermatologists can exhibit poor intraobserver and interobserver reproducibility. In general, this test should be confirmed by a culture, biopsy (which also does not differentiate herpes simplex from herpes zoster), or direct viral identification (immunofluorescent antibody testing, in situ hybridation, or polymerase chain reaction technique) if there is any question as to the correct diagnosis.

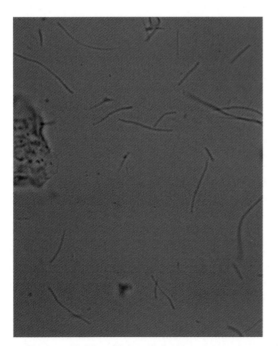

FIG. 3-9. The long, delicate filaments in this wet mount were formerly called Leptothrix, and these were believed to be a marker for *Trichomonas.* More recent information indicates that these are actually lactobacilli that have lined up from end to end.

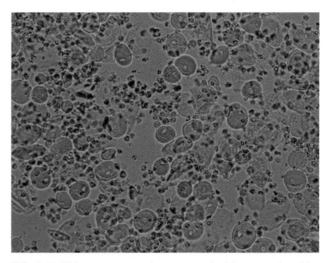

FIG. 3-10. This wet mount shows a marked increase in white blood cells, far more than the normal ratio of one white blood cell per epithelial cell. Also seen are parabasal cells, a regular finding in the presence of inflammation.

Gram Stains

When treating genital disease, Gram stains are used primarily to differentiate the clustered gram-positive cocci of staphylococcal folliculitis from sterile folliculitis. Most clinicians do not use Gram stain for vaginal secretions or skin afflicted by other common diseases, because a culture is generally required for identification of less common genital pathogens.

Polymerase Reaction Technique

More recently, very sensitive laboratory testing for organisms with polymerase chain reaction technique has moved from the research arena to the practitioner's office as availability and expense concerns have improved remarkably. A simple swab of the base of an erosion of possible herpes simplex virus or varicella-zoster virus infection can produce a simple and reliable answer; cervical swabs for *Chlamydia* or gonorrhea, a swab of an ulcer for syphilis, chancroid, lymphogranuloma venereum, vaginal secretions for trichomonas, swabs of skin for human papillomavirus (HPV) detection and typing are additional tests that are available. Costs are usually under $100, generally covered by insurance, and results are available in about a week.

Microscopic Examination for Infestations

The most important aspects of an evaluable scabies preparation are the selection of a burrow and the aggressive removal of the affected upper epidermis. The microscopic confirmation of scabies is often difficult and requires practice. The average patient with scabies has few mites despite widespread rash; most of which results from the immunologic response to the mite and due to inflammation produced by itching and rubbing. For scraping the skin for microscopic diagnosis, only an edematous, unscratched, oval papule should be selected. The nodules

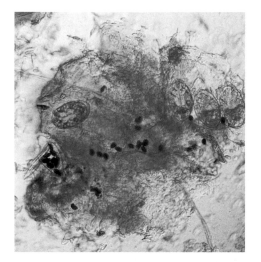

FIG. 3-11. A skin scraping for scabies can yield the mite itself, which is almost impossible to overlook. However, ova and golden brown globules of feces (scybala) seen here are also pathognomonic.

of scabies most common on the penis are not the lesions best selected for sampling. Rather, burrows in web spaces between the fingers or on the wrists are best for microscopic evaluation. A thin layer of epidermis is shaved with a number 15 scalpel blade, and the skin specimen is laid flat on a glass slide. A drop of normal saline or immersion oil is applied to the material, and a coverslip is affixed. The presence of ova, feces (scybala), or the mite itself is definitive evidence of infestation (Fig. 3-11). The mite, if present, is not subtle and is rarely missed. Eggs are regular, smooth, and fairly large, so they are usually identified without difficulty. Scybala, however, are regular, clustered, small, golden brown globules that require some experience to identify with confidence. A negative scraping does not eliminate scabies as a diagnosis; sometimes a biopsy adds information in the absence of a positive scraping, by either identification of the mite or by the presence of eosinophils, suggesting a parasite.

Although pubic lice are large enough for a suspicious clinician to identify in situ without magnification, an infested pubic hair examined microscopically reveals obvious nits and mites in more detail.

Nocturnal perianal pruritus suggests pinworm infestation. Before the patient arises in the morning, the perianal skin is stretched to evert the distal mucosa slightly. The sticky side of cellophane tape is applied to the anus to affix ova deposited during the night. The tape is then stuck to a glass slide and is examined microscopically under low power. Multiple, monomorphous ova are generally easily identified when pinworms are present.

Dermoscopy

Dermoscopy is a newer means of evaluating the epidermis and upper dermis with a dermatoscope, a hand-held magnifier which, when touched to the skin, reveals otherwise invisible structures. Dermoscopy is especially useful for the evaluation of pigmented lesions, sometimes allowing avoidance of a biopsy (2). Dermoscopy also can be useful in the diagnosis of scabies (3), and it may aid in the identification of pediculosis pubis (4), although this organism also can be seen with simple magnification. Dermoscopy can also confirm a diagnosis of molluscum contagiosum in the occasional patient without pathognomonic lesions (5).

Genital Skin Biopsies

Inflammatory, infectious, and neoplastic conditions may be clinically similar or may exhibit nonspecific morphology. Therefore, a histologic evaluation of the skin may be indicated in an attempt to render a definitive diagnosis. Because skin and mucosa are relatively superficial, obtaining a specimen for evaluation is simple, quick, safe, and relatively painless when done properly. However, inflammatory dermatoses that present with nonspecific morphology in a patient are likely to exhibit nonspecific histology on biopsy. An understanding of the classification of dermatoses as determined by the International Society for the Study of Vulvovaginal Disease allows the clinician to formulate a differential diagnosis in the absence of a definitive histologic diagnosis (see Appendix 1).

Anesthesia

Whatever the skin biopsy technique, local anesthesia is indicated. This can be achieved quickly by infiltrating skin under the biopsy site with 0.5 to 1.0 mL of lidocaine 1% with epinephrine, using a 30-gauge needle. The epinephrine produces vasoconstriction within about 10 minutes and helps to prevent hemorrhage and bruising in this area of loose connective tissue. Epinephrine should be avoided in deep injections such as blocks on the penile shaft, to prevent ischemia, but superficial anesthesia that includes epinephrine for skin biopsies is well tolerated.

Patients who are especially anxious can be pretreated with a newer-generation potent topical anesthetic such as lidocaine 2.5%/prilocaine 2.5%, or 10% lidocaine cream. A very thick layer of cream applied to genital skin and modified mucous membranes for 20 to 30 minutes partially anesthetizes the skin. When properly used, these topical anesthetics render the definitive anesthesia of injected lidocaine much less painful. These agents should not be inserted into the vagina because of the increased risk of absorption. Keratized, hairbearing skin is less well anesthetized by these topical agents.

Biopsy Techniques

The choice of technique depends on the diseases being considered and the location. Tissue is most often removed by shave biopsy, excision by curved iris scissors, or punch biopsy. Vaginal biopsies are procured with the use of instruments developed for the cervical biopsy, such as the Kevorkian biopsy forceps. Although some clinicians use these cervical biopsy forceps for the vulva, the shave biopsy and punch biopsy techniques allow for a smaller specimen and more precise sampling.

A shave biopsy or snip with curved iris scissors is used when a disease occurring primarily superficially, such as lichen sclerosus or lichen planus, is contemplated, as well as for the removal of an exophytic lesion. It is also used when fragile bullae or the edge or an erosion would be traumatized by the rotary motion of punch biopsy procedures (see below). Pigmented lesions should not be obtained with this technique because the base of the lesion, which is critical in both diagnosing a melanoma and assessing the prognosis of the patient, sometimes cannot be evaluated. An advantage of shave biopsies is that they do not require suturing, but a disadvantage is the technical difficulty in performing a shave biopsy on the very thin, fragile, and slippery skin of the non–hair-bearing portion of the vulva or the uncircumcised glans or inner foreskin. After local anesthesia has been established, a number 15 scalpel blade or a razor blade is used to shave the lesion from the skin (Fig. 3-12). Because shave biopsy is indicated only in superficial conditions, the sample should be obtained well into but not through the dermis; the wound does not gape open and require suturing, and scarring is minimized. Aluminum chloride, ferric chloride, or ferric subsulfate is applied to the base of the shave biopsy site as a chemical cautery agent, to produce less tissue damage than electrocautery or silver nitrate.

A snip with curved iris scissors is variation of a shave biopsy, which is useful on the thin, slippery skin of the

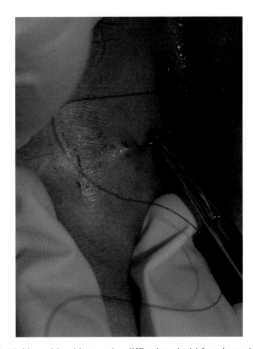

FIG. 3-13. Very thin skin can be difficult to hold for shave biopsy, so stabilizing the skin with a suture avoids crushing the tissue by grasping with forceps.

clinically non–hair-bearing skin of the vulva, glans, or inner prepuce. To avoid crush injury by forceps to this fragile skin, any 5-0 or 6-0 suture is placed through the lesional skin (Fig. 3-13). The skin is then lifted by the suture, and the now exophytic skin is snipped off with curved iris scissors (Fig. 3-14).

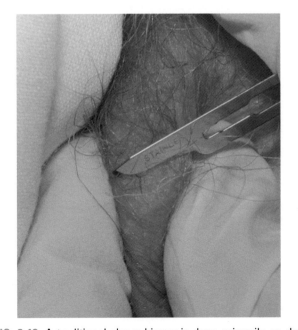

FIG. 3-12. A traditional shave biopsy is done primarily on dry, keratinized skin that can be grasped and gently pinched with fingers into a tense fold of skin.

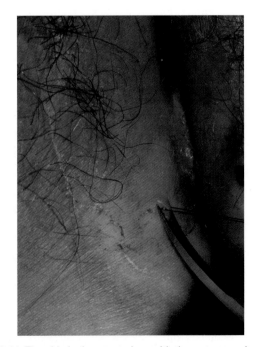

FIG. 3-14. The skin is then tented up with the suture, and curved iris scissors are able to snip the exact place and depth desired.

A punch biopsy is preferred for tumors, pigmented lesions, indurated ulcers, or when the process obviously extends into the submucosal or subcutaneous tissues. A punch biopsy samples epidermis, dermis, and some fat. Small lesions can be completely excised with a punch that is greater in diameter than the lesion. A punch instrument is a cylindrical blade (3 to 5 mm) that is applied to anesthetized tissues and, with both a rotary motion and gentle downward pressure, cuts through the epidermis and into fat, up to the hub of the punch biopsy instrument (Fig. 3-15). Often, the biopsy sample remains attached at the base, and care should be taken not to crush the tissue as it is lifted out and the base is snipped. The retained tissue can be snagged and lifted with a needle, rather than crushed with forceps, while curved iris scissors pointed toward the base of the defect detach the specimen at the base (Fig. 3-16).

Many clinicians close punch biopsy sites with suture, whereas others leave small defects open. The suture material used is dependent on the location and the size of the lesion. Generally, keratinized, clinically hair-bearing skin is closed with fairly stiff nonabsorbable suture such as nylon. However, moist mucosa and modified mucous membrane can be closed with more comfortable, soft, absorbable sutures such as glycoprotein acid. Soft, nonabsorbable suture such as silk that requires removal may also be used. However, the braiding of silk predisposes to bacterial infections, and nonabsorbable sutures require a return visit for removal.

For deep processes such as large-vessel vasculitis, necrotizing fasciitis, or panniculitis (inflammation of the fat), deep incisional biopsy or surgical exploration is indicated.

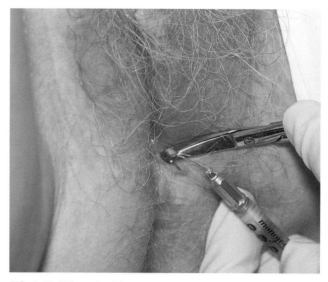

FIG. 3-16. When the biopsy specimen remains tethered to the skin at the base, the specimen can be stabilized with needle rather than crushed with forceps, and then the base is snipped with curved iris scissors.

Acetic Acid Examination

The application of 5% acetic acid (white vinegar) produces whitening of any thick or hyperkeratotic epithelium. This technique originally was used to allow for identification of subtle HPV and to allow for early and complete treatment (Fig. 3-17). However, all hyperkeratotic or inflammatory epithelial conditions whiten in response to the application of acetic acid, thus making this a

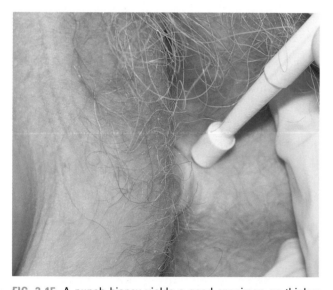

FIG. 3-15. A punch biopsy yields a good specimen on thicker skin and is obtained by twisting the punch instrument up to the hub.

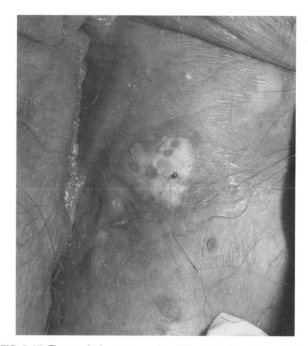

FIG. 3-17. Flat genital warts can be difficult to visualize, and the application of acetic acid makes these lesions turn white and more distinct.

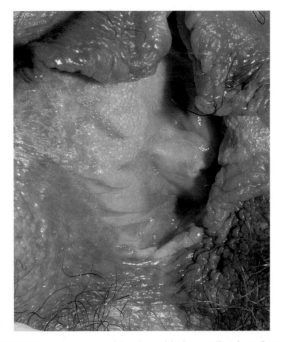

FIG. 3-18. Unfortunately, whitening with the application of acetic acid to the vulva is a nonspecific finding, and most patients exhibit white epithelium if acetic acid is left on for prolonged periods or is applied to any thickened or irritated skin. This patient had no specific lesions, but all areas touched by acetic acid turned white nonspecifically.

nonspecific finding, and normal women exhibit vulvar acetowhitening after prolonged application of acetic acid (Fig. 3-18) (2). The application of acetic acid produces burning, and many clinicians believe that this acetic acid test should not be performed because of its poor specificity. Visual inspection alone is accurate in evaluating clinical HPV infection, and the value of the identification and treatment of subclinical infection has not been shown. Clearly, any "subclinical" HPV infection identified by acetowhitening should be confirmed by a biopsy or direct viral studies.

Wood Light Examination

The Wood light is a handheld apparatus that contains a filter that blocks all low-intensity ultraviolet light except for a band of light between 320 and 400 nm. The Wood light initially was used in detecting fungal infections of the scalp, but it can aid also in the identification of other conditions. This is a procedure only occasionally useful to the genital clinician. A Wood light is used most often in the genital area to evaluate infections of erythrasma. However, a Wood light examination of tinea corporis, tinea versicolor, and epidermal disorders of pigmentation is occasionally helpful.

Erythrasma, an intertriginous infection caused by *Corynebacterium minutissimum*, produces a bright coral red fluorescence. This fluorescence is the result of a water-soluble porphyrin, and this fluorescence can be negative if the area was recently washed.

Uncommon dermatophyte fungi such as *Microsporum audouinii*, *M. canis*, and *Trichophyton schoenleinii* produce a blue-green fluorescence, although most superficial fungal infections do not fluoresce, so a lack of fluorescence is usual for tinea cruris.

Pityriasis "tinea" versicolor, which characteristically presents as either hypopigmented or hyperpigmented scaly patches on the trunk, can be seen occasionally on the abdomen and thighs. A Wood light accentuates the lesions, and a dull green fluorescence is sometimes evident as well.

Localization of melanin pigment is facilitated with a Wood light examination. Melanin in the epidermis absorbs long-wave ultraviolet light, so that epidermal pigmentation is accentuated, whereas dermal pigment is relatively inapparent. In postinflammatory hyperpigmentation, the localization of melanin beneath the epidermis and in melanophages results in little color contrast with surrounding skin. However, the epidermal pigment occurring in melanoma, physiologic hyperpigmentation, and lentigines is accentuated. In addition, the depigmentation of vitiligo is accentuated by loss of melanin in the epidermis, whereas hypopigmented processes such as postinflammatory hypopigmentation show little contrast with surrounding skin.

Unfortunately, common foreign bodies such as lint and some topical medications fluoresce, so that the simple presence of fluorescence is unhelpful. Only when a characteristic pattern of fluorescence is correlated with the clinical appearance of a disease is this test helpful.

THERAPEUTIC PROCEDURES

Unlike bedside diagnostic procedures, which require experience to interpret, common office therapeutic procedures are usually simple and safe in the hands of careful generalists. Intralesional corticosteroid administration and cautious cryotherapy belong in the domain of the primary care provider.

Cryotherapy

Cryotherapy consists of destruction of tissues by freezing. The crystallization of intracellular fluid and subsequent thaw results in cell death. Rapid freezing and slow thawing maximize destruction. Melanocytes are the most sensitive cells in the skin to low temperatures, followed by keratinocytes and, finally, fibroblasts. As a result, hypopigmentation may be a permanent consequence of vigorous cryotherapy, although posttreatment hyperpigmentation sometimes occurs but usually is transient. Cryotherapy is generally considered simple, safe, and effective even when performed by inexperienced clinicians, but the variable freezing duration required for ablation of different skin lesions depending on location, size, and cells of origin makes this a therapy that requires experience to perform well. Both inadequate treatment and overly aggressive freezing producing ulceration and permanent scarring are common.

Liquid nitrogen, the most common cryogen used in dermatology, has a temperature of −196°C. Liquid nitrogen is delivered most often with either a cotton-tipped swab gently touched to the lesion or a handheld spray unit. The nozzle is directed at the center of the lesion, and short bursts of spray are applied.

Cryotherapy of the external genitalia is limited to the treatment of warts, molluscum contagiosum, seborrheic keratoses, and, by very experienced clinicians and under some circumstances, vulvar intraepithelial neoplasia (3). This therapy is generally avoided in patients with Raynaud disease and cold urticaria; unbiopsied pigmented lesions and most malignant or destructive tumors are usually poor candidates for cryotherapy rather than removal techniques that allow for the evaluation of surgical margins.

Intralesional Corticosteroid Therapy

Inflammatory processes such as an inflamed epidermal cyst or an aphthous ulcer are too deep to respond to topical corticosteroids, but these often clear quickly with the injection of a corticosteroid. Intralesional corticosteroids also have the advantage of avoiding exposure to significant amounts of systemic medication or risking the surrounding skin to the atrophy caused by a steroid cream that spreads from treated skin. In addition, thickened areas such as hypertrophic scars or prurigo nodules thin more rapidly in response to injections of a corticosteroid than the application of topical medications.

For inflammatory processes, triamcinolone acetonide 10 mg/mL is diluted with normal saline to a concentration of about 3.3 mg/mL (0.6 mL normal saline and 0.3 mL triamcinolone acetonide) and 0.2 to 0.5 mL is injected into the inflamed area with a 30-gauge needle, depending on the area treated; this generally produces improvement in symptoms within 24 hours. Hypertrophic lesions require undiluted triamcinolone acetonide, 10 mg/mL, to decrease the thickness and itchiness. Possible adverse reactions include temporary atrophy of the overlying skin and hypopigmentation, which is unusual but can be permanent.

REFERENCES

1. Micheletti L, Bogliatto F, Lynch PJ. Vulvoscopy: review of a diagnostic approach requiring clarification. *J Reprod Med.* 2008; 53:179–182.
2. Lin J, Koga H, Takata M, et al. Dermoscopy of pigmented lesions on mucocutaneous junction and mucous membrane. *Br J Dermatol.* 2009. [Epub ahead of print].
3. Dupuy A, Dehen L, Bourrat E, et al. Accuracy of standard dermoscopy for diagnosing scabies. *J Am Acad Dermatol.* 2007; 56:53–62.
4. Budimci_ D, Lipozenci_ J, Pastar Z, et al. Pediculosis pubis and dermoscopy. *Acta Dermatovenerol Croat.* 2009;17:77–78.
5. Panasiti V, Devirgiliis V, Roberti V, et al. Molluscum contagiosum on a tattoo: usefulness of dermoscopy. *Int J Dermatol.* 2008; 47:1318–1319.

CHAPTER 4

Genital Pruritus and the Eczematous Diseases

PETER J. LYNCH

The sensation of pruritus (itching) is carried from mucocutaneous tissue to the sensory cortex by unmyelinated type C sensory nerve fibers. These same fibers also carry certain types of pain. It is not known precisely why triggering of these twig-like nerve endings, which are located in the epidermis and upper dermis, sometimes results in the perception of itching and at other times the perception of pain. However these sensations are qualitatively different. That is, a quantitative increase in stimulation does not convert itching to pain. Moreover, since the impulses transmitted by these nerves are interpreted in the brain within the sensory cortex, it is apparent that both itch and pain can have a peripheral component, a central component or a mix of these two components.

Genital pruritus occurs in two settings. It may arise from apparently normal appearing tissue ("primary" pruritus) or it may occur as a part of separate disease process on visibly abnormal tissue ("secondary" pruritus). Conceptually it is worth trying to separate the two forms of pruritus, but since scratching occurs in both settings, the clinical appearance at the time of examination often does not allow one to separate the two processes. When that is the case, treatment specifically directed toward the cessation of scratching and/or rubbing will usually allow for separate identification. That is, when the scratching completely stops, the skin will return to its normal appearance if the process is primary or will reveal an underlying disorder if the process is secondary. In both instances, adverse environmental factors in the anogenital area, such as heat, sweating, friction, and irritation from urine, feces, and vaginal secretions, will often initiate or aggravate the degree of pruritus.

When skin is scratched or rubbed on a continual basis over a period of days or weeks, the tissue takes on an appearance classical for the eczematous (dermatitic) diseases. For this reason, "eczema" and "dermatitis" (which are synonyms) can be defined morphologically. The morphologic pattern for the eczematous diseases is represented by the presence of red papules and plaques with poorly marginated borders, overlying scale, and evidence of epithelial disruption and/or lichenification. *Epithelial disruption* is most often recognized by the presence of excoriations, but other signs of epithelial disruption can include weeping, crusting, fissuring, or the presence of yellow-colored scale. This yellow color is due to the presence of small amounts of plasma that coats and covers the otherwise gray, white, or silver color of scale. When rubbing is more prominent than scratching, the callus-like response of lichenification may supplant much of the evidence for epithelial disruption. *Lichenification* is recognized clinically by three features: palpably thickened skin, exaggerated skin markings, and lichen-type scale. Note that lichen-type scale, because of its adherence to the epithelium, is more or less colorless when dry but becomes quite white when it absorbs moisture as is likely to happen in the genital area.

Lesions possessing an eczematous clinical appearance as described in the paragraph above have a characteristic histological appearance on biopsy. This microscopic appearance demonstrates spongiotic inflammation (inflammatory cells accompanied by intercellular and intracellular edema within the epithelium) when the process is acute and by acanthosis (epithelial thickening often termed "psoriasiform dermatitis") when the process is chronic. This is the histological appearance of all of the disorders discussed in this chapter. Since all of these diseases share a common histologic appearance, pathologists are usually unable to separately identify each of the disorders that exist within the general category of eczematous disease. For this reason, when a pathologist makes a diagnosis of "spongiotic dermatitis" or "psoriasiform dermatitis" it is necessary for the clinician to make a clinical–pathologic correlation in order to arrive at a more specific diagnosis (1).

IDIOPATHIC ("ESSENTIAL") PRURITUS

When itching occurs but leads to only a little rubbing or scratching, the involved tissue may look quite normal on clinical examination. This process, when it develops in the anogenital area, is sometimes termed "pruritus ani," "pruritus vulvae," or "pruritus scroti." However when biopsies are obtained from this normal appearing tissue, there is almost always some evidence of spongiotic dermatitis and/or psoriasiform dermatitis. This microscopic finding, together with the regularly present evidence of the "itch–scratch" cycle, leads me to believe that this represents a subclinical variant of atopic dermatitis (see below).

ATOPIC DERMATITIS AND LICHEN SIMPLEX CHRONICUS

The nomenclature regarding atopic dermatitis and its variants is somewhat complex and controversial. The term "atopy" has been defined in many ways, but most often the definition includes a genetic predisposition for the development of hypersensitivity allergic IgE reactions to common environmental antigens. Thus, atopic individuals frequently develop allergic rhinitis (hay fever), asthma, or atopic dermatitis. A semantic problem arises when an eczematous eruption occurs in an individual who lacks a personal or prominent family history of hay fever or asthma. In this setting the eczematous process has alternatively been called neurodermatitis, infantile eczema, childhood eczema, and lichen simplex chronicus (LSC). Given the lack of consensus regarding the diagnostic criteria for atopic dermatitis (2) and in view of the fact that all of these eczematous eruptions share the presence of the "itch–scratch cycle," I believe it is appropriate to use the term atopic dermatitis (for the generalized form) and LSC (for the localized form) of the disease regardless of whether or not the individual has other clinical evidence of atopy. Moreover, since genital involvement very often occurs in the absence of eczematous disease elsewhere, it will be referred to as LSC for the purposes of this chapter.

Clinical Presentation

Atopic dermatitis is an extremely common disorder affecting about 15% of the population in Western countries. The localized form of atopic dermatitis, genital LSC, occurs in both sexes and at all ages. It is commonly encountered in those who are adults and in this group it is found in women a little more frequently than in men. In children, boys are affected somewhat more often than girls. The prevalence and incidence of genital LSC are unknown but based on a few older studies and discussion at conferences, it is probably the single most common symptomatic condition involving the anogenital area.

History

Possibly because of embarrassment, patients with genital LSC rarely seek medical attention until the problem has been present for weeks or months. Often the itching arises subtly, but in women a specific event, most often vaginal discharge (perceived to be a yeast infection), will be identified by the patient as the initial trigger. In either setting, once itching has occurred, scratching almost inevitably follows. Most patients describe the itching as severe and find that nothing in terms of home remedies or over-the-counter medications will relieve it. In the most intractable cases, patients will scratch until pain caused by excoriation replaces the pruritus. In instances of long-standing duration, patients

will often shift from scratching to rubbing since they find they can alleviate some of the itching without causing the pain and tissue damage that arises with excoriation.

In time, a vicious circle of itching followed by scratching, followed by more itching and more scratching, develops. This is termed the "itch–scratch cycle" and its presence is the pathognomonic and defining characteristic of atopic dermatitis and LSC. Sometimes the patients are conscious of the scratching and many such individuals continue on with the scratching "because I can't make myself stop" or "because it feels so good to scratch." Others are unaware of scratching and tend to think that they scratch very little. This is quite analogous to the personal unawareness that develops with fingernail biting, knuckle cracking, and other such "habit tics."

Scratching during the daytime primarily occurs after using the toilet, when changing clothes after work, and in the evening when one gets undressed for bed. Scratching almost always also occurs episodically at night during the lighter stages of non-REM sleep and it is associated with an abnormal increase in the number of partial awakenings (3,4). I have termed this nocturnal scratching the "Penelope phenomenon" based on Homer's tale of Odysseus (Ulysses) and his wife Penelope (5). When Odysseus tarried for many years on his voyage home from the Trojan War, Penelope was urged to declare him deceased and marry one of her many suitors. She agreed to do so once she had completed weaving a funeral shroud for her dying father-in-law. During the day she wove the shroud, but at night when everyone was sleeping she would undo most of the previous day's weaving. The Penelope phenomenon thus represents the nighttime scratching that undoes the benefits of a good daytime therapeutic program.

Examination

As indicated above, LSC shares the morphological characteristics of all eczematous diseases. This includes erythematous, poorly marginated, scaling papules and plaques with evidence of epithelial disruption and/or lichenification (Figs. 4-1 through 4-6). But in contrast to other eczematous diseases, the severity of excoriation and/or lichenification often allows for correct clinical identification. This may not be true in mild cases because the warm, moist environment of the anogenital area may obscure some of the characteristic morphological features. First, scale may not be as visibly apparent (though it can still be recognized by roughness on palpation) as it is with LSC in other locations (Figs. 4-7 and 4-8). Second, scale is hydrophilic and when it takes up water it turns white. This white color can be fairly prominent when a patient first undresses but decreases as evaporation reduces the moisture content (Fig. 4-9). Third, deep scratching may destroy or remove melanocytes, leaving hypopigmented areas when the scratch marks heal (Fig. 4-10). Fourth, the anogenital area pigments easily. When LSC has been

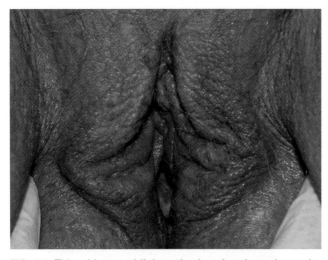

FIG. 4-1. This widespread lichen simplex chronicus shows the classic signs of poorly demarcated thickened lichenification, erythema, and excoriations.

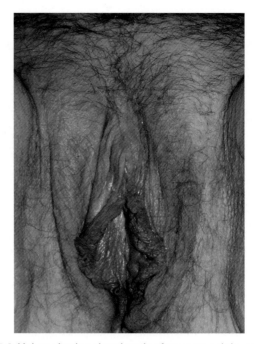

FIG. 4-3. Lichen simplex chronicus is often more subtle, as seen in the less erythematous lichenification of the right anterior labium majus. The severity of pruritus does not necessarily correlate with the extent of skin findings.

present for a long time, postinflammatory hyperpigmentation often develops. This can decrease the apparentness of erythema, leading one to underestimate the amount of inflammation that is present (Figs. 4-11 and 4-12). This is especially likely in patients with naturally dark skin.

Diagnosis

The diagnosis of LSC is usually made on the basis of the clinical findings. In some instances it is not clear whether the LSC is arising de novo or is superimposed

on another underlying dermatological problem. This is particularly likely to happen with genital psoriasis but is also common with tinea cruris in men and lichen sclerosus in women. One might think that biopsy could identify the underlying problem in the setting of secondary LSC, but this is often not true. In the acute phase of LSC, spongiotic inflammation will be prominent and this finding may obscure the presence of an associated disorder.

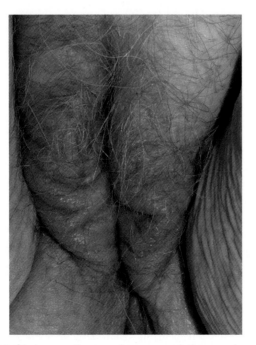

FIG. 4-2. Obvious erythema, edema, excoriations, and scale of this vulva are produced by chronic rubbing and scratching.

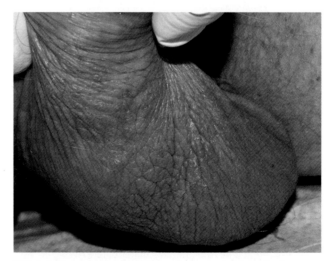

FIG. 4-4. Remarkable erythema, edema, and the marked accentuation of skin markings of lichenification indicate a diagnosis of lichen simplex chronicus. This location of the posterior scrotum is the most common on the male genitalia.

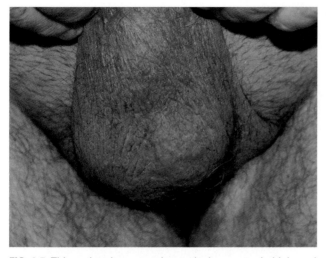

FIG. 4-5. This patient has not only poorly demarcated, thickened skin as a result of rubbing, but also excoriations produced by scratching.

Even more confusion generally occurs when chronic LSC is biopsied. In this situation, the report is often signed out as "psoriasiform dermatitis," which will not offer the clinician much help in trying to determine whether or not psoriasis is present. If this occurs, the clinician will have to undertake a clinical–pathologic correlation (1). Because candidiasis is the condition most commonly associated with the development of LSC in women, culture and/or KOH examination for associated candidiasis will be worthwhile. In both sexes, if the

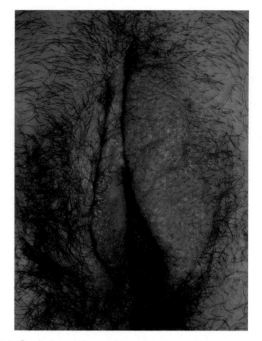

FIG. 4-7. Scale is subtle on this vulva due to the moist environment, although thickening from rubbing is remarkable; LSC can sometimes be remarkably unilateral.

upper inner thighs are involved it may be useful to obtain a KOH and/or culture for dermatophyte fungi associated with tinea cruris.

Psoriasis can be very similar in appearance to LSC, especially in the anogenital area where LSC may be

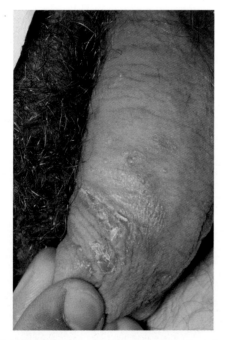

FIG. 4-6. Although the poorly demarcated redness and scale/crust on this penile shaft is characteristic of eczema/LSC, this is an unusual location. However, a close examination of the skin shows mollusca contagiosa, a virus infection that can precipitate pruritus and secondary eczematization.

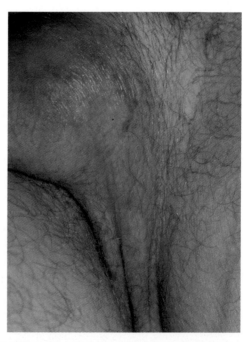

FIG. 4-8. Although scale seems absent on this scrotum because of the moist environment, the shiny character of the epithelium is indicative of lichenoid scale. Lichenoid scale is adherent scale from rubbing, and it appears shiny, rather than flaky.

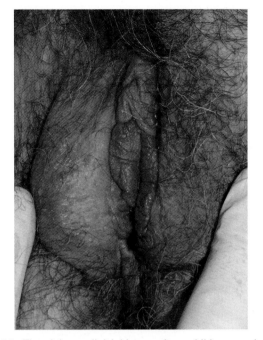

FIG. 4-9. The right medial labium majus exhibits excoriations from scratching and thickened epithelium from rubbing; this thick skin appears white due to hydration of this thick epithelium

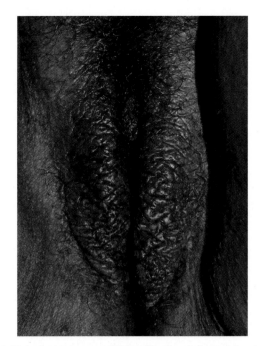

FIG. 4-11. In the presence of lichenification, inflammation in dark complexioned people appears hyperpigmented rather than red. Once again, lichenoid scale appears shiny rather than flaking.

superimposed over psoriasis. Helpful clues to the presence of psoriasis would be the presence of more typical psoriatic plaques in characteristic sites elsewhere, the identification of typical psoriatic nail changes, and the presence of psoriatic arthritis. Unfortunately, as noted above, biopsy may not be helpful in separating psoriasis from LSC.

In women, LSC frequently overlies vulvar lichen sclerosus and may obscure the typical clinical characteristics of this condition. However, architectural damage such as the presence of clitoral hooding, loss of the labia minora, or the presence of purpura would help to identify associated lichen sclerosus. Biopsy is helpful in this situation.

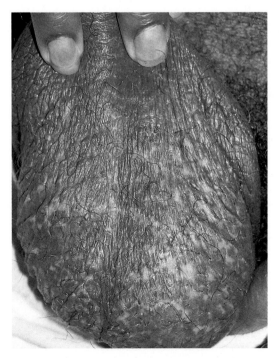

FIG. 4-10. Scratching has destroyed and removed melanocytes, so that the skin has areas of hypopigmentation and depigmentation.

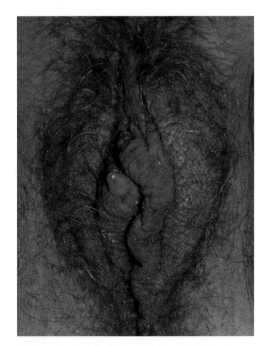

FIG. 4-12. Even patients who are not naturally dark sometimes exhibit hyperpigmentation that obscures the inflammation of lichen simplex chronicus, as seen on this left labium majus.

At the histological level, LSC can be confused with the often rather mundane appearance of the differentiated (non-HPV related) squamous cell intraepithelial neoplasia (6,7). Moreover the frequent histological presence of epithelial acanthosis, similar to that seen in LSC, immediately adjacent to the carcinoma raises a question of what, if any, relationship might exist between LSC and the development of genital squamous cell carcinoma.

Pathophysiology

The cause of LSC is not known. A large proportion of the patients who develop LSC have a personal or immediate family history of hay fever, asthma, or earlier eczematous skin disease and thus are presumably atopic. But, it is still not clear just how atopy results in the development of LSC. There is increasing appreciation that many, if not most, patients with atopic dermatitis possess genetic defects (notably mutations in the fillagrin gene) that interfere with the normal development of the outer layer of the epidermis ("the barrier layer"). These barrier layer defects allow easier exposure and processing of both irritants and allergens. Presumably these defects in the barrier layer also allow easier triggering of the terminal branches of sensory nerves that carry itch and light pain. Even though peripheral eosinophilia and elevated serum IgE levels are frequently present, atopic dermatitis is different from other atopic disorders in that the immune dysfunction associated with it is T-cell mediated rather than occurring as a type 1 IgE–related humoral dysfunction as occurs in hay fever and asthma. Atopic dermatitis appears to involve the TH2 component of the cell-mediated immune system and this process is presumably responsible for the increased serum IgE levels and peripheral eosinophilia.

In addition to such peripheral abnormalities, it seems likely that there are also important central aspects. Possibly there is a heightened appreciation for itching at the level of the sensory cortex and maybe an innate tendency for the development of an obsessive–compulsive-like scratching that characterizes the itch–scratch cycle in LSC. Some clinicians also believe that patients with atopic dermatitis, and by extrapolation, some of those with LSC, have mild-to-moderate psychological abnormalities such as heightened anxiety levels and stress vulnerability that may lead to worsening of the disease (8,9). Moreover some clinicians, including myself, believe that there is a predilection for internalization of anger and hostility that is distinctive for patients with atopic dermatitis.

At the clinical level it is apparent that factors in the local environment, such as heat and sweating, trigger both the initiation and the continuation of the process. As opposed to this important role for contact irritants, the role of contact allergens is much more controversial. A significant proportion of patients with anogenital dermatitis are reported to have positive patch tests (10,11) that were considered to be clinically relevant. However data indicating that removal of the offending agent leads to resolution of the problem are lacking. Based on our personal experience, patch testing in patients with LSC is rarely necessary or justifiable.

Management

LSC is a chronic disease. Left untreated, the itch–scratch cycle persists indefinitely, although it can be somewhat episodic rather than consistently present. This process is extremely discomforting for the patient and it may lead to a significant decrement in quality of life (12). Other troublesome sequelae may include hyperpigmentation and hypopigmentation due to activation or destruction of melanocytes, respectively. At the hypothetical level it has been suggested that chronic scratching might lead to hyperproliferation-type cell signaling for epithelial cells and that in turn might act as "promoter" for the development of squamous cell carcinoma if previous "initiating" events such as genetic mutations should have occurred (6,7,13).

Treatment for LSC can be extremely effective. Approach to therapy includes five basic steps: (1) improvement in the local environment to reduce the triggering that leads to itching and scratching, (2) restoration of normal barrier layer function, (3) reduction in inflammation, (4) cessation of the itch–scratch cycle, (5) identification and treatment for any detrimental psychological factors that may be present.

Improvement in the Local Environment

As mentioned previously, heat and sweat act as provoking factors for the development of both itching and inflammation. Removing or reducing these factors is certainly desirable but is more difficult to do than one might expect. Immediate steps include a change to less occlusive, tight fitting clothing and the use of materials (such as cotton and cotton-blends) that allow for better movement of air. Contrary to decades of physician recommendations, however, the avoidance of dyes in underwear ("use white underwear only!") lacks any scientific merit. Other approaches include the avoidance of prolonged sitting, the use of cloth rather than vinyl for seating-surfaces, and the use of cooler temperatures in the workspace or home. Weight loss can help those who are particularly obese by way of decreasing intertriginous surface area and reducing frictional rubbing. Note that the use of hair dryers, even on their lowest temperature settings, in an attempt to dry the area is not helpful and in most instances is actually detrimental.

Other irritants include fecal contamination, and for women, the chronic presence of urine and vaginal secretions. Discussion of approaches to fecal and urinary incontinence is outside the scope of this chapter, but additional medical consultation will probably be necessary for ameliorating these two factors. Vaginal discharge needs to be properly diagnosed and treated (see Chapter 15) and the use of regular panty liners can be discouraged.

Excess hygiene, by way of removing natural skin lubricants, can also be irritating. Asking the patient about the frequency and nature of anogenital hygiene is important because many patients, especially women, think of the anogenital area as a site that is "especially dirty." Again, contrary to popular opinion, laundering practices for underwear (number of rinses, use of certain detergents, use of antistatic dryer strips, etc.) are for practical purposes never an important triggering factor.

Restoration of Barrier Layer Function

Barrier layer function is never intact in patients with atopic dermatitis and LSC. Dysfunction occurs as a result of genetic factors interfering with epithelial cell differentiation, the irritant factors mentioned above, and the physical disruption of the surface epithelium due to scratching and rubbing. The approach to all three of these factors involves the use of lubrication. Since lubricants are covered in detail in Chapter 2, this material will not be repeated here. Irritants can be dealt with as described in the preceding two paragraphs and the reduction of scratching is covered below.

Reduction in Inflammation

Steroids, used topically or systemically, are the sine qua non for the treatment of inflammation. This subject is covered in Chapter 2 in the section "Anti-inflammatory Therapy" and, other than discussion of a few important principles, will not be repeated here. First, the strength of the topical steroid must be appropriate for the task at hand. Low and mid potency steroids such as hydrocortisone and triamcinalone are usually ineffective. Second, an ointment vehicle, rather than a cream, will be better tolerated and adds a bit of lubrication. Third, topical steroids must be continued for a month or more after the clinical symptoms and signs have regressed. This duration of therapy is necessary because microscopic evidence of inflammation remains for a considerable period of time after clinical improvement is noted. Fourth, if topical steroids have not been effective after a month of treatment, consider the use of systemic steroid therapy. While a "burst" of prednisone can work, it is often too short to be maximally effective and in addition rebound often occurs shortly after the last pills are administered. For this reason, consider the use of intramuscularly administered triamcinalone (Kenalog) as described in Chapter 2. The indications and directions for use of the nonsteroidal calcineurin inhibitors tacrolimus and pimecrolimus are also discussed in Chapter 2.

Breaking the Itch–Scratch Cycle

This is the single most important aspect in the treatment of LSC. Unfortunately, it is also the most often overlooked. The presence of clothing, a conscious attempt to control scratching and embarrassment over scratching the genitalia, prevents most daytime scratching. However, none of these constraints are present at night while the patient is sleeping and thus do not prevent the nighttime scratching that characteristically is present with the itch-scratch cycle. Approaches for the treatment of nighttime rubbing and scratching are thoroughly covered in Chapter 2, but several major principles will be reviewed here. First, nighttime scratching occurs periodically while the patient is in the lighter stages of sleep (3,4). Nonhabituating medications with a sedative effect such as the first generation of antihistamines and certain tricyclics work well for this purpose. Second, the dose of the medication chosen should be increased until nighttime scratching ceases or until the risks of side effects caution against any further increase. Third, the medication should be taken about 2 hours before the expected hour of sleep to prevent morning "hangover." Fourth, the medication should be taken every evening rather than on an "as necessary" basis.

In many instances, sedating therapy for nighttime scratching obviates the need to treat daytime itching with medications such as hydroxyzine that can cause sleepiness or dangerous operation of machinery. However, some patients will still experience significant daytime pruritus. Many clinicians prescribe nonsedating antihistamines for these individuals. Unfortunately, this approach does not work well probably because histamine plays only a minor role in the itching associated with atopic dermatitis and LSC. In this situation, I prefer the use of selective serotonin reuptake inhibitors (SSRIs). It is not clear whether these agents work because of their beneficial effect on anxiety and depression or whether they diminish the obsessive–compulsive component of chronic scratching. Further information on the use of SSRIs can be found in Chapter 2.

Identification and Treatment of Detrimental Psychological Components

Anxiety and/or depression are regularly present in patients with LSC (8,9). Most patients will not volunteer this information unless it is directly sought by a clinician. Even then, the importance of psychological factors tends to be minimized by patients and thus questioning in this area should occur not just initially but also periodically at the time of return visits.

Some controversy exists as to whether these psychological factors play a role in the etiology of the LSC or whether they occur secondary to the presence of LSC. It is my opinion, supported by some published data, that they are frequently important in causation (14,15). But, either way, once identified, treatment, generally with SSRIs as described in Chapter 2, is very helpful.

In addition to the common problems of anxiety and depression, patients with eczematous disease such as LSC may also experience sexual dysfunction (16). Although most of us would not consider ourselves as expert in the area of sexual counseling, giving patients an opportunity to discuss this aspect of their lives can also be quite beneficial in the treatment of patients with LSC.

IRRITANT CONTACT DERMATITIS

Irritant contact dermatitis is an eczematous reaction that develops in response to an exogenous substance that can cause an inflammatory reaction when applied to the skin of any individual. Thus all individuals have the potential for developing irritant contact dermatitis, whereas only patients specifically sensitized to an allergen develop allergic contact dermatitis (see next section).

Clinical Presentation

The prevalence of irritant contact dermatitis involving the anogenital area is unknown, although one major study indicated that irritant·contact dermatitis accounted for about 20% of all patients with anogenital problems referred to dermatologists for patch testing (11). Almost no data exist regarding the development of anogenital irritant contact dermatitis in men, but in this same study, and somewhat counterintuitively, it appears as though it occurs appreciably more frequently in men than in women (11). Irritant contact dermatitis is often divided into two categories: chronic and acute irritant contact dermatitis.

Chronic irritant contact dermatitis is usually manifested by symptoms of irritation, pain, soreness, or rawness. Note that if the patient is atopic, the irritant can also cause itching and can initiate an itch–scratch cycle. Morphologically, the area affected in irritant contact dermatitis depends on where the contact occurred. Generally, this is manifested by a poorly demarcated slightly scaly erythematous patch or slightly elevated plaque. Little or no edema is present (Fig. 4-13). The red hues sometimes occur at the dusky red or brown-red end

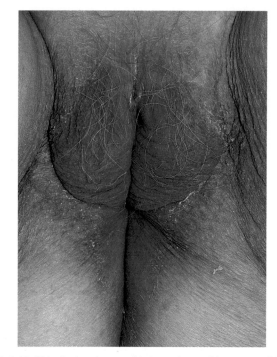

FIG. 4-14. This dusky plaque of irritant dermatitis occurred from frequent use of topical antifungal creams.

of the erythema spectrum (Fig. 4-14). Often there is a dry, glazed, fissured, chapped appearance (Figs. 4-15 and 4-16). If the irritant in question triggered itching and scratching, the morphology will be indistinguishable from that of atopic dermatitis.

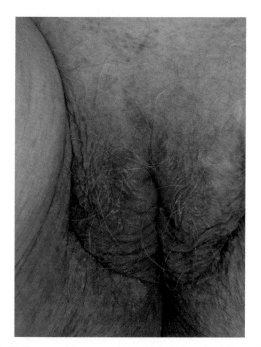

FIG. 4-13. Overwashing, together with harshness of the antibacterial soap, has produced this poorly demarcated, red plaque.

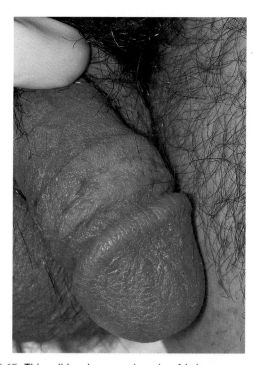

FIG. 4-15. This mild redness and scale of irritant contact dermatitis was caused by frequent washing with povidone–iodine solution.

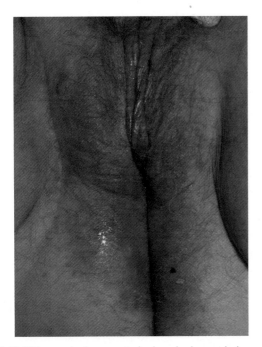

FIG. 4-16. This poorly demarcated, glazed, chapped plaque was produced by chronic irritation of urine in this incontinent woman.

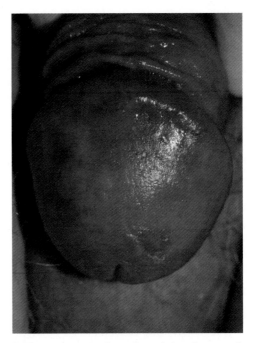

FIG. 4-18. The redness and erosion of the glans penis of this patient resulted from frequent soaks in an antibacterial mouthwash.

Acute irritant contact dermatitis is essentially a chemical "burn." The rapid appearance of erythema, edema, and sometimes blistering is typical (Fig. 4-17). Poorly keratinized skin, such as the modified mucous membranes of the vulva, the glans penis, and the inner aspect of the prepuce, is very fragile, and blister roofs are shed quickly,

forming erosions or even ulcers (Fig. 4-18). On the more resilient keratinized skin, blisters may remain visible for a day or two before they too become unroofed, leaving erosions or ulcers (Fig. 4-19).

Diagnosis

The diagnosis of *chronic* irritant contact dermatitis is made on the appearance as described above, together with a history that suggests undue exposure to soap, water, sweat, urine, feces, vaginal discharge, or less

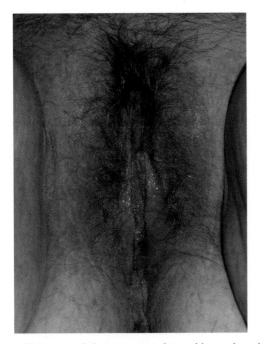

FIG. 4-17. This acute irritant contact dermatitis produced by a reaction to an azole cream exhibits erythema and edema sufficient to produce exudation.

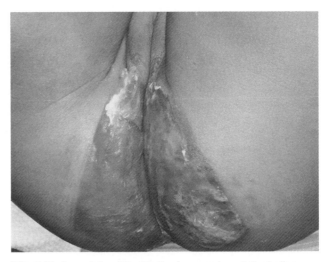

FIG. 4-19. One night of liquid diarrhea produced the bulla seen on the right buttock, and the erosion from an unroofed bulla on the left.

frequently encountered irritants as listed under the section "Pathogenesis." Biopsy is rarely necessary and if carried out, provides only the spongiosis and acanthosis that are characteristic of all eczematous diseases. That is, the histology only indicates that the problem is an eczematous process without specifically pointing toward an irritant contact etiology. The differential diagnoses are primarily the other eczematous diseases, especially LSC, as described above. Differentiation from allergic contact dermatitis can be problematic. Patch testing may be helpful in this regard (11), but all too often a positive result may not correlate with documentable exposure to that chemical or product. Uncommon and rare conditions that can mimic chronic irritant contact dermatitis include candidiasis, extramammary Paget disease, Hailey–Hailey disease, and Darier disease.

The diagnosis of *acute* contact dermatitis is made easier because of the short interval between exposure and development of inflammation. Thus patients can almost always identify the contactant that caused the problem. Most often the products responsible are medications that usually have been recently applied by medical personnel (Table 4-1). On the rare occasions where such a history is not forthcoming, one should consider the possibility of obsessive–compulsive disorder or factitial disease caused by the patient or the patients' care takers. Biopsy is not useful in acute irritant contact dermatitis as the histology only shows disruption or destruction of the epithelium without pointing to a specific cause.

TABLE 4.1	Common causes of irritant contact dermatitis

Weak irritants (as a cause of chronic irritant dermatitis)
Excessive hygiene with soap and water
Sweat
Urine
Feces
Depilatories
Vaginal lubricants
Panty liners
Menstrual pads
Spermicides
Preservatives and stabilizers used in
    Some topical creams, gels, and solutions
Candida sp. proteins
Strong irritants (as a cause of acute irritant dermatitis)
Salicylic acid
Podophyllin and podophyllotoxin products
Imiquimod
Fluorouracil
Cantharidin
Trichloroacetic and bichloroacetic acid
Laser and electrosurgical therapy

Pathophysiology

Irritant contact dermatitis can be caused either by repeated exposure to a weak irritant (chronic irritant contact dermatitis) or by one, or only a few, exposures to a very strong irritant (acute irritant contact dermatitis) (Table 4-1).

The most common causes of *chronic* irritant contact dermatitis are overexposure to soap and water and chronic exposure to urine or feces in a diapered infant or an incontinent adult (Figs. 4-13 and 4-16). Other chronic irritants include douches, feminine hygiene products, depilatories, personal lubricants, and spermicides (Fig. 4-14). An often overlooked irritant is the presence of candidiasis where the candidal proteins can cause irritation quite apart from true infection. Because repeated exposure is necessary for the development of irritant contact dermatitis and because the symptoms and signs develop gradually, the patient is frequently unaware that the offending substance is irritating and is thus playing a role as a cause of his or her problem.

Because *acute* irritant contact dermatitis is produced by one or only a few exposures to a very strong irritant, this exposure is often accompanied by a very short duration of time before pain, burning, and stinging are noted. For this reason, the patient usually knows what caused the problem, although he or she frequently misinterprets this as allergy rather than irritation. The most common causes of acute irritant contact dermatitis include various treatments for genital warts, such as trichloroacetic and bichloroacetic acids, podophyllin products, imiquimod, and cantharidin. Some patients with very sensitive skin can experience acute irritant contact dermatitis to the cream, gel, or solution vehicles used in topical medications and lubricants. This is probably the result of chemicals such as alcohol, propylene glycol, and polyethylene glycol. This type of problem is frequently experienced with the "azole" group of anticandidal/antifungal creams. Lastly, keep in mind that patients will sometimes apply very unorthodox products to their genitalia in misguided attempts to clean an area that is perceived to be "dirty" or "odorous." We have seen reactions to things such as lye, kerosene, and bleach.

Management

The most important aspects of therapy are the identification and elimination of all irritants. Irritant contact dermatitis in the genital area is often multifactorial, so all medications, soaps, antiseptics, douches, powders, and vigorous washing should be discontinued. However keep in mind that some patients become "addicted" to certain behaviors and as a result there may be very poor compliance with instructions to cease these ritualistic behaviors. After the offending agent(s) are discontinued, chronic irritant contact dermatitis improves quickly with the use of a mid potency topical corticosteroid ointment, such as triamcinolone 0.1% applied twice a day. If the skin is dry and chapped, lubricants (see Chapter 2) may be useful. Infants and diapered adults may require the use of a "barrier" product such as zinc oxide ointment to keep urine and feces away from the skin. In those instances where itching or pain is really troublesome, prednisone, at a dose of 40 mg each morning for a few days, can improve this symptom until healing is well underway, at which point topical corticosteroid can be substituted.

The pain and burning of acute irritant contact dermatitis can be minimized through the use of tepid tap water bathtub soaks several times a day for the first few days. Lubrication with a thin layer of petrolatum should be applied immediately following each soak. Nighttime sedation and oral analgesics may be necessary for several days. Topical analgesics should be avoided as they may cause additional discomfort.

ALLERGIC CONTACT DERMATITIS

As opposed to irritant contact dermatitis wherein all individuals are potentially capable of developing the problem, allergic contact dermatitis requires immunological processing. This is a more restrictive process and only certain individuals exposed to a potential allergen will develop allergic contact dermatitis at the time of their next contact with the allergen.

Clinical Presentation

Controversy exists regarding the frequency with which allergic contact dermatitis of the genitalia occurs. Nearly all of the published material on prevalence deals primarily with contact dermatitis of the vulva in women. The excellent review article by Warshaw et al. summarizes this work and also adds new information regarding contact dermatitis in men (11). The information contained in this review suggests that one or more clinically relevant positive patch test will be found in 15% to 40% of women with vulvar dermatoses and that the frequency in men is roughly similar. This study also suggests that allergic contact dermatitis occurs approximately twice as frequently as does irritant contact dermatitis (11). These observations are not consistent with our own clinical experience that suggests a frequency of allergic contact dermatitis appreciably less than that of irritant contact dermatitis and one accounting for no more than a few percent of our patients with genital dermatitis. This discrepancy probably revolves around two potential problems. First, there is considerable difficulty in determining which positive patch tests are truly clinically

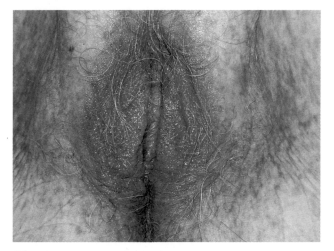

FIG. 4-20. Benzocaine obtained over the counter and applied for itching has resulted in these tiny, coalescing vesicle of allergic contact dermatitis.

relevant. Second, patients with rigorously defined atopic dermatitis have an extraordinarily high frequency of positive patch tests to common environmental allergens and it is not known what role, if any, these allergens play in the pathogenesis of their atopic dermatitis (17).

Allergic contact dermatitis is characterized by the presence of poorly marginated, bright red, edematous patches and plaques. Scale is generally less prominent than it is in atopic dermatitis and irritant contact dermatitis. Pruritus is regularly present and in some instances can be quite problematic. Not surprisingly, this frequently results in the development of the itch–scratch cycle and the clinical signs of LSC. Sometimes minute vesicles, representing macroscopic evidence of spongiosis, stud the surface of the erythematous plaques (Fig. 4-20). Occasionally odd shapes (linear or angular) are found (Fig. 4-21). These generally occur as a result through the irregular application

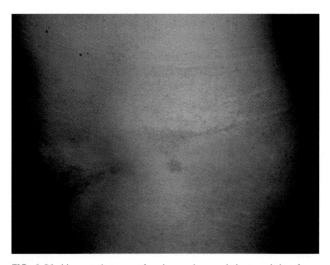

FIG. 4-21. Linear plaques of red papules and tiny vesicles from allergic contact with poison ivy that brushed against the skin during a camping trip.

of medications applied with the finger tips. The labia majora are usually involved in women and both the penis and the scrotum may be affected in men. Perianal involvement is found in both sexes.

Allergic contact *urticaria* is rarely encountered and is a separate and distinct disorder from allergic contact dermatitis. The appearance can be that of tissue swelling (angioedema) or can develop as urticarial papules (wheals, hives) and plaques that are entirely similar to those that occur with garden-variety urticaria. Unlike the situation with allergic contact *dermatitis*, there is no evidence of epithelial abnormalities. Such reactions are usually easy to recognize because of the development of the urticarial reaction within minutes after contact has taken place.

Diagnosis

The diagnosis of allergic contact dermatitis is most often made on a clinical basis. The role of patch testing for patients with eczematous disease of the genitalia is controversial. Some clinicians believe that a diagnosis of allergic contact dermatitis is often missed unless all patients presenting with an eczematous morphology are tested. Others, like ourselves, believe that, in accordance with Bayes theorem, testing is best carried out only in highly selected patients so as to reduce the large number of false-positive results that occur when testing is carried out in a relatively unselected population. Moreover, the simple presence of a positive patch test does not prove that the disease in question is due to that allergen. It is necessary first to identify the presence of that allergen in one or another of products being applied to the anogenital tissue and, second, to obtain marked clinical improvement when use of the offending product is discontinued.

Biopsy is not likely to be helpful because the principle findings of spongiosis and acanthosis are essentially identical to those in all of the other eczematous diseases. In spite of this, some believe that the presence of eosinophils in the inflammatory infiltrate suggests a high likelihood of allergic contact dermatitis.

All of the eczematous disorders, as described in this chapter, need to be considered in one's list of differential diagnoses. In addition one should bear in mind the possibility of candidiasis and the dermatophyte fungal infection, tinea cruris.

Pathophysiology

Allergic contact dermatitis represents a cell mediated delayed-type (type IV) hypersensitivity reaction. It arises when a chemical, acting as an antigen, is processed by macrophages (Langerhans cells) in the epidermis and is then presented to the T-cell immune system. This results in the development, activation, and proliferation of antigen-specific T cells. These cells return to the skin at the time of the next contact with allergen, resulting in the clinical development of allergic contact dermatitis.

The most common causes of allergic contact dermatitis in the anogenital area are either prescription or over-the-counter topical medications. The agent most often incriminated is benzocaine, which is a component of Vagisil and some other topical analgesics (18). In addition to these products, clinicians who frequently carry out patch testing identify numerous other substances that are potential offenders (11,19–23). The most common of these substances are listed in Table 4-2. Note specifically that positive patch tests occur quite often with several topically applied corticosteroids and with vehicles, preservatives, and stabilizers found in almost all cosmetic and medical products. Our experience suggests that these infrequently cause problems, but in instances of recalcitrant anogenital dermatitis, discontinuation of all topically applied agents including corticosteroids and all lubricants other than petrolatum is warranted. If this is followed by improvement, agents can be added back one at a time in an attempt to identify the culprit.

A special situation occurs in patients who are allergic to seminal fluid and latex. These represent a type I, IgE-mediated, immediate reaction in which angioedema and urticarial papules and plaques arise within minutes of contact. These occur very infrequently but are mentioned because of the potential for development of anaphylaxis.

A number of commonly used products are not listed here because of controversy about their ability to cause either allergic or irritant reactions. These include soaps, laundry detergents, fabric softeners, antistatic sheets, medicated wipes, toilet paper (scented or not scented), menstrual pads, and other feminine hygiene agents (24–27). In

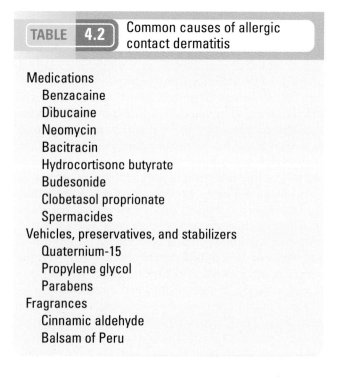

TABLE 4.2	Common causes of allergic contact dermatitis

Medications
    Benzacaine
    Dibucaine
    Neomycin
    Bacitracin
    Hydrocortisone butyrate
    Budesonide
    Clobetasol proprionate
    Spermacides
Vehicles, preservatives, and stabilizers
    Quaternium-15
    Propylene glycol
    Parabens
Fragrances
    Cinnamic aldehyde
    Balsam of Peru

our opinion, normal use of these products rarely leads to anogenital dermatitis.

Management

Most important in the treatment of contact dermatitis is the identification and elimination of the offending contactant. If the contactant can be identified either clinically or through patch testing, the patient needs to be instructed regarding avoidance. This can be difficult because some allergens can be found in multiple, often apparently innocuous and unsuspected sources. Information regarding these potential sources can be found in standard dermatological textbooks. In instances of suspected allergic contact dermatitis where a specific contactant cannot be identified, it may be necessary to counsel the patient to avoid all topical agents other than clear water and petrolatum.

After the elimination of the contactant, the symptoms of itching and discomfort that are present in allergic contact dermatitis can be improved with cool soaks or sitz baths for the first few days. Oral prednisone, at a dose of 40 mg for 5 days will bring rapid improvement in severe allergic contact dermatitis and if the correct allergen has been identified and removed, rebound is unlikely to occur when the steroids are stopped. If the reaction is milder, a topical corticosteroid such as fluocinonide 0.05% ointment can be applied twice daily until healing is complete. Nighttime sedation can be added if itching and scratching are problematic.

Once a patient has become sensitized to an allergen, re-exposure will quickly lead to reappearance of the contact dermatitis. Patients should be made aware that this immunological memory can last for many years and that contact with even a very small quantity of the antigen can result in allergic reaction.

SEBORRHEIC DERMATITIS AND INTERTRIGO

Clinical Presentation

Seborrheic dermatitis is easily identified because of the presence of characteristic yellow scale when it occurs in hairy areas such as the scalp. On the other hand it is controversial as to whether a similar eruption, but with little or no scale, occurring in nonhairy intertriginous folds should be termed intertrigo or seborrheic dermatitis. For the purposes of this chapter, intertriginous redness and no scale will be termed intertrigo. The term seborrheic dermatitis will be used for the occurrence of intertriginous redness accompanied by scale.

The clinical appearance is that of poorly marginated, erythematous patches, or very slightly raised plaques, occurring in folded areas where moisture such as sweat or urine is retained. Early on, scale will not be apparent (intertrigo) but, left untreated and with the passage of time, the chronic inflammation will result in epithelial proliferation and the gradual development of scale (seborrheic dermatitis) (Figs. 4-22 through 4-24). Often the scale

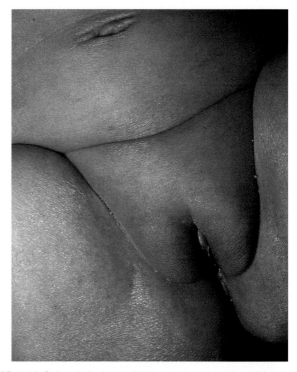

FIG. 4-22. Seborrheic dermatitis is most common in children and is manifested by skin fold redness and scale; cradle cap is also often present in infants with anogenital seborrheic dermatitis.

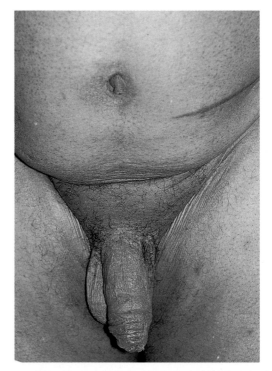

FIG. 4-23. Seborrheic dermatitis is characterized by prominent skin fold involvement to include the crural crease, umbilicus, and axillae. Inflammation is obscured in this patient by his dark skin color, so that the plaques appear hyperpigmented rather than red.

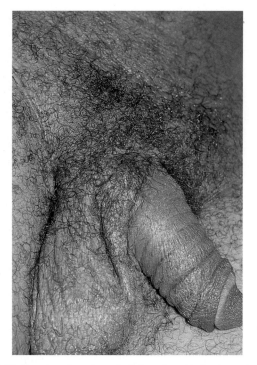

FIG. 4-24. Prominent scale on hair-bearing skin is characteristic of seborrheic dermatitis.

is not loose but rather more attached, resulting in a glazed, shiny, or chapped appearance. If itching is present, resultant scratching may lead to the superimposition of excoriations and the appearance of LSC.

Not surprisingly, because of anatomic differences, this process is encountered more frequently in women than in men and in those who are obese rather than those who are slender. Other environmental irritation such as high ambient temperature, high relative humidity, and occlusive clothing will also increase the frequency with which this phenomenon occurs. The diagnosis of anogenital seborrheic dermatitis is rarely made in adults but is often identified in infants when it is accompanied by additional sites of seborrheic dermatitis in the scalp, retroauricular folds, and axillae.

Diagnosis

The diagnosis is made on a clinical basis; biopsy reveals only the generic changes found in all eczematous diseases. The major consideration in differential diagnosis is psoriasis of the inverse type. This condition is sometime called "sebo-psoriasis" to indicate the possible overlap of these conditions and the difficulty in differentiating between them. In most instances this differentiation will be based on whether or not other more classical lesions of psoriasis can be found elsewhere. Superimposition of candidiasis occurs with some frequency in intertrigo and seborrheic dermatitis. The presence of minute pustules either disseminated throughout the main portion of the patches or occurring at the periphery as "satellite" lesions suggest that candidiasis is present.

Pathophysiology

The pathogenesis of intertrigo and seborrheic dermatitis relates to maceration, defined as the presence of too much moisture for too long a time. The viability of epithelial cells depends on, among other constraints, an appropriate amount of water in and around them. When the immediate environment around epithelial cells is either too wet or too dry, they can perish. The resultant disruption of the epithelial barrier incites inflammation and the presence of chronic inflammation creates epithelial proliferation and the consequent development of scale. This warm moist environment, when it occurs in the anogenital area, often leads to the development of secondary candidiasis which in turn causes further, persistent inflammation. Dermatology textbooks usually indicate that seborrheic dermatitis occurs directly as an overgrowth of the yeasts, *Malassezia* sp., that are normally resident in hair follicles. However it seems likely to me that this overgrowth occurs as a result of, rather than the cause of, the seborrheic dermatitis.

Management

Left untreated, seborrheic dermatitis becomes a chronic condition that waxes and wanes. On the other hand, there is usually an excellent and rapid response to therapy. The first step in treatment is to improve the environment as much as possible through the reduction of retained heat and moisture. But even when this cannot easily be achieved (such as in diapered infants or incontinent adults), marked improvement can be obtained with topical agents. Topically applied "azoles," such as ketoconazole, usually represent the initial approach by most clinicians. These products are recommended based on the belief that the process is caused by *Malassezia* sp. and by a desire to avoid topical steroids in intertriginous sites. However, in our experience the use of low potency (2.5% hydrocortisone) or mid potency (triamcinolone 0.1%) steroids in either a cream or ointment vehicle sting less, work faster, and are equally safe when used for relatively short periods of time.

Topical calcineurin inhibitors such as tacrolimus and pimecrolimus can be used for their steroid-sparing effects, although stinging and burning somewhat limit patient acceptability (28). If response is inadequate, consider the possibility that candidiasis is also present and consider adding one or another of the "azoles." Because of the difficulty in achieving long-term improvement in the environmental conditions that precipitated the condition in the first place, recurrences are common and retreatment is often necessary. Treatment of seborrheic dermatitis of the scalp, if such is present, seems to be helpful both in improving anogenital disease and preventing recurrences.

REFERENCES

1. Lynch PJ, Moyal-Barracco M, Bogliatto F, et al. 2006 ISSVD classification of vulvar dermatoses: pathologic subsets and their clinical correlates. *J Reprod Med.* 2007;52:3–9.
2. Brenninkmeijer EEA, Schram ME, Leeflang MMG, et al. Diagnostic criteria for atopic dermatitis: a systematic review. *Br J Dermatol.* 2008;158:754–765.
3. Koca R, Altin R, Konuk N, et al. Sleep disturbance in patients with lichen simplex chronicus and its relationship to nocturnal scratching: a case control study. *South Med J.* 2006;99:482–485.
4. Bender BG, Ballard R, Canono B, et al. Disease severity, scratching and sleep quality in patients with atopic dermatitis. *J Am Acad Dermatol.* 2008;58:415–420.
5. Lynch PJ. Lichen simplex chronicus (atopic/neurodermatitis) of the anogenital region. *Dermatol Ther.* 2004;17:8–19.
6. Nascimento AF, Granter SR, Cviko A, et al. Vulvar acanthosis with altered differentiation: a precursor to verrucous carcinoma? *Am J Surg Pathol.* 2004;28:638–643.
7. Lee ES, Allen D, Scurry J. Pseudoepitheliomatous hyperplasia in lichen sclerosus of the vulva. *Int J Gynecol Pathol.* 2003;22:57–62.
8. Buske-Kirschbaum A, Ebrecht M, Kern S, et al. Personality characteristics in chronic and non-chronic allergic conditions. *Brain Behav Immun.* 2008;22:762–768.
9. Pavlovic S, Danitchenko M, Tobin DJ, et al. Further exploring the brain-skin connection: stress worsens dermatitis via substance P-dependent neurogenic inflammation in mice. *J Invest Dermatol.* 2008;128:434–446.
10. Virgili A, Bacileri S, Corazzo M. Evaluation of contact sensitization in vulvar lichen simplex chronicus. *J Reprod Med.* 2003;48:33–36.
11. Warshaw EM, Furda LM, Maibach HI, et al. Anogenital dermatitis in patients referred for patch testing. *Arch Dermatol.* 2008;144:749–755.
12. Higaki Y, Kawamoto K, Kamo T, et al. Measurement of the impact of atopic dermatitis on patients quality of life: a cross-sectional and longitudinal questionnaire study using the Japanese version of Skindex-16. *J Dermatol.* 2004;31:977–982.
13. Hsieh MY, Kuo HW. The simplex (differentiated) variant of vulvar intraepithelial neoplasia. *Dermatol Surg.* 2004;30:948–951.
14. Konuk N, Koca R, Atik L, et al. Psychopathology, depression and dissociative experiences in patients with lichen simplex chronicus. *Gen Hosp Psychiatry.* 2007;29:232–235.
15. Lotti T, Buggiani G, Prignano F. Prurigo nodularis and lichen simplex chronicus. *Dermatol Ther.* 2008;21:42–46.
16. Mercan S, Altunay IK, Demir B, et al. Sexual dysfunction in patients with neurodermatitis and psoriasis. *J Sex Marital Ther.* 2008;34:160–168.
17. Ponyai G, Hidvegi B, Nemeth I, et al. Contact and aeroallergens in adult atopic dermatitis. *J Eur Acad Dermatol Venereol.* 2008;22:1346–1355.
18. Margesson LJ. Contact dermatitis of the vulva. *Dermatol Ther.* 2004;17:20–27.
19. Bauer A, Rodiger C, Greif C, et al. Vulvar dermatoses–irritant and allergic contact dermatitis of the vulva. *Dermatology.* 2005;210:143–149.
20. Vermaat H, Smienk F, Rustemeyer T, et al. Anogenital allergic contact dermatitis, the role of spices and flavour allergy. *Contact Dermatitis.* 2008;59:233–237.
21. Nardelli A, Degreef H, Goossens A. Contact allergic reactions of the vulva: a 14-year review. *Dermatitis.* 2004;15:131–136.
22. Utas S, Ferahbas A, Yildiz S. Patients with vulvar pruritus: patch test results. *Contact Derm.* 2008;58:296–298.
23. Haverhoek E, Reid C, Gordon L, et al. Prospective study of patch testing in patients with vulval pruritus. *Australas J Dermatol.* 2008;49:80–85.
24. Farage MA, Stadler A, Chassard D, et al. A randomized prospective trial of the cutaneous and sensory effects of feminine hygiene wet wipes. *J Reprod Med.* 2008;53:765–773.
25. Farage M, Elsner P, Maibach H. Influence of usage practices, ethnicity and climate on the skin compatibility of sanitary pads. *Arch Gynecol Obstet.* 2007;275:415–427.
26. Wakashin K. Sanitary napkin contact dermatitis of the vulva: location-dependent differences in skin surface conditions may play a role in negative patch test results. *J Dermatol.* 2007;34:834–837.
27. Zoli V, Tosti A, Silvani S, et al. Moist toilet papers as possible sensitizers: review of the literature and evaluation of commercial products in Italy. *Contact Dermatitis.* 2006;55:252–254.
28. Cook BA, Warshaw EM. Role of topical calcineurin inhibitors in the treatment of seborrheic dermatitis: a review of pathophysiology, safety and efficacy. *Am J Clin Dermatol.* 2009;10:103–118.

SUGGESTED READINGS

Bauer A, Rodiger C, Greif C, et al. Vulvar dermatoses–Irritant and allergic contact dermatitis of the vulva. *Dermatology.* 2005;210:143–149.

Lynch P. Lichen simplex chronicus (atopic/neurodermatitis) of the anogenital region. *Dermatol Ther.* 2004;17:8–19.

Naidi L, Rebora A. Clinical practice. Seborrheic dermatitis. *N Eng J Med.* 2009;360:387–396.

Siddiqi S, Vijay V, Ward H, et al. Pruritus ani. *Ann R Coll Surg Engl.* 2008;90:457–463.

Warshaw EM, Furda LM, Maibach HI, et al. Anogenital dermatitis in patients referred for patch testing. *Arch Dermatol.* 2008;144:749–755.

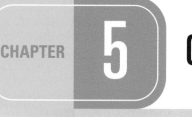

Genital Pain Syndromes

LIBBY EDWARDS

Most chronic external or lower genital symptoms fall into one of two main categories: those who describe itching and scratching and those who report symptoms of pain, burning, rawness, irritation, aching, soreness, or hypersensitivity. Most chronic itching with scratching results from dermatoses. Chronic superficial burning, soreness, and pain, as distinct from pelvic pain, can result from a number of conditions. Pain syndromes rather than specific, observable abnormalities represent the largest proportion of these patients, and most women with self-reported chronic pain were found to have vulvodynia on further evaluation (1). Idiopathic vulvovaginal pain is extremely common, with as many as 1 in 20 women each year developing unexplained, chronic vulvovaginal pain (2). However, there is very little data on pain syndromes in men, although these certainly are recognized by clinicians. The diagnosis and therapy of superficial male genital pain is extrapolated from data and experience with vulvovaginal pain and anecdotal reports regarding experience of a very few individual clinicians.

The International Society for the Study of Vulvovaginal Disease has classified vulvar pain into several main categories (see Table 5-1 and Appendix 1). In the absence of a similar classification for male genital pain, these categories can be used for both genders. This classification serves as a differential diagnosis for patients with superficial genital pain.

The categories of disorders producing genital pain are skin disease, infection, and specific neurological disorders such as diabetic neuropathy, pudendal neuralgia, or postherpetic neuralgia. Those patients who have no observable skin disease, no infection, and no specific neurologic abnormality fall into the category of genital pain syndrome: vulvodynia, penodynia, scrotodynia, and anodynia.

The patient who presents with burning, irritation, and pain-type symptoms should be evaluated in an organized fashion (see Table 5-2). The skin should be examined carefully, using simple magnification if needed. Most patients who report symptoms of burning, irritation, or rawness also report redness and, often, edema. Redness that is mild, poorly demarcated, and without scaling or thickening is frequently within the range of normal, as genital skin is frequently red in asymptomatic individuals (Fig. 5-1).

At times, patients present with objective skin disease or infection, but discomfort is disproportionate to the degree of skin disease noted, the skin disease may be in a different location than the pain, or pain may persist after the infection or skin disease is cleared. These patients have an underlying pain syndrome either unassociated with the skin disease or triggered by it. The skin disease or infection must be controlled but without clearing of the symptoms before a pain syndrome is definitively diagnosed.

CAUSES OF GENITAL PAIN

Many clinicians and most patients initially assume that genital pain without obvious clinical findings is due to infection, either yeast or sexually transmitted disease. Chronic, unremitting pain is not due to infection, and negative cultures and a lack of response to antimicrobial therapy also signifies a different diagnosis. Most yeast infections are primarily pruritic rather than painful, with the character and degree of vulvovaginal discomfort different as measured on the McGill scale (Fig. 5-2) (3). Sexually transmitted diseases generally either do not cause superficial genital pain (gonorrhea, syphilis, Chlamydia, warts) or they produce intermittent symptoms with visible skin findings (herpes simplex virus in-

---

TABLE 5.1 Causes of chronic genital pain

Infection, especially herpes simplex infection, rubbed/scratched yeast infection, trichomonas, fissures associated with infection

Dermatoses (noninfectious skin disease), especially lichen planus, excoriated/eroded lichen simplex chronicus or lichen sclerosus, irritant contact dermatitis, cicatricial pemphigoid, pemphigus vulgaris, desquamative inflammatory vaginitis, atrophic vaginitis, fissures unassociated with infection, and malignancies/eroded tumors

Neuropathy, including diabetic neuropathy, postherpetic neuralgia, multiple sclerosis, pudendal neuralgia, herniated disc disease

Vulvodynia, Penodynia, Scrotodynia, Anodynia— multifactorial pain syndromes

TABLE 5.2	Evaluation of the patient with genital pain

History
Neurologic history; diabetes, herpes zoster in the
genital distribution
    Agents applied to the genital skin include soaps,
medications, pads/liners
    Washing techniques, frequency, etc.
    Estrogen status
Physical Examination
    Evaluation of affect
    Inspection of mucous membranes for evidence of
subtle erosive mucosal disease, especially
lichen planus
    Gross neurologic examination for allodynia, numb-
ness, paresthesias of the anogenital skin and
proximal medial thighs.
    Examination of the external genitalia with magnifica-
tion if required for subtle fissures, erosions, signs
of scarring/agglutination, or other specific lesions
    Assessment of vaginal mucosa for redness,
erosions, etc.
Microscopic examination of vaginal secretions for
signs of infection, inflammation, and atrophic
changes (in addition to yeast forms, evaluation
for white blood cells, parabasal cells, lack of
lactobacilli)
Culture if examination is suspicious for infection
Biopsy of any specific skin lesion; no biopsy of redness
alone or of painful area in normal-appearing skin

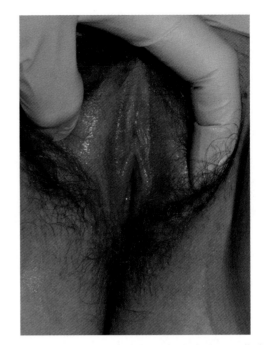

FIG. 5-1. The vulva is normally red, particularly the vestibule and the modified mucous membranes; this patient has no symptoms.

pain symptoms are erosive lichen planus and desquamative inflammatory vaginitis (Fig. 5-7), both of which are characterized by purulent vaginal secretions which irritate the modified mucous membranes of the vulva (Fig. 5-8). Because the vaginal mucosa can be difficult to visualize, especially in the patient with pain, a wet mount can be crucial to rule out inflammatory vaginal disease (Fig. 5-9).

The patient with pain and visible erosions does not present a diagnostic dilemma. However, erosions can be subtle at times; vaginal and introital erosions can be missed in women, and fissures are overlooked easily in

fection.) However, trichomonas, particularly in women, certainly produces irritation and burning, although often accompanied by itching.

The most common skin disease that causes symptoms of burning is irritant contact dermatitis, especially due to overwashing and medications (Figs. 5-3 and 5-4). Allergic contact dermatitis more often produces itching than burning and irritation. Erosive dermatoses most often produce pain and burning as well as itching. Lichen planus is often erosive (Fig. 5-5), as are other blistering diseases such as pemphigus vulgaris or cicatricial pemphigoid (see Chapter 9). However, dermatoses that are primarily pruritic also can be painful when patients have rubbed and scratched the skin; this is usually clear from the history of itching and the findings of excoriations (Fig. 5-6). In women, skin disease causing vulvar burning includes skin disease of the vagina. Even in the face of negative cultures, vaginal inflammation (not infection) can produce introital symptoms. The vaginal skin conditions that most often produce

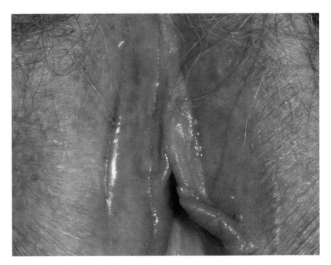

FIG. 5-2. Although Candidiasis is more pruritic than painful, yeast is the most common cause of fissures, which burn and are often described as "paper cuts." See Chapter 9.

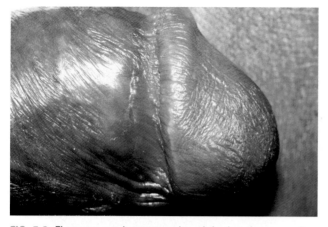

FIG. 5-3. Fissures can be extremely subtle, but they are often very uncomfortable, producing stinging and burning. This patient had irritant contact dermatitis from overwashing as a cause of his fissure and burning.

both men and women. Specific skin lesions other than poorly demarcated, nonscaling redness that are not morphologically diagnosable should be biopsied.

Specific neurologic disease can sometimes be identified by history. For example, a diabetic with burning of the feet and genitalia most likely has diabetic neuropathy, and the patient with past herpes zoster of the genital area has postherpetic neuralgia. Postherpetic neuralgia only follows herpes zoster, not herpes simplex virus infection. Multiple sclerosis is sometimes associated with pain syndromes.

Pudendal nerve entrapment syndrome is an occasional cause of anogenital pain (4,5). This can be difficult to di-

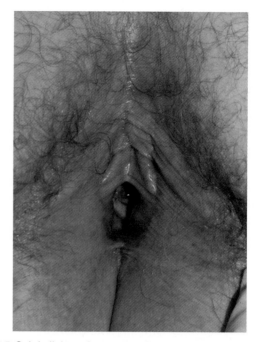

FIG. 5-5. Subtle lichen planus can mimic vestibulodynia (vestibulitis); the well-demarcated nature of the vestibular erythema in this patient is the clue that the redness is abnormal. A biopsy of the edge of this red plaque showed lichen planus.

agnose, at least partly because there are several types, and there is considerable individual variation in the anatomy and course of this nerve. There is no one standard evaluation and diagnostic regimen. This condition is suggested by sensory abnormalities in the saddle distribution of the pudendal nerve. There is pain or numbness of the genitalia and adjacent buttock, the proximal, medial thigh, and/or rectal area. Classically, the pain is worst when sitting and minimized by standing or lying. The diagnosis can be implicated further by a careful physical examination,

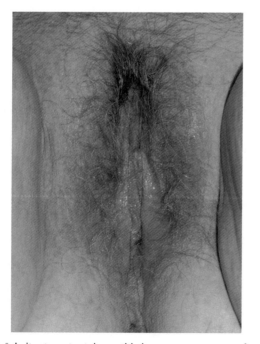

FIG. 5-4. Irritant contact dermatitis is a common cause of poorly demarcated redness and burning; this was contact dermatitis to a panty liner.

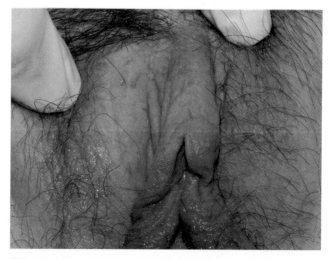

FIG. 5-6. Although excruciating itching was a presenting complaint of this patient, burning and rawness as a result of excoriations followed bouts of scratching. The lichenified skin and excoriations are typical for lichen simplex chronicus.

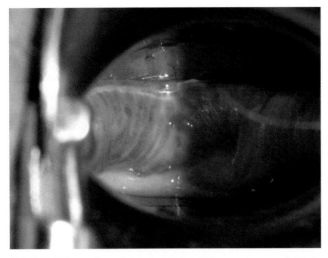

FIG. 5-7. This vagina of desquamative inflammatory vaginitis is diffusely red or speckled with monomorphous red, tiny macules/papules, whereas vaginal lichen planus usually shows patchy redness.

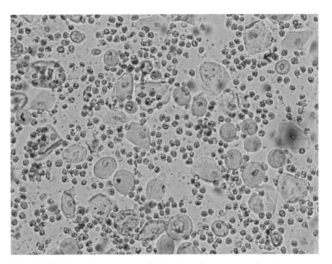

FIG. 5-9. Inflammatory vaginal disease of any cause is characterized by grossly and microscopically purulent vaginal secretions; increased numbers of white blood cells, either neutrophils or lymphocytes occur, usually in a setting of parabasal cells and absent lactobacilli. These nonspecific findings are common to desquamative inflammatory vaginitis, atrophic vaginitis, and any erosive vaginal disease, including lichen planus, cicatricial pemphigoid, and pemphigoid vulgaris.

magnetic resonance imaging examination performed by specialists in this disease, and magnetic resonance neurography. Management consists of injections of botulinum toxin, anesthetics, and corticosteroids. Some find benefit from medications for neuropathy and pelvic floor therapy. Those patients who do not improve with these therapies require surgical release of the entrapped nerve.

Patients with normal genital skin, to include the vagina, negative cultures, and no specific diagnosable neuropathy, are diagnosed as vulvodynia, penodynia, scrotodynia, or penodynia.

Vulvodynia

Vulvodynia is defined as vulvar discomfort characterized by chronic burning, stinging, rawness, irritation, aching, soreness, or throbbing in the absence of objective findings of skin disease, infection, or specific neurologic disease. Itching is not a prominent symptom.

Clinical Presentation

Vulvodynia is an extraordinarily common condition. Several studies report a life-time incidence of 10% to 17% and a current prevalence of 3.8% to 7% (1,6,7). Although initially believed to occur most often in Caucasians, these studies have indicated that patients of African genetic background experience vulvodynia at the same rate as white patients (6), and Hispanics may have an increased risk of developing this disease. The risk of Asian individuals is not known. Vulvodynia is most often reported after the age of 20, but this may simply correlate with the increasing numbers of sexually active people about that age. However, the onset of vulvodynia occurs fairly frequently after menopause as well, independent of atrophic changes. Vulvodynia is found uncommonly in prepubertal girls (8).

Women often report that symptoms began with a yeast infection, although idiopathic vulvar symptoms are frequently empirically treated as yeast. The most common and most troublesome symptom is superficial dyspareunia, often described as sensations of burning, rawness, tearing, or aching. As noted above, other factors that commonly produce discomfort include tight clothing, wiping after urination, tampon use, and gynecologic examinations.

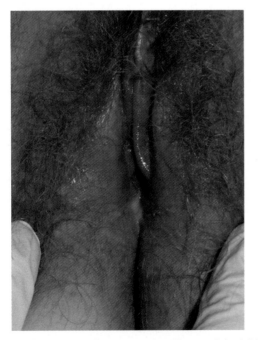

FIG. 5-8. Redness of the introitus and puffiness of the labia minora result from an irritant contact dermatitis to the purulent vaginal secretions of vaginal skin disease.

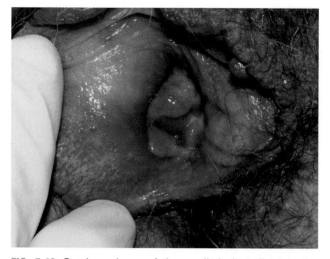

FIG. 5-10. Patchy redness of the vestibule just distal to the hymeneal ring is common in women with vestibulodynia.

Most women indicate the vestibule as the area of greatest discomfort, although extension beyond the vestibule, either by touch/pressure in the office or by history, is usual. At times, pain symptoms extend to the perianal area.

A physical examination reveals no skin changes except for variable erythema, especially in the vestibule, and pain to touch with a cotton-tipped applicator that typically is either limited to, or worst, in the vestibule (Fig. 5-10). A vaginal wet mount and fungal preparation are normal. On evaluation of the pelvic floor, tightness to insertion of a finger, tenderness to palpation of the pelvic floor muscles, and overall weakness of these muscles are common.

Vulvodynia occurs most often in women with other chronic pain syndromes, including headaches, fibromyalgia, irritable bowel syndrome, interstitial cystitis, and temporomandibular joint syndrome. Other pelvic floor symptoms are common as well, to include incontinence, frequency, urgency, and constipation. Depression and anxiety are generally prominent, and sexual dysfunction is universal.

Diagnosis

The diagnosis of vulvodynia is made by the presence of pain in the absence of objective, definable causes of vulvovaginal pain, other than, at times, minor redness, pain to touch, or abnormal pelvic floor examinations. Skin disease is excluded by a careful examination, and, when indicated by the presence of specific lesions, a biopsy. Vaginal secretions must be normal, without signs of inflammation, atrophy, or infection on wet mount (see Chapter 15). A routine culture to exclude infection as a major or minor factor should be performed for most patients. A history to explore the possibility of neurologic disease as a factor must be done, with referral to a specialist gynecologist in the occasional instance of

pudendal neuralgia or a neurologist in the unlikely event of serious considerations of other specific neurologic disease such as multiple sclerosis.

Most women with vulvodynia experience pain to pressure with a cotton tipped applicator; this pain is nearly always present in the vestibule, but sometimes extends beyond this area. In addition to pain with touch and pressure, most patients with vulvodynia also report discomfort in the absence of touch or friction, at least occasionally with flares. The occasional patient describes only background burning and irritation but no pain with touch or pressure.

Appendix 1 reports the classification of recognized patterns of vulvodynia. There are two major patterns of vulvodynia; those patients with pain to pressure in the vestibule and no extension beyond this area are said to have vestibulodynia (previously called the vulvar vestibulitis syndrome, vestibular adenitis, or infection of the minor vestibular glands). Those patients who have more generalized or migratory discomfort are diagnosed with generalized vulvodynia. However, vulvodynia can be localized to other areas, such as the clitoris, and pain can be either spontaneous or occurring in response to touch, pressure, or friction. This author believes that a careful history and examination shows overlap among the patterns of vulvodynia in most patients, and several studies support this contention (9,10). The importance of differentiation among the patterns lies in a search for differing etiologies, the allowance for studies with uniformity in patient population, and the success of excisional surgery only in patients with vestibulodynia pattern. Otherwise, treatments are the same for all groups.

An examination of pelvic floor muscles usually reveals tightness of the introitus with insertion of a finger or a speculum (variable degrees of vaginismus), but with overall weakness, including an inability both voluntarily to contract firmly and to hold the contraction. There is often tenderness to palpation of these pelvic floor muscles.

Pathophysiology

Vulvodynia is a symptom rather than a specific disease. As more research and experience explore the causes of vulvodynia, this syndrome should become less often diagnosed. At this time, however, vulvodynia appears to be multifactorial in origin (see Table 5-3).

Pelvic floor muscle abnormalities have recently been recognized as a crucial factor (11,12). The introital tightness and pain to insertion of a speculum, finger, penis, or tampon originally was assumed to be solely an expected reflex to pain and tenderness. However, this tightness, in combination with overall weakness and muscular irritability on electromyographic studies, now is thought to be a constitutional abnormality that predisposes to vulvodynia. Despite a lack of research, this assumption is supported

TABLE 5.3 Etiologic factors in vulvodynia

Pelvic floor muscle abnormalities
  Increased muscle tension
  Muscle irritability
  Weakness
  Myofascial pain
Neuropathic pain
  Peripheral neuropathy
  Complex regional pain syndrome
  Regional pain referred from bladder or intestinal
    origin
  Central pain syndromes
  Increased nerve fiber generation in the presence
    of injury
Psychological factors
  Depression of chronic pain, endogenous, or
    situational
  Anxiety
  Psychosexual issues, either primary or secondary
    from pain-induced sexual dysfunction
Other possible factors
  Inflammatory mediators from fibroblasts
  Estrogen influences on pain
  Pain susceptibility genes

by the regular, marked improvement in vulvodynia with pelvic floor physical therapy.

Neuropathic pain appears to be a major factor in the pain of vulvodynia, and until recently it was believed to be the primary etiology, substantiated by the good response of discomfort to medications regularly used for neuropathy, such as the tricyclics and anticonvulsants approved for the neuropathy of postherpetic neuralgia and diabetic neuropathy (13,14). The recent discovery that VGLUT3 sensory neurons in the dorsal root ganglia play a role in the pathophysiology of pain to light touch following injury or inflammation has implications for the etiology of vulvodynia as well (15). In addition, increased numbers of nerve fibers have been reported in the vestibule (16).

Estrogen issues are believed by some to be operative in a portion of patients. Clearly, patients with estrogen deficiency as the sole factor in pain do not have vulvodynia but rather atrophic vagina/vaginitis. However, some clinicians and researchers believe that insensitivity to normal levels of estrogen produce or worsen vulvar burning and pain (17).

Vestibulodynia (vulvar vestibulitis) was initially believed to represent infection of the vestibular glands. When organisms were not identified, this condition was still assumed to be an inflammatory process, hence the name vulvar vestibulitis. More recently, all subsets of vulvodynia to include vestibulodynia are generally accepted as noninflammatory conditions (18,19). Recently, the name vulvar vestibulitis was changed to vestibulodynia to reflect this noninflammatory nature of vestibulodynia. However, several researchers have found evidence for inflammation playing a role, leaving inflammation as a possible factor in some patients (20,21).

Finally, all patients with chronic pain experience anxiety and depression that worsen symptoms, and this is magnified in women with genital pain and the additional impact of pain with sexual activity on isolation, relationships, and self-image. Psychological abnormalities are recognized in women with vulvodynia (22,23). A distinct minority of vulvodynia clinicians, including Peter Lynch, believe that psychosexual dysfunction is the sole etiologic factor (see discussion in Chapter 16) (24,25). Evidence for this consists of studies reporting depression and dysfunction in these women and a trial showing equal improvement in women with vulvodynia who were treated with surgery, biofeedback, or cognitive-behavioral therapy (26). Vulvologists agree that women with vulvodynia experience depression, anxiety, and sexual dysfunction that should be addressed for maximal improvement. Whether this dysfunction is the entire cause of pain, one aspect present at varying degrees in the pathogenesis, or is a result of unremitting and unexplained pain is fiercely debated. Most vulvologists believe that anxiety and depression are but a piece of the vulvodynia picture, either as one underlying factor or as a result of genital pain that exacerbates the symptoms.

The Vulvodynia Workshop at the National Institutes of Health (Bethesda, MD, April 14 and 15, 2003) included pain and vulvodynia clinicians and scientists, with discussion of new and leading theories on the causes of vulvodynia at that time. Another conference tentatively is planned for 2011. Regional pain with bladder or intestinal pain producing vulvar pain by cross-sensitization and cross-talk between one or more of these nerves and others were discussed as likely factors. Altered central sensitization (27) and increased nerve fiber generation in the presence of injury were discussed as producing allodynia (16). A pain susceptibility gene and gender factors causing or worsening pain were reported. Influences by inflammatory mediators from a subgroup of fibroblasts may play a role (20). Some women exhibit trigger points, suggesting myofascial pain. Data were presented at this workshop showing that estrogen can both lower the pain threshold and also act as a mediator of peripheral nerve remodeling. In addition, information regarding pharmacologic therapy to include the use of selective serotonin reuptake inhibitors was discussed, and capsaicin as a depletor of substance P was presented. Visceral K opioid and K agonists were discussed, and there were suggestions that combining analgesic therapies may be beneficial.

Previous theories of etiologies for vulvodynia have been generally discredited; these include chronic yeast infection, subclinical human papillomavirus infection (28), and oxaluria (29). Critical and common exacerbating factors in many women with vulvodynia include irritant (and, less so, allergic) contact dermatitis to overwashing, topical medications, lubricants, and panty liners/pads.

Management

Although up to 22% of patients in a 2-year study experienced spontaneous resolution of symptoms in one study, most women have ongoing symptoms and require therapy (30). There are three primary specific treatments for vulvodynia: pelvic floor physical therapy, oral medication for neuropathy/pain syndromes, and attention to anxiety/depression/psychosexual dysfunction (see Table 5-4). In addition, women with vestibulodynia pattern of vulvodynia can be treated with surgical removal of the area of pain, generally with excellent results. Also, there are nonspecific, general therapies that are important for all patients, including patient education, topical anesthetics, and avoidance of irritants. There are also alternative, anecdotal therapies that may be useful for the patient who is intolerant or unresponsive of standard therapies.

Optimal therapy requires attention to all factors producing discomfort. A prescription for a medication for neuropathic pain without attention to psychological factors, discontinuation of irritants, treatment of accompanying abnormalities, and education regarding vulvodynia rarely produces adequate improvement on a patient who takes the medication.

Attention to *patient education/psychological factors* is paramount. Vulvodynia is not a concept in the lexicon of the average layperson. A handout (see Appendix 2) is extremely useful not only to serve as a reminder of the facts regarding vulvodynia but also as confirmation of the very real nature of the condition and as a reminder that the patient is not alone in her experience with this pain syndrome. A brief discussion of pelvic floor abnormalities, neuropathy, and anxiety/depression as major factors is important, as well as the nonrole of infection, malignancy, and sexually transmitted diseases. Avoidance of unnecessary irritants such as soap, topical medications, panty liners, some irritating lubricants, and douches should be advised. Correction of any abnormalities can improve symptoms in some women. For example, management of estrogen deficiency, clearing of inflammatory vaginitis, and control of any skin disease may minimize symptoms of pain in patients with vulvodynia.

All patients experience anxiety and depression associated with their discomfort, and psychosexual factors are universal. This must be acknowledged, and most patients require therapy. This can be achieved by referral for professional counseling, sex therapy, and antidepressants that double as medication for neuropathic pain (31). Although these psychological factors are paramount, pa-

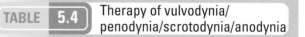

TABLE 5.4 Therapy of vulvodynia/penodynia/scrotodynia/anodynia

General, nonspecific measure
  Patient education, handouts
  Counseling for most
  Evaluation for and correction of coincidental abnormalities; irritant contact dermatitis, estrogen deficiency, infections, etc.
  Topical lidocaine
Pelvic floor evaluation and physiotherapy (not studied in men)
Neuropathic pain/pain syndrome, oral (see individual patient handouts)
  Tricyclic medications beginning at 5 to 10 mg, titrating as high as 150 mg hs
  Gabapentin beginning at 100 mg, titrating as high as 1200 mg t.i.d.
  Pregabalin beginning at 25 mg, titrating as high as 300 mg b.i.d.
  Venlafaxine sustained/extended release, beginning at 37.5 mg, titrating as high as 150 mg q.d.
  Duloxetine, beginning at 20 mg titrating as high as 60 mg b.i.d.
Psychological factors
  Psychological counseling/sex therapy
  Antidepressant therapy
Vestibulectomy in women with vestibulodynia (pain strictly localized to the vestibule)
Other therapies (only reported in women)
  Topical therapies
    Lidocaine 5% ointment at introitus under occlusions hs
    Estradiol cream at introitus under occlusion hs
    Amitriptyline 2%/baclofen 2% compounded
    Amitriptyline 2%/baclofen 2%/ketamine 2% compounded
    Nitroglycerin 0.2% compounded, three times a week and 5 to 10 minutes before sexual activity
    Gabapentin compounded
  (botulinum toxin, hypnotherapy, acupuncture used for vulvodynia by some)

tients often respond best if these issues are discussed toward the end of a visit, after a relationship is achieved.

Pelvic floor physical therapy is an exceptionally useful therapy for patients with vulvodynia (32,33). This treatment not only treats the pelvic floor abnormalities but also provides desensitization for patients who are afraid of the pain that occurs with touch and serves as emotional support for the patient who is depressed, anxious, frightened, and isolated. The goal of physical therapy includes strengthening the pelvic floor muscles that, in turn, produce a background of relaxed and quiet muscles that lack the irritability of that found in women with vulvodynia. There is little research in this area of pelvic floor physical therapy for vulvodynia, and individual therapists use different methods for achieving these goals, with individualization of therapy depending upon the patient's needs and the therapist's training and experiences. Some women exhibit sufficient muscle rigidity that therapy begins with relaxation techniques of the hips and other joints even before the pelvic floor muscles are addressed. Other procedures include pelvic floor exercises to strengthen the pelvic floor, which also helps train these muscles to relax. Also, soft tissue mobilization and myofascial release of the pelvic girdle, pelvic floor, and associated structures are used by most. Bowel and bladder retraining is used in some patients. The importance of meeting with a compassionate physical therapist on a regular basis for an hour for psychological benefit is enormous. Many women are unwilling to seek formal psychological counseling because of expense, stigma, and the implication that their pain is not real but rather psychosomatic. But the psychological benefit through physical therapy is usually acceptable to the patient and very useful.

Oral therapy for neuropathic pain/pain syndromes usually produces significant improvement. These medications either belong to the antidepressant or to the anticonvulsant class of medication. Dosage of each is normally begun low, and the dose is gradually increased to allow the body to acclimate to these medications in a patient population that tends to be intolerant of medication. Improvement is delayed with these medications, as they do not function as pain suppressants, but rather from management of neuropathy. Improvement may require 2 to 4 weeks after reaching an optimal dose. Partial improvement with one medication often can be maximized by the addition of a medication of a different class.

The tricyclic medications, to include amitriptyline, desipramine, and imipramine, have the longest history of use as well as the added benefit of antidepressant actions (13,34). Common side effects include dry mouth and eyes, sedation, constipation, increased appetite; less often, free-floating anxiety, palpitations, tremor, and sleeplessness occur. Amitriptyline exhibits the most sedating effects and highest likelihood of increased appetite. Desipramine is most likely to produce tremor and anxiety. Imipramine is available in a sustained released preparation that is extremely well tolerated. Many women object to being on antidepressants "on principle." Careful explanation for the reasons for these medications (for neuropathic pain as the primary objective and the fortuitous secondary effects as an antidepressant) most often reassures patients that the clinician is not using the tricyclic medication because the pain is "all in her head."

Gabapentin, originally developed as an anticonvulsant, is approved by the Food and Drug Administration for the treatment of neuropathic pain of postherpetic neuralgia and diabetic neuropathy. This is a medication regularly used for vulvodynia as well (14). Side effects include fatigue and dependant edema, but generally it is much better tolerated than the tricyclic medications. If ineffective or not tolerated, pregabalin is a similar medication that can be substituted.

An additional medication used is venlafaxine, which, like the tricyclic medications, exerts antidepressant effects as well. This medication is used regularly for vulvodynia although data reporting efficacy are lacking. Nausea is common except in the extended/sustained release forms. Discontinuation of this medication must be by gradual tapering, because abrupt withdrawal can sometimes produce severe constitutional symptoms. The closely related medication duloxetine usually is very well tolerated but should also be discontinued by taper.

A *vestibulectomy* is the most effective therapy available for women with vestibulodynia, vulvodynia that is strictly localized to the vestibule. This surgery consists of excision of the area of pain to include the hymeneal ring, with advancement of the vagina to cover the defect. From 61% to 94% of patients who are good candidates for this treatment experience clearing or remarkable improvement in the hands of an experienced surgeon (35). Many clinicians believe that the degree of success is higher in women who have received the oral medications discussed above for pain syndromes and who have participated in physical therapy (36).

Beyond these therapies, management is more individualized. An occasional patient experiences pain that is extremely localized. These women sometimes benefit from intralesional corticosteroids into this area of point tenderness. Triamcinolone acetate 10 mg/cc, 0.2 to 1.0 cc injected with a 30 gauge needle into the area occasionally, produces remarkable improvement.

For patients who either do not benefit from or do not tolerate these treatments, topical medications can be used. None is well studied, but these include topical estrogen applied nightly to the vestibule or into the vagina thrice weekly, lidocaine 2% jelly or 5% ointment applied nightly (37), and the use of compounded gabapentin (38), amitriptyline/baclofen (39), amitriptyline/baclofen/ketamine, or nitroglycerin (40). One proposed therapy is capsaicin, but this is an extraordinarily irritating substance and should be used with great care (41).

An additional therapy widely studied for other pain syndromes is the injection of botulinum toxin A (42). Only anecdotal reports and small series are available for its use in vulvodynia, but the injection of botulinum toxin A (20 to 40) units into the levator ani muscles, vestibule, or perineal muscles may be useful. This is likely most useful in combination with pelvic floor physiotherapy.

One open series each suggests that lamotrigine or montelukast may be useful (43,44). There are therapies that have been used for vulvodynia which, over time, have been found to be ineffective. These include oral and topical corticosteroids, systemic and intralesional interferon alpha, oral and topical antifungal medications in the absence of documented yeast infections, laser ablation, therapies for human papillomavirus, and the low oxalate diet. When women with vulvodynia experience a flaring of symptoms, prescribing therapy for yeast or bacterial vaginosis is the easiest path for the provider. However, these additional irritants are not needed, and this only reinforces the patient's impression that her underlying problem is one of resistant or recurrent infection. Rather, reassurance, bland emollients such as petroleum jelly, cool compresses, and topical lidocaine should be advised.

Scrotodynia, Penodynia

Scrotodynia (red scrotum syndrome) and penodynia can be defined as pain symptoms rather than itching, to include burning, soreness, aching, hypersensitivity, or other pain symptoms in the absence of relevant skin disease, infection, or definable neuropathy such as postherpetic neuralgia or diabetic neuropathy. This definition has been extrapolated from that of vulvodynia, because idiopathic pain of the male genitalia is much less often recognized, and there is almost no information available.

I believe that scrotodynia and penodynia are generally male equivalents of vulvodynia. These pain syndromes are nearly unreported in the literature, and this section is based upon my and Peter Lynch's experience with patients who report anogenital pain in the absence of objective physical or laboratory findings.

Clinical Manifestations

The frequency of scrotodynia and penodynia is not known. Like the initial impressions of vulvodynia, the frequency of male genital pain is probably under-recognized. Penodynia and scrotodynia have been reported only in adult men. Patients complain of penile or scrotal pain or swelling, often with a perception of redness and burning (Fig. 5-11). As for women with vulvodynia, perianal skin can be affected. This generally interferes with sexual activity and exercise. Often, the patient has consulted multiple clinicians, and, like women with vulvodynia, has been treated with many topical antifungal therapies. At times, topical corticosteroids have been used, sometimes producing redness of steroid dermatitis or atrophy, which exacerbates symptoms.

Peter Lynch feels strongly that scrotodynia and penodynia are accompanied by, and produced by, psychosexual dysfunction (see discussion in Chapter 16). He reported a series of 13 men who displayed an unusual degree of psychosexual dysfunction. These men ranged from 35 to 70 years, with an average of 50 years. Eight had never been married, but three of four of the older men were married. When pain was associated with a pre-

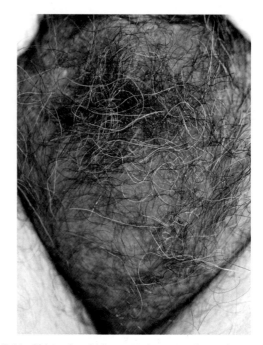

FIG. 5-11. Although within normal range, the redness of this scrotum leads to the name "red scrotum syndrome" as a term for scrotodynia.

cipitating event, the event was most often a sexual contact that produced feelings of guilt or anxiety. Nine men had only penile pain, whereas two had only scrotal pain; two had both. The penile pain was either solely or primarily of the glans in all patients. All patients perceived redness, although most exhibited normal degrees of erythema on examination; several who showed greater redness were using topical steroids. Patients improved but did not clear with antidepressants, including amitriptyline. I have seen 11 men recently, and my patients followed a similar pattern, with all having been seen by multiple physicians. Ages ranged from 23 to 75 years, with most between 37 and 55 years. Five were married, and six were single (including two patients in their twenties). Patients reported the onset of pain occurring from 3 months to 10 years earlier, with five being less than a year and four being 2 to 4 years. Four patients related their symptoms to a sexual encounter. In addition to redness, several patients reported new findings of lesions of the skin that were recognizable to me on examination as pearly penile papules, prominent sebaceous glands, normal pigment changes, and, sometimes, lesions I could not see. Five men reported penile pain only, three described scrotal pain only, and three reported scrotal, penile, and anal pain, occasionally with radiation into the legs. All penile pain was localized to the glans except one patient who also experienced pain of the shaft. One patient reported pain only with intercourse, one reported post voiding incontinence, and one reported urinary frequency and pain with defecation. All were treated with oral medications for neuropathy: tricyclic medications, gabapentin, pregabalin, or venlafaxine. Of those men who returned to the office, three reported clearing of their symptoms, three reported marked improvement, one experienced no improvement, and one was intolerant of amitriptyline. Those patients who did not derive benefit did not follow-up in the office after an alternative medication was prescribed. Three patients never followed up in the office after their first visit.

Diagnosis

The diagnosis of scrotodynia and penodynia is, like vulvodynia, made by the presence of chronic pain in the absence of objective, definable causes of pain. Background redness is sometimes present, and this should be differentiated from irritant contact dermatitis. Deeper genital pain can be due to testicular abnormalities, prostatitis, or an inguinal hernia, requiring evaluation by an urologist. Patients with urinary or colon symptoms should have these addressed as well.

Pathophysiology

The pathophysiology is unknown. Peter Lynch believes that all genital pain syndromes are due to psychosexual dysfunction and that men with genital pain display more severe dysfunction than most patients with vulvodynia. I believe that scrotodynia and penodynia are most likely produced by the same neuropathic and psychological factors as are operative in vulvodynia, as patients improve with medications such as gabapentin and tricyclic medications; however, I believe that both psychological and physical factors can trigger this syndrome.

The issue of pelvic floor abnormalities as a cause of penodynia and scrotodynia has not been reported although pelvic floor dysfunction is known to be a factor in pelvic pain and chronic prostatitis symptoms in men (45).

Management

As for vulvodynia, patient education, discontinuation of irritants, and psychological support are crucial (Table 5-4). Otherwise, oral medications for pain syndromes, to include tricyclic medications, gabapentin, pregabalin, venlafaxine, and duloxetine, often are useful for those who are willing to take them. Pelvic floor therapy, both for the correction of hypothesized muscle dysfunction and for the psychological benefits, is an untried treatment, although a series is currently underway. Topical therapies have not been reported.

As for women with vulvodynia, these patients should be referred for counseling. Genital pain syndromes can be life-ruining and careful and compassionate care of these patients can remarkably improve their quality of life, and, at least theoretically, improve symptoms in some patients.

Anodynia

Like scrotodynia and penodynia, anodynia is a rarely reported symptom. Anodynia is defined as idiopathic pain syndrome of the anus, and, also like scrotodynia and penodynia, the causes and treatment must be extrapolated from information derived from experience with vulvodynia. In my experience, anodynia is seen most often in combination with scrotodynia or vulvodynia.

Patient education, avoidance of irritants, psychological support and therapy, oral medications for neuropathic pain, and pelvic floor evaluation and therapy are potential therapies.

REFERENCES

1. Reed BD, Haefner HK, Harlow SD, et al. Reliability and validity of self-reported symptoms for predicting vulvodynia. *Obstet Gynecol.* 2006;108:906–913.
2. Sutton JT, Bachmann GA, Arnold LD, et al. Assessment of vulvodynia symptoms in a sample of U.S. women: a follow-up national incidence survey. *J Womens Health (Larchmt).* 2008;17: 1285–1292.
3. Saunders NA, Reed BD, Haefner HK. McGill pain questionnaire findings among women with vulvodynia and chronic yeast infection. *J Reprod Med.* 2008;53:385–389.
4. Beco J, Climov D, Bex M. Pudendal nerve decompression in perineology: a case series. *BMC Surg.* 2004;4:15.
5. Filler AG. Diagnosis and treatment of pudendal nerve entrapment syndrome subtypes: imaging, injections, and minimal access surgery. *Neurosurg Focus.* 2009;26:1–14.
6. Harlow BL, Stewart EG. A population-based assessment of chronic unexplained vulvar pain: have we underestimated the prevalence of vulvodynia? *J Am Med Womens Assoc.* 2003;58: 82–88.
7. Arnold LD, Bachmann GA, Rosen R, et al. Assessment of vulvodynia symptoms in a sample of US women: a prevalence survey with a nested case control study. *Am J Obstet Gynecol.* 2007;196:128.e1–128.e6.
8. Reed BD, Cantor LE. Vulvodynia in preadolescent girls. *J Low Genit Tract Dis.* 2008;12:257–261.
9. Edwards L. Subsets of vulvodynia: overlapping characteristics. *J Reprod Med.* 2004;49:883–887.
10. Masheb RM, Lozano C, Richman S, et al. On the reliability and validity of physician ratings for vulvodynia and the discriminant validity of its subtypes. *Pain Med.* 2004;5:349–358.
11. Butrick CW. Pelvic floor hypertonic disorders: identification and management. *Obstet Gynecol Clin North Am.* 2009;36: 707–722.
12. Glazer HI, Jantos M, Hartmann EH, et al. Electromyographic comparisons of the pelvic floor in women with dysesthetic vulvodynia and asymptomatic women. *J Reprod Med.* 1998;43: 959–962.
13. Reed BD, Caron AM, Gorenflo DW, et al. Treatment of vulvodynia with tricyclic antidepressants: efficacy and associated factors. *J Low Genit Tract Dis.* 2006;10:245–251.
14. Harris G, Horowitz B, Borgida A. Evaluation of gabapentin in the treatment of generalized vulvodynia, unprovoked. *J Reprod Med.* 2007;52:103–106.

15. Seal RP, Wang X, Guan Y, et al. Injury-induced mechanical hypersensitivity requires C-low threshold mechanoreceptors. *Nature.* 2009;10:651–655.

16. Tympanidis P, Terenghi G, Dowd P. Increased innervation of the vulval vestibule in patients with vulvodynia. *Br J Dermatol.* 2003;148:1021–1027.

17. Eva LJ, MacLean AB, Reid WM, et al. Estrogen receptor expression in vulvar vestibulitis syndrome. *Am J Obstet Gynecol.* 2003;189:458–461.

18. Eva LJ, Rolfe KJ, MacLean AB, et al. Is localized, provoked vulvodynia an inflammatory condition? *J Reprod Med.* 2007;52: 379–384.

19. Halperin R, Zehavi S, Vaknin Z, et al. The major histopathologic characteristics in the vulvar vestibulitis syndrome. *Gynecol Obstet Invest.* 2005;59:75–79.

20. Foster DC, Piekarz KH, Murant TI, et al. Enhanced synthesis of proinflammatory cytokines by vulvar vestibular fibroblasts: implications for vulvar vestibulitis. *Am J Obstet Gynecol.* 2007;196:346.e1–346.e18.

21. Lev-Sagie A, Prus D, Linhares IM, et al. Polymorphism in a gene coding for the inflammasome component NALP3 and recurrent vulvovaginal candidiasis in women with vulvar vestibulitis syndrome. *Am J Obstet Gynecol.* 2009;200:303. e1–303.e16.

22. Desrochers G, Bergeron S, Khalifé S, et al. Fear avoidance and self-efficacy in relation to pain and sexual impairment in women with provoked vestibulodynia. *Clin J Pain.* 2009;25:520–527.

23. Jantos M. Vulvodynia: a psychophysiological profile based on electromyographic assessment. *Appl Psychophysiol Biofeedback.* 2008;33:29–38.

24. Lynch PJ. Vulvodynia as a somatoform disorder. *J Reprod Med.* 2008;53:390–396.

25. Mascherpa F, Bogliatto F, Lynch PJ, et al. Vulvodynia as a possible somatization disorder. More than just an opinion. *J Reprod Med.* 2007;52:107–110.

26. Bergeron S, Khalifé S, Glazer HI, et al. Surgical and behavioral treatments for vestibulodynia: two-and-one-half year follow-up and predictors of outcome. *Obstet Gynecol.* 2008;111:159–166.

27. Foster DC, Dworkin RH, Wood RW. Effects of intradermal foot and forearm capsaicin injections in normal and vulvodynia-afflicted women. *Pain.* 2005;117:128–136.

28. Gunter J, Smith-King M, Collins J, et al. Vulvodynia: in situ hybridization analysis for human papillomavirus. *Prim Care Update Ob Gyns.* 1998;5:152.

29. Harlow BL, Abenhaim HA, Vitonis AF, et al. Influence of dietary oxalates on the risk of adult-onset vulvodynia. *J Reprod Med.* 2008;53:171–178.

30. Reed BD, Haefner HK, Sen A, et al. Vulvodynia incidence and remission rates among adult women: a 2-year follow-up study. *Obstet Gynecol.* 2008;112(2 Pt 1):231–237.

31. Masheb RM, Kerns RD, Lozano C, et al. A randomized clinical trial for women with vulvodynia: cognitive-behavioral therapy vs. supportive psychotherapy. *Pain.* 2009;141:31–40.

32. Hartmann D, Strauhal MJ, Nelson CA. Treatment of women in the United States with localized, provoked vulvodynia: practice survey of women's health physical therapists. *J Reprod Med.* 2007;52:48–52.

33. Forth HL, Cramp MC, Drechsler WI. Does physiotherapy treatment improve the self-reported pain levels and quality of life of women with vulvodynia? A pilot study. *J Obstet Gynaecol.* 2009;29:423–429.

34. Munday PE. Response to treatment in dysaesthetic vulvodynia. *J Obstet Gynaecol.* 2001;21:610–613.

35. Landry T, Bergeron S, Dupuis MJ, et al. The treatment of provoked vestibulodynia: a critical review. *Clin J Pain.* 2008;24: 155–171.

36. Goetsch MF. Surgery combined with muscle therapy for dyspareunia from vulvar vestibulitis: an observational study. *J Reprod Med.* 2007;52:597–603.

37. Zolnoun DA, Hartmann KE, Steege JF. Overnight 5% lidocaine ointment for treatment of vulvar vestibulitis. *Obstet Gynecol.* 2003;102:84–87.

38. Boardman LA, Cooper AS, Blais LR, et al. Topical gabapentin in the treatment of localized and generalized vulvodynia. *Obstet Gynecol.* 2008;112:579–585.

39. Nyirjesy P, Lev-Sagie A, Mathew L, et al. Topical amitriptyline-baclofen cream for the treatment of provoked vestibulodynia. *J Low Genit Tract Dis.* 2009;13:230–236.

40. Walsh KE, Berman JR, Berman LA, et al. Safety and efficacy of topical nitroglycerin for treatment of vulvar pain in women with vulvodynia: a pilot study. *J Gend Specif Med.* 2002;5:21–27.

41. Murina F, Radici G, Bianco V. Capsaicin and the treatment of vulvar vestibulitis syndrome: a valuable alternative? *MedGenMed.* 2004;6:48.

42. Yoon H, Chung WS, Shim BS. Botulinum toxin A for the management of vulvodynia. *Int J Impot Res.* 2007;19:84–87.

43. Meltzer-Brody SE, Zolnoun D, Steege JF, et al. Open-label trial of lamotrigine focusing on efficacy in vulvodynia. *J Reprod Med.* 2009;54:171–178.

44. Kamdar N, Fisher L, MacNeill C. Improvement in vulvar vestibulitis with montelukast. *J Reprod Med.* 2007;52:912–916.

45. Anderson RU, Sawyer T, Wise D, et al. Painful myofascial trigger points and pain sites in men with chronic prostatitis/chronic pelvic pain syndrome. *J Urol.* 2009;182:2753–2758.

The usually characteristic appearance of individual skin diseases is modified by the environment in skin folds, so that diagnosis by morphology is challenging. Moisture and heat obscure scale. Subtle lichenification (thickening from rubbing) sometimes appears white due to hydration. Normally well-demarcated borders of lesions may appear fuzzy as friction irritates the skin. Also, genital skin, even more than dry, keratinized skin, often is affected by more than one disease process, so secondary infection and irritation from sweat, urine, feces, and overwashing can change the appearance of the skin. In addition, redness is difficult to detect when occurring in a patient with a naturally dark complexion; erythema is generally perceived as hyperpigmentation in this population.

Often, the correct diagnosis of red genital plaques and patches depends on the identification of more typical morphology on other areas of the body, and, when in doubt, a skin biopsy is sometime helpful. Unfortunately, a skin biopsy of nonspecific erythema often yields a nonspecific result. Often, empiric corticosteroid therapy while monitoring or treating for likely infections is necessary. Red plaques and patches that are not diagnosed clinically or do not respond to therapy as expected should be biopsied to rule out the occasional extramammary Paget disease or intraepithelial neoplasia (also known as squamous cell carcinoma in situ, Bowen disease, or erythroplasia of Queyrat).

ATOPIC DERMATITIS, ECZEMA, AND LICHEN SIMPLEX CHRONICUS (discussed primarily in Chapter 4)

Because rubbing and scratching produce the visible signs of eczema, the appearance varies, depending on the individual tendency to rub, scratch, or both, and any tendency of the patient's skin to thicken in response to rubbing or scratching. A person who rubs exhibits thickened, lichenified skin with increased skin markings or occasionally excessive smoothness, as though the skin has been polished by rubbing (Figs. 6-1 through 6-3). Skin that has been scratched is red with excoriations (Fig. 6-4). Usually, the plaques are poorly demarcated since a general area is rubbed or scratched, and the area may simply show a generalized area of irritation.

Scale and excoriation are often subtle because of moisture and thin skin, and erythema may be relatively unremarkable because the genitalia are frequently pink normally. Erythema can be especially difficult to detect in patients with normally dark skin, when inflammation often appears hyperpigmented rather than red.

The diagnosis of eczema in the genital area is normally made by a combination of a history of itching with intense pleasure on scratching, morphology, and the exclusion of infection that can produce itching, especially candidiasis and dermatophytosis. The diagnosis is confirmed by the excellent response to standard therapy.

A mainstay in the treatment of eczema includes the elimination of irritants, especially overwashing; protection from urine, feces, and perspiration; avoidance of irritating lubricants and topical medications; and the discontinuation of panty liners. Scratching is a potent irritant, and bedtime sedation to prevent nighttime scratching is crucial. The specific medication of choice is the application of a potent topical corticosteroid ointment such as clobetasol sparingly twice daily initially, tapering the frequency or the potency when the skin becomes normal. Topical tacrolimus (Protopic) ointment 0.1% and pimecrolimus (Elidel) cream are calcineurin inhibitors approved for use in eczema (1,2). These can be irritating on the genitalia, are expensive, and are less effective than potent corticosteroids for eczema. Although these characteristics make these medications second-line therapy for genital eczema after corticosteroids, these can be useful for some patients who require chronic therapy. As with other chronic skin diseases, an ongoing high index of suspicion for and therapy of infection is important (3). Finally, patient education is extremely important in the treatment of eczema. Patients must realize that this is a chronic skin disease that often requires chronic or intermittent therapy.

CONTACT DERMATITIS (discussed primarily in Chapter 4)

Contact dermatitis is an eczematous reaction in response to either an irritant or an allergen. Although any patient will develop skin changes and symptoms after contact with a sufficiently irritating substance, only patients specifically sensitized to an allergen develop allergic contact dermatitis. The poorly keratinized nature of much of the genitalia and the damp environment result in increased permeability of the skin, and a resulting

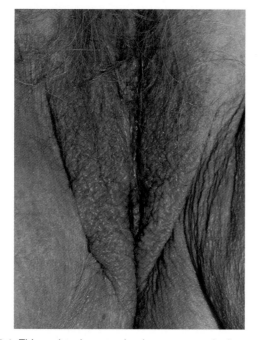

FIG. 6-1. This patient has a red, edematous poorly demarcated plaque with lichenification.

increased risk for contact dermatitis compared to other skin surfaces (4).

Irritant Contact Dermatitis

This extremely common dermatitis is a frequent secondary factor in patients with genital symptoms, often associated with overwashing, use of topical medications, and chronic moisture from incontinence or sweat.

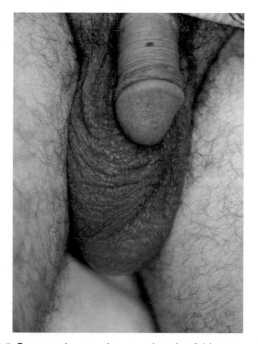

FIG. 6-2. Deep erythema, edema, and scale of this eczematized scrotum are characteristic of chronic rubbing and scratching.

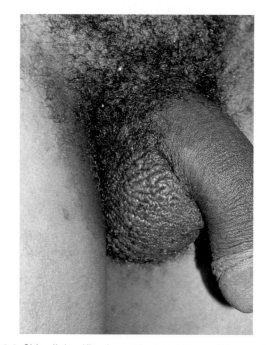

FIG. 6-3. Shiny lichenification with excoriations of the scrotum is a common manifestation of lichen simplex chronicus. Individuals with dark complexions exhibit hyperpigmentation rather than redness.

Chronic irritant contact dermatitis is usually manifested by symptoms of irritation, soreness, or rawness. If the patient is atopic, the irritant can precipitate itching and can initiate an itch–scratch cycle. Morphologically, the area affected depends on where the contact occurred. Generally, this is manifested by a poorly demarcated

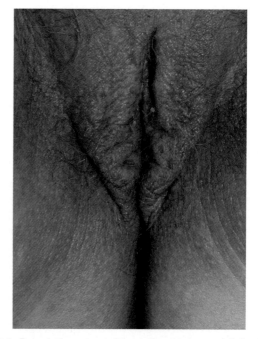

FIG. 6-4. Excoriations as well as inflammation and lichenification are additional signs of scratching.

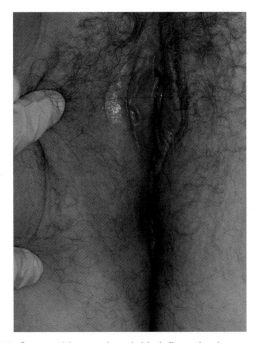

FIG. 6-5. Overwashing produced this inflamed, edematous, red plaque of irritant contact dermatitis with interlabial fissures.

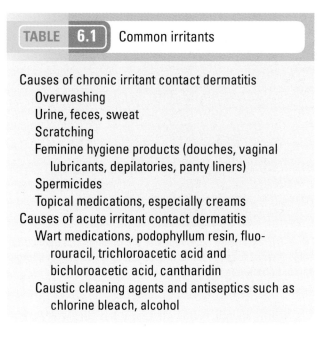

TABLE **6.1**	Common irritants

Causes of chronic irritant contact dermatitis
  Overwashing
  Urine, feces, sweat
  Scratching
  Feminine hygiene products (douches, vaginal
    lubricants, depilatories, panty liners)
  Spermicides
  Topical medications, especially creams
Causes of acute irritant contact dermatitis
  Wart medications, podophyllum resin, fluo-
    rouracil, trichloroacetic acid and
    bichloroacetic acid, cantharidin
  Caustic cleaning agents and antiseptics such as
    chlorine bleach, alcohol

erythematous or dusky plaque with scale that may be subtle (Fig. 6-5). Patients who have experienced itching frequently have superimposed excoriations or lichenification. In these patients, the morphology is indistinguishable from that of atopic dermatitis, and indeed the irritant can be viewed simply as a precipitating factor for atopic dermatitis or eczema. Acute irritant dermatitis is essentially a chemical burn. The rapid appearance of erythema, edema, and blistering is typical. Poorly keratinized skin such as the modified mucous membranes of the vulva, the glans penis, and the inner aspect of the prepuce is very fragile, and blister roofs are shed quickly, forming erosions.

Irritant contact dermatitis can be caused either by repeated exposure to a weak irritant or by one or few exposures to a very strong irritant. Common irritants are listed in Table 6-1. A diaper rash is a typical example of chronic irritant contact dermatitis, although in this case superimposed candidiasis is sometimes a complicating factor. Because repeated exposure is often necessary for the development of irritant contact dermatitis and the symptoms and signs occur gradually, the patient is frequently unaware that the substance is irritating and is playing a role in symptoms.

Acute irritant contact dermatitis, however, is produced by one or a few exposures to a very strong irritant, and this exposure is often accompanied by immediate burning and stinging. The patient usually is aware of the cause of the symptom and frequently misinterprets this as allergy. The most common causes of acute irritant contact dermatitis include treatment for external genital warts, such as trichloroacetic and bichloroacetic acids, podophyllum

resin, and cantharidin. Some patients with very sensitive skin can experience acute irritant contact dermatitis to alcohol-containing creams, most often antifungal medications used in a setting of pre-existing inflamed skin.

The diagnosis of irritant contact dermatitis is made by correlation of the symptoms and physical findings with a history of possible contactants. The diagnosis is confirmed when the contactants are eliminated and the eruption and symptoms resolve. Dermatoses with similar morphology include eczema/lichen simplex chronicus and allergic contact dermatitis. Psoriasis, vulvar/penile/anal intraepithelial neoplasia (Bowen disease) and Paget disease can also resemble irritant contact dermatitis. Acute irritant dermatitis can be confused with other blistering or ulcerative conditions, including acute allergic contact dermatitis, herpes simplex virus infection, a fixed drug eruption, or candidiasis. Autoimmune blistering diseases are slower in onset and are less likely to produce diagnostic confusion.

The most important aspects of therapy are the identification and elimination of all irritants. A midpotency topical corticosteroid ointment, such as triamcinolone 0.1% twice a day is often useful. The pain and burning of acute irritant contact dermatitis are minimized by cool or tepid tap water sitz baths several times a day for the first few days, followed by the application of petrolatum on open erosions. Nighttime sedation provides comfort and sleep to those with pain and itching and minimizes ongoing irritation from nighttime scratching.

Allergic Contact Dermatitis

Allergic contact dermatitis occurs as a result of contact of an allergen to the skin of a patient who has specifically developed a hypersensitivity to that allergen.

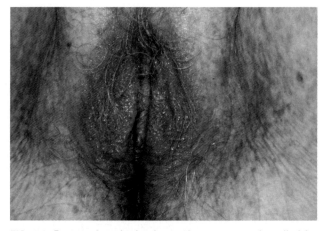

FIG. 6-6. Benzocaine obtained over the counter and applied for itching has resulted in these tiny, coalescing vesicles of allergic contact dermatitis.

Chronic allergic contact dermatitis is characterized by itching as well as by a poorly demarcated erythematous, scaling plaque that often shows linear erosion from scratching and lichenification. Often, chronic allergic contact dermatitis cannot be distinguished clinically from irritant contact dermatitis and atopic dermatitis and its variants. Acute allergic dermatitis, however, presents with cutaneous edema that produces tiny, monotonous, closely set vesicles in the areas of the contact (Fig. 6-6). Often, there are linear or irregular plaques in which the contactant was spread on the skin, such as by fingers for medication or brushed on by the leaves of a plant.

The allergen is rarely recognized by the patient, because symptoms follow exposure by one or several days. Allergic contact dermatitis has been found by European clinicians to play a significant role in chronic vulvovaginal symptoms, whereas American physicians have not found allergy to be a common factor (5). More common allergens are listed in Table 6-2.

The diagnosis of allergic contact dermatitis is made by correlation of symptoms and physical findings with a history of a likely contactant. The diagnosis is confirmed when the contactant is eliminated and the eruption and symptoms resolve. Sometimes, allergic contact dermatitis is suspected when atopic dermatitis does not respond to

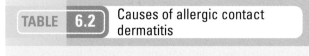

TABLE 6.2	Causes of allergic contact dermatitis

Topical medications, especially benzocaine, neomycin, diphenhydramine; anticandidal medications are less common
Spermicides
Preservatives in feminine hygiene products
Latex (condoms, diaphragms, elastic bands)

therapy, but an allergen is not identified. In these cases, patch testing by a dermatologist is warranted to identify any offending allergens.

The differential diagnosis of chronic allergic contact dermatitis includes irritant contact dermatitis, atopic dermatitis/lichen simplex chronicus, psoriasis, secondarily rubbed or scratched tinea cruris, candidiasis, seborrheic dermatitis, vulvar/penile/anal intraepithelial neoplasia (Bowen disease), and Paget disease. Acute allergic contact dermatitis can be confused with other blistering or erosive diseases, especially acute irritant contact dermatitis, candidiasis, and herpes simplex virus infection.

Most important in the treatment of contact dermatitis is the elimination of the contactant. Sometimes, the contactant cannot be identified, and the patient is counseled to avoid all topical agents other than clear water and petrolatum (petroleum jelly). After the elimination of the contactant, acute, blistering, or exudative contact dermatitis can be improved with cool soaks or sitz baths for the first few days. Oral prednisone for severe disease and topical corticosteroids for less erosive dermatitis are useful as well. Topical corticosteroids should be continued until symptoms are clear and the skin is normal. Nighttime sedation and control of secondary infection are important to minimize symptoms while the skin heals.

SEBORRHEIC DERMATITIS (also discussed in Chapter 4)

Seborrheic dermatitis is an uncommon cause of genital skin disease in adults, although seborrhea of the scalp is extraordinarily common (see also Chapter 12).

Clinical Presentation

Seborrheic dermatitis of the scalp is a common disease, occurring at all ages. However, seborrheic dermatitis is most common in newborns and after puberty. In addition, this condition is most severe in those who cannot shampoo regularly, such as the homeless and those with neurologic disease or other infirmities that interfere with activities of daily living. Finally, patients of African background cannot shampoo daily because of the excessive dryness of their hair with frequent washing.

Seborrheic dermatitis generally affects the scalp first and most remarkably. Erythematous plaques at the hairline exhibit yellowish scale with a slightly greasy texture, hence the term seborrhea. As the disease worsens, the entire scalp becomes involved, and erythema and scale spread to other areas, preferentially affecting the ears, posterior auricular folds, eyebrows, and the nasolabial folds. Most often, seborrheic dermatitis does not extend beyond these areas. Occasionally, however, severe seborrheic dermatitis can involve the entire face, and the eruption can spread to the chest and to skin folds including the axillae, umbilicus, and genital skin (Fig. 6-7).

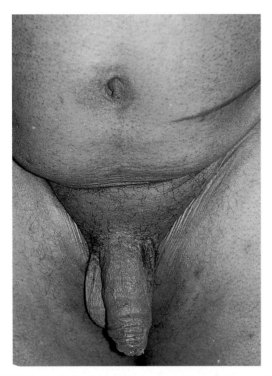

FIG. 6-7. Seborrheic dermatitis is characterized by prominent skin fold involvement including the crural crease, umbilicus, and axillae. Erythema in a darkly pigmented person regularly appears as hyperpigmentation.

Seborrheic dermatitis of the genital area is accentuated within the skin folds. A classic but not unique characteristic of genital seborrheic dermatitis is a glazed, shiny texture to the affected skin.

Infants often develop seborrhea of the scalp, also called cradle cap. Spread of the eruption to the face, trunk, and genitalia is much more common in infants than in adults.

Diagnosis

The diagnosis of seborrheic dermatitis can generally be made by the pattern of red, scaling plaques that include the scalp, central face, and other skin folds and by the absence of negative culture or skin scrapings for candidiasis. A biopsy is generally not required to make this diagnosis, but histology is characterized by varying degrees of acanthosis and elongation of the rete ridges, with hyperkeratosis and spongiosis. There is an underlying perivascular lymphocytic infiltrate, with some migration into the epidermis. Neutrophils can be seen in the stratum corneum. The diagnosis of seborrheic dermatitis is confirmed by the rapid and complete response to therapy.

Most causes of generalized red patches and plaques of the genitalia are in the differential diagnosis. This includes atopic dermatitis and its variants, allergic and irritant contact dermatitis, fungal infection, and psoriasis. The accentuation of disease in the skin folds especially

mimics cutaneous candidiasis. Generally, these diseases can be differentiated by their pattern of involvement on other parts of the body, as well as by the characteristic yellowish, greasy scale on the scalp and face seen in seborrhea. Psoriasis, however, frequently exhibits the same distribution, but the thicker nature of the plaque, the more discrete rather than generalized scalp plaques, the psoriatic nail changes, and the typical lesions of psoriasis of other skin surfaces usually differentiate these two diseases.

SEBORRHEIC DERMATITIS:	Diagnosis

- Morphology of red plaques in skin folds in a setting of red plaques in a typical distribution for seborrhea; scalp, central face, ears, chest, axillae
- Patient who is an infant or unable to wash regularly; homeless, debilitated

Pathophysiology

The cause of seborrheic dermatitis is not known. Some evidence suggests that *Malassezia* yeasts, the causative organism of pityriasis (tinea) versicolor, play a role in the development of seborrheic dermatitis. Unencapsulated yeast forms stimulate cytokine production by keratinocytes (6). This yeast has been identified in the scalp of patients with seborrhea, and the antifungal cream ketoconazole topically is effective for the treatment of pityriasis versicolor and scalp seborrheic dermatitis. However, this organism is a frequent colonizer, and other equally effective antifungal medications have not been reported to be beneficial for the treatment of seborrhea; both of these facts suggest an alternate or additional etiology. Other clinicians believe that seborrhea is an inflammatory response to perspiration, heat, and sebum trapped under normal stratum corneum that is not normally shed from skin folds and hairy areas because of anchoring hair shafts. This theory is also used to explain the distribution of seborrhea, which includes the scalp, eyebrows, beard area, nasolabial and retroauricular folds on the head and neck, and other skin folds such as the axillae and groin (Fig. 6-7). Inflammation from heat, sweat and scale held against the skin by scale result in increased epidermal turnover and the production of even more scale.

Management

The treatment of anogenital seborrheic dermatitis requires the control of disease on the scalp and other areas as well. This involves the removal of scale from the scalp and any other affected hairy areas, as well as administration of topical corticosteroids. Vigorous and irritating means of scale removal is not indicated in the much more sensitive skin folds and genital regions.

Brisk shampooing of the adult scalp with antiseborrheic shampoos containing antiproliferative agents such as tar zinc pyrithione or selenium sulfide or keratolytic substances such as salicylic acid aids in the debridement of scale from the scalp. Medication is scrubbed into the scalp and is allowed to stay on the skin for 5 to 10 minutes before it is rinsed. Generally, use of these shampoos in the genital area is not recommended because of their irritant properties and because they are not required for clearing. Again, because of the irritant properties of these shampoos, infant seborrhea is not treated with these agents. The scalp scale is softened with baby oil or mineral oil and is then removed with a soft brush or gentle use of fingernails.

Otherwise, topical corticosteroids are primary therapy for seborrhea, both on the scalp and on genital skin. Patients with mild disease and infants are easily treated with a low-potency medication such as hydrocortisone 1% or 2.5%. For more severe disease, a midpotency topical corticosteroid such as triamcinolone 0.1% cream generally produces marked improvement quickly. An inexpensive, cosmetically pleasing, and effective corticosteroid for use in the scalp is betamethasone valerate 0.01% lotion, but this alcohol-based therapy should not be used on easily irritated genital skin.

For those patients who do not improve adequately with this safe and relatively inexpensive therapy, ketoconazole (Nizoral) cream or shampoo can be a beneficial treatment. The cream is applied twice a day, and the shampoo is used daily on the scalp.

The treatment of seborrheic dermatitis in patients of African descent must be modified because of the tendency for the hair of these patients to dry excessively and to break with overwashing. Twice-weekly vigorous shampooing of the scalp initially with careful attention to moisturizing the hair afterward is usually a reasonable compromise. However, moisturizers should be applied to the hair only, with the patient's taking care to avoid application to the scalp itself because this can exacerbate retention of scale and occlusion.

Scalp seborrheic dermatitis is a chronic skin condition with a tendency to wax and wane in severity. Usually, the regular and proper use of an antiseborrhic shampoo controls scalp disease, although some patients require intermittent application of a corticosteroid solution to the scalp. Because the groin generally is the last area involved with severe seborrhea, control of scalp disease usually prevents the recurrence of anogenital seborrheic dermatitis.

SEBORRHEIC DERMATITIS: **Management**

- Ongoing removal of excess scale of the scalp by shampooing with keratolytic (salicylic acid) or tar shampoos
- Topical corticosteroid cream (triamcinolone 0.1%) very sparingly twice a day until clear

---

PSORIASIS

Psoriasis is a relatively common skin disease that frequently affects genital skin in addition to the elbows, scalp, and knees as classic locations.

Clinical Presentation

Psoriasis is a very common skin condition, occurring in 2% to 3% of people. Males and females are affected equally, and persons of African ancestry are less often affected than white individuals. This condition occurs at all ages but begins most often in young adults. There is a familial predisposition, with one in three patients reporting a family history of psoriasis.

Classic psoriasis vulgaris (common psoriasis) exhibits well-demarcated thickened, red plaques with dense, silvery scale (Figs. 6-8 through 6-10). Often, patients report severe itching, but this is not universal. Plaques typically occur on the scalp, elbows, knees, umbilicus, and gluteal cleft. Genital involvement is common, and plaques are more generalized in patients with more severe disease. The face is usually relatively spared.

About 20% of patients exhibit Koebner phenomenon, in which psoriasis is precipitated in skin by irritation or injury. This partially explains the distribution of lesions, including the elbows and knees, as well as the frequent involvement of the genitalia, an area subject to friction and occlusion.

A variant of psoriasis that presents with prominent genital involvement is inverse psoriasis (Figs. 6-11 through 6-13, 6-15, 6-17 through 6-19). Inverse psoriasis involves skin folds preferentially and often spares the classic dry, keratinized knees, elbows, and scalps. The axillae, inframammary skin, umbilicus, gluteal cleft, crural creases, and genitalia are affected. Psoriasis occurring in skin folds exhibits very subtle scale as well as plaques that are far

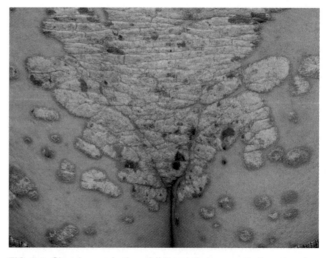

FIG. 6-8. Classic psoriasis exhibits well-demarcated coalescing plaques with distinctive, heavy, silvery scale.

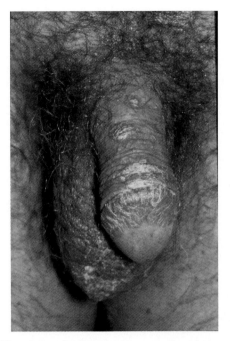

FIG. 6-9. The circumcised penis shows scaling plaques that are thinner than those occurring on dry, fully keratinized skin.

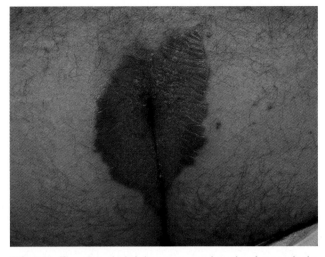

FIG. 6-11. The gluteal cleft is a common location for psoriasis; redness is often marked in skin folds.

thinner than psoriasis on other skin surfaces (Figs. 6-14 through 6-17). In addition, the borders frequently are less well demarcated (Fig. 6-18). Not uncommonly, yeast or dermatophyte infection may coexist with or may mimic intertriginous psoriasis (Fig. 6-19). Psoriasis predominantly affects the hairbearing vulva of women, mostly sparing the modified mucous membranes and vagina. However, psoriasis often is located on the glans penis in addition to the penile shaft, scrotum, and groin.

Psoriasis sometimes can become generalized, so that confluent erythema, scale, and sometimes exudation are indistinguishable from generalized eczema or generalized seborrhea. A final form of psoriasis, pustular psoriasis, is characterized by plaques of pustules or crusting. This variant is discussed in Chapter 8.

Psoriasis produces nail abnormalities in addition to inflammatory skin lesions (Fig. 6-20). Most common are small nail pits, not to be confused with simple irregularity or rippling of the surface. Also fairly specific are "oil-drop spots." These are brownish-red discolorations of the nail plate. A third form of nail psoriasis, onycholysis, is much

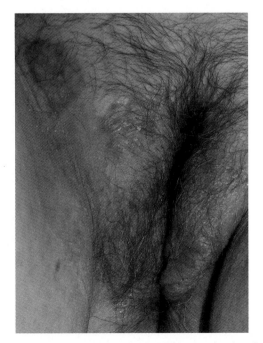

FIG. 6-10. Genital psoriasis often exhibits scale that is less dense than psoriatic scale on dry extragenital skin.

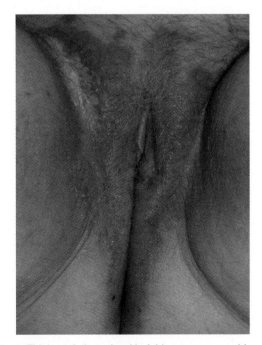

FIG. 6-12. Thick scale in moist skin folds appears as white, macerated skin, whereas the shiny, glazed red skin of the labia majora actually represents adherent scale.

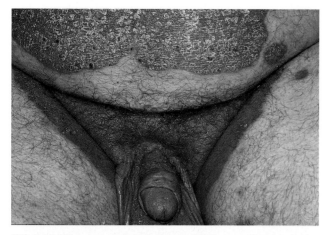

FIG. 6-13. Whereas truncal lesions exhibit more classic psoriasis with prominent scale, genital lesions often show more subtle scale. The presence of the truncal lesions is helpful in making the diagnosis.

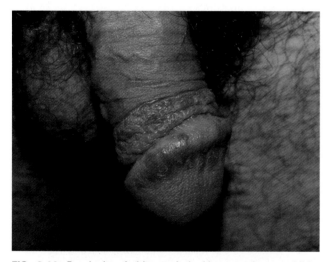

FIG. 6-14. Psoriasis of thin genital skin sometimes exhibits erosions as well as scale, which can be yellowish from serous exudate.

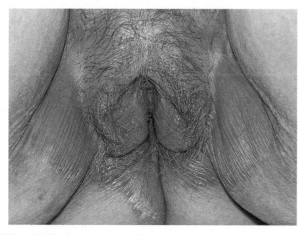

FIG. 6-15. Genital psoriasis often shows glazed erythema rather than flaky scale.

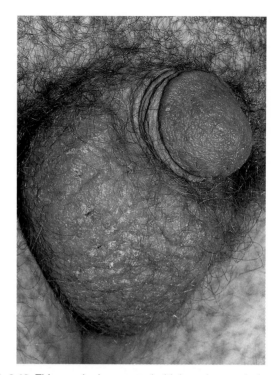

FIG. 6-16. This poorly demarcated, thickened scrotal plaque is consistent with lichen simplex chronicus; however, the white, dense quality of the scale suggests the correct diagnosis of psoriasis.

less specific. Onycholysis refers to lifting of the nail from the underlying surface, in this case from psoriasis of the nail bed. The scale and keratin debris collect under the nail, with the final picture nearly identical to that of a fungal nail infection.

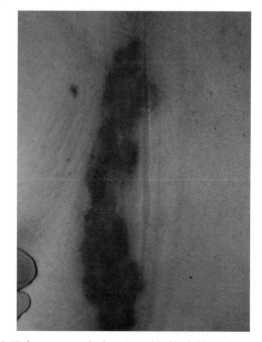

FIG. 6-17. Inverse psoriasis occurs in skin folds and lacks obvious clinical scale.

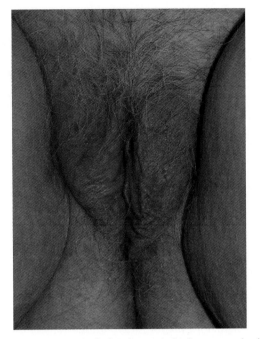

FIG. 6-18. Vulvar psoriasis is often poorly demarcated without psoriasiform scale, mimicking lichen simplex chronicus or contact dermatitis.

The primary extracutaneous manifestation of psoriasis is arthritis. A significant minority of patients experience joint disease that ranges from pain with minimal inflammation to severe, deforming, and mutilating arthritis.

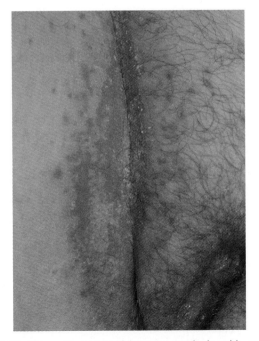

FIG. 6-19. This red plaque of inverse psoriasis with surface white, moist scale can be indistinguishable from intertriginous Candidiasis. Even the satellite papules do not guarantee a diagnosis of yeast; a culture for yeast was negative, and the plaque resolved with a topical corticosteroid.

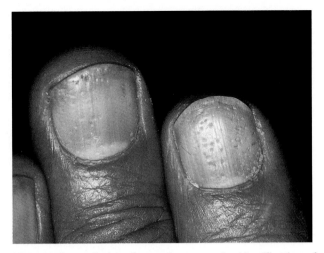

FIG. 6-20. In confusing diagnostic cases, the identification of typical psoriasis on other skin surfaces such as the scalp, elbows, or nail pits, such as these, can be very useful.

There are also several comorbidities associated with psoriasis, suggesting that psoriasis is actually a complex constellation of systemic conditions. Patients with psoriasis are more likely to be obese, and alcoholism and depression are recognized as common occurrences. Cardiovascular disease, inflammatory bowel disease, and even osteoporosis have been reported more recently to occur more often (7,8). Autoimmune diseases also are increased in this group (9).

Diagnosis

Psoriasis of the genitalia can be diagnosed with confidence when morphologically consistent plaques in this area are associated with typical psoriasis of the elbows and knees, scalp, and nails. If the distribution and morphology are atypical, the diagnosis can often be confirmed on biopsy, but a nondiagnostic biopsy does not rule out psoriasis as a cause of the eruption.

The classic but nonspecific histologic picture of psoriasis includes marked thickening of the epidermis with regular elongation of the rete pegs and suprapapillary thinning. Hyperkeratosis and parakeratosis are prominent, and there is an absence of the granular layer. More specific histologic findings are collections of neutrophils just under the stratum corneum of the thinned suprapapillary epidermis (spongiform pustules of Kogoj) and in the overlying parakeratotic layer (Munro microabscesses). A biopsy of an older lesion is often nonspecific and may be interpreted as psoriasiform dermatitis.

Tinea cruris is the most common disease confused with psoriasis, and they often coexist. However, in immunocompetent patients, tinea cruris usually spares the scrotum and penis, whereas these structures are often prominently affected with psoriasis. In addition, tinea cruris is uncommon in women. Cutaneous candidiasis frequently shows satellite pustules or erosions but can also resemble and coexist with psoriasis. Lichen simplex chronicus, Bowen disease (also called squamous cell carcinoma in situ, as well as erythroplasia of Queyrat in men and vulvar intraepithelial neoplasia on the vulva), and Paget disease are all red, scaling diseases that can be confused with psoriasis, and lichen planus on the glans penis is sometimes indistinguishable from smaller papules of psoriasis of this area. Seborrheic dermatitis, especially in infants, can appear very similar to psoriasis and shows the same pattern of distribution as inverse psoriasis.

PSORIASIS :	**Diagnosis**

- Presence of well-demarcated red plaques in skin folds
- Usually, more typical, heavily scaling plaques on other skin surfaces including elbows, knees, and scalp
- Negative scrapings or cultures for *Candida* and dermatophytosis
- In the absence of classic extragenital disease, biopsy, which shows acanthosis with regular elongation of the rete pegs and suprapapillary thinning, hyperkeratosis, parakeratosis are prominent, absence of the granular layer. More specific are collections of neutrophils just under the stratum corneum of the thinned suprapapillary epidermis and within parakeratotic stratum corneum. Nonspecific "psoriasiform dermatitis" result is common
- Nonresponse to antifungal therapy

Pathophysiology

The thickened plaques of psoriasis result from unusually rapid proliferation of the epidermis. The usual transient time from the basal cell layer of the epidermis to the mature stratum corneum is about 20 days. However, psoriatic epithelium turns over in 5 days. This produces much thicker skin with more remarkable scale. The underlying etiology is multifactorial, with autoimmune features, genetic predisposition, and environmental issues serving as factors (10). Other factors include smoking, obesity, and alcohol (11,12). In addition, classic triggers for the development of psoriasis include streptococcal disease, sunburn, and human immunodeficiency virus infection. Some medications are associated with the development or worsening of psoriasis, including lithium and nonsteroidal anti-inflammatory medications.

Management

First-line therapy for genital psoriasis is topical corticosteroid administration. Potent steroids such as fluocinonide 0.05% (Lidex) or ultrapotent medications such as clobetasol propionate (Temovate) can be used initially, with tapering of potency as tolerated to preparations that can be used more safely for long periods of time, such as triamcinolone 0.1% or desonide 0.05%. Sometimes, the intermittent use of corticosteroids provides benefits while minimizing tachyphylaxis (the tendency of psoriasis to become resistant to long-term corticosteroid use) and side effects.

For genital psoriasis not adequately controlled with this treatment, addition of calcipotriene (Dovonex) is effective in many patients, but there is a 1- to 2-month delay before improvement is evident. This medication is no longer available in an ointment base, so the cream vehicle must be substituted. However, a similar medication, calcitriol (Vectical) is now approved and available in an ointment formulation (13). Alternatively, a combination of betamethasone dipropionate and calcipotriene ointment (Taclonex) can be used once daily (14). However, this expensive and potent medication used chronically in skin folds can produce thinning and striae. If the patient is not irritated by the calcipotriene in the cream base, best results often are obtained by the addition of twice-daily calcipotriene cream if tolerated, or calcitriol ointment to intermittent topical corticosteroid ointment twice daily. Topical tar can be useful on some skin surfaces, but are irritating on genital skin, as are topical retinoids and anthralin.

There are conflicting reports on the potential usefulness of topical tacrolimus ointment for psoriasis (15). This immunomodulator sometimes stings with application, especially on the genitalia.

Although ultraviolet light is frequently used for psoriasis, this treatment is of little use on the genitalia. First, the delivery of ultraviolet light to this area is logistically difficult. Second, an increase in penile squamous cell carcinomas is known to occur in patients treated on a long-term basis with ultraviolet light.

Severe genital psoriasis often is not adequately controlled with topical medications. These patients frequently require systemic therapy with oral methotrexate, retinoids such as acitretin, or cyclosporine. More recently, immunosuppressive biologic agents administered by self-injection at home (etanercept, adalimumab) are convenient and effective, although extremely expensive.

In addition to specific therapy for psoriasis as discussed earlier, control of irritants such as bacterial and fungal infection, maceration from moisture, and irritation from overwashing and topical medications can remarkably improve symptoms. Nighttime sedation for patients with significant itching can also improve quality of life.

Psoriasis is a chronic disease for which there is no cure, although control is usually effected. Many patients with psoriasis are psychologically incapacitated by their disease (16). The constant production of scale, the disfigurement of their skin, and the incurable nature of the disease are hard for many patients to tolerate. People with genital psoriasis must also deal with the sexual ramifications of this chronic genital abnormality, so aggressive treatment of their psoriasis as well as counseling can be crucial. Patients should be urged to join the National Psoriasis Foundation, which provides information and support to those living with psoriasis. Also, patients with significant psoriasis should be made aware of the comorbidities of the disease and referred to a primary care physician for evaluation and treatment of any obesity or alcoholism and for counseling regarding the prevention of cardiovascular disease.

PSORIASIS:	**Management**

- Topical corticosteroid (triamcinolone 0.1%) ointment sparingly twice a day; for poor response, increase potency to clobetasol but follow nearby skin for atrophy and steroid dermatitis. Taper frequency as possible
- Calcipotriene cream or calcitriol ointment twice daily in addition to corticosteroid if needed
- For severe disease, add systemic therapy; methotrexate, acitretin, adalimumab, etanercept, etc.

TINEA CRURIS (JOCK ITCH)

This common disease is often assumed by male patients to be the cause of any genital itching.

Clinical Presentation

Tinea cruris occurs far most often in men. There is no predisposition for any race, but the most common age is middle age and is extremely uncommon in children. Tinea cruris is usually associated with tinea pedis and onychomycosis, which serve as a reservoir for the organism, and recurrence is common.

Most often, the visible lesions of tinea cruris are limited to the proximal, medial thighs. Classically, plaques are erythematous and well demarcated, with accentuation of scale peripherally (Figs. 6-21 through 6-24). Many patients, particularly those with prominent hair in the area, exhibit red papules, nodules, or pustules within the plaque that represent extension of the infection to the follicular epithelium (fungal folliculitis).

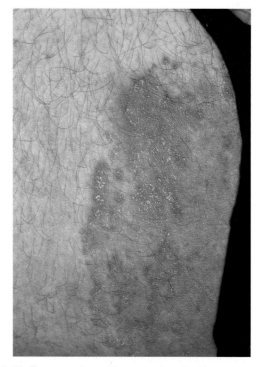

FIG. 6-21. Tinea cruris, a disease primarily of men, generally shows sharply demarcated borders with scale.

Occasionally, the plaque extends to the scrotum, and in women the plaque may extend to the labia majora and mons pubis. This is most likely to occur when patients are immunosuppressed or have been using a topical corticosteroid for the itching. Immunocompetent patients not using topical corticosteroids do not experience dermatophyte infections of the shaft or glans of the penis.

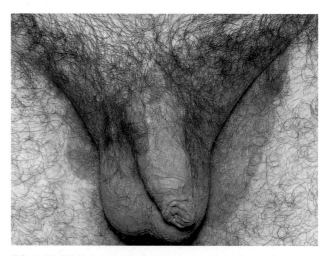

FIG. 6-22. Well-demarcated erythema and scale on the proximal, inner thighs are classic signs of tinea cruris. The penis and scrotum are classically spared.

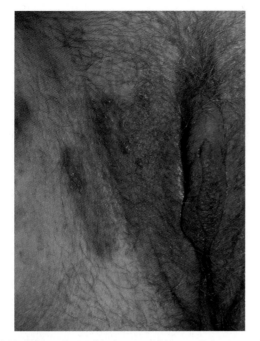

FIG. 6-23. This patient with tinea cruris treated the area with a topical antifungal agent, thus clearing the surface infection, encouraging the dermatophyte to invade the follicles, producing nodules of superimposed fungal folliculitis.

Diagnosis

The diagnosis of tinea cruris is made by the morphologic features and is confirmed by the identification of hyphae on microscopic examination of scales scraped from the affected skin. A biopsy is performed in patients with tinea cruris only if the diagnosis is unsuspected or a fungal preparation is negative. The specific findings are those of hyphae in the stratum corneum, best visualized with special stains, usually periodic acid–Schiff reaction or the methenamine silver nitrate method. Otherwise, the findings are those of eczema.

The diseases most often confused with tinea cruris are eczema (lichen simplex chronicus) and psoriasis. Eczema generally is less well demarcated, and it usually prominently affects the scrotum and labia majora. Psoriasis can be nearly indistinguishable, but an examination of other skin surfaces usually reveals typical scalp psoriasis, involvement of elbows or knees or nail pits. Seborrheic dermatitis, irritant and allergic contact dermatitis, Paget disease, and Bowen disease (also known as vulvar intraepithelial neoplasia in women, or squamous cell carcinoma in situ) should also be considered.

TINEA CRURIS:	**Diagnosis**

- Presence of well-demarcated red plaques with peripheral accentuation/scale on the proximal, medial thighs; occasionally extending to the scrotum or vulva; often coexisting onychomycosis
- Skin scraping that shows dermatophyte on microscopic examination, or positive culture
- Prompt improvement with antifungal therapy

Pathophysiology

Dermatophyte fungi infecting the stratum corneum of keratinized skin of the genital area result in the eruption of tinea cruris. The predominant species are *Epidermophyton floccosum* and *Trichophyton rubrum*, with *T. mentagrophytes* and *T. verrucosum* responsible at times. These organisms are ubiquitous, and even immunocompetent patients sometimes experience recurrent infection. Usually, these patients also exhibit tinea pedis and onychomycosis, which serve as a source for autoinoculation. Fomites also contribute to the spread of this fungal infection.

Management

Oral or topical antifungal medications are the mainstay of treatment for tinea cruris. Generally, tinea cruris, exhibiting only erythema and scale and lacking pustules and firm papules within the plaque, can be cleared with a topical medication. Any of the topical azoles are effective, including clotrimazole, miconazole, econazole, and ketoconazole. Terbinafine (Lamisil) is also effective. Azoles exhibit good coverage against yeast as well as the dermatophyte fungi that cause tinea cruris, whereas the allylamines terbinafine and naftifine are less effective against yeast infection. Although quite useful in the treatment of genital

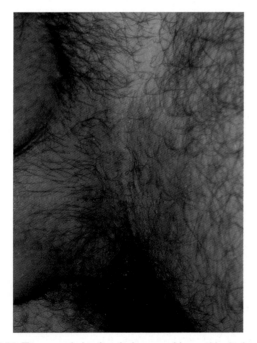

FIG. 6-24. Tinea cruris is often itchy, as evidenced by its lay term "jock itch." This well-demarcated plaque of fungal infection exhibits superimposed lichenification.

candidiasis, nystatin has no activity against the dermatophyte fungi of tinea cruris. Other effective but less often used medications include ciclopirox, haloprogin, and iodoquinol, as well as tolnaftate.

Patients with follicular involvement characterized by papules or pustules within the plaque require oral therapy because topical medication does not penetrate sufficiently to eradicate organisms within follicles. Similarly, tinea cruris of skin containing dense, thick hair often is incompletely treated with a topical medication. There are several effective and safe oral medications for patients with very widespread disease, plaques within very hairy areas, and patients with pustules or nodules within plaques indicating follicular involvement. A time-honored and effective therapy is griseofulvin at 500 mg twice a day. Unfortunately, nausea and headache are very common with this medication. Although hepatotoxicity was a concern of many clinicians in the past, this is very uncommon, and laboratory testing is no longer the standard of care with this medication.

The newer oral antifungal are better tolerated by patients. Fluconazole at a dose of 100 to 200 mg/day, itraconazole at 200 mg/day, or terbinafine at 250 mg/day is very effective and is usually well tolerated. For the length of time (1 to 2 weeks) required to treat tinea cruris, laboratory testing is not required for patients without pre-existing liver disease. Coadministration of itraconazole with cisapride (Propulsid), pimozide, and quinidine can precipitate cardiac arrhythmia, and this medication has multiple other interactions that require careful monitoring. Similarly, fluconazole should not be administered concomitantly with cisapride, and fluconazole can increase levels or actions of coumarin-type anticoagulants, phenytoin, cyclosporine, theophylline, terfenadine, and tacrolimus. Oral ketoconazole (Nizoral) currently is avoided because of the occasional occurrence of severe, idiosyncratic hepatotoxicity as well as medication interactions.

Some patients are unusually inflamed and red or extremely itchy. These patients improve more quickly if a topical corticosteroid such as triamcinolone 0.1% cream is used concomitantly for the first few days. Some clinicians use a commercial combination of clotrimazole and betamethasone dipropionate (Lotrisone). Although this combination is very convenient for the first few days, it contains a high-potency cortisone that should not be used on the proximal, medial thighs for a prolonged period because of the propensity to develop striae. In addition, a topical corticosteroid slightly decreases the effectiveness of the antifungal medication and is generally needed only for the first few days of therapy. A rational approach to this problem is the addition of a midpotency corticosteroid to the antifungal medication just for the first few days so those early anti-inflammatory actions are provided without a significant decrease in the cure rate, and the topical antifungal medication is used until the skin is clear.

Often, tinea cruris is recurrent, with the reservoir being a dermatophyte infection of the toenails. Patients with tinea cruris may benefit from a longer course of an oral antifungal to clear the nail disease. The most common regimens consist of terbinafine at 250 mg/day for 3 months or itraconazole at 200 mg twice daily for 1 week of each month for 3 months. Fluconazole at 200 mg/week until the nail grows out (about 1 year) is also effective. Alternatively, patients can simply reapply a topical antifungal cream immediately with a recurrence.

TINEA CRURIS: **Management**

- Any topical azole once or twice daily until clear; miconazole, clotrimazole, terconazole, econazole, ketoconazole, etc; also, terbinafine, tolnaftate, ciclopirox, haloprogin, and iodoquinol
- In the presence of papules within the plaque (fungal folliculitis) or extensive disease, oral therapy is needed until clear; griseofulvin 500 mg b.i.d., fluconazole 100 to 200 mg q.d., itraconazole 200 mg q.d., terbinafine 250 mg q.d.

ERYTHRASMA

Erythrasma is a genital skin infection that is found most often in men and mimics tinea cruris.

Clinical Presentation

Most common in men in warm climates, erythrasma shows no tendency for particular races or populations. Erythrasma affects the proximal, medial thighs and crural crease. Tan-pink, lightly scaling or finely wrinkled, well-demarcated plaques are characteristic. Patients with dark complexions often exhibit hyperpigmentation rather than erythema (Figs. 6-25 and 6-26). These plaques are solid, without peripheral scale or central clearing. The scrotum, penis, and vulva are generally not affected.

Diagnosis

The diagnosis is made principally by the appearance of the skin and with confirmation either by characteristic coral-pink fluorescence when examined with Wood's light or by response to therapy.

Tinea cruris is the disease most likely to be confused with erythrasma. Tinea cruris, also seen primarily in men, shares the same location and pattern. However, tinea cruris usually exhibits peripheral scaling and some degree of central clearing. In addition, the dermatophyte often extends down follicles of some of the coarser hairs and produces red papules or nodules within the plaque. A

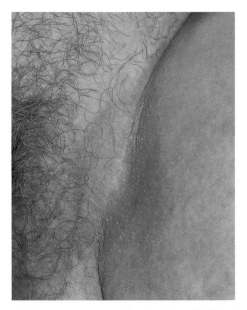

FIG. 6-25. Erythrasma presents as tan-pink, solid, lightly scaling plaques on the proximal, medial thighs.

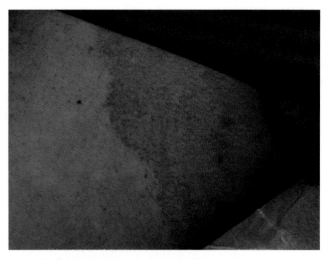

FIG. 6-26. Like tinea cruris, erythrasma occurs most often in men; however, it lacks the peripheral scale and exhibits a negative fungal microscopic preparation.

fungal preparation of peripheral scale in a patient with tinea cruris shows branching long hyphae. Diseases that less often mimic erythrasma include eczema, which is characterized by prominent involvement of the scrotum or vulva with poorly demarcated plaques and is extremely pruritic. Psoriasis also frequently affects the genitalia itself and usually is associated with other signs of psoriasis, such as knee, elbow, and scalp involvement and nail pits.

ERYTHRASMA:	Diagnosis

- Presence of well-demarcated pink or pink/tan plaques without peripheral accentuation/scale on the proximal, medial thighs
- Negative microscopic examination of skin scraping; coral-pink fluorescence with Wood's lamp
- Response to therapy

Pathophysiology

Erythrasma is caused by the bacterium *Corynebacterium minutissimum*. Found on the feet and in skin folds such as the axillae, inframammary skin, and genital area, it is most prevalent in warmer, more humid environments.

Management

Erythrasma is generally cleared by erythromycin at 500 mg two times daily for 1 to 2 weeks. Topical erythromycin twice daily has also been used, as has fusidic acid.

Recurrence and a need for retreatment or even long-term application of erythromycin, clindamycin, or azoles are fairly common.

ERYTHRASMA:	Management

- Erythromycin 500 mg twice a day; also topical erythromycin, fusidic acid, clindamycin
- Suppressive therapy often needed because of frequent recurrences

CANDIDIASIS

Both the cause and the treatment of this genital fungal dermatosis are often confused with those of a dermatophyte infection (see also Chapters 8, 9, and 15).

Clinical Presentation

Cutaneous candidiasis consists of red plaques predominantly in skin folds such as the crural crease (Figs. 6-27 through 6-29). These plaques are often moist and classically exhibit satellite pustules or collarettes that represent unroofed pustules, and peripheral peeling (Fig. 6-30). This infection is almost always accompanied by *Candida* vaginitis in women. Most often seen in premenopausal women, vulvar candidiasis is manifested by edema and redness of the modified mucous membranes, and often fissuring of skin folds (Fig. 6-31). Occasionally, however, *Candida* vulvovaginitis is treated with an intravaginal preparation only, thus allowing yeast on the external genitalia to persist, especially if the patient is also using a topical corticosteroid on the external genitalia.

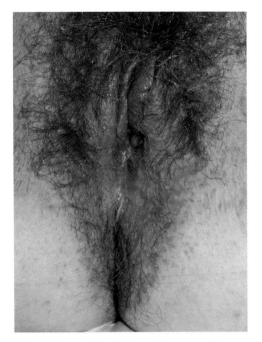

FIG. 6-27. Genital candidiasis is most common in women and presents as redness with peripheral peeling when occurring on the keratinized skin of the vulva.

In addition to the crural crease, the glans penis is prominently affected in uncircumcised men (Fig. 6-32). Penile candidiasis is very uncommon in immunocompetent, circumcised men. However, following intercourse with women with *Candida* vaginitis, some men experience transient, poorly demarcated patchy erythema of the glans.

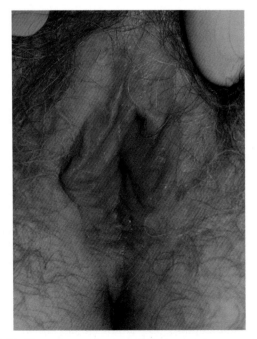

FIG. 6-28. Most often, vulvar candidiasis presents as erythema and edema of the modified mucous membranes of the vulva.

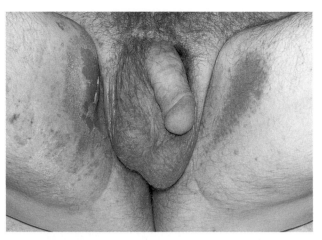

FIG. 6-29. Genital candidiasis in men occurs most often in those who are incontinent, obese, or diabetic.

Diagnosis

The diagnosis is made by the clinical findings and is confirmed by the identification of hyphae, pseudohyphae, and budding yeasts on a microscopic smear of scale from the periphery of the plaques or of a pustule roof. A biopsy is neither necessary nor desirable for the diagnosis. However, the histologic findings of cutaneous candidiasis are those of pseudohyphae and hyphae invading the stratum corneum and infiltration of the epidermis with neutrophils that form subcorneal pustules.

Candida can both be mistaken for and coexist with atopic dermatitis, lichen simplex chronicus, irritant and allergic contact dermatitis, psoriasis, and tinea cruris. The lack of symmetry and the pattern of Paget disease and Bowen disease make both conditions less likely to produce confusion in women, but Bowen disease of the glans penis can be nearly indistinguishable from *Candida* balanitis.

CANDIDIASIS:	Diagnosis

- Morphology:
  - Presence of red plaques with satellite papules, superficial pustules, or collarettes; common on the vulva and scrotum and in the crural creases, especially in overweight, diabetic and/or incontinent individuals
  - Red, puffy, modified mucous membranes and mucous membranes of the vulva and vagina
  - Red, flat papules on the glans primarily of uncircumcised males
- Microscopic examination of skin scrapings shows mycelia and budding yeast; positive culture
- Confirmed by response to antifungal therapy

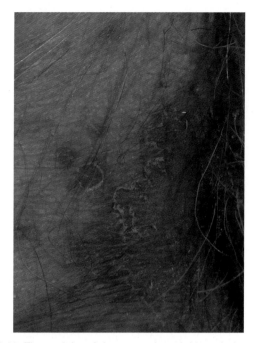

FIG. 6-30. The peripheral desquamation of this red plaque is a very strong sign of probable cutaneous candidiasis.

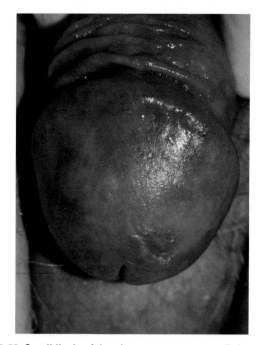

FIG. 6-32. Candidiasis of the glans presents as a red plaque that sometimes is erosive.

Pathophysiology

Cutaneous candidiasis is produced by the yeast *Candida albicans*. Local factors such as incontinence, retention of sweat, and heat provide a favorable environment for this fungus. In addition, obesity, diabetes mellitus, immunosuppression, and the administration of systemic antibiotics also predispose to infections with *C. albicans*.

Management

Topical therapy is very effective for cutaneous candidiasis. Nystatin and all of the topical azoles are beneficial for

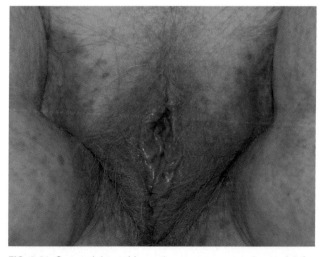

FIG. 6-31. Overweight and incontinent women are also at risk for genital yeast, which is characterized in this setting by red plaques that extend up the crural creases and exhibit satellite papules.

this problem. Evaluation of the vagina for candidiasis is important for women, since treatment of the vulva without treatment of the vagina often results in relapse. One oral dose of fluconazole (Diflucan), 150 mg, treats both the vagina and minor skin involvement, and this is effective for *Candida* balanitis.

The occasional patient with very inflammatory, exudative cutaneous disease is likely to experience burning and stinging with the use of creams. Because there are no azoles available in a nonirritating ointment base, these patients should receive either nystatin ointment or an oral therapy such as fluconazole 100 mg/day, or itraconazole 200 mg/day. Ketoconazole sometimes produces

---

CANDIDIASIS:　　　**Management**

- Any topical azole once or twice daily until clear; miconazole, clotrimazole, terconazole, econazole, ketoconazole, etc.
- Vulvar candidiasis is generally accompanied by vaginal yeast as well and should be treated with oral fluconazole 150 mg once, or any intravaginal azole
- For very inflammatory skin disease, fluconazole 100 to 200 mg/day, econazole 200 mg/day
- Suppressive therapy often needed because of frequent recurrences in obese, immunosuppressed, diabetic patients with crural crease and external cutaneous candidiasis

severe idiosyncratic liver disease, and terbinafine is less useful for yeast than for dermatophyte forms of fungus. Griseofulvin is not effective against yeast forms. Alleviation of chronic moisture, control of diabetes, and improvement in immunosuppression help to prevent recurrent or chronic disease.

PERIANAL STREPTOCOCCAL DISEASE (PERIANAL STREPTOCOCCAL CELLULITIS)

Perianal streptococcal dermatitis is a superficial infection of perianal skin that sometimes affects the penis/scrotum or vulva and vagina (see also Chapter 14). Although the causative organism is most often group A *Streptococcus*, group B *Streptococcus* and *Staphylococcus aureus* have been reported as well. This is most often a pediatric disease affecting young children, but it can also affect both the genitalia and perianal skin of adults.

Symptoms include persistent pruritus or pain that has been unresponsive to antifungal and corticosteroid medications frequently used by the patient. The disease consists of redness, fissuring, fragility, crusting, exudation, and erosion of the perianal skin (Figs. 6-33 through 6-36). Occasionally, the scrotum and penis are involved, and the vulva may also exhibit similar abnormalities, usually associated with an erythematous vaginal mucosa and a purulent vaginal discharge.

The skin should be cultured to confirm the diagnosis and to ensure that other organisms, especially *S. aureus*, are not present as well. The treatment consists of oral penicillin (unless *S. aureus* is present), often in conjunction with a

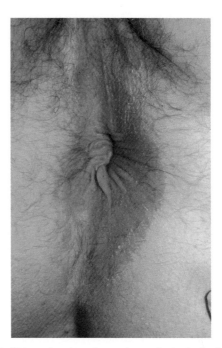

FIG. 6-34. This red, edematous plaque is typical of perianal streptococcal disease.

topical medication such as mupirocin (Bactroban) ointment several times a day. Recurrences are common.

LICHEN PLANUS

Lichen planus exhibits many different morphologic appearances and symptoms (see also Chapters 9, 11, and 15). This variation is partially dependent on the location of the disease, and many patients exhibit several different forms of lichen planus. The least common form in women and the most common form in circumcised men is that of red plaques and papules.

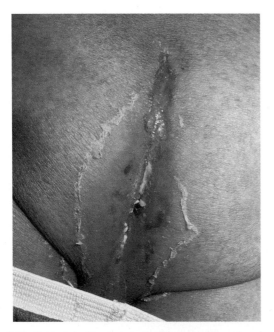

FIG. 6-33. Perianal streptococcal disease, although primarily seen in children, can happen at any age, such as in this 58-year-old man.

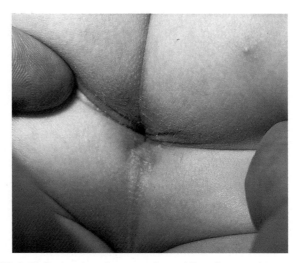

FIG. 6-35. Perianal erythema, scale, and fissuring are characteristic of perianal streptococcal disease.

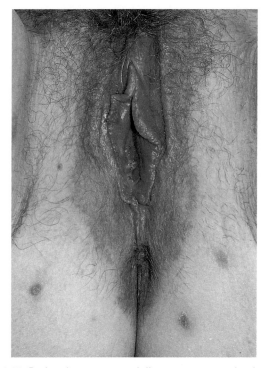

FIG. 6-36. Perianal streptococcal disease can extend to involve both the vulva and vagina.

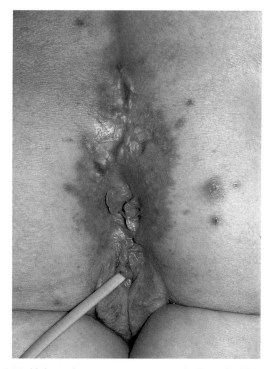

FIG. 6-38. Lichen planus can present as dusky red, shiny, well-demarcated, thickened, and fissured plaques.

Clinical Presentation

Lichen planus is a relatively common skin disease. Although once believed to be uncommon on the genitalia of women, this recently has become more often recognized. Lichen planus of dry, keratinized skin is most often manifested by violaceous or dusky red-brown, well-demarcated, flat-topped, shiny papules (Figs. 6-37 through 6-40). Although most common on the ventral aspect of the wrist, this form of lichen planus can be seen on any dry skin surface.

A common place for genital papular lichen planus is the glans penis. These lesions are usually well demarcated, red, flat topped, and shiny. Occasionally, the lesions are annular, hypopigmented, or hyperpigmented. Other areas of the external genitalia are not commonly affected by this form of lichen planus, although the proximal medial thighs are sometimes involved. Papular lichen planus occurring in women is found most often on the hairbearing labia majora, crural creases, and proximal, medial thighs.

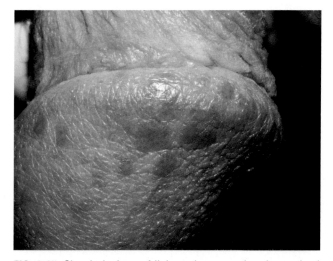

FIG. 6-37. Classic lesions of lichen planus on the circumcised glans are red, well demarcated, and flat topped.

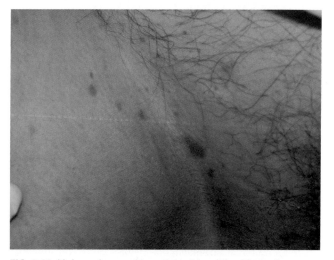

FIG. 6-39. Lichen planus of keratinized but thin skin is often nondescript, such as these red papules in the crural crease.

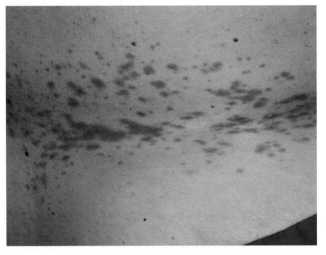

FIG. 6-40. This dusky red color is typical of lichen planus on dry keratinized skin.

Papular lichen planus of the genitalia is often accompanied by erosive, atrophic, or white, reticulate mucous membrane lichen planus. This is most easily evaluated by examining the buccal mucosa. Characteristic papular lesions are white, linear, branching papules that often form a fernlike or lacy pattern (Chapter 11), red, atrophic, smooth patches, or red erosions (Chapter 6). Sometimes, superficial erosions of these modified mucous membranes can be difficult to differentiate from atrophic patches of mucous membranes (Fig. 6-41). Even when the vaginal epithelium appears generally normal, nonspecific inflammatory vaginitis characterized by a large number of white cells and an increased proportion of parabasal (immature epithelial) cells is common (see Chapter 13).

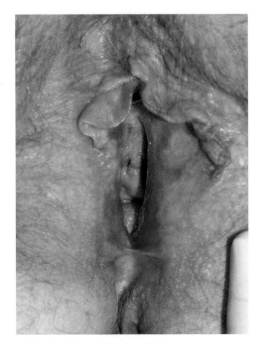

FIG. 6-41. Erosive lichen planus of mucous membranes often exhibits accompanying atrophic red plaques.

Diagnosis

The diagnosis of lichen planus is made on the basis of clinical morphology and is confirmed either by finding pathognomonic white, reticular or fernlike papules on mucous membranes or modified mucous membranes, or by characteristic histology on biopsy. A biopsy of papular lichen planus shows thickening of the epidermis in a regular, saw-toothed pattern. In addition, there is prominence of the granular cell layer and an absence of parakeratosis. A bandlike mononuclear infiltrate present in the upper epidermis tightly hugs the dermal–epidermal junction and produces some areas of vacuolar degeneration of the basal cell layer. Scattered within the epidermis are individual dyskeratotic keratinocytes.

Papular lichen planus of the glans penis can be indistinguishable from Bowen disease (erythroplasia of Queyrat), psoriasis, and candidiasis. Papular lichen planus of the vulva should be differentiated from flat warts and VIN (squamous cell carcinoma in situ). The white and eroded patches and plaques on the modified mucous membranes of the vulva or the uncircumcised glans can be mistaken for pemphigus vulgaris, cicatricial pemphigoid, herpes simplex virus infection, or candidiasis.

PAPULAR LICHEN PLANUS: **Diagnosis**

- Presence of well-demarcated, dusky, flat-topped papules on keratinized skin of the vulva and anogenital area or on the circumcised glans penis; atrophic red patches on the mucous membranes skin of the vulva and the uncircumcised glans
- Oral typically white, lacy lichen planus is common
- Biopsy that shows acanthosis in a regular, saw-toothed pattern with prominent granular cell layer with no parakeratosis; a thinned and flattened epithelium occurs with atrophic mucous membrane lichen planus. A bandlike mononuclear infiltrate in the upper epidermis abuts and disrupts the basal layer

---

Pathophysiology

Lichen planus is believed to be a disease of cell-mediated autoimmunity. In addition to data suggesting this origin, the histologic findings of lichen planus are similar to those of graft versus host disease. Also, lichen planus responds to immunosuppressant medications.

Management

Generally, papular lichen planus is self-limited, and resolution usually occurs within several years, unlike the chronic course of erosive disease. Papular lichen planus on keratinized skin is usually adequately treated with a topical corticosteroid. However, the lesions usually do not resolve but only fade somewhat and itch less. Unfortunately, a rather high-potency preparation is required, and spread of this medication to the surrounding inner thighs and crural crease is likely to produce atrophy.

Other therapies include a short burst of oral prednisone at 40 to 60 mg/day, oral retinoids, and oral hydroxychloroquine. Careful attention to the vagina is imperative, since erosive disease can occur and eventuate in permanent obliteration of the vaginal space. Vaginal lichen planus is discussed in Chapter 15. Management of lichen planus is discussed in detail in Chapters 8 and 6.

PAPULAR LICHEN PLANUS:	**Management**

- Topical corticosteroids (clobetasol 0.05% b.i.d.) tapering frequency when possible
- Chronic or intermittent therapy often needed because of frequent recurrences

PITYRIASIS ROSEA

This is a very common skin disease, which does not preferentially affect the genital skin, but typically involves the trunk, where it often extends to the bathing trunk area. Adolescents and young adults are most often affected. Sometimes pruritic, pityriasis rosea is typically characterized by 0.5- to 1.5-cm, oval, pink papules with subtle scale. These papules are usually aligned with the long axis of the oval lesion lying along skin lines. Often, several lesions will demonstrate a collarette of scale (Figs. 6-42 and 6-43). Most often, one initial, larger (and sometimes round rather than oval) lesion, the herald patch, is noted by the patient.

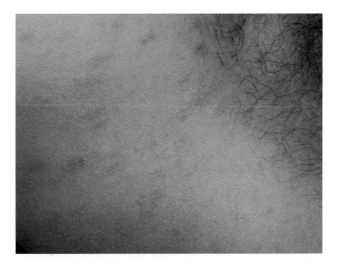

FIG. 6-42. Pink, finely scaling, oval papules are characteristic of pityriasis rosea; a collarette is a classic finding but is often absent.

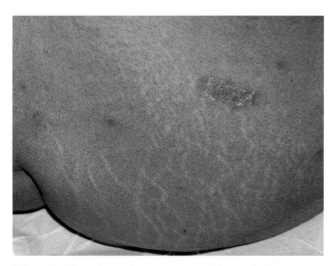

FIG. 6-43. Like other inflammatory conditions, pityriasis rosea appears more brown-red in patients of color; the oval shape and collarette are again distinctive.

The cause of pityriasis rosea is unknown, but many believe it is a reaction to a mild viral infection. There is no treatment, but topical corticosteroids are useful for reducing itching. Exposure to sunlight may shorten the course, which is usually 1 to 2 months. Pityriasis rosea is self-limited but can recur.

PITYRIASIS (TINEA) VERSICOLOR

Although called *tinea versicolor* in the past, this fungus infection is not produced by a dermatophyte (tinea), but rather by a yeast form. Pityriasis versicolor does not often affect the genital skin, but sometimes extends from its usual location from the upper trunk to the lower trunk and keratinized genital skin. More common in teenagers and young adults, pityriasis versicolor is usually asymptomatic. Lesions are pink, tan, or hypopigmented, hence the name "versicolor." Individual papules are well demarcated and usually affect the upper chest and back most prominently, with coalescence of 2 to 10 mm papules into larger plaques (Figs. 6-44 and 6-45). Although the surface is lightly scaling, this scaling is so subtle that the skin surface must be scratched to raise visible scale.

The cause of pityriasis versicolor is *Malassezia furfur*, an organism that is ubiquitous. This infection is not generally spread from person to person, but rather contracted from the environment by a host whose immune system does not mount an adequate defense. These are not patients with clinically significant immune suppression, but treatment of pityriasis versicolor is regularly followed by recurrence.

Therapy consists of any topical azole, including clotrimazole, miconazole, or econazole once or twice daily; ketoconazole 200 mg daily for 5 days for more extensive disease is effective. Either regular use of an azole cream to prevent recurrence or the prompt institution of therapy with new lesions is usual therapy.

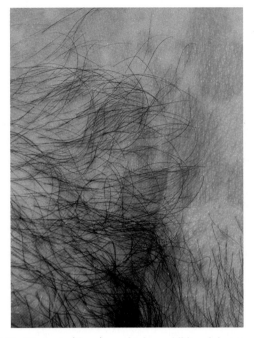

FIG. 6-44. Pityriasis (tinea) versicolor exhibits pink, tan, or hypopigmented, well-demarcated, coalescing, very finely scaling papules that incidentally involve the keratinized skin of the bathing trunk area.

PLASMA CELL MUCOSITIS (PLASMA CELL VULVITIS AND BALANITIS, ZOON MUCOSITIS, VULVITIS, AND BALANITIS CIRCUMSCRIPTA PLASMACELLULARIS)

This is a rare, poorly understood disease of anogenital skin and, probably less often, oral mucosa that is defined by its morphologic appearance and histology.

Clinical Presentation

The prevalence of plasma cell mucositis is not known, but is low. This disease is found at all postpubertal ages, and there seems to be no racial predilection. Plasma cell mucositis has been reported more often in men than in women. Although believed to be rare, it is probably more common than realized. For example, few women with plasma cell mucositis have been reported. However, this author has treated over 20 women with this condition in the past 10 years in her solo practice and observed the development of plasma cell vulvitis in existing patients.

Plasma cell mucositis presents as a glistening deep red to rusty red, well-demarcated, usually solitary plaque that is easily eroded and may bleed (Figs. 6-46 through 6-48). This is generally stable, without spontaneously waxing, waning, or migrating to other areas. When occurring on the glans, it is seen only in uncircumcised men. Lesions of plasma cell mucositis have no obvious scale, and they may be characterized by itching, soreness, or burning, but they are often asymptomatic. This condition is not related to any other skin or systemic disease.

Diagnosis

The diagnosis of plasma cell mucositis is made by the presence of the typical deep red, well-demarcated color change and histologic confirmation. A biopsy is required to rule out other red patches and erosions. A biopsy is characterized by a thinned and flattened epidermis composed of keratinocytes that are diamond shaped,

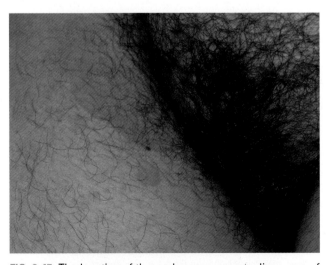

FIG. 6-45. The location of these plaques suggests diagnoses of tinea cruris or erythrasma, and the color is consistent with both erythrasma and pityriasis versicolor; a fungal preparation provides the correct diagnosis of pityriasis versicolor.

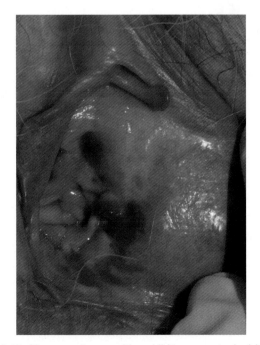

FIG. 6-46. Plasma cell mucositis exhibits a very typical lesion that is deep red, glistening, and well demarcated.

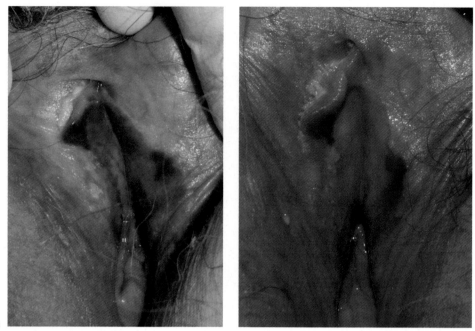

FIG. 6-47a&b. Deep redness of plasma cell mucositis is improved and less symptomatic, although not clear, following treatment with clobetasol ointment twice daily for 6 weeks.

A

B

sometimes necrotic, and separated by intercellular edema. There is an upper dermal infiltrate of plasma cells (17,18).

Any red, well-demarcated plaque should be considered, including lichen planus, psoriasis on moist skin, candidiasis, and VIN or PIN (squamous cell carcinoma in situ).

PLASMA CELL MUCOSITIS (ZOON BALANITIS/VULVITIS):	Diagnosis

- Presence of well-demarcated deep red or rusty red patches on mucous membranes or modified mucous membranes
- Confirmed on biopsy, which shows a dense upper dermal infiltrate of plasma cells under a thinned and flattened epidermis composed of keratinocytes that are diamond shaped, sometimes necrotic, and separated by intercellular edema

Pathophysiology

The cause of plasma cell mucositis is unknown, and some do not believe that this represents a specific entity, but rather a nonspecific inflammatory reactive pattern. However, plasma cell mucositis is a useful term to indicate this very characteristic presentation.

Some have postulated an association with lichen planus and, anecdotally, two women with vulvar lichen planus treated successfully by this author later developed plasma cell mucositis.

Management

There is no satisfactory therapy, and there are no studies that evaluate therapies. Circumcision is the overwhelming treatment of choice for plasma cell balanitis in uncircumcised men. Anecdotal reports have shown potent topical steroids to be useful, and intralesional corticosteroids sometimes clear lesions (19). Imiquimod and the calcineurin inhibitors tacrolimus ointment and pimecrolimus cream have been reported to be variably useful (20–22). Carbon dioxide laser has been used by some

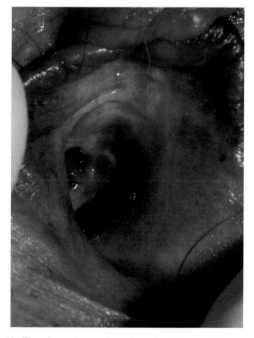

FIG. 6-48. The deep purpuric color of plasma cell mucositis is correlated by the red cells noted on a typical biopsy.

(23), and there is one report of success with erbium: YAG laser ablation. A compounded topical therapy consisting of clobetasol, oxytetracycline, and nystatin has been found useful by some, but there is no supporting data (personal communication, Lynne Margesson, MD). There is one case of Zoon balanitis and penile intraepithelial neoplasia, so surveillance is suggested (24).

PLASMA CELL MUCOSITIS: **Management**

- Topical corticosteroids (clobetasol 0.05% b.i.d., tapering frequency when possible). Alternatively, intralesional triamcinolone 3 to 5 mg/cc, small amounts injected into the underlying dermis
- Other, less well-described therapies include CO_2 laser, imiquimod

---

VESTIBULODYNIA (VULVAR VESTIBULITIS SYNDROME, VESTIBULAR ADENITIS)

Vestibulodynia is a localized pain syndrome, which is primarily discussed in Chapter 5. This condition is defined as sensations of pain, including burning, stinging, rawness, soreness, irritation, tearing, aching—itching is generally absent or a minor symptom—in the absence of objective relevant physical findings and laboratory abnormalities. However, most patients describe redness and swelling. These are abnormalities that are difficult to gauge in a setting of an area that normally shows variable degrees of redness and puffiness.

The classic finding in vestibulodynia is redness of some of the ostia of vestibular glands located adjacent to the external aspect of the hymeneal caruncles (Fig. 6-49).

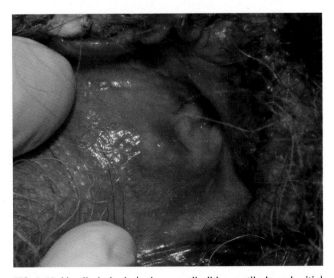

FIG. 6-49. Vestibulodynia (vulvar vestibulitis, vestibular adenitis) often exhibits redness of the vestibular gland ostia, but this can be a normal finding as well.

On biopsy, however, the mild chronic nonspecific inflammation is the same as that found in the normal, nonpainful vestibule.

The diagnosis of this syndrome is one of exclusion, with correction of any infection, estrogen deficiency, cutaneous abnormalities, and specific neuropathic syndromes such as postherpetic neuralgia. Then, treatment consists of oral medication for neuropathic pain, pelvic floor physical therapy for the usually occurring pelvic muscle dysfunction, and attention to psychologic aspects including anxiety, depression, and sexual dysfunction. The last therapy, also the most effective when performed in a setting of adequate oral medication and physical therapy, is the surgical removal of affected skin, when the pain is absolutely localized to the vestibule.

RED SCROTUM SYNDROME

Red scrotum syndrome (discussed primarily in Chapter 5) is one name for the sensation of scrotal burning or rawness in the absence of objective skin disease other than variable degrees of erythema. This is a condition in which the patient describes burning and redness, which is often not visible to the examiner or which is within the range of normal (Fig. 6-50).

The syndrome being likely analogous to vestibulodynia, some clinicians believe that it is especially influenced by anxiety and depression and may be primarily a

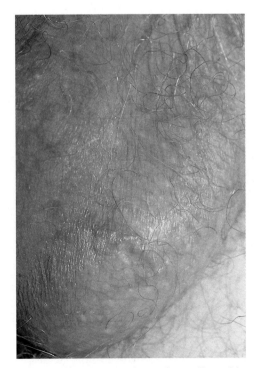

FIG. 6-50. The red scrotum syndrome is manifested by sensations of burning or rawness, with physical findings limited to redness of variable degrees, which includes the normal range of redness.

manifestation of sexual dysfunction. This author believes that there is an enormous range of dysfunction in these men, with some responding promptly to oral therapy for neuropathy and others either unwilling to accept this diagnosis and therapy or unresponsive to treatment.

EXTRAMAMMARY PAGET DISEASE

Paget disease is an uncommon malignancy occurring on genital or breast skin. Although its appearance on the breast is always indicative of underlying breast carcinoma, extramammary Paget disease can be primary or associated with underlying carcinoma of urothelial origin (24).

Clinical Presentation

Extramammary Paget disease presents most often in people over 50 years of age and much more often in women than in men. Pruritus is the most common initial symptom, occurring in most patients. Pain and exudation are less common complaints. Generally, there is an indolent history rather than one of rapid growth or change and a history of poor response to topical corticosteroids.

The most common location for extramammary Paget disease is on the vulva, both the keratinized skin and modified mucous membrane surfaces, as well as the perianal skin. Less common are the perineum, scrotum, mons, and penis. Extramammary Paget disease presents as a well-demarcated red plaque with a scaling or moist surface, often with islands of whitened epithelium (Figs. 6-51 through 6-53). Erosions are common as well, and occasionally plaques exhibit hyperpigmentation.

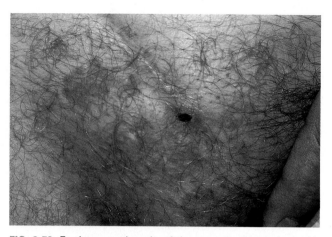

FIG. 6-52. Erythema and scale of the mons in this patient with extramammary Paget disease can be nearly indistinguishable from the lesions of psoriasis or lichen simplex chronicus.

Ten to twenty percent of patients exhibit an underlying genitourinary or gastrointestinal malignancy on specific evaluations. Much less commonly, breast carcinoma is associated.

Diagnosis

The diagnosis of Paget disease is made by clinical suspicion and is confirmed on biopsy. Most patients experience delayed diagnosis because the appearance mimics several benign skin diseases. A skin biopsy of Paget disease shows an epidermis with scattered large clear cells that exhibit nuclear atypia. These cells are often seen in

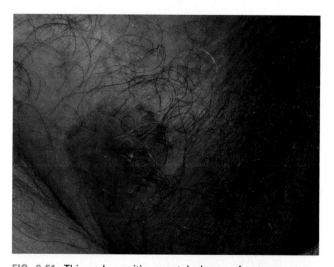

FIG. 6-51. This red, pruritic, scrotal plaque of extramammary Paget disease shows superficial white hyperkeratosis and erosions that would be consistent with the much more common lichen simplex chronicus, but the well-demarcated borders and poor response to topical corticosteroids suggested the correct diagnosis.

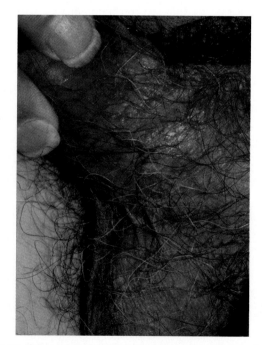

FIG. 6-53. This moist, red, fissured plaque of the proximal penis is characteristic of extramammary Paget disease, but a biopsy is required to differentiate this from other red, scaling plaques.

hair follicles and sweat gland ducts. Often, there is an underlying chronic inflammatory infiltrate.

Paget disease closely resembles Bowen disease (VIN, squamous cell carcinoma in situ) psoriasis, or eczema, including lichen simplex chronicus, atopic dermatitis and irritant, or allergic contact dermatitis. Paget disease also can exhibit similar morphology to tinea cruris, and pigmented disease can mimic superficial spreading melanoma.

EXTRAMAMMARY PAGET DISEASE: **Diagnosis**

- Red plaques with rough surface, often with erosions or white, thickened islands; most often on keratinized genital epithelium
- Biopsy is primary diagnostic tool, which shows an epidermis with scattered large clear cells that exhibit nuclear atypia. These cells are often seen in hair follicles and sweat gland ducts. Often, there is an underlying chronic inflammatory infiltrate

---

Pathophysiology

Extramammary Paget disease is a malignancy whose cause is controversial. The etiology likely differs between the primary and secondary forms. The primary form appears to arise from the epidermis; the cell being of sweat gland origin or from Toker cells (25). Toker cells are epidermal cells that share characteristics with Paget cells; both stain for mucin and positive for CK 7 (26,27). Toker cells also share the same distribution as apocrine glands; the breasts, milk line, and anogenital skin. Secondary extramammary Paget disease arises from cells that migrate from the underlying adenocarcinoma (28). There are no known precipitating causes for Paget disease other than the underlying adenocarcinoma of secondary Paget disease.

Management

The primary treatment of Paget disease consists of excision. This allows not only for removal of the tumor, but for evaluation of the entire lesion for dermal invasion; those patients with <1mm of invasion rarely die of their disease or experience metastasis. Histology showing greater than 1 mm of dermal invasion justifies lymph node evaluation. Local recurrences are usual and expected for both invasive and in situ Paget disease, even with substantial margins or Mohs surgery. These recurrences, again, can be treated with conservative surgical excision. Alternatively, laser surgery and radiation therapy have also been used, and several case reports suggest that topical fluorouracil may be beneficial. Imiquimod applied topically has been reported to be useful (29).

Extramammary Paget disease extending more than 1 mm into the dermis can be rapidly progressive and metastasize. The prognosis of disease associated with underlying adenocarcinomas is also dependent upon the state of this related malignancy. Patients should undergo screening evaluation for genitourinary carcinoma or a gastrointestinal malignancy because these can certainly cause death if they are not detected and treated adequately. Immunohistochemical investigations can help to differentiate between primary and secondary Paget disease.

EXTRAMAMMARY PAGET DISEASE: **Management**

- Excision
- Laser ablation
- Reports of imiquimod topically

INTRAEPITHELIAL NEOPLASIA (BOWEN DISEASE, SQUAMOUS CELL CARCINOMA IN SITU, AND ERYTHROPLASIA OF QUEYRAT)

Intraepithelial neoplasia is the proper term for noninvasive full-thickness dysplasia of the epidermis. Intraepithelial neoplasia has many different morphologic appearances, and Bowen disease refers to the morphologic variant of one or a few red plaques. This condition is discussed in more detail in Chapters 11 and 12.

Clinical Presentation

Although squamous intraepithelial neoplasia is often associated with human papillomavirus (HPV) infection, that form is most often manifested by multiple small, skin-colored, red, or white papules in younger patients. When presenting as larger plaques, Bowen disease is seen in an older age group. This well-demarcated plaque is often solitary, with a scaling, hyperkeratotic, or exudative surface (Figs. 6-54 through 6-56). Occasionally, hyperpigmentation

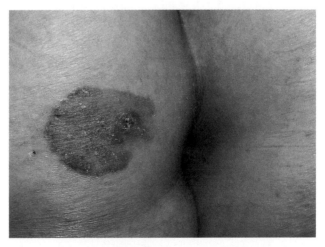

FIG. 6-54. Intraepithelial neoplasia, often called Bowen disease when occurring on dry, keratinized skin, is characterized by well-demarcated erythema and scale similar to the lesions of psoriasis, tinea, or eczema.

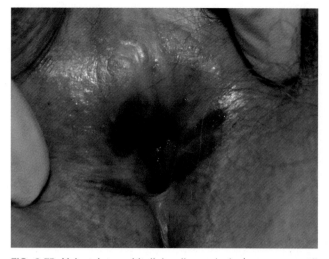

FIG. 6-55. Vulvar intraepithelial cell neoplasia (squamous cell carcinoma in situ) of the mucous membranes of the vulva consist of red, glistening papules and plaques that mimic lichen planus and plasma cell mucositis

can occur, suggesting a diagnosis of melanoma. The perianal area, perineum, glans penis (in which this condition is called erythroplasia of Queyrat), and vulva are common areas.

Diagnosis

Bowen disease is diagnosed on clinical suspicion and is confirmed by skin biopsy. A skin biopsy of Bowen disease shows full-thickness dysplasia of the epithelium, but there

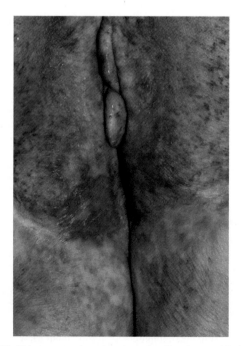

FIG. 6-56. This woman has developed vulvar intraepithelial cell neoplasia on the basis of lichen sclerosus and past radiation for uterine carcinoma.

is no invasion of these cells through the basement membrane into the dermis, as occurs in invasive squamous cell carcinoma.

Bowen disease can be difficult to distinguish from Paget disease and contact dermatitis. Psoriasis, lichen simplex chronicus, tinea cruris, and candidiasis are usually more widespread and exhibit symmetric patterns.

INTRAEPITHELIAL NEOPLASIA (VIN, PIN, AIN) BOWEN MORPHOLOGY:	Diagnosis

- Well-demarcated red plaques, scaling on keratinized skin
- Biopsy is primary diagnostic tool, which shows full-thickness squamous dysplasia without invasion into the dermis

Pathophysiology

Bowen disease (vulvar intraepithelial neoplasia, penile intraepithelial neoplasia, anal intraepithelial neoplasia) is a low-grade squamous cell carcinoma. Although VIN, PIN, and AIN often are associated with HPV infection and chronic dermatoses such as lichen sclerosus and lichen planus, the morphologic form of intraepithelial neoplasia referred to as Bowen disease often is unassociated with any of these factors. There is no known cause for this dysplasia in most patients, although chronic arsenic exposure, as from drinking contaminated well water, can result in Bowen disease. In other areas of the body, chronic sun exposure can produce Bowen disease.

Treatment

Bowen disease is treated by conservative surgical excision or ablation. More recently, topical imiquimod cream has shown in small series to sometimes clear Bowen disease.

INTRAEPITHELIAL NEOPLASIA (VIN, PIN, AIN) BOWEN MORPHOLOGY:	Management

- Excision
- Laser ablation
- Topical imiquimod

REFERENCES

1. Reitamo S, Rustin M, Ruzicka T, et al. Efficacy and safety of tacrolimus ointment compared with that of hydrocortisone butyrate ointment in adult patients with atopic dermatitis. *J Allergy Clin Immunol.* 2002;109:547–555.

2. Ho VC, Gupta A, Kaufmann R, et al. Safety and efficacy of nonsteroid pimecrolimus cream 1% in the treatment of atopic dermatitis in infants. *J Pediatr.* 2003;142:155–162.

3. Abeck D, Mempel M. *Staphylococcus aureus* colonization in atopic dermatitis and its therapeutic implications. *Br J Dermatol.* 1998;139(suppl 53):13–16.

4. Farage MA. Vulvar susceptibility to contact irritants and allergens: a review. *Arch Gynecol Obstet.* 2005;272:167–172.

5. Haverhoek E, Reid C, Gordon L, et al. Prospective study of patch testing in patients with vulval pruritus. *Australas J Dermatol.* 2008;49:80–85.

6. Thomas DS, Ingham E, Bojar RA, et al. In vitro modulation of human keratinocyte pro- and anti-inflammatory cytokine production by the capsule of *Malassezia* species. *FEMS Immunol Med Microbiol.* 2008;54:203–214.

7. Prodanovich S, Kirsner RS, Kravetz JD, et al. Association of psoriasis with coronary artery, cerebrovascular, and peripheral vascular diseases and mortality. *Arch Dermatol.* 2009;145:700–703.

8. Nijstem T, Wallee M. Complexity of the association between psoriasis and comorbidities. *J Invest Dermatol.* 2009;129:1601–1603.

9. Makredes M, Robinson Jr D, Bala M, et al. The burden of autoimmune disease: a comparison of prevalence ratios in patients with psoriatic arthritis and psoriasis. *J Am Acad Dermatol.* 2009;61:405–410.

10. Smith RL, Warren RB, Griffiths CE, et al. Genetic susceptibility to psoriasis: an emerging picture. *Genome Med.* 2009;22(1):72.

11. Wolk K, Mallbris L, Larsson P, et al. Excessive body weight, and smoking associates with a high risk of onset of plaque psoriasis. *Acta Derm Venereol.* 2009;89:492–497.

12. Dediol I, Buljan M, Buljan D, et al. Association of psoriasis and alcoholism: psychodermatological issue. *Psychiatr Danub.* 2009;21:9–13.

13. Sigmon JR, Yentzer BA, Feldman SR. Calcitriol ointment: a review of a topical vitamin D analog for psoriasis. *J Dermatolog Treat.* 2009;20:208–212.

14. Saraceno R, Andreassi L, Ayala F, et al. Efficacy, safety and quality of life of calcipotriol/betamethasone dipropionate (Dovobet) versus calcipotriol (Daivonex) in the treatment of psoriasis vulgaris: a randomized, multicentre, clinical trial. *J Dermatolog Treat.* 2007;18:361–365.

15. Bissonnette R, Nigen S, Bolduc C. Efficacy and tolerability of topical tacrolimus ointment for the treatment of male genital psoriasis. *J Cutan Med Surg.* 2008;12:230–234.

16. Magin P, Adams J, Heading G, et al. The psychological sequelae of psoriasis: results of a qualitative study. *Psychol Health Med.* 2009;14:150–161.

17. Virgili A, Levratti A, Marzola A, et al. Retrospective histopathologic reevaluation of 18 cases of plasma cell vulvitis. *J Reprod Med.* 2005;50:3–7.

18. Alessi E, Coggi A, Gianotti R. Review of 120 biopsies performed on the balanopreputial sac. from Zoon's balanitis to the concept of a wider spectrum of inflammatory non-cicatricial balanoposthitis. *Dermatology.* 2004;208:120–124.

19. Tseng JT, Cheng CJ, Lee WR, et al. Plasma-cell cheilitis: successful treatment with intralesional injections of corticosteroids. *Clin Exp Dermatol.* 2009;34:174–177.

20. Frega A, Rech F, French D. Imiquimod treatment of vulvitis circumscripta plasmacellularis. *Int J Gynaecol Obstet.* 2006;95:161–162.

21. Virgili A, Mantovani L, Lauriola MM, et al. Tacrolimus 0.1% ointment: is it really effective in plasma cell vulvitis? Report of four cases. *Dermatology.* 2008;216:243–246.

22. Stinco G, Piccirillo F, Patrone P. Discordant results with pimecrolimus 1% cream in the treatment of plasma cell balanitis. *Dermatology.* 2009;218:155–158.

23. Retamar RA, Kien MC, Chouela EN. Zoon's balanitis: presentation of 15 patients, five treated with a carbon dioxide laser. *Int J Dermatol.* 2003;42:305–307.

24. Starritt E, Lee S. Erythroplasia of Queyrat of the glans penis on a background of Zoon's plasma cell balanitis. *Australas J Dermatol.* 2008;49:103–105.

25. Willman JH, Golitz LE, Fitzpatrick JE. Vulvar clear cells of Toker: precursors of extramammary Paget's disease. *Am J Dermatopathol.* 2005;27:185–188.

26. Liegl B, Leibl S, Gogg-Kamerer M, et al. Mammary and extramammary Paget's disease: an immunohistochemical study of 83 cases. *Histopathology.* 2007;50:439–447.

27. Di Tommaso L, Franchi G, Destro A, et al. Toker cells of the breast. Morphological and immunohistochemical characterization of 40 cases. *Hum Pathol.* 2008;39:1295–1300.

28. Yanai H, Takahashi N, Omori M, et al. Immunohistochemistry of p63 in primary and secondary vulvar Paget's disease. *Pathol Int.* 2008;58:648–651.

29. Mirer E, El Sayed F, Ammoury A, et al. Treatment of mammary and extramammary Paget's skin disease with topical imiquimod. *J Dermatolog Treat.* 2006;17:167–171.

SUGGESTED READINGS

Brix WK, Nassau SR, Patterson JW, et al. Idiopathic Lymphoplasmacellular mucositis-dermatitis. *J Cutan Pathol.* 2009. [Epub ahead of print].

Gupta AK, Cooper EA. Update in antifungal therapy of dermatophytosis. *Mycopathologia.* 2008;166:353–367.

Kalb RE, Bagel J, Korman NJ, et al. National Psoriasis Foundation. Treatment of intertriginous psoriasis: from the Medical Board of the National Psoriasis Foundation. *J Am Acad Dermatol.* 2009;60:120–124.

Margesson LJ. Contact dermatitis of the vulva. *Dermatol Ther.* 2004;17:20–27.

Menter A, Korman NJ, Elmets CA, et al. American Academy of Dermatology. Guidelines of care for the management of psoriasis and psoriatic arthritis. Section 3. Guidelines of care for the management and treatment of psoriasis with topical therapies. *J Am Acad Dermatol.* 2009;60:643–659.

Red Papules and Nodules

PETER J. LYNCH

Genital disorders that present as red papules or nodules are most often either neoplasms or inflammatory lesions. Vascular neoplasms present as bright red, dusky red, or violaceous papules and nodules with sharply demarcated borders. Nonvascular neoplasms are also sharply marginated but tend to be lighter red in color. Inflammatory papules and nodules are most often medium to dark red toward the center and fade to light red or pink at their less distinctly marginated borders. Most of the lesions considered in this chapter lack scale and therefore are smooth surfaced. Many skin-colored papules and nodules appear pink or red at times because of secondary inflammation or increased vascularity. This is particularly notable in patients with a light complexion. Therefore, when encountering pink or red papules or nodules, the clinician may also need to consider lesions from Chapter 12. The lesions in the first part of this chapter represent the smaller lesions (the red papules) and those in latter part represent the larger lesions (the red nodules). Note, however, that this is not a hard and fast distinction since some of the conditions discussed may present with a mixture of papules and nodules.

FOLLICULITIS

Both bacterial and dermatophyte fungal folliculitis can present as small red papules. (Figs. 7-1 and 7-2). Generally, multiple, often clustered, lesions are present. At least a few of these lesions will have a white or yellow-white pustule at the summit. This distinguishing feature, followed by appropriate culture, allows for establishment of the correct diagnosis. The primary discussion of these conditions can be found in Chapter 8, The Purulent and Pustular Disorders.

KERATOSIS PILARIS

Clinical Presentation

Keratosis pilaris (KP) is a noninfectious form of folliculitis. It is a very common condition with a prevalence of about 10% in children and 2 or 3% in adults (1). The prevalence of KP gradually decreases with age and it is not often seen after the fourth decade. The clinical appearance is that of minute (1 to 2 mm) closely set, clustered papules. Some, but not all of the papules will have a small hair emerging from the summit of the papule. All of the lesions are approximately the same size and are equidistant from one another (Fig. 7-3). This lends a monomorphic appearance to the process.

In those individuals with the least severe involvement the papules may be skin-colored or pink, but in most patients, both the papules and a narrow halo around them are distinctly red. A few of the larger lesions may be capped by a firm, solid, white summit (pseudopustule) consisting of compacted keratin retained in the follicular orifice. If this solid white "ball" of keratin is scraped away, it sometime contains a fine, rolled-up hair within it. The most commonly involved sites are the upper arms, thighs, and buttocks. There is a sandpaper-like, slightly rough, feel when the fingertips are lightly passed over clustered lesions of KP. KP is usually asymptomatic though mild pruritus is sometimes present.

Diagnosis

KP is diagnosed on a clinical basis. The key features include (i) a large number of closely set homogeneous papules, (ii) location on lateral, upper arms, thighs, and buttocks, (iii) long duration with little or no change in clinical appearance, and (iv) failure to respond to antibiotic therapy.

KERATOSIS PILARIS:	Diagnosis

- Clustered, small (1 to 2 mm) red papules
- Hairs emerging from the summit of some papules
- Location on the arms, thighs, and/or buttocks
- Rough, sandpaper-like feel on palpation
- Failure to respond to antibiotics

Pathophysiology

KP is caused by excess keratinization (keratin plugging) of the outermost portion of hair follicles. The cause of this accumulation of keratin is unknown but it is likely related to an abnormality of keratinocyte differentiation since KP occurs primarily in those with ichthyosis vulgaris and atopic dermatitis, two conditions that are

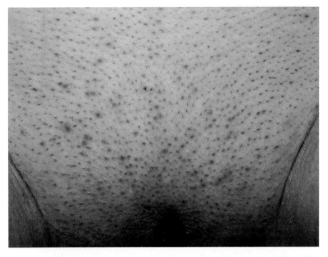

FIG. 7-1. Shaving is a very common cause of bacterial folliculitis and is manifested by follicular papules, small crusts, and occasional pustules in the area recently shaved.

almost always associated with keratinocyte differentiation abnormalities secondary to mutations in the filaggrin gene.

Management

No therapy is necessary. This is fortunate as no treatment is very effective. Patients who are bothered by the appearance or the pruritus may periodically undertake a

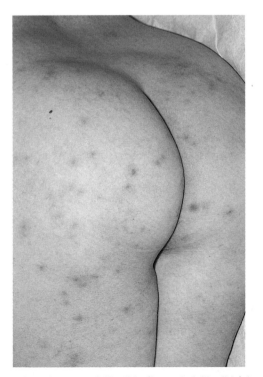

FIG. 7-2. Pseudomonas folliculitis (hot tub folliculitis) is seen preferentially in the genital area, where swimsuits hold contaminated water next to the skin. The individual lesions are tender, pink, follicular papules.

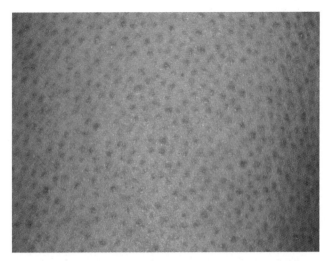

FIG. 7-3. Keratosis pilaris exhibits monomorphous, follicular papules with a keratotic plug that gives the skin a sandpapery texture; although sometimes skin-colored, many patients exhibit erythema as seen on the buttocks of this patient. This patient also had typical keratosis pilaris on the lateral, upper arms.

prolonged bathtub soak followed by the use of light abrasion with a loofah sponge or soft brush. Lubrication, especially with products containing humectants such as urea or alpha hydroxy acids, improves the textural feel of the skin. Topical retinoids, while theoretically attractive as therapeutic agents, tend to increase the inflammation and thus are not routinely useful.

KERATOSIS PILARIS:	Management

- 20-minute bathtub soak
- Light scrubbing with a soft brush or loofah
- Application of a moisturizer after soak and scrub
- Cautious trial of topical tretinoin

NODULAR SCABIES

The primary discussion of scabies can be found in Chapter 14. Only the nodular form of the infestation will be considered here. Nodular scabies occurs as a hypersensitivity reaction to mite proteins. It occurs weeks or months after the initial lesions of scabies are first noted and often develops after successful treatment of more generalized disease. The lesions contain no live organisms and thus are not a cause of transmission to others.

Nodular scabies occurs almost solely in males. The reason for this site and gender predilection is unknown. The lesions of nodular scabies may be papules or nodules or a mixture of both. These dome-shaped, red to brown-red lesions are usually 5 to 20 mm in diameter (Figs. 7-4 and 7-5). The surface of some of the lesions may demonstrate erosions occurring as a result of excoriation. Nodular scabies

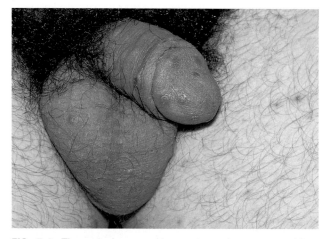

FIG. 7-4. These lesions on the penis and scrotum, with a predilection for the glans, are typical of nodular genital scabies.

has a special predilection for the glans penis, penile shaft, and scrotum but occasionally lesions are found in the pubic region, groin, buttocks, and axillae. The clinical features overlap appreciably with the lesions of prurigo nodularis. The correct diagnosis is usually established on the basis of clinical features, but when uncertainty is present, biopsy, while not usually revealing the presence of mites, ova, or feces, does demonstrate a characteristic heavy infiltrate of eosinophils.

Left untreated, the lesions of nodular scabies may persist for months but do eventually resolve spontaneously. Assuming that the patient has been successfully treated for more generalized infestation, repeated applications of scabicides are not helpful. The use of high-potency topical steroids does little to improve the situation. However, improvement in both the pruritus and appearance of the lesions can be obtained with intralesional injections of 0.2 to 0.4 mL of triamcinolone acetonide (Kenalog), 10 mg/mL, into each lesion.

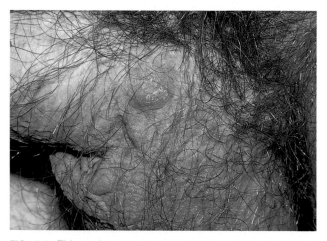

FIG. 7-5. This typical scabetic lesion on the penis is an indurated, pink, dome-shaped nodule.

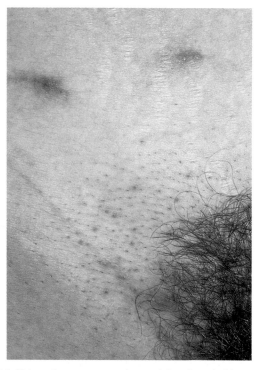

FIG. 7-6. This patient was camping and developed chigger bites, excruciatingly itchy red papules with a surrounding pink flare. In general, these are concentrated at the panty line.

MISCELLANEOUS BITES AND INFESTATIONS

Insect bites in the genital area are uncommon because this area is usually protected by clothing. However, such bites do occur in campers and hikers who expose the genital area when urinating, defecating, or having intercourse alfresco. The most common of these bites are due to chiggers. Chiggers, also called harvest mites, bite and fall off, rather than burrowing into the skin as occurs with the scabies mite. In nonsensitized people, chigger bites are tiny red papules that are minimally symptomatic and resolve quickly. However, those patients who are allergic to chigger proteins develop extremely pruritic, pink, nonscaling, dome-shaped 0.5- to 1.5-cm papules, occasionally with a central vesicle (2) (Fig. 7-6). Such bites are particularly likely to occur where clothing binds against the skin such as at waistbands. Lesions due to chigger bites resolve spontaneously in about 2 weeks. Oral antihistamines and topical steroids provide some symptomatic improvement. The best approach is to avoid the possibility of chigger bites through the use of standard insect repellents.

Lesions due to other biting insects (Fig. 7-7) also appear as pruritic red papules. While there is nothing that clinically identifies which insect is responsible, the likelihood that a given red papule is due to some type of insect bite can be ascertained by the presence of numerous eosinophils within the inflammatory infiltrate in a biopsy specimen.

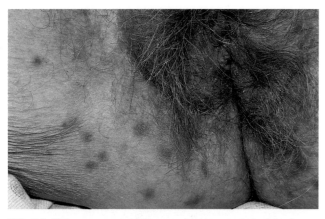

FIG. 7-7. This woman exhibits poorly demarcated pink, dome-shaped papules of insect bites on buttocks and medial thighs.

CHERRY ANGIOMA

Cherry angiomas (Campbell de Morgan spots) represent a benign neoplasm of clustered capillary blood vessels. They first appear in young adult life and generally increase with age. These angiomas occur as sharply marginated dome-shaped papules that are bright red, dusky red, or even violaceous in color (Fig. 7-8). They vary in size from nearly flat, pinpoint lesions to 3- to 6-mm papules. The majority of light-skinned persons will have developed at least one by age 40 and the average adult has 30 to 50 scattered lesions. Cherry angiomas are most commonly found on the trunk and proximal extremities but occasionally are also noted on the pubis and genitalia.

The cause of cherry angiomas is not known though the frequency of familial development suggests a genetic predisposition. The diagnosis is made on a clinical basis. The differential diagnosis is that of angiokeratomas. Since both are asymptomatic and benign it is not really necessary to differentiate these lesions. No treatment is necessary.

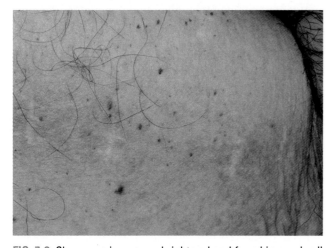

FIG. 7-8. Cherry angiomas are bright-red and found in nearly all white people on the trunk by age 40; the tendency to have large numbers, as seen in this patient, is inherited.

Lesions that bleed frequently with trauma may be excised or may be destroyed with electrosurgery or laser ablation.

ANGIOKERATOMA

Angiokeratomas represent clusters of ectatic superficial cutaneous blood vessels. These asymptomatic papules are sometimes given the eponymous epithet of Fordyce but should not be confused with Fordyce spots referring to prominent sebaceous glands on the lip or genitalia.

Angiokeratomas are sufficiently common to be considered as a normal variant rather than a disease. The prevalence is not known, but based on our experience they develop in early adulthood in about 10% of men but less that 1% of women. In men they appear as 1- to 2-mm red, smooth-surfaced, dome-shaped papules occurring primarily on the scrotum and, rarely, on the penile shaft (Fig. 7-9). Sometimes they are lined up as minute ("beads on a string") outpouchings along a linear telangiectatic vessel. Generally 10 to 30 papules are present. In women, the lesions are found on the labia majora where they are fewer in number (often solitary), larger in size (3 to 8 mm), and darker in color (dusky red, violaceous, or blue) (Fig. 7-10). In both sexes, they are asymptomatic.

The diagnosis is made on a clinical basis. In men they may resemble benign cherry angiomas (Campbell de Morgan spots). The angiokeratomas found in the extremely rare condition, angiokeratoma corporis diffusum (Anderson–Fabry disease), are similar in appearance but in this life-threatening systemic disorder they are more numerous and occur throughout the lower

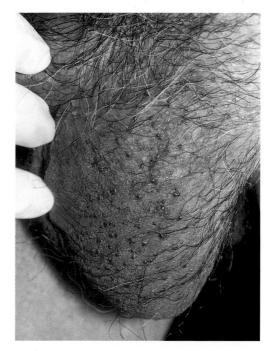

FIG. 7-9. Some patients exhibit large numbers of angiokeratomas, such as these tiny dark purple scrotal lesions.

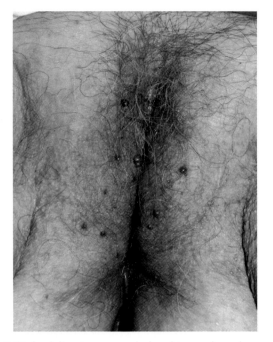

FIG. 7-10. Angiokeratomas are dark red to purple and occur on both the modified mucous membranes of the vulva and hair-bearing skin.

trunk and upper thighs. In women, darker lesions may be confused with nevi or even melanoma. Histologically, clustered, dilated vessels are noted in the upper dermis. The overlying epidermis is slightly thickened and elongated rete ridges usually extend into the dermis around the vessels, sometimes entirely encircling them. The cause of these lesions is unknown. However, based on their frequent occurrence along a dilated vessel in men, it is possible that they develop as saccular varices in aging, weak-walled capillaries.

PRURIGO NODULARIS (PICKER'S NODULE)

Clinical Presentation

Prurigo nodules occur in patients who chronically pick or scratch at a small area of skin. This produces a callus-like reaction as the epithelial cells proliferate and produce increased amounts of keratin in response to chronic trauma (3). Individual lesions are 0.5- to 1.5-cm pink, red, or brown-red papules usually with overlying excoriation (Figs. 7-11 and 7-12). The surface is palpably rough due to the presence of compacted scale. Generally no primary lesions are seen, but occasionally a coexisting underlying problem such as folliculitis is present and serves as a focus for the initial scratching. Prurigo nodules may occur anywhere on the body but are fairly common on the labia majora in women, on the scrotum in men, and in the pubic area in both sexes. Picking may start as a result of pruritus, but habitual picking, often at

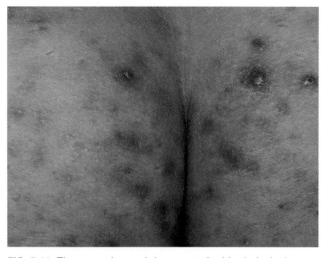

FIG. 7-11. These prurigo nodules are typical in their dusky erythema and superficial erosion from picking.

the subconscious level, plays the major role in the perpetuation of these lesions.

Diagnosis

The diagnosis is made by the clinical appearance and history of scratching or picking. If biopsy is carried out, the histological features are those of epidermal hyperkeratosis with acanthosis and irregular downward proliferation of the rete ridges. Secondary nonspecific inflammation is present and there is usually a proliferation of nerve endings. Nodular scabies, particularly in males, and pseudowarts are the main conditions to be considered in differential diagnosis.

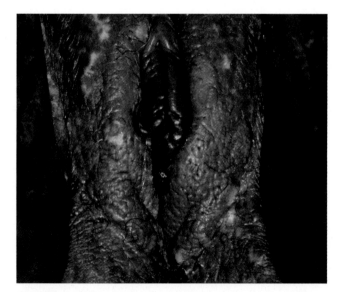

FIG. 7-12. Patients of color with prurigo nodules are less likely to show redness; however, these irregularly eroded nodules in a background of thickened lichen simplex chronicus and scarring are typical of this diagnosis.

PRURIGO NODULARIS: **Diagnosis**

- Excoriated, rough-surfaced papules or nodules
- History of habitual scratching or picking
- In some patients there is a belief that "something is in the skin and must be removed"
- Confirmation by biopsy, if necessary

Pathophysiology

These nodules arise as a protective, callus-like response of the epithelial cells to the chronic trauma of picking, scratching, and rubbing. The process is analogous to that occurring with the itch–scratch cycle that results in lichenification (see Chapter 4) but is restricted to a much smaller area of skin. Some degree of psychological dysfunction is regularly present. The intensity and repetitiveness of the picking has many features of an obsessive–compulsive disorder.

Management

Treatment consists of the identification and elimination of any underlying pruritic condition such as folliculitis that initiates the picking. Patients with anxiety or depression, a common occurrence, should have these psychological issues addressed. Individual lesions can be treated fairly effectively by intralesional injections of 0.2 to 0.5 mL of triamcinolone acetonide 10 mg/mL. A light freeze with liquid nitrogen may help temporarily because cold temperatures selectively destroy nerve endings before causing other types of tissue damage. High-potency topical steroid therapy is usually prescribed but, used alone, this approach is rarely of help. Nighttime sedation with a tricyclic medication such as doxepin or amitriptyline can minimize scratching during sleep. An orally administered selective serotonin reuptake inhibitor (SSRI), used in doses recommended for the treatment of obsessive–compulsive disease, can be very helpful. In the most severe cases, use of one of the atypical antipsychotic agents may be worth trying. Additional approaches to help break up the itch–scratch cycle are covered in Chapter 4.

PRURIGO NODULARIS: **Management**

- Intralesional steroid injection, triamcinolone 10 mg/mL, 0.2 to 0.5 mL each lesion
- Trial of light, liquid nitrogen therapy
- Hydroxyzine or doxepin, 25 mg 2 hours before bedtime. Increase weekly to 75 mg, if necessary
- SSRI, such as citalopram, if daytime therapy is necessary

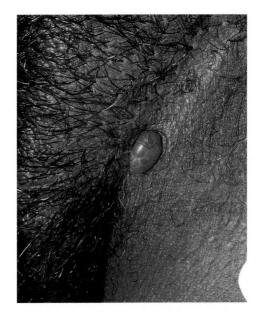

FIG. 7-13. Sometimes called the tumor of pregnancy, pyogenic granuloma presents as a pedunculated, red, glistening nodule.

PYOGENIC GRANULOMA

This reactive neoplasm is most commonly encountered in children and pregnant women. The genitalia are not a usual site of predilection but there have been a few reported cases involving these areas (4) (Figs. 7-13 and 7-14). Clinically, pyogenic granuloma presents as a red papule or small nodule that is often slightly pedunculated ("pinched in" at the base). Because the surface epithelium of these lesions is markedly thinned, a glistening surface that bleeds easily following minimal trauma is often noted. The diagnosis is generally apparent on clinical examination but many of the lesions discussed in this chapter should be considered in the list of differential diagnoses. Importantly, amelanotic melanoma can closely mimic the appearance of

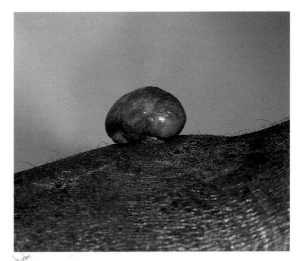

FIG. 7-14. This pyogenic granuloma has occurred on a thigh in a background of unrelated lichenification from rubbing.

pyogenic granuloma. For this reason histologic confirmation of a clinical diagnosis is usually warranted.

Pyogenic granuloma is a benign reactive neoplasm. Bleeding represents the only important complication of these lesions. The cause of pyogenic granuloma is not known but in many cases they arise after trauma, perhaps developing as a result of disturbed normal reparative angiogenesis. Since these lesions occur with much increased frequency during pregnancy and in the prepubertal years of childhood, it is possible that hormonal factors play a role in pathogenesis.

The treatment of choice is shave excision at the level of the surrounding skin. This provides a specimen for histological examination. The base of the excision should be treated with electrosurgery as otherwise the recurrence rate is unacceptably high.

URETHRAL CARUNCLE

Urethral caruncle occurs in middle-aged and elderly women where it appears as a solitary red papule at the urethral meatus (Figs. 7-15 and 7-16). These caruncles are less than 1 cm in diameter and usually occur as pedunculated or dome-shaped lesions. The surface is friable and for this reason they usually come to the attention of the patient because of mild hematuria or the presence of blood on the toilet tissue after wiping. Microscopic features include vascular dilatation and an infiltration of neutrophils in a loose connective tissue stroma. The cause is unknown. Asymptomatic small lesions may be left untreated. If treatment is desirable, the lesion can be removed by shave excision at the base of the lesion. Light electrosurgery may be necessary to achieve hemostasis and prevent recurrence. The removed specimen should be submitted for histological examination to rule out other types of urethral tumors.

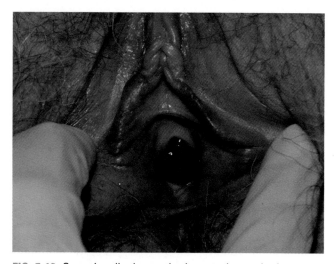

FIG. 7-16. Occasionally the urethral caruncle can be large and very red.

URETHRAL PROLAPSE

Prolapse of the urethra occurs primarily in premenarchal girls (especially those of African descent) and post-menopausal women (5). It presents as a red, edematous cuff, partially or completely, surrounding the urethral meatus (Fig. 7-17). This condition may be asymptomatic in children but in adult women dysuria and symptoms of local discomfort (especially on walking) are often present. In more severe instances with marked edema, patients may have difficulty voiding. Biopsy is rarely necessary but if carried out, the histological features are those of normal urethral epithelium with a variable amount of underlying inflammation. The cause of urethral prolapse is unknown. Rarely, it occurs as a congenital abnormality but in most instances, it seems to be related to pelvic straining, especially in those who are overweight. As ex-

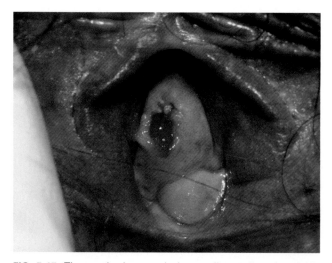

FIG. 7-15. The urethral caruncle is usually small and variably red, emanating from the urethral orifice.

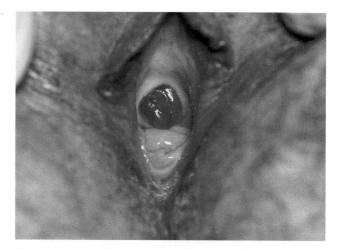

FIG. 7-17. Although urethral prolapse resembles a urethral caruncle, the erythematous nodule is circumferential around the meatus, thus making a doughnut shape with the urethral opening in the center.

emplified by its occurrence principally in premenarchal girls and postmenopausal women, estrogen deficiency may play a role. Topical estrogen therapy (6) and manual reduction of the prolapse are often successful but relapse is common. Surgical excision, ligation, or electrosurgical destruction is sometimes necessary.

VULVAR ENDOMETRIOSIS

Clinical Presentation

Cutaneous endometriosis is an uncommon condition that presents with papules or nodules of variable size and color. These are usually located in the vulvar vestibule but occasionally are found on the keratinizing epithelium of the perineum and labia majora. Smaller, superficial lesions occur as a solitary pink, red, violaceous, brown or skin-colored, smooth-surfaced papule or nodule. The average size is 1 to 2 cm. Larger and deeper lesions are usually skin-colored, blue, or violaceous (Fig. 7-18).

Diagnosis

Recognition is usually easy because, characteristically, these nodules enlarge and become painful at the time of menstruation. Regression then occurs after menstruation. Biopsy will confirm a clinically suspected diagnosis. Conditions included in the differential diagnosis include hidradenoma papilliferum, pyogenic granuloma, vascular tumors, and inflamed cysts. Other secondarily inflamed tumors may also mimic vulvar endometriosis.

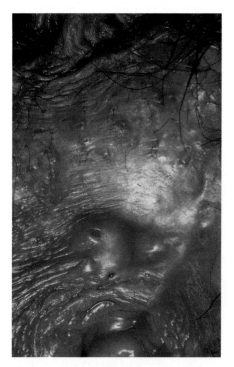

FIG. 7-18. Deeper nodules of cutaneous endometriosis are dome-shaped and nondescript, requiring a biopsy for diagnosis. (Courtesy of Raymond Kaufman.)

ENDOMETRIOSIS:	Diagnosis

- Usually a solitary lesion located within the vulva
- Color variable
- Surface intact
- Enlargement during menses; regression afterwards

Pathophysiology

Vulvar endometriosis develops when endometrial tissue is accidentally implanted in the vulva at the time of parturition or during surgical procedures (7). Even more rarely, implantation can occur if vulvar erosions are present during menstrual flow. Development of vulvar endometriosis may lag behind endometrial implantation by months to years.

Management

Surgical excision or laser destruction may be adequate for small lesions but recurrences, which are common, and larger or more widespread lesions of endometriosis may require hormonal suppression of ovulation.

ENDOMETRIOSIS:	Management

- Surgical excision
- Laser ablation is possible after biopsy
- Expect a high rate of recurrence
- Hormonal suppression of ovulation for extensive disease

HEMATOMA

Hematomas represent a loculated collection of blood. They occur rather easily within the vulva and scrotum because of the loose connective tissue at these sites and the dependent location of the genitalia. They usually occur following accidental, incidental, or sexual trauma (Fig. 7-19). The clinical appearance is that of acute or subacute swelling accompanied by poorly demarcated, nonblanching purple discoloration. After the first few days, the purple color is replaced by hues of yellow, green, and brown.

Depending on the nature of the trauma, the possibility of urethral rupture and intrapelvic tissue damage should be considered. In a different form of hematoma, nontraumatic loculation of blood occurs in hematocolpos where menstrual blood is trapped within the vagina by an imperforate hymen. Treatment of genital hematoma is usually expectant and conservative. Soaks and pain control can be useful. Surgical incision and evacuation of a clot may be necessary in instances of rapidly enlarging hematomas.

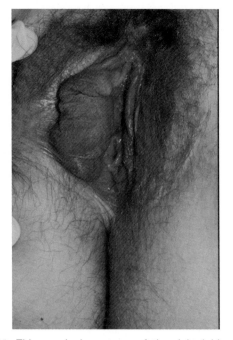

FIG. 7-19. This purple hematoma of the right labium minus occurred following relatively minor trauma of a fall onto a boy's bicycle.

HIDRADENOMA PAPILLIFERUM (MAMMARY-LIKE GLAND ADENOMA)

Hidradenoma papilliferum is an uncommon adnexal neoplasm of the female anogenital area (8). It develops primarily in middle-aged and older women and appears clinically as a solitary, small (15 to 30 mm), hemispherical nodule. The lesion is most often pink, red, or skin-colored. Some appear cystic and others appear solid. The surface may be smooth but about one third ulcerate with attendant bleeding (Fig. 7-20). Most lesions are asymptomatic. The diagnosis may be suspected clinically but biopsy is necessary for confirmation.

Hidradenoma papilliferum was originally thought to be an apocrine gland tumor but recent studies suggest that it is an adenoma derived from anogenital mammary-like glands (9). Hidradenoma papilliferum is a benign neoplasm. The treatment is surgical excision and recurrences are infrequent after removal. Hidradenoma papilliferum should be differentiated from another somewhat similarly named adnexal neoplasm, syringocystadenoma papilliferum that is located primarily on the face and scalp.

KAPOSI SARCOMA

Kaposi sarcoma is a low-grade malignancy of blood vessel origin. The lesions of Kaposi sarcoma are dome-shaped, dusky red-brown, or purplish papules, nodules, or plaques (Figs. 7-21 and 7-22). The color may be dusky-red or violaceous. There are several forms of Kaposi sarcoma

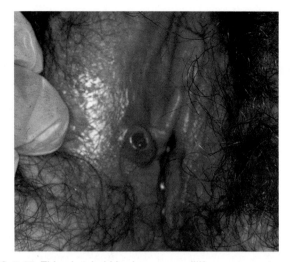

FIG. 7-20. This classic hidradenoma papilliferum presents as a red nodule with a central ulceration. (Courtesy of Raymond Kaufman.)

all of which appear to be caused by Kaposi sarcoma–associated herpes virus, which is also known as human herpes virus type 8. The most common type of Kaposi sarcoma found in Western countries is the one that is associated with severe immune suppression, especially as occurring in patients with HIV/AIDS. Not surprisingly, the prevalence of Kaposi sarcoma has decreased by about 90% since the advent of highly active antiretroviral therapy.

In this form of Kaposi sarcoma, lesions are most commonly found on the trunk and on mucosal surfaces of the mouth. There is no particular predilection for the genital area but lesions occasionally do occur at this location. There are only a few case reports involving the female genitalia but, presumably because Kaposi sarcoma in general occurs more frequently in men, at least 50 cases of penile involvement have been reported (10). Treatment is unnecessary for small tumors, but if therapy is desired, individual lesions can be treated with cryotherapy, surgical excision, or intralesional vinblastine or vincristine. Systemic

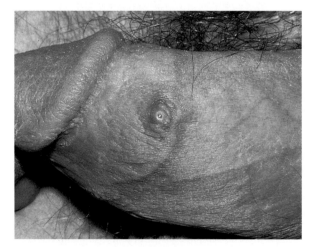

FIG. 7-21. Although Kaposi sarcoma is a vascular malignancy, it often appears as a dusky red violaceous, or even brown nodule, as seen here on the shaft of the penis.

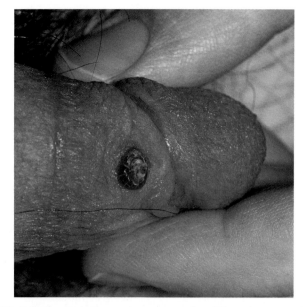

FIG. 7-22. Purple is the most common color of Kaposi sarcoma in a white patient. The setting of HIV makes the diagnosis much easier.

chemotherapy for Kaposi sarcoma falls outside the scope of this book.

PSEUDOWARTS (DIAPER DERMATITIS OF JACQUET, GRANULOMA GLUTEALE INFANTUM)

The entities listed in the title, together with those known as erosive diaper dermatitis and pseudoverrucous papules, are probably minor variants of a single disorder (11). The lesions in this condition occur as discreet flat-topped or somewhat dome-shaped, pink, red or violaceous papules and nodules (Fig. 7-23). Most are about 1 cm in diameter but larger lesions are also fairly common. Because the surface is made up of a thickened stratum corneum that is markedly hydrophilic, they may even appear white when they are wet and macerated. Often some of the lesions have an eroded surface. This condition presumably arises as a callus-like, protective reaction to the chronic irritation of continually present moisture. For that reason the lesions occur almost solely in diapered infants and in incontinent (and usually diapered) elderly men and women. Conditions such as HPV infection (warts), condyloma lata, and prurigo nodularis should be considered in the list of differential diagnoses. Secondary colonization or infection with *Candida* sp. is common.

Treatment requires improvement in the local environment notably obtaining a reduction in the amount and duration of retained urine, sweat, or feces. Skin protective products such as zinc oxide ointment or sucralfate are modestly helpful (12). Controversy exists regarding the usefulness of topical steroids as some clinicians believe that these agents actually worsen the problem and may even play a

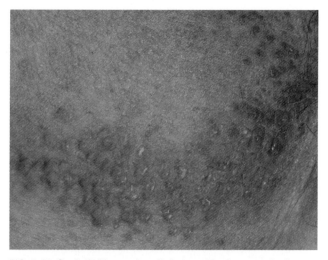

FIG. 7-23. Genital skin continually irritated by feces and urine reacts by developing red, discrete, flat-topped irritant papules sometimes called pseudowarts.

role in its etiology. This author, however, has found time-limited use of high-potency topical steroids to be helpful. Rarely, systemic steroids, administered either orally or intramuscularly, are necessary. Concomitant anticandidal therapy is usually warranted.

FURUNCULOSIS

Furuncles develop as a deep form of bacterial folliculitis and usually present as a solitary, red, dome-shaped nodule (Fig. 7-24). Most are 2 to 4 cm in diameter. They are

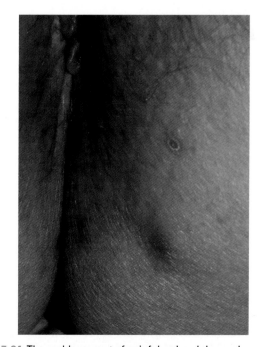

FIG. 7-24. The sudden onset of painful red nodules and a culture showing a heavy growth of *Staphylococcus aureus* differentiates this furuncle from hidradenitis suppurativa.

painful, warm, and tender to touch. On palpation they may be firm or have a central soft area of fluctuance. The term "abscess" is used for similar infections, presenting with a similar appearance, occurring at an extrafollicular site. Untreated lesions may undergo necrosis, breaking through the overlying skin and draining pus.

Furuncles and abscesses are almost always caused by *Staphylococcal aureus* infection. The warm, moist environment of the anogenital area facilitates the development of these lesions as does sexual activity and other forms of frictional trauma. Debility, immunocompromise, diabetes, and topical and systemic steroids may act as cofactors in causation. Individuals who are chronic nasal carriers of *S. Aureus* tend to have frequently recurring lesions.

The inflammatory nodules of hidradenitis suppurativa (HS) are regularly confused with furuncles, but the presence of multiple nodules, location at multiple sites along the milk line, recovery of more than a single species of bacteria, and the failure to quickly and fully respond to antibiotic therapy allow for correct identification of HS. Inflamed cysts are also similar in appearance to furuncles. For these lesions, there is generally a history of a pre-existing noninflamed nodule at that site. This bit of history together with a poor response to antibiotic therapy allows for correct identification. Other conditions to consider in the list of differential diagnoses include pilonidal cysts and Crohn disease. If the lesion is very large, cellulitis and the early stage of necrotizing fasciitis, should also be considered.

The diagnosis is generally made on a clinical basis; confirmation by bacterial culture is possible if the lesion is fluctuant and is incised. Small, relatively asymptomatic lesions may clear spontaneously. Larger lesions should be treated with oral antibiotics such as dicloxacillin or cephalexin in doses of 260 to 500 mg q.i.d. Today one should also consider the possibility of methicillin-resistant *S. aureus* infection in which case alternative antibiotics, depending on local resistance patterns, should be chosen. Small firm lesions do not benefit from incision and drainage but larger, fluctuant lesions do. Although warm, wet compresses are often recommended, there is little factual evidence to support their use.

INFLAMED CYSTS

Most cysts occurring in the anogenital region are skin-colored and asymptomatic. As such, the primary discussion of these lesions can be found in Chapter 12. However, sometimes these cysts become painfully inflamed. In this situation, a patient may present for the first time with a red, tender nodule. Inflammation occurring in or around a cyst develops as the result of cyst wall leakage or rupture with release of cyst contents into the surrounding connective tissue. These cyst contents subsequently induce a foreign body-type inflammatory reaction. It should be noted that many clinicians speak of these inflamed cysts as being infected but, in fact, infection is a most unlikely event for intact cysts. Infection can, however, occur after a cyst has undergone necrosis and drains to the skin surface.

Noninflamed cysts are usually asymptomatic but inflamed cysts are generally tender and painful. When a patient initially presents with an inflamed cyst, the first consideration is usually that of a furuncle. However, a diagnosis of an inflamed cyst is usually possible based on the history of a pre-existing, nontender, skin-colored lesion. This observation together with an unchanging size of 10 days or more and a failure to respond quickly and completely to antibiotic therapy allows for correct clinical identification. The type of cysts most like to become inflamed include epidermoid ("sebaceous") cysts (Fig. 7-25), pilonidal cysts (Fig. 7-26), and Bartholin duct cyst (Fig. 7-27). Other conditions to be considered in the list of differential diagnoses include cutaneous Crohn disease and HS.

The treatment of inflamed cysts depends partly on the type of cyst involved. But in most instances incision and drainage with bacterial culture of the contents is a desirable first step. If the cyst cavity is quite large, packing it with sterile iodoform gauze may be warranted. Antibiotics are often administered even though infection is rarely present in intact cysts. Often there is some improvement with antibiotics but this is probably more related to the anti-inflammatory property of most antibiotics rather than to any direct antimicrobial effect.

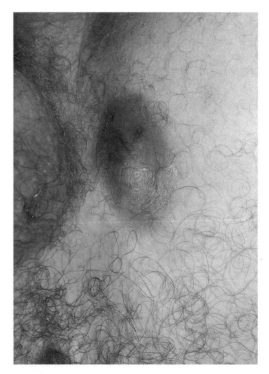

FIG. 7-25. An inflamed epidermal cyst is morphologically indistinguishable from a furuncle, but there is a history of a preceding nodule; inflamed cysts are usually solitary lesions.

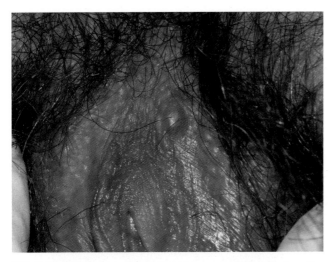

FIG. 7-26. Although a pilonidal cyst is normally located on the sacral skin, vulvar pilonidal cysts occur as well, and are generally periclitoral in location.

Soaks and sitz baths with warm tap water are often recommended but there are few data to support their use.

Not all cysts need to be completely excised though the recurrence rate is fairly high if this is not carried out. In any event, definitive, complete excision of the cyst is best delayed until the initial inflammation has resolved as this leads to a reduced size of the lesion to be removed. The excision of pilonidal and Bartholin cysts requires special expertise and discussion of this topic lies beyond the scope of this chapter.

HIDRADENITIS SUPPURATIVA (ACNE INVERSA)

HS is a chronic disfiguring disease that is difficult to treat successfully. It is often accompanied by pain, drainage, and odor. As such it has the potential to materially reduce the quality of life for patients affected by it. Two general reviews of this disease have recently been published (13,14).

Clinical Presentation

HS is a relatively common problem with an estimated prevalence of about 1% in Western countries (15). It affects women appreciably more often than men, but severity of the disease, when it occurs in men, appears to be greater. In women, it most commonly develops after menarche, usually during the second and third decade of life. New onset after menopause is unusual and disease activity tends to decrease slowly over time. Cigarette smoking and obesity are predisposing factors for the development of the disease. Most clinicians believe that HS is more common in Africans and African-Americans, but data to support this supposition are lacking. A positive family history for HS (or for the facial equivalent, acne conglobata) is found in a significant minority of patients.

HS begins with painful, red nodules, many of which eventually rupture to form chronic, draining sinus tracts (Figs. 7-28 through 7-31). The inflammatory nodules greatly resemble furuncles and are often initially misdiagnosed as such. Less often chronic ulcers develop. Both the sinuses

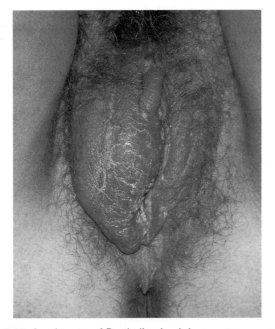

FIG. 7-27. An abscess of Bartholin gland duct cyst presents as a diffuse, painful, red swelling of the vulva underlying the posterior vestibule and labium majus. (Courtesy of Raymond Kaufman.)

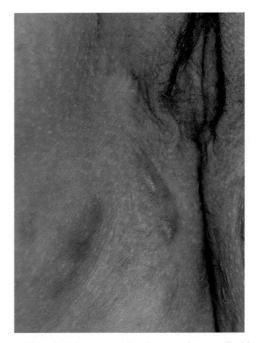

FIG. 7-28. Hidradenitis suppurativa is sometimes called inverse acne and consists of inflamed acne-type cysts that evolve into chronic draining sinuses.

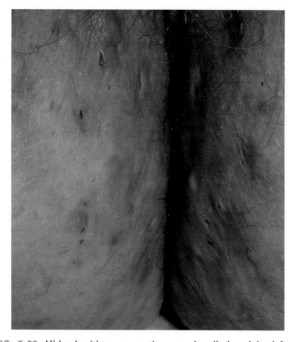

FIG. 7-29. Hidradenitis suppurativa can be distinguished from furunculosis by the presence of comedones that may be subtle or marked, as well as poor response to antibiotics, and nondiagnostic cultures.

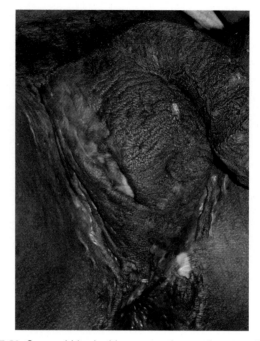

FIG. 7-31. Severe hidradenitis suppurativa produces mutilating scarring, and the ongoing inflammation should be monitored for malignant transformation.

and the ulcers tend to heal with thick, rope-like scars. Comedones are regularly found in the areas around the inflammatory lesions. These comedones are larger than normal. The presence of two comedones separated by only 1 to 2 mm ("twin" comedones) is so distinctive as to represent a pathognomonic sign of the disease. These twin black heads occur as a result of a bifurcated follicular outlet suggesting that anatomic follicular abnormalities play a role in the development of the disease. Similar atypical comedones at flexural sites have also been

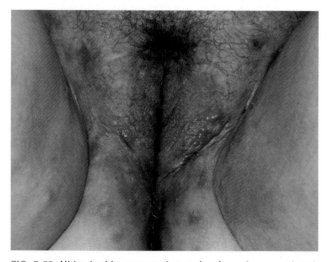

FIG. 7-30. Hidradenitis suppurativa varies from the occasional, annoying inflamed cyst, to continually draining, painful, and foul-smelling nodules.

reported to occur in the absence of inflammatory lesions (16), and it is possible that children with such lesions are predisposed to the development of HS.

The inflammatory lesions of HS occur almost solely at sites possessing hair follicles with associated apocrine glands. Because of the relationship between mammary glands and apocrine glands, it is not surprising that nearly all of the lesions of HS will occur along the "milk line" that runs from the axillae through the mammary area and extends into the pubic, inguinal, genital, perineal, and perianal area. Scattered lesions (presumably related to ectopically located apocrine gland-related follicles) may be found on the buttocks and thighs. The axillae are the locations most often affected and in many instances represent the site of initial involvement before further dissemination is noted.

Two systems for judging the severity of HS have been proposed: the Hurley and the Sartorius staging systems (13). Both are useful for purposes of clinical studies but it is generally unnecessary to utilize either one in routine clinical practice.

Diagnosis

A diagnosis of HS is made on a clinical basis. The clinical features that lead to the diagnosis include (i) the presence of multiple lesions, (ii) the location of lesions within the milk line, (iii) recurrence at the same site, (iv) long duration (weeks to months) of individual lesions, (v) bacterial cultures that are either negative or demonstrate the presence of multiple bacterial species, and (vi) failure to respond quickly and completely to antibiotic therapy. A diagnostic algorithm that includes many of these features has recently been proposed (13). Biopsy is rarely indicated, and because of the nonspecific inflammation that is found, it is usually not helpful if it is carried out. However, when Crohn disease is a consideration in the differential diagnosis, a biopsy may be helpful for the identification of this disorder.

Two common diseases should be considered in the list of differential diagnoses. Furunculosis is the condition with which HS is most often confused. Several clinical features are useful in identifying furunculosis: (i) only one or two nodules are usually present at any given time, (ii) additional lesions, if they occur at all, are found at random sites rather than solely within the milk line, (iii) culture reveals only a single bacterial species, *S. aureus*, and (iv) there is a complete response to antibiotic therapy within 7 to 10 days. Anogenital Crohn disease can look very much like HS. A history of bowel symptoms and signs, absence of lesions in the axillae, the presence of anal fistulae, the lack of twin comedones, and the somewhat more distinctive histological findings on biopsy would point toward a diagnosis of Crohn disease. Note, however, that even though they appear to be entirely separate entities, there are several reports indicating that the two diseases coexist with a greater frequency than would be expected by chance (17). Other rare disorders that may appear similar to the inflammatory lesions of HS include deep fungal infections (especially in the immunosuppressed), mycobacterial infections, granuloma inguinale, and inflamed cysts of various types. HS can also be encountered in association with acne conglobata and dissecting cellulitis of the scalp (the follicular retention triad) as well as with several very uncommon syndromes involving acne, arthropathy, fever, and bone lesions (13).

HIDRADENITIS SUPPURATIVA: **Diagnosis**

- Multiple lesions are present
- Lesions located within the milk line
- Recurrence of lesions at the same site
- Long duration with little spontaneous regression
- Cultures sterile or contain multiple species of bacteria
- Slow and incomplete resolution with antibiotics

Pathophysiology

Although the inflammatory lesions of HS occur in apocrine gland-associated hair follicles, HS is not a disease of the apocrine gland itself. Instead, the lesions arise because of anatomic or keratinous plugging of the apocrine duct and/or hair follicle. Once the blockage is in place, activity of the apocrine gland leads to a damming effect with subsequent follicular dilatation and, eventually, follicular leakage or rupture. This results in extravasation of follicular contents into the surrounding connective tissue where they induce a foreign body inflammatory response. This inflammatory response, consisting of neutrophils, lymphocytes and macrophages, creates a sterile abscess. If abscess-related necrosis breaks through the skin, secondary bacterial colonization and/or infection may occur. This process can be viewed as analogous to the pathophysiology of cystic acne and hence the alternative name for HS is "acne inversa."

Environmental factors such as obesity with attendant intertriginous friction and sweat retention presumably contribute to occlusion of apocrine gland-related follicles. The frequent occurrence of familial cases is best explained by an inherited pattern of anatomically malformed apocrine gland-related hair follicles. Hormonal factors probably play some role as evidenced by the greater incidence in women, the usual onset after menarche, worsening at the time of menstruation, and a tendency for improvement during pregnancy (18). Obesity could also play a role hormonally by way of obesity-related reduction in sex-hormone-binding globulin and attendant increase in circulating free androgens. On the other hand, data regarding abnormal serum levels of hormones have been variable with no consistent elevation in sex hormones having been reported. Finally, there is an unequivocal association between smoking and the development of HS (15). The mechanism accounting for this relationship remains unknown and it appears that cessation of smoking has little or no beneficial effect on the course of the disease.

Management

HS is an extraordinarily chronic disease extending over many years or even decades. When HS is untreated or is treated inadequately, *nondraining abscesses* eventually resolve spontaneously over the course of several months. Unfortunately, recrudescence at the same sites occurs frequently. *Draining sinuses* remain in place even longer, sometimes for years. And, of course, scars, often with contractures, last for a lifetime. Overall, in the untreated state, there is a tendency for the process to extend locally. This probably occurs because of inflammatory cytokine release with resultant extension of inflammation-related destruction of adjacent follicles. Eventually, after years of activity, scarring causes obliteration of apocrine gland-related hair follicles and the process gradually "burns" itself out.

The quality of life for patients with HS is very seriously impaired, perhaps more so than for patients with any other common dermatologic disease (19). Patients are hindered socially and at work because of odor and drainage. Sexual intimacy becomes impossible for many patients. Some patients are even rejected by physicians from whom they seek therapy. Severe psychological disability develops and most patients with moderate to severe disease develop debilitating anxiety and/or depression.

The clinical sequelae of long-standing disease include hypertrophic, rope-like scarring, architectural distortion of involved tissue (especially of the genitalia), and moderate to severe limitation in limb mobility. Massive, persistent vulvar and scrotal edema may occur. Moreover, by analogy with the development of carcinoma in long-standing stasis ulcers (Marjolin ulcers), squamous cell carcinoma, mostly in the anogenital area, has been reported in more than 60 patients with HS (20).

Medical therapy, despite its limitations, represents the initial approach for nearly all patients (21). Improving the local environment through reduction in sweat retention and weight loss is modestly helpful, though difficult to achieve. Patients with nondraining abscesses can be treated with long-term topical antibiotic solutions such as 1% clindamycin or 2% erythromycin. Individual abscesses can be injected intralesionally with triamcinolone acetonide (Kenalog) in a concentration of 10 mg/mL. Small nodules will require 0.1 to 0.5 mL and larger ones may benefit from 0.5 to 1.0 mL. Patients with numerous lesions should be placed on long-term oral antibiotic therapy. This treatment, as well as the topical antibiotic therapy mentioned above, utilizes the anti-inflammatory properties of antibiotics rather than their direct antimicrobial effect. The products most often used are equally effective and include tetracycline 250 mg q.i.d., doxycycline 100 mg b.i.d., and minocycline 100 mg b.i.d. Antibiotic therapy usually leads to only mild to moderate improvement but recent reports suggest a greater degree of success when combination therapy with clindamycin (300 mg b.i.d.) and rifampin (600 mg/day) is instituted (22,23).

Hormonal therapy may be considered for women with HS even though there are only meager data published regarding efficacy. This is initiated with oral contraceptives (especially with those incorporating drospirenone or cyproterone as the progestational agent) and is followed, if necessary, by spironolactone or finasteride. A recent small retrospective review suggested that antiandrogen therapy was superior to the use of antibiotics (18).

Oral retinoids, primarily isotretinoin, have very limited value in the treatment of HS. This is somewhat unexpected given their highly beneficial effect in cystic acne. Perhaps this relative lack of efficacy is due to the minimal effect of retinoids on apocrine gland activity. Currently there is great enthusiasm for the use of tumor necrosis factor alpha (TNF-α) inhibitors such as infliximab, etanercept, and adalimumab (24). However these early reports of success in small trials with limited follow-up must be balanced against both the known and the unknown adverse effects of this relatively new class of medications. Other anecdotally supported therapies include dapsone, cyclosporine, zinc gluconate, and systemic steroids (13,21).

Given the significant limitations of medical therapy, many clinicians consider HS to be a disease for which surgery represents the best approach. Multiple surgical procedures have been used. Incision and drainage of individual lesions offers little of long-term value and is no longer often recommended. Marsupialization, likewise, has fallen out of fashion. Surgical excision is extremely effective for limited areas of disease. It is somewhat less successful for widespread disease where the appearance of new lesions at the margins of excision represents the rule rather than the exception (13,14). When excisional surgery is carried out, controversy exists as to the best technique to be used. Some favor extensive surgery with grafting, others allow for healing by secondary intention, and still others prefer staged removal with primary closures.

Unfortunately, many surgeons are hesitant to perform surgery for HS because of two concerns. First, they fear the development of wound infection because of the draining pus in and around the surgical field. Second, they view the development of new lesions at the surgical margin as surgical failure. In answer to these concerns it should be noted that the pus is usually sterile and there is no reported increase in wound infections beyond that which might occur in a "clean" field. Moreover, the new lesions that occur at the surgical margin represent "new" lesions rather than "recurrences" and these may be excised at a later date on an "as necessary" basis. Most importantly, patient satisfaction with surgical procedures for HS is really quite high and, in reported series, is almost always higher than the satisfaction expressed by the surgeons.

HIDRADENITIS SUPPURATIVA: **Management**

- Intralesional steroids for lesions small in size or number
- Prolonged oral antibiotics for their anti-inflammatory effect
- Consider hormonal therapy for women
- TNF-α inhibitors for severe disease
- Surgical excision of involved areas if possible and available

---

MISCELLANEOUS RED PAPULES AND NODULES

Langerhans cell histiocytosis. Two varieties of this condition occur. The more common, disseminated type (Letterer-Siwe disease) occurs in infancy and frequently involves the anogenital area. It is discussed in Chapter 14. In the less common adult form, papules, nodules, and plaques, often with linear "knife cut" ulcers, can develop in the genital area. They may arise in the setting of already existent systemic disease or they may occur as primary in the skin. However, some of the reported cases thought to be primary subsequently developed systemic disease. Of the approximately 25 cases thought to be primary in the genital area, about 20 occurred on the vulva and about 5 occurred on the penis (25,26). The lesions are very pleomorphic in appearance. Evaluation and treatment of this condition is outside the scope of this chapter.

Sarcoidosis. About 25% of patients with systemic sarcoidosis have, or will develop, skin lesions. Not surprisingly, a handful of cases have been reported as occurring on the genitalia (27,28). The cutaneous lesions of sarcoid can occur as smooth-surfaced papules, nodules, and plaques. Rarely these may ulcerate. These lesions may be skin-colored, red, brown-red, or even darkly pigmented. Sarcoidosis occurring as primary in the skin, without systemic involvement, has been reported for extragenital sites but the cases reported as occurring on the genitalia appear to be secondary to spread from systemic disease. However, it is possible that the form of idiopathic genital edema with granuloma formation (Melkersson–Rosenthal granulomatosis) as discussed in Chapter 12, is an example of unrecognized sarcoidosis confined to the skin.

Crohn Disease. Crohn disease in the anogenital area generally presents with ulcers (often linear), fistulae, and edema (Figs. 7-32 through 7-34). The primary coverage for

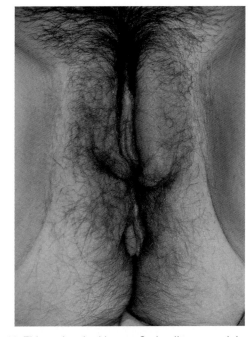

FIG. 7-33. This patient had known Crohn disease and developed mild, asymptomatic edema of the left labium majus that showed changes consistent with cutaneous Crohn disease on biopsy.

this disease is in Chapter 10 but intermingled with these lesions there may be erythematous perianal skin tags and friable red papules and nodules. These latter lesions are often similar in appearance to those of HS from which they must be differentiated.

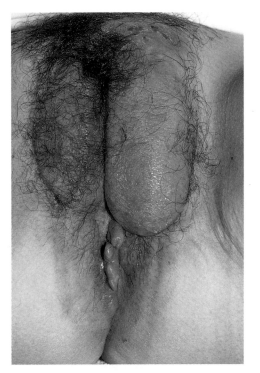

FIG. 7-32. Crohn disease presented in this 13-year-old girl as a painless, enlarged, and indurated right labium majus, followed over the next several years by perianal, fibrotic skin tags and a perianal fistula.

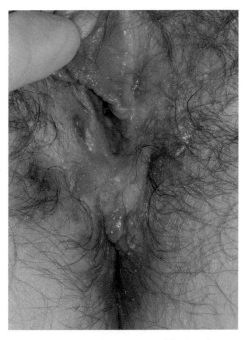

FIG. 7-34. These draining sinus tracts of Crohn disease are indistinguishable from those of hidradenitis suppurativa. The absence of comedones and the presence of inflammatory bowel disease usually clarify the diagnosis.

REFERENCES

1. Hwang S, Schwartz RA. Keratosis pilaris: a common follicular hyperkeratosis. *Cutis.* 2008;82:177–180.
2. Elston DM. What's eating you? *Cutis.* 2006;77:350–352.
3. Lee MR, Shumack S. Prurigo nodularis: a review. *Australas J Dermatol.* 2005;46:211–218.
4. Kaur T, Gupta S, Kumar B. Multiple pyogenic granuloma involving the female genitalia: a rare entity? *Pediatr Dermatol.* 2004;21:614–615.
5. Hillyer S, Mooppan U, Kim H, et al. Diagnosis and treatment of urethral prolapse in children: experience with 34 cases. *Urology.* 2009;73:1008–1011.
6. Abouzeid H, Shergill IS, Al-Samarrai M. Successful medical treatment of advanced urethral prolapse. *J Obstet Gynaecol.* 2007;27:634–635.
7. Buda A, Ferrari L, Marra C, et al. Vulvar endometriosis in surgical scar after excision of the Bartholin gland: report of a case. *Arch Gynecol Obstet.* 2008;277:255–256.
8. Virgilli A, Marzola A, Corazza M. Vulvar Hidradenoma papilliferum. A review of 10.5 years' experience. *J Reprod Med.* 2000;45:616–618.
9. Scurry J, van der Putte SC, Pyman J, et al. Mammary-like gland adenoma of the vulva: a review of 46 cases. *Pathology.* 2009; 41:372–378.
10. Pacifico A, Piccolo D, Fargnoli MC, et al. Kaposi's sarcoma on the glans penis in an immunocompetent patient. *Eur J Dermatol.* 2003;13:582–583.
11. Van L, Harting M, Rosen T. Jacquet erosive diaper dermatitis: a complication of adult urinary incontinence. *Cutis.* 2008;82: 72–74.
12. Paradisi A, Capizzi R, Ghitti F, et al. Jacquet erosive dermatitis: a therapeutic challenge. *Clin Exp Dermatol.* 2009;34(7):e385–e386. [Published online in advance of print: 22 June 2009].
13. Alikhan A, Lynch P, Eisen DB. Hidradenitis suppurativa: a comprehensive review. *J Am Acad Dermatol.* 2009;60:539–561.
14. Buimer MG, Wobbes T, Klinkenbijl JH. Hidradenitis suppurativa. *Br J Surg.* 2009;96:350–360.
15. Revuz JE, Canoul-Poitrine F, Wolkenstein P, et al. Prevalence and factors associated with hidradenitis suppurativa: results from two case-control studies. *J Am Acad Dermatol.* 2008;59: 596–601.
16. Larralde M, Abad ME, Munoz AS, et al. Childhood flexural comedones: a new entity. *Arch Dermatol.* 2007;143:909–911.
17. Nassar D, Hugot JP, Wolkenstein P, et al. Lack of association between CARD15 gene polymorphisms and hidradenitis suppurativa: a plot study. *Dermatology.* 2007;215:359.
18. Kraft JN, Searles GE. Hidradenitis suppurativa in 64 female patients: retrospective study comparing oral antibiotics and antiandrogen therapy. *J Cutan Med Surg.* 2007;11:125–131.
19. Wolkenstein P, Loundou A, Barrau K, et al. Quality of life impairment in hidradenitis suppurativa: a study of 61 cases. *J Am Acad Dermatol.* 2007;56:621–623.
20. Lavogiez C, Delaporte E, Darras-Vercambre S, et al. Clinicopathological study of 13 cases of squamous cell carcinoma complicating hidradenitis suppurativa. *Dermatology.* 2009 Dec 23. [Epub ahead of print]
21. Lam J, Krakowski AC, Friedlander SF. Hidradenitis suppurativa (acne inversa): management of a recalcitrant disease. *Ped Dermatol.* 2007;24:465–473.
22. van der Zee HH, Boer J, Prens EP, et al. The effect of combined treatment with oral clindamycin and oral rifampicin in patients with hidradenitis suppurativa. *Dermatology.* 2009;219(2): 143–147. [Epub ahead of print July 8].
23. Gener G, Canoui-Poitrine F, Revuz JE, et al. Combination therapy with clindamycin and rifampicin for hidradenitis suppurativa: a series of 116 consecutive patients. *Dermatology.* 2009; 219(2):148–154. [Epub ahead of print July 8].
24. Haslund P, Lee RA, Jemec GB. Treatment of hidradenitis suppurativa with tumor necrosis factor-alpha inhibitors. *Acta Derm Venereol.* 2009;89:595-600.
25. Pan Z, Sharma S, Sharma P. Primary Langerhans cell histiocytosis of the vulva: report of a case and brief review of the literature. *Indian J Pathol Microbiol.* 2009;52:65–68.
26. Hagiuda J, Ueno M, Ashmine S, et al. Langerhans cell histiocytosis on the penis: a case report. *BMC Urol.* 2006;11:28.
27. Wei H, Friedman KA, Rudikoff D. Multiple indurated papules on penis and scrotum. *J Cutan Med Surg.* 2000;4:202–204.
28. Decavalas G, Adonakis G, Androutsopoulos G, et al. Sarcoidosis of the vulva: a case report. *Arch Gynecol Obstet.* 2007;275:203–205.

CHAPTER 8

Yellow and Pustular Lesions

LIBBY EDWARDS

Yellow lesions primarily result from purulent material. These can occur as intact pustules, or as yellow crusting, when pustules rupture. On occasion, desquamated, hydrated stratum corneum that obstructs or distends follicles form can appear somewhat yellow and mimic pustules.

TRUE PUSTULAR DISEASES

Folliculitis

Folliculitis is a common pustular eruption resulting from the inflammation or infection of the superficial portion of hair follicles (Figs. 8-1 through 8-4). This can be bacterial, fungal, or irritant.

Clinical Presentation

Folliculitis occurs in all age groups, and the affected population depends on the underlying etiology. Fungal folliculitis occurs primarily in middle-aged or older men, especially those with fungal toenail infection. Irritant folliculitis occurs in women who shave the area and in overweight individuals at risk for prominent friction and chronic moisture. There is no particular patient at risk for Staphylococcal folliculitis, whereas hot tub folliculitis is found in individuals exposed to inadequately treated hot tubs or those who use washcloths or sponges that do not completely dry from day-to-day.

Staphylococcus aureus folliculitis usually presents with symptoms of mild tenderness and pruritus. On examination, there are red papules and variable numbers of small yellow pustules 1 to 5 mm in size with a surrounding red flare. The pustule is short-lived and leaves a residual red papule with crust or a fine collarette of scale. Individual lesions heal within 7 to 10 days. Many patients have associated folliculitis with furunculosis, representing a deeper infection of the follicle. These tender, red nodules often suppurate and drain. Frequent sites include the mons pubis, buttocks, and thighs.

Pseudomonas folliculitis presents as tender, red, non-scaling papules and occasional pustules concentrated in areas where contaminated water has been held against the skin, such as intertriginous skin and under wet swimsuits. Sometimes, patients exhibit constitutional symptoms such as fever, malaise, ear pain, and sore throat.

Follicular pustules within scaly, annular, pink-red plaques of tinea cruris characterize fungal folliculitis (Fig. 8-5). However, women with tinea pedis sometimes develop scattered single papules or pustules of fungal folliculitis on their lower legs and thighs by inoculating fungi into follicles when they shave their legs.

Noninfectious, irritant folliculitis is most often asymptomatic. Shaving folliculitis is a very common form of irritant folliculitis, as increasing numbers of women shave the vulva. Either the shaved, short, curly hair curves back and pierces the skin, producing an inflammatory reaction (Fig. 8-6) or the prominent tips of follicles are removed by the razor, again causing an irritant reaction. In addition, follicular occlusion from pressure, friction, and moisture often produces folliculitis that is often indistinguishable from Staphylococcal folliculitis. Small pustules surrounded by a thin rim of erythema characterize these almost ubiquitous lesions. These occur primarily on those areas of friction and pressure, such as the medial thighs and the buttocks.

Diagnosis

The diagnosis of folliculitis is usually made clinically. A bacterial or fungal culture is often helpful to identify any causative organisms and to guide the treatment course. A potassium hydroxide preparation sometimes reveals hyphae in dermatophyte folliculitis. Histopathology shows neutrophils within the hair follicle with abscess formation. Special stains may reveal the causative organism.

Folliculitis can be confused with scabies, pustular miliaria, *Candida* infection, eosinophilic folliculitis of human immunodeficiency virus (HIV) infection, arthropod bites, keratosis pilaris, and herpes simplex virus (HSV) infection.

FOLLICULITIS: **Diagnosis**

- Morphology of red papules, pustules, and/or crusts, often with a hair piercing some lesions
- Culture showing causative organism, or fungal preparation showing branching hyphae should reveal infectious causes

---

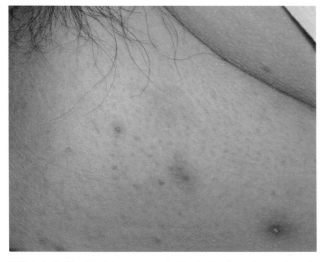

FIG. 8-1. Folliculitis is common on the buttocks, where chronic pressure and occlusion promote follicular obstruction.

Pathophysiology

Bacterial folliculitis is most often caused by *S. aureus*, but it can be caused by gram-negative bacteria, especially *Pseudomonas aeruginosa*, the cause of hot tub folliculitis. Folliculitis may also be caused by dermatophytes and is most often seen in men in association with tinea cruris. Chemical, mechanical, or frictional irritation are also very common causes of superficial folliculitis.

Management

The treatment of folliculitis depends on the etiology. Staphylococcal folliculitis can be treated with oral and topical antibiotics. Oral antibiotics with past predictable coverage include dicloxacillin and cephalexin at 500 mg twice a day for 7 to 10 days. Recently, a large proportion of community-acquired *S. aureus* is resistant to methicillin, dicloxacillin, and cephalexin. From 4% (France) to 76% (North Carolina) of community-acquired *S. aureus* is

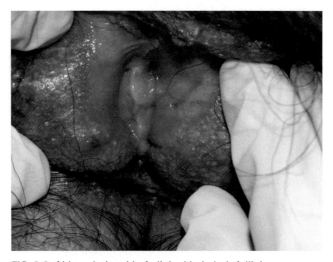

FIG. 8-3. Although devoid of clinical hair, hair follicles are present on the modified mucous membranes of the vulva. This patient exhibited the red papules and pustules of irritant folliculitis on both the clinically hair-bearing skin and the medial aspects of the labia minora.

resistant to methicillin (1,2). Clindamycin at 150 mg twice daily is somewhat more likely to be effective, and trimethoprim-sulfamethoxazole double strength is nearly always efficacious. Linezolid, daptomycin, and tigecycline are advanced agents available for the rare infection resistant to the older oral medications (3). Treatment with clindamycin 1% topical solution twice a day in conjunction with antibacterial soaps is also useful. Mupirocin cream and ointment are extremely effective for the first week of use but resistance occurs quickly.

Recurrence of Staphylococcal folliculitis is common. Nasal staphylococcal carriage is common in affected individuals with chronic and recurrent folliculitis. These patients benefit by the application of mupirocin ointment to the anterior nares twice a day for 5 days. Because carriers often have recurrent colonization of *S. aureus* within their

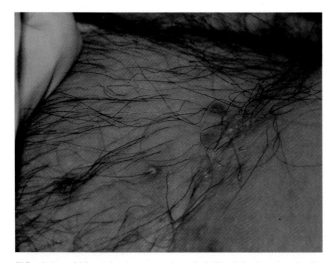

FIG. 8-2. Although the pustule of folliculitis is classically pierced by a hair as seen here, this is often not seen.

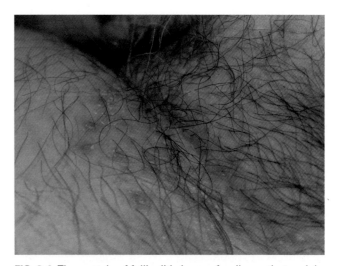

FIG. 8-4. The pustule of folliculitis is very fragile, so that peripheral collarettes, the remaining, circular edge of a ruptured pustule roof, and desquamation are often the predominant lesions.

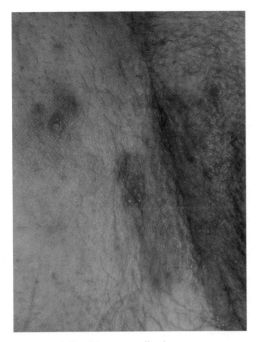

FIG. 8-5. Fungal folliculitis gnereally does not present as isolated, scattered pustules, but rather occurs within plaques of tinea cruris, in which infection extends down follicles to produce pustules or red papules. Often, this occurs in a setting of topical corticosteroids, so that scale is sometimes subtle.

nares, some clinicians recommend that these patients apply the mupirocin treatment for 5 days every 1 to 6 months indefinitely to prevent recurrent folliculitis.

Pseudomonas folliculitis (hot tub folliculitis) requires no treatment because it resolves when exposure ceases. Therefore, identification of the source of the organism and avoidance of reinoculation are most important. Emptying and cleaning the spa or hot tub and proper maintenance of bactericidal chemicals is also important. However, those patients who exhibit constitutional symptoms may improve more rapidly if they receive oral ciprofloxacin at 500 mg twice a day or levofloxacin 500 mg per day.

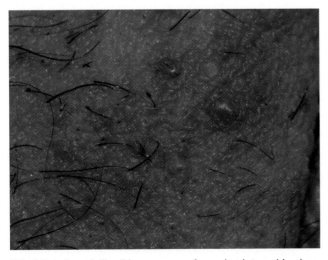

FIG. 8-6. Irritant folliculitis can occur from shaving and is characterized by red papules and pustules limited to the area of shaving, and produced by stiff, curled hairs piercing the skin.

Fungal folliculitis requires oral therapy because the organism extends into the follicle where topical antifungal creams cannot penetrate. Therapies include oral griseofulvin 500 mg twice daily until the eruption resolves. Alternatively, oral fluconazole or itraconazole may also be prescribed at doses of 100 mg/day orally for 15 days or until the skin is clear. Finally, oral terbinafine at 250 mg/day until the skin is clear is effective, and it is the least expensive solution because this medication is available generically. After treatment, the daily use of an antifungal cream or powder to the groin area helps to prevent recurrences.

Irritant folliculitis can be improved by minimizing irritants. Avoiding shaving clears shaving folliculitis; laser hair removal may be preferable. Cool, nonocclusive clothing, weight loss, and powders may prevent chronic moisture, pressure, and friction. Otherwise, the chronic administration of anti-inflammatory antibiotics such as doxycycline or minocycline 100 mg b.i.d. or clindamycin 150 mg b.i.d. can improve irritant folliculitis, although improvement generally requires about a month and entails ongoing administration.

FOLLICULITIS:	**Management**

- Depends on the underlying cause:
  - Bacterial folliculitis: treat according to culture results. For suspected Staphylococcal folliculitis, oral clindamycin 150 mg b.i.d., trimethoprim-sulfamethoxazole double strength b.i.d.
  - Fungal folliculitis: terbinafine 250 mg daily, griseofulvin 500 mg b.i.d., fluconazole 100 to 200 mg daily, or itraconazole 200 mg a day until clear
  - Irritant folliculitis: minimize irritants. Discontinue shaving, add powders to reduce friction and moisture. When required, chronic anti-inflammatory antibiotics such as doxycycline 100 mg b.i.d. can be taken chronically

Furunculosis

While folliculitis is characterized by inflammation of the superficial portion of the hair follicle, furunculosis involves the deeper follicle, producing a red "boil."

Clinical Presentation

Furunculosis occurs in all patient populations. It is somewhat more common in patients who are immunosuppressed, diabetic, or who exhibit scaling dermatoses that are likely to be colonized with *S. aureus*.

A furuncle is a red, usually painful nodule that typically suppurates and drains (Figs. 8-7 and 8-8). Patients experience evolving lesions, with some appearing as others heal. Often, there is associated staphylococcal folliculitis. Uncommonly, patients develop associated fever and malaise.

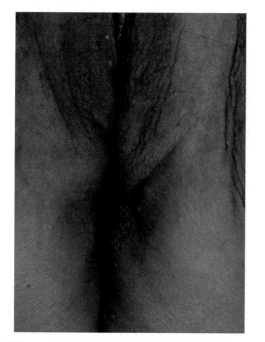

FIG. 8-7. Furunculosis is a deeper and larger infection than folliculitis and exhibits associated induration.

Diagnosis

The diagnosis is made on clinical grounds, and it is confirmed by a culture that usually yields *S. aureus*. A biopsy is generally not performed, but it reveals a dermal and subcutaneous abscess with surrounding cellulitis. Special stains show organisms consistent with *S. aureus*.

A furuncle occurring in the genital area is indistinguishable from an inflamed cyst of hidradenitis suppurativa (Fig. 8-8), which is a form of deep cystic acne. However, furuncles are not confined to the genital and

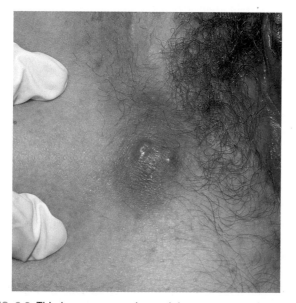

FIG. 8-8. This large, suppurative nodule represents a furuncle, but it is clinically indistinguishable from a ruptured, inflamed epidermal ("sebaceous") cyst.

axillary area as is hidradenitis, and comedones and scarring from recurrent draining abscesses are characteristic only of hidradenitis suppurativa. Cultures of hidradenitis suppurativa usually show normal skin organisms or a multitude of bacteria rather than a pure growth of a pathogen. Hidradenitis suppurativa occasionally is secondarily infected by *S. aureus*, but oral antistaphylococcal agents at most improve, but never eliminate, hidradenitis. Other possible diagnostic challenges include other inflamed cysts, especially an epidermal cyst, but inflamed Bartholin's gland duct cysts or vestibular cysts can also mimic a furuncle. Occasionally, inflamed tumors such as a basal cell carcinoma can mimic a furuncle.

FURUNCULOSIS: **Diagnosis**

- By morphology and acute onset of red painful nodules, often with rupture and draining
- Confirmed by culture and complete response to therapy

Pathophysiology

Furunculosis represents a bacterial infection, usually with *S. aureus*, of the deep portion of the follicle, with a resulting inflammatory nodule.

Management

Oral antistaphylococcal antibiotics are effective in clearing furunculosis. Previous first-line medications such as cephalexin, dicloxacillin, and methicillin are often ineffective due to the increase in community-acquired methicillin *S. aureus* (see above). Trimethoprim-sulfamethoxazole double strength or antibiotics according to culture results are preferable. Unfortunately, recurrent disease after discontinuation of medication is common. Some patients require prolonged oral therapy of weeks to months, in addition to the insertion of mupirocin ointment to the anterior nares twice a day for the first 5 days of therapy to reduce the carrier state.

FURUNCULOSIS: **Management**

- Oral antibiotics, choice by culture and sensitivities. Initial choices include clindamycin 300 mg b.i.d., trimethoprim-sulfamethoxazole double strength b.i.d.; cephalexin/dicloxacillin/methicillin 500 mg b.i.d. is no longer a good choice in most areas because of high resistance
- Warm soaks, incision and draining if fluctuant
- For recurrent disease, apply mupirocin ointment or cream in the nose two times a day for 5 days each month for 3 to 6 months to eliminate the carrier state.

Hidradenitis Suppurativa (Acne Inversa)

(see also Chapter 7)

This relatively common eruption is often misdiagnosed as furunculosis, but actually represents cystic acne of skin folds rather than an infectious process.

Clinical Presentation

Hidradenitis suppurativa is an inflammatory condition of skin folds that presents with a remarkable variability of severity. Hidradenitis suppurativa generally occurs after puberty, and this condition is worse in overweight individuals (4). There is a strong association with smoking as well (4). Painful, firm, red nodules occur in the axillae and/or the genital area, including the crural crease, proximal inner thighs, scrotum, and vulva (Fig. 8-9). Occasionally, the buttocks and lower abdomen can be involved. These nodules become fluctuant and drain. Some draining tracts become chronic. Although others heal, reaccumulation of keratin and purulent debris generally occurs, and the process repeats, eventually leaving multiple sinus tracts and scars (Fig. 8-10). A careful examination usually yields some comedones and follicles with more than one outlet to the surface (Fig. 8-11). Patients with hidradenitis suppurativa exhibit disease that ranges from an occasional comedone to confluent firm scars with painful, ulcerated nodules, chronic sinus tracts, and foul-smelling drainage (Fig. 8-12).

Other areas of the body that exhibit apocrine glands are the face and scalp. Some unfortunate patients have associated cystic acne and dissecting cellulitis of the scalp, which are also sterile pustular diseases preceded by keratin obstruction of follicles. Cystic acne, dissecting cellulitis, and hidradenitis suppurativa are sometimes referred to as the follicular retention triad.

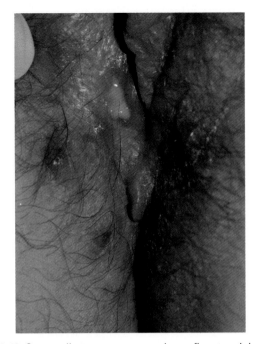

FIG. 8-10. Severe disease causes nearly confluent nodules and comedones.

As occurs with other chronic inflammatory dermatoses, squamous cell carcinoma is a rare, late complication (5).

Diagnosis

The diagnosis is made on the basis of the history of chronic or recurrent draining nodules in the axillae and/or groin and the presence of comedones. A biopsy,

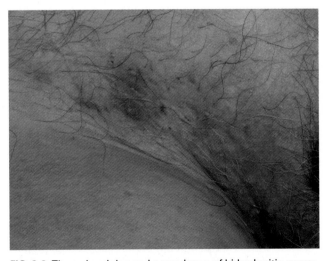

FIG. 8-9. The red nodules and comedones of hidradenitis suppurativa can occur on the buttocks, genital skin, proximal medial thighs, and, occasionally, on the abdomen.

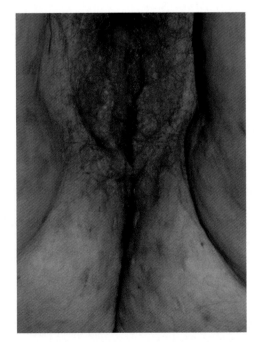

FIG. 8-11. Hidradenitis suppurativa is characterized by red nodules and purulent, draining sinuses, often with surrounding irritant dermatitis from the chronic exudative material.

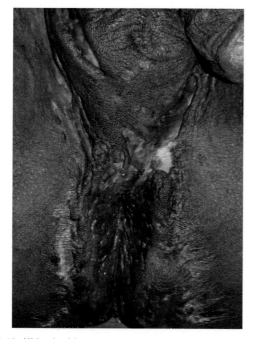

FIG. 8-12. Hidradenitis suppurativa is a disease well known to produce scarring, which can be severe.

which is not indicated, reveals a distended follicle with surrounding inflammation consisting of neutrophils, lymphocytes, and histiocytes. Abscesses form and destroy pilosebaceous units, with resulting granulation tissue and epithelialized sinus tracts.

Staphylococcal furunculosis is the disease most easily confused with hidradenitis suppurativa. However, furunculosis is usually not limited to the axillae and groin. In addition, furuncles resolve quickly and completely with antistaphylococcal antibiotics although recurrence after discontinuation of antibiotics is common. In addition, comedones are not seen in association with furunculosis. A solitary inflamed epidermal cyst can mimic mild hidradenitis and may, in fact, represent mild hidradenitis.

HIDRADENITIS SUPPURATIVA:	**Diagnosis**

- Morphology of inflamed nodules, comedones, scarring of genitalia and/or axillae; scrotum, vulva, crural creases, perianal skin; sometimes medial thighs and buttocks
- Location of the groin, buttocks, medial thighs, vulva, scrotum, lower abdomen, breast areas, and/ or axillae
- Chronicity
- Cultures that show normal skin flora or mixed bacteria;
- Incomplete response to antibiotics

Pathophysiology

Sometimes called inverse acne, or apocrine acne, hidradenitis suppurativa represents a foreign body inflammatory reaction to keratin within the dermis. The initial lesion is a comedone, in which the follicle is obstructed by keratin debris from desquamated stratum corneum of the follicular epithelium. This occurs primarily in those people who, as an inherited characteristic, exhibit follicles that have two or more rather than one outlet to the surface of the skin in areas containing apocrine glands. After the follicle is obstructed, it is then distended by keratin shed from deeper portions of the follicle to form an epidermal cyst. Eventually, the stretched, thin walls of the follicle rupture, allowing keratin to extrude into the surrounding dermis and to produce an inflammatory reaction.

Cultures often reveal multiple organisms, and although some physicians believe that bacteria play a pathogenic role, others believe that these organisms act as irritants. Clearly, lesions sometimes become secondarily infected.

Hormonal influence plays a role as well, with hidradenitis rarely occurring before puberty and often flaring premenstrually and postpartum.

Management

Weight loss can be helpful in many patients, and discontinuation of smoking is important.

Although incision and drainage of tense, fluctuant lesions make the patient more comfortable, this approach provides only temporary improvement of individual lesions. The intralesional injection of triamcinolone acetonide 3 mg/mL into acutely inflamed nodules can produce marked, although temporary, improvement.

Oral antibiotics with direct anti-inflammatory effects can inhibit the appearance of new nodules. These antibiotics include tetracycline 500 mg, erythromycin 500 mg, doxycycline or minocycline 100 mg, clindamycin 150 mg, or double-strength trimethoprim-sulfamethoxazole, all prescribed to be taken twice daily on a long-term basis. More recently, the combination of clindamycin and rifampin has been reported to be beneficial (6,7).

For those who do not improve adequately after several months with an antibiotic, surgical removal of the affected skin should be considered when practical and has the highest cure rate (8). The removal of apocrine gland-containing skin is curative. Excision is the most common mode of removal, but hidradenitis suppurativa occurring in the groin can be too extensive for excision. Alternatives include carbon dioxide laser ablation with healing by secondary intention, excision of only the most involved areas, and excision of individual fistulas (8).

Women with hidradenitis sometimes derive benefit from hormonal therapy. High-estrogen oral contraceptives such as those with ethinyl estradiol 0.035 mg or higher and antiandrogens such a spironolactone can sometimes be useful.

Many patients' disease is not controlled with the foregoing measures. More recently, marked improvement of hidradenitis suppurativa has been reported with tumor necrosis factor alpha (TNF-α) antagonists such as infliximab (9), etanercept (10,11), and adalimumab (12). These extremely expensive medications are approved by the Food and Drug Administration for rheumatoid arthritis and psoriasis. Although infliximab must be given by intravenous infusion, etanercept and adalimumab are self-administered at home, with minimal monitoring. These medications may well become the treatment of choice in the future if early experience is confirmed.

Other therapies that have been used include oral retinoids, such as isotretinoin, which are primarily used for cystic acne of the face and trunk. Although a 4- to 5-month course of isotretinoin normally induces long-term remission of acne, incomplete clearing and prompt relapse of hidradenitis suppurativa is usual (13).

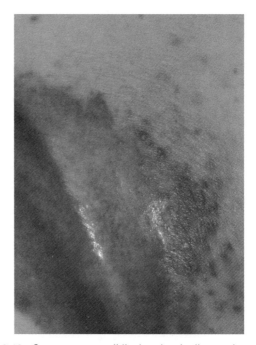

FIG. 8-13. Cutaneous candidiasis classically produces red plaques with peripheral pustules and erosions.

HIDRADENITIS SUPPURATIVA:	Management

- Mild disease (often, multiple concomitant medications)
  - oral anti-inflammatory antibiotics: doxycycline or minocycline 100 mg b.i.d., clindamycin 150 mg b.i.d., trimethoprim-sulfamethoxazole double strength b.i.d.
  - High-estrogen oral contraceptives (women)
  - Spironolactone 50 to 200 mg as anti-androgen (women)
  - Topical anti-inflammatory antibiotics: clindamycin or erythromycin solution twice a day.
  - Antiperspirants
- Severe disease
  - Excision of affected skin: total excision or individual cysts
  - TNF-α antagonists – etanercept, adalimumab, infliximab

Mucocutaneous Candidiasis (see also Chapter 15)

Clinical Presentation

Cutaneous candidiasis occurs in women with severe vaginal candidiasis, but more often in individuals who are overweight, diabetic, and/or incontinent so that there is a warm, wet environment. Immunosuppression can be a major factor.

Although cutaneous candidiasis classically presents as a red plaque with surrounding satellite pustules,

pustules actually are observed only rarely (Figs. 8-13 and 8-14). The extremely superficial nature of the pustules and the fragile character of the modified mucous membrane that covers part of the external genitalia result in early rupture of pustules. Therefore, the usual morphology is that of superficial collarettes or round erosions surrounding the typical intertriginous red plaque.

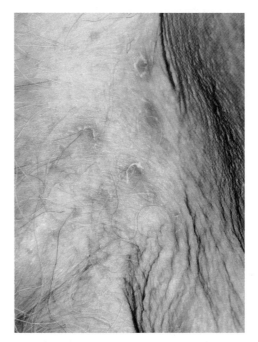

FIG. 8-14. Despite the initial lesion of a pustule, the pustule roof of *Candida albicans* is extremely fragile, so desquamation is more prominent than pustules.

Candida vaginitis usually accompanies the skin disease in women. In men, intertriginous candidiasis presents with red, well-demarcated, polycyclic plaques in the crural crease, and multiple satellite l- to 3-mm papulo-pustules, erosions, or collarettes at the periphery. Eventually, the disease may spread to the scrotum and the proximal, medial thighs. Uncircumcised men often develop balanitis or balanoposthitis with flat, delicate, white-yellow, discrete 1-mm pustules, and surface erosions on the glans penis.

Diagnosis

The diagnosis of candidiasis is confirmed by direct microscopic examination of the skin scrapings or purulent exudate, using potassium hydroxide. A fungal culture may be performed from skin pustules as well as vaginal secretions to confirm candidal infection. Because the diagnosis of candidiasis can be confirmed by a microscopic examination of skin scrapings, a biopsy is not indicated. However, histology shows a subcorneal pustule although some pustules are spongiform, showing also basophilic hyphae with a periodic acid–Schiff stain within the upper layers of the epithelium.

The differential diagnosis includes psoriasis, seborrheic dermatitis, tinea cruris, and folliculitis. Intertrigo dermatitis can mimic and coexist with candidiasis.

CANDIDIASIS: **Diagnosis**

- Morphology of red intertriginous plaques with satellite pustules, collarettes, or papules
- Confirmed by microscopic fungal preparation or culture

Pathophysiology

Candidiasis is a superficial yeast infection that occurs on mucosal and cutaneous surfaces (see Chapters 3 and 15 for primary discussion). Although there are several pathogenic species of *Candida*, *Candida albicans* is by far the most likely to affect the external genitalia and produce pustules or crusting.

Management

Maceration and exudation are initially managed with cool soaks. Tap water is adequate for this, with no allergens or irritants. Although topical azoles such as miconazole, clotrimazole, terconazole, econazole, and ketoconazole are the most commonly prescribed anti-candidal agents, those patients who exhibit pustules, erosions, or crusting may experience local irritation or maceration with these topical, alcohol-containing creams. Fluconazole 150 mg once is the only oral medication that has indication approval by the United

States Food and Drug Administration for the treatment of vulvovaginal candidiasis. Patients with prominent involvement of keratinized skin may require more than single-dose therapy, and 100 mg daily for several days until the skin is clear or healed sufficiently so that a topical therapy can be substituted is a common regimen. This oral medication avoids the problem of local irritation and stinging, as well as exacerbation of maceration from agents that add moisturization. Those patients without excessive exudation and erosion can also be treated effectively and comfortably with nystatin, which is available in a nonirritating ointment base if the cream stings. Acute inflammation and pruritus can be rapidly improved by the addition of topical hydrocortisone ointment 1% or 2.5% twice daily for the first 2 or 3 days.

Treatment of recurrent intertriginous candidiasis requires drying of the skin by minimizing occlusion, applying drying antifungal powders, and separating skin folds of obese patients with soft cloth. Oral fluconazole given weekly can also help to control this problem in those with recalcitrant disease (14). Once clear, antiperspirants help to maintain dryness in skin folds.

Cutaneous anogenital candidiasis is often recurrent, since common underlying risk factors of obesity, incontinence, and diabetes are difficult to control. The time-honored prevention of lactobacilli administered by mouth or, sometimes, by insertion into the vagina to control recurrent disease has not shown proven benefit (15).

CANDIDIASIS: **Management**

- Mild disease
  - any topical azole (clotrimazole, miconazole, terconazole, ketoconazole, etc.) once or twice daily
  - topical terbinafine twice daily
  - nystatin cream or ointment four times daily
- Exudative or eroded candidiasis
  - oral fluconazole or itraconazole 100 to 200 mg daily until clear

---

Pustular Psoriasis

Psoriasis is a disease that exhibits several very disparate morphologies. This disease is discussed primarily in Chapter 6; the pathogenesis and therapies are similar for all varieties of psoriasis.

Clinical Presentation

Pustular psoriasis occurs when the neutrophilic histologic inflammation is sufficiently marked as to aggregate into clinically apparent, small abscesses, changing the morphologic character from the classic red, scaling, well-demarcated plaques into plaques of pustules. Pustular psoriasis occurs in two broad categories: a localized form that is sometimes disabling and may run a chronic course and an acute, generalized form associated with constitutional symptoms. The form of pustular psoriasis most likely to produce diagnostic and therapeutic problems in the genital area is localized disease, because generalized psoriasis usually provides more clues to the diagnosis and requires systemic therapy that incidentally clears the genital area.

Localized pustular psoriasis frequently occurs on the palms and soles, sometimes accompanied by genital involvement. Crops of pustules within well-demarcated red plaques occur, but these rupture quickly to produce well-demarcated, coalescing erosions with scale or crust (Fig. 8-15).

Generalized pustular psoriasis is characterized by more widespread, confluent, red psoriatic plaques covered with pustules that rupture to form scale or crust. Severe generalized pustular psoriasis can be a life-threatening disease, accompanied by weakness, leukocytosis, weight loss, myalgias, fevers, chills, and hypocalcemia. Within red skin, pinpoint pustules appear in clusters and become confluent lakes of yellow pus. Lesions are accentuated in the flexural and anogenital regions and are accompanied by burning and tenderness.

Genital pustular psoriasis of either form is manifested by crops of superficial, subcorneal pustules that generally rupture immediately, leaving round, coalescing erosions and collarettes. Individual pustules or collarettes are about 1 to 10 mm in diameter. On dry, keratinized skin, ruptured pustules become plaques of crust with yellow scale (Fig. 8-15). Macerated lesions also occur on the glans of the uncircumcised penis, whereas scaling occurs on the circumcised glans. On occasion, arcuate white/yellow papules occur on the glans, mimicking balanitis circinata of the very closely related disease, Reiter syndrome (16). In skin folds, red plaques occur, with satellite papules and pustules that mimic Candidiasis (Figs. 8-16 and 8-17).

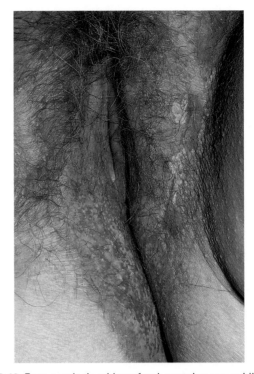

FIG. 8-16. Even psoriasis without frank pustules can exhibit red plaques with macerated yellow-white epithelium suggestive of Candida infection.

Psoriasis is associated with obesity, anxiety and depression, alcoholism, arthritis, and metabolic syndrome, particularly in those individuals who exhibit widespread or severe disease (17,18).

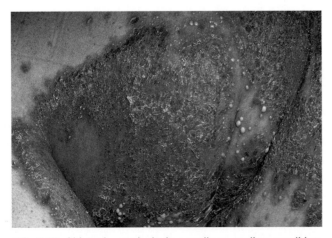

FIG. 8-15. Although psoriasis is usually a scaling condition, intensely inflammatory pustular psoriasis is manifested by well-demarcated plaques with scale or crust and pustules. This morphology can be nearly indistinguishable from cutaneous candidiasis.

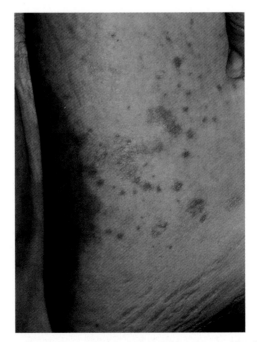

FIG. 8-17. This patient with psoriasis exhibits plaques identical to Candida. Negative culture and poor response to therapy prompted a biopsy that showed the correct diagnosis of psoriasis.

Diagnosis

The diagnosis is usually suspected from the clinical appearance, and it is confirmed by microscopic smears and cultures that are negative for infection, and by biopsy. A biopsy shows neutrophils that collect in the tips of the papillary dermis and migrate into the epidermis to form spongiform degeneration with numerous neutrophils. Neutrophilic abscesses collect just under the stratum corneum. Psoriasiform acanthosis is usual in developed disease.

Localized pustular psoriasis must be distinguished from Reiter disease, tinea cruris with pustular follicular involvement, impetigo, and acute candidiasis. At times, localized pustular psoriasis cannot be distinguished from the very closely related Reiter disease. The skin lesions are identical clinically and histologically, and differentiation rests with the more common occurrence of arthritis, inflammatory eye changes, and urethritis in patients with Reiter syndrome. However, these abnormalities can occur with pustular psoriasis as well, and these closely related diseases exist on a spectrum. Acute exanthematous pustular dermatosis is morphologically identical to generalized pustular psoriasis, but it occurs acutely in response to medication, usually an antibiotic. Subcorneal pustular dermatosis resembles pustular psoriasis and may, in fact, be a form of psoriasis. Discrete larger pustules with "lakes of pus" that exhibit a fluid-pus level characterize subcorneal pustular dermatosis.

Tinea cruris with follicular involvement and candidiasis can be differentiated by the identification of fungal organisms on microscopic smears or culture and by complete resolution with therapy. Impetigo is less symmetric and much less inflammatory, and it does not affect the modified mucous membranes of the vulva. A pustular drug eruption is a generalized eruption, an extremely rare condition that is morphologically and histologically indistinguishable from generalized pustular psoriasis. The explosive onset of rash in association with recent institution of a possible offending medication suggests this diagnosis, and rapid improvement in the skin after discontinuation of the medication confirms the diagnosis of a pustular drug eruption. Chronic generalized pustular psoriasis generally does not exhibit prominent pustules but rather generalized erythema and exudation. This form of psoriasis can be confused with any cause of exfoliative erythroderma, especially when it is superinfected. This includes generalized eczema, a medication reaction, and cutaneous T-cell lymphoma.

PUSTULAR PSORIASIS: **Diagnosis**

- Identification of red plaques of superficial pustules, crusting, scale, and collarettes
- Negative microscopic examinations and cultures
- Confirmed by the identification of classic extragenital lesions, such as pustular plaques of the hands and feet, otherwise;
- Biopsy

Pathophysiology

The underlying cause of psoriasis is unknown although immunologic and hereditary factors play a role (see also Chapter 3). Acute precipitating factors include various drugs such as corticosteroids, TNF antagonists (19), diltiazem, lithium, nonsteroidal anti-inflammatory medications, β-blockers, terbinafine, and hydroxychloroquine. Acute infections such as dental and upper respiratory infections, and the chronic infection of acquired immunodeficiency syndrome (AIDS) are also well known to trigger psoriasis. Pregnancy is associated with the onset of psoriasis in some patients.

Management

The presence of superimposed infection should be investigated at the outset, because specific therapy for psoriasis is often immunosuppressive and can exacerbate unrecognized and untreated infection. In addition, those patients with extremely inflamed, exudative disease often benefit from prophylactic oral antimicrobial therapy until the skin begins to improve. Fluconazole 150 mg/week, as well as twice-daily administration of a broad-spectrum antibiotic such as cephalexin, generally prevents secondary infections as topical corticosteroid therapy is added.

Patients with localized, mild disease can be treated with a mid-potency or high-potency topical corticosteroid such as triamcinolone 0.1% or fluocinonide 0.05% with a variable measure of prompt improvement. However, satisfactory and long-lasting benefit of significant pustular psoriasis from topical corticosteroids is rare, and specific systemic therapy is generally required. Topical calcipotriene (Dovonex) cream and calcipotriol (Vectical) ointment, applied twice a day, can improve the skin, and the combination medication calcipotriene and betamethasone dipropionate ointment applied daily can be useful. Other standard antipsoriasis topical therapies including tars, retinoids, and anthralin are too irritating for use in the genital area.

There are several systemic therapies for pustular psoriasis. These medications are quite effective, but because they exhibit important adverse reactions, they should be used only with great care and by physicians knowledgeable about their use and necessary monitoring. Acitretin (Soriatane) is an oral aromatic retinoid that is very useful for many patients with erythrodermic or pustular psoriasis (20). This medication often produces rapid cessation of new pustules with substantial clearing of the skin within a few weeks. However, this potent medication has several major adverse reactions. It is a formidable teratogen that can be stored for years in body fat if it is ingested with alcohol. In addition, retinoids raise serum triglyceride levels and sometimes produce exostoses that can even progress to ankylosis of the vertebrae. More common and sometimes incapacitating symptoms are skin fragility, dryness, and arthralgias. The usual dose of acitretin is 0.5 to 1.0 mg/kg/day, generally given as 25 to 50 mg once a day.

Methotrexate is a folic acid analog that usually is very effective for pustular psoriasis. It has the advantage over acitretin of improving rather than exacerbating arthritis. This antimetabolite has potent acute bone marrow toxicity, and it can produce fibrosing liver disease when it is given on a long-term basis. Nausea and phototoxicity occur at times. Methotrexate is contraindicated in pregnant or lactating women and in patients with cirrhosis, alcohol abuse, chronic renal failure, hepatitis or other liver disease, psychiatric illness, or in patients with disorders of platelets, white blood cells, or red blood cells.

Systemic corticosteroids produce a fast and dramatic improvement in disease, but the withdrawal of corticosteroids can precipitate a flare of the disease (21). Therefore, this medication is used with care, and the patient is advised of this possibility. Cyclosporine is approved for the treatment of psoriasis as well, and this is a good medication for quick improvement. However, potential nephrotoxicity dictates that this agent be reserved for severe, recalcitrant disease or to gain temporary control while safer but slower therapy is begun. Newer biologic therapies including infliximab, etanercept, and adalimumab are immunosuppressive medications with potent effects on psoriasis, although there are several reports of flaring of psoriasis with these medications (19).

Ultraviolet B light or ultraviolet A light in combination with the photosensitizing medication psoralen is not particularly useful for genital psoriasis, in which exposure to light is not practical. In addition, ultraviolet light is associated with an increase in penile carcinoma.

Generalized pustular psoriasis sometimes is a life-threatening disease. Patients who are toxic should be hospitalized for supportive care including, at times, cardiac monitoring, antibiotic therapy, and fluid and electrolyte replacement. A complete chemistry profile is indicated because abnormally low levels of calcium, albumin, and zinc levels can occur.

PUSTULAR PSORIASIS: **Management**

- Mild disease
  - topical corticosteroid ointment and/or
  - topical calcipotriol ointment
- Moderate to severe disease
  - oral acitretin, methotrexate, or cyclosporine and/or
  - the biologics: infliximab, etanercept, adalimumab

Reiter Syndrome

Reiter syndrome is an uncommon triad of conjunctivitis, nongonococcal urethritis, and oligoarthritis that is often associated with skin lesions identical to those of pustular psoriasis (see also Chapter 15).

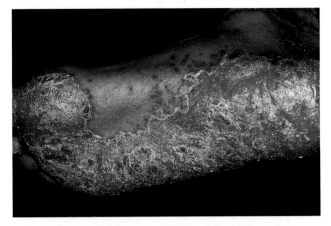

FIG. 8-18. The genital disease of Reiter syndrome is generally accompanied by keratoderma blennorrhagica, well-demarcated red, scale or crust of the palms and soles.

Clinical Presentation

Reiter syndrome is a condition that predominately affects men in a ratio of 20:1. This occurs most often in those who are human leukocyte antigen (HLA)-B27 positive, and it is diagnosed most often in the third decade.

Reiter syndrome is defined as noninfectious arthritis, urethritis, and conjunctivitis of at least 1 month's duration. However, most patients with Reiter syndrome initially present without all these features (incomplete Reiter syndrome), and the picture becomes complete over time. Skin lesions are morphologically indistinguishable from those of psoriasis. Patients with Reiter syndrome present with well-demarcated, red, scaly, crusted, or pustular papules or plaques on the palms and soles and on dry, hair-bearing, keratinized genital skin. As palm and sole plaques become chronic, hyperkeratosis occurs, resulting in the typical lesions of keratoderma blennorrhagicum (Fig. 8-18).

The uncircumcised glans penis typically shows circinate balanitis, with white, circinate, well-demarcated papules and superficial red erosions (Fig. 8-19). In the rare case of Reiter syndrome in women, the hydrated skin of the labia minora and vestibule can exhibit similar erosions or white solid, annular, or arcuate papules (Fig. 8-20). Hair-bearing vulvar skin and the dry skin of the penis exhibit well-demarcated, crusted, red, scaly papules, and plaques. Other genitourinary features include urethritis, prostatitis, seminal vesiculitis, hemorrhagic cystitis, and urethral stricture. The cervix may demonstrate white, arcuate, interlacing papules.

The arthritis of Reiter syndrome is an asymmetric arthritis of the large, weight-bearing joints such as the back, knee, or ankle. Heel pain from inflammation at the insertion of the Achilles tendon is also characteristic. Patients may develop anterior uveitis, conjunctivitis, and iritis necessitating close ophthalmologic management.

Diagnosis

A high degree of suspicion is required to make the diagnosis of Reiter syndrome, because patients usually do

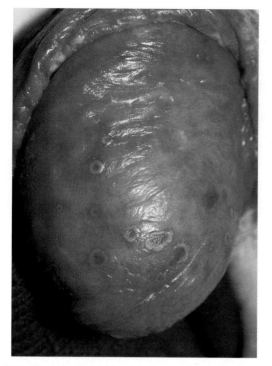

FIG. 8-19. Circinate balanitis of Reiter syndrome is manifested by annular yellow-white papules on glans of uncircumcised male patients.

not develop all the defining clinical features at the outset. The American Rheumatism Association adopted the diagnostic criteria of peripheral arthritis of more than 1 month's duration in association with urethritis and/or cervicitis and inflammatory eye disease. Infectious causes of

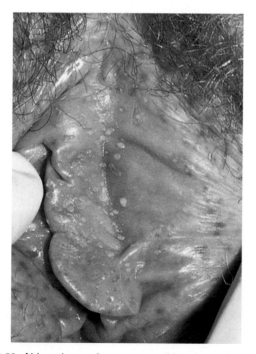

FIG. 8-20. Although rare in women, solid and annular yellow-white papules of the vulva are nearly indistinguishable from lesions of circinate balanitis.

symptoms, especially gonorrhea, must be ruled out. Radiographs of joints can show periarticular osteoporosis and enthesopathy, a combination of erosions around the insertion of tendons and ligaments, bone lucency, and new bone formation to include spurs. Serum studies for HLA typing typically reveal the presence of the HLA-B27 antigen in patients with Reiter syndrome. The histologic features of an established lesion are analogous to those of pustular psoriasis. The stratum corneum is thick and parakeratotic, and there is psoriasiform hyperplasia of the underlying epidermis. Neutrophils collect in the papillary dermis, migrate into the epidermis, and form subcorneal abscesses. In addition, underlying chronic dermal inflammation is usual.

The skin diseases to be differentiated from Reiter syndrome are candidiasis and pustular psoriasis. Psoriasis is a closely related disease that exists on a spectrum with Reiter syndrome, and these two diseases cannot always be distinguished. The diagnosis cannot be made from skin lesions alone, and the clinician must follow the American Rheumatism Association diagnostic criteria. *Candida* can be eliminated by culture or microscopic smear, as well as by nonresponse to therapy. Tinea cruris, impetigo, and superinfected eczema can also be occasionally confused with the genital lesions of Reiter syndrome.

REITER SYNDROME:	**Diagnosis**

- Identification of red plaques of superficial pustules, scale, crusting on hands, feet, and genitalia; uncircumcised glans penis with annular, white, coalescing papules
- Accompanying chronic arthritis, conjunctivitis, urethritis, or cervicitis. Negative microscopic examinations and cultures
- Confirmed by characteristic biopsy when required

Pathophysiology

Reiter syndrome results from a reactive immune response that is triggered in a genetically susceptible individual (22). The most common infections reported to precipitate Reiter syndrome are with those organisms that cause dysentery or urethritis such as *Yersinia enterocolitica, Shigella flexneri, Neisseria gonorrhoeae, Chlamydia trachomatis, Ureaplasma urealyticum, Campylobacter fetus,* and, more recently, *Borrelia burgdorferi* and HIV. It is not known whether HIV directly provokes the disease or whether the immune changes associated with the human immunodeficiency syndrome causes an individual to become more susceptible to Reiter syndrome.

Reiter syndrome and pustular psoriasis share many common features and exist on a spectrum. Reiter syndrome has occasionally been reported to be familial, and HLA-B27 positivity is common.

Management

Reiter syndrome is a chronic and difficult disease to treat. It is of foremost importance to treat any precipitating underlying infection. All patients should be tested for HIV and *Chlamydia*, which are the most notable infectious agents. When diarrhea is present, the stool should be cultured and evaluated for those organisms known to precipitate Reiter syndrome and produce diarrhea. It is recommended that vaginal secretions and white adherent lesions be cultured for yeast or examined by potassium hydroxide microscopically to rule out a superimposed candidal infection.

Methotrexate is a treatment of choice for both Reiter syndrome and pustular psoriasis, especially if there is an arthritis component (see earlier). Oral acitretin also produces excellent results. However, it often exacerbates arthritis, and it is a teratogen that should be avoided in women of childbearing potential.

REITER SYNDROME:	Management

- Mild disease
  - topical corticosteroid ointment
- Moderate to severe disease
  - oral methotrexate or cyclosporine, or
  - the biologics, infliximab, etanercept, adalimumab

Subcorneal Pustular Dermatosis (Sneddon–Wilkinson Disease)

Subcorneal pustular dermatosis is a rare skin disease of unknown origin characterized by very superficial pustules containing neutrophils.

Clinical Presentation

Found primarily in middle-aged or older women, subcorneal pustular dermatosis is characterized by discrete fragile pustules that are primarily truncal, with a strong predilection for the skin folds, including the neck, inframammary skin, axillae, and crural creases. Purulent material fills these very fragile pustules, creating a pus-fluid level. Because the pustule is located just below the stratum corneum, the roof is easily denuded, and the resulting lesion may be simply a collarette (Fig. 8-21). Itching and pain are not remarkable.

Diagnosis

The diagnosis is made by morphology, by biopsy, and by culture to rule out bullous impetigo. Histologically, pustules containing neutrophils and occasional eosinophils and mononuclear cells are identified just beneath the

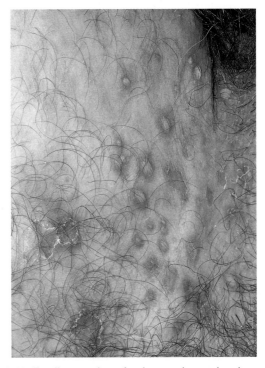

FIG. 8-21. Fragile pustules of subcorneal pustular dermatosis quickly erode, leaving fine collarettes overlying intact epithelium.

stratum corneum that overlies fairly normal epidermis. Neutrophils can be seen migrating upward through this epidermis, and there is a perivascular neutrophilic infiltrate that may contain occasional eosinophils. Sometimes, direct immunofluorescent studies show immunoglobulins, especially IgA, in these patients in the intercellular spaces of the epidermis. Other diseases to be considered include pemphigus foliaceus and pustular psoriasis.

SUBCORNEAL PUSTULAR DERMATOSIS:	Diagnosis

- Identification of fragile, superficial pustules in skin folds, including the crural creases, with collarettes
- Negative microscopic examinations and cultures for yeast
- Characteristic biopsy showing subcorneal pustule with neutrophils, some of which are migrating through the epidermis. There is a perivascular neutrophilic infiltrate that may contain occasional eosinophils.

Pathophysiology

The nature of subcorneal pustular dermatosis is not known. Some physicians have postulated this disease to represent a form of pustular psoriasis, and others believe this is a form of immunoglobulin A (IgA) pemphigus.

Many patients develop monoclonal gammopathies, especially with IgA and lymphoproliferative disorders, particularly myeloma. Also, this disease is sometimes associated with autoimmune diseases such as rheumatoid arthritis. Subcorneal pustular dermatosis probably contains several subgroups of patient with different etiologies.

Management

First-line treatment is dapsone, 50 to 200 mg/day, and other sulfonamides can be tried in nonresponding patients. Oral corticosteroids, oral retinoids, and ultraviolight therapy have also been reported useful. Most recently, the biologic agents TNF-α antagonists have been shown in case reports to be effective in some (23,24).

SUBCORNEAL PUSTULAR DERMATOSIS:	Management

- Dapsone 50 to 200 mg per day, otherwise
  - oral corticosteroids
  - retinoids acitretin, isotretinoin

Bullous Impetigo

Bullous impetigo consists of flaccid blisters or pustules resulting from a toxin produced by some types of *S. aureus*. Although impetigo can occur on any area of the body, the warmth and moisture of the genital area and proximal thighs provide an especially favorable environment for this disease.

The individual lesions are extremely fragile so, as in subcorneal pustular dermatosis, collarettes are frequently the primary lesion noted (Fig. 8-22). Bullous impetigo most closely resembles subcorneal pustular dermatosis, but the correct diagnosis is made by a culture showing *S. aureus*. Treatment consists of antibiotic therapy. Very limited disease can be treated topically with mupirocin cream or ointment, but otherwise an antistaphylococcal antibiotic is required, keeping in mind that *S. aureus* often is now resistant to historically effective antibiotics such as cephalexin, dicloxacillin, and erythromycin. Culture is

now important, with clindamycin and trimethoprim-sulfamethoxazole often as better choices.

SOLID LESIONS THAT SOMETIMES APPEAR PUSTULAR

Keratosis Pilaris

Keratosis pilaris is a common condition consisting of superficial keratin plugs occurring primarily on the lateral arms and buttocks (see Chapter 12 for full discussion). However, the anterior thighs and even the cheeks are sometimes affected. This problem is generally asymptomatic, but it produces a rough, sandpapery texture to the skin. Most often, individual lesions are small, skin-colored, acuminate papules (Fig. 8-23). However, associated follicular erythema occurs in some patients, and this finding with an associated keratin plug sometimes resembles a pustule. In addition, patients sometimes experience significant secondary inflammation and actual pustules (Fig. 8-24).

Therapy is not needed, and it is unsatisfactory. Patients who want treatment for cosmetic reasons can soften keratin plugs by soaking in warm water, and they can subsequently scrub them out with an abrasive sponge. Lactic acid 12% lotion, salicylic lotions, or tretinoin

KERATOSIS PILARIS:	Diagnosis

- The identification of monomorphous, less than 1 mm acuminate skin-colored and sometimes red papules, sometimes with pustules or keratin plug resembling pustules
- Sandpapery texture
- Location on lateral upper arms; sometimes on buttocks, anterior thighs, face

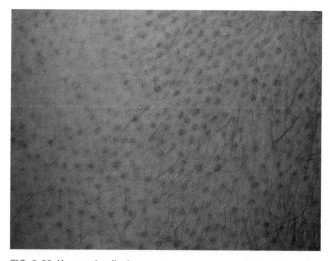

FIG. 8-23. Keratosis pilaris appears as monomorphous pink, skin-colored, or yellowish, rough papules with a sandpapery texture.

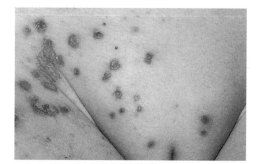

FIG. 8-22. The superficial blisters of impetigo rupture almost immediately leaving yellow crusts and superficial erosions.

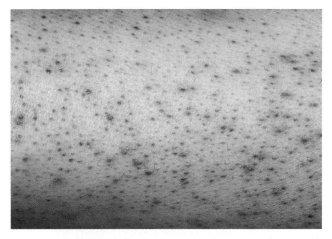

FIG. 8-24. Follicular inflammation sometimes associated with keratosis pilaris is manifested by red papules with occasional crusts and pustules.

Keratosis Pilaris:	**Management**

- No therapy needed, but when desired, mechanical removal of keratin plugs by
  - tub soaks to soften keratin plugs, followed by scrubs with loofah, or
  - lactic acid or salicylic acid containing over-the-counter lotions to dissolve plugs, or
  - tretinoin cream 0.025% to loosen plugs

cream 0.025% may help to dissolve these plugs in some patients, but these can also be irritating.

Fordyce Spots (Ectopic Sebaceous Glands)

Clinical Presentation

Numerous ectopic sebaceous glands appear on the medial aspect of the labia minora and less commonly on the lateral surface of the labia minora, the labia majora, the prepuce of the clitoris, or the prepuce and the shaft of the penis. They appear as pinpoint, lobular, and/or flat, irregular, yellowish to skin-colored papules that may be discrete or confluent (Fig. 8-25). The abundance of large sebaceous glands, called Fordyce condition, is a normal variant and is asymptomatic, although this finding was once believed to produce pruritus.

Diagnosis

The diagnosis is made on the basis of the location and the morphologic appearance. A biopsy is rarely necessary. If Fordyce spots are examined by biopsy inadvertently, histology reveals enlarged but normal sebaceous glands. Normally, sebaceous glands are associated with and secrete into hair follicles, yet on the labia minora where hairs are scant, they open freely on the surface.

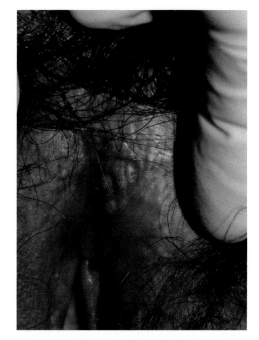

FIG. 8-25. Enlarged sebaceous glands appear as lobular, yellowish papules.

Fordyce spots may be easily confused with condylomata acuminata, tiny epidermal cysts or milia, and mollusca contagiosa. Unlike warts, Fordyce spots are yellowish rather than skin-colored and are distributed symmetrically. Milia are usually more white than yellow, fewer in number, and firmer. In addition, unlike milia, individual Fordyce spots are often subtly multilobular. Mollusca contagiosa are more discrete, less symmetrical, shiny, and more nodular and dome-shaped.

Pathophysiology

These ectopic sebaceous glands are normal structures, but the larger size may be related to hormonal influences. Visible Fordyce spots on the female genitalia rarely occur before puberty or following the climacteric.

Management

Ectopic sebaceous glands are a normal anatomic variant, and medical or surgical treatment is unwarranted.

Molluscum Contagiosum (see also Chapters 11 and 12 for full discussion)

Clinical Presentation

This highly infectious disease is found in two major populations: young children and young sexually active individuals. Children exhibit lesions on any skin surface, but when occurring on the genitalia, lesions do not imply sexual contact. Mollusca contagiosa of adults is most often a sexually transmitted disease, with lesions found primarily on the vulva, penis, scrotum, proximal, medial

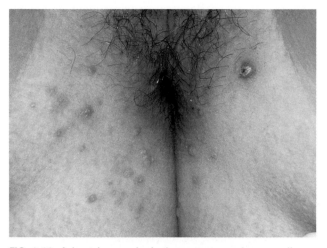

FIG. 8-26. A host immunological response produces mollusca that are red and pustular.

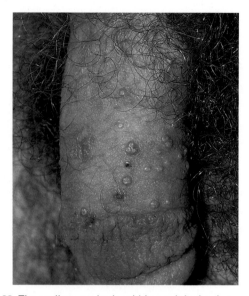

FIG. 8-28. The molluscum body within each lesion is sometimes visible as white or yellowish lobular nodules.

thighs, and perineal skin. Individual mollusca are usually skin-colored or white, dome-shaped papules, some with a tiny central depression. However, they can occasionally appear slightly yellow or even become inflamed and frankly pustular (Figs. 8-26 through 8-28). Although mollusca contagiosa are generally asymptomatic, inflamed, pustular lesions are often pruritic.

Diagnosis

The diagnosis is usually made on the basis of the clinical appearance, but when the diagnosis is not clear, a microscopic examination of a curetted lesion with Tzanck's

smear usually demonstrates the typical Henderson–Patterson inclusion bodies, also called molluscum bodies. Mollusca contagiosa can mimic tumors, Fordyce spots, milia, or genital warts. When inflamed, mollusca can be confused with folliculitis, but the usual presence of surrounding, typical lesions generally indicates the diagnosis.

MOLLUSCUM CONTAGIOSUM:	**Diagnosis**

- Identification of white, skin-colored dome-shaped, shiny nodules, usually some with a central dell; at times, some lesions become inflamed and pustular
- When required, curettage reveals a molluscum body, a white core with a characteristic appearance microscopically

Pathophysiology

Molluscum contagiosum is caused by a DNA poxvirus. Cellular immunodeficiency as seen in AIDS is associated with recrudescent, large, recalcitrant lesions (see Chapter 16).

Management

Mollusca contagiosa in an immunocompetent person resolves spontaneously. The presence of pustular lesions can indicate a host immunological response to the infection with imminent eradication of the virus. Otherwise, cryotherapy (25), curettage (26) podophyllin resin, podofilox, trichloroacetic acid (27), cantharidin (28,29), and salicylic acid preparations have been used successfully (30). Imiquimod has been reported to be beneficial as

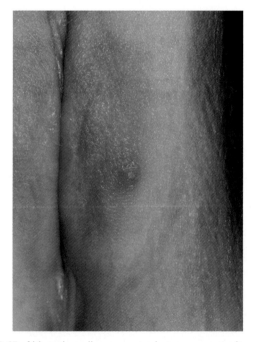

FIG. 8-27. Although mollusca contagiosa are most often skin-colored and may mimic vesicles, they can precipitate an immune response that produces inflamed and pustular lesions.

well (25,30). Even pulse-dye laser has been reported as useful (31). Many clinicians believe that daily application of tretinoin cream 0.05% helps to minimize recurrences and gradually eliminate small lesions.

MOLLUSCUM CONTAGIOSUM:	Management

- Options include
  - no treatment as these are self-resolving, especially in children
  - physical removal with curettage or needle
  - physical destruction by cryotherapy, cantharidin, or trichloroacetic acid
  - imiquimod topically as immune-enhancer

Epidermal Cysts

Epidermal cysts, sometimes erroneously called sebaceous cysts, are extremely common on the labia majora and scrotum (see also Chapters 11 and 12). Epidermal cysts arise from hair follicles that become obstructed and distended with keratin. The hydrated keratin within the cyst gives the lesion its white-yellow color (Figs. 8-29 and 8-30). This hydrated keratin is a tallowy, cheesy, crumbly, malodorous material. Many of these cysts demonstrate a follicular opening that manifests as a small punctum or black dot centrally on the surface of the cyst. If the cyst is traumatized, keratin leaks through its capsule of follicular epithelium into the dermis, thus producing a brisk inflammatory response. The nodule becomes painful and purulent as a result of this foreign body response rather than from infection (Fig. 8-31). Sometimes, especially on the modified mucous membranes of the vulva, multiple tiny

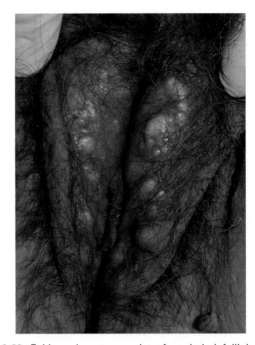

FIG. 8-30. Epidermal cysts consist of occluded follicles distended by an accumulation of keratin shed from the follicular epithelium. The keratin debris can appear yellow through the stretched and thinned overlying skin, and cysts sometimes become frankly pustular when ruptured and inflamed.

epidermal cysts (milia) occur and can be frequently and recurrently inflamed.

An inflamed epidermal cyst is most often confused with furunculosis, a deep follicular infection with *S. aureus*. However, an inflamed cyst is usually an isolated inflammatory lesion, and, unlike in bacterial furunculosis, erythema generally is limited to the nodule and does not

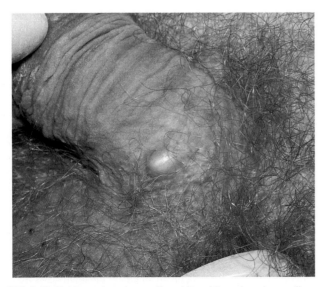

FIG. 8-29. Epidermal cysts can be white, skin-colored, or yellow, as seen on the shaft of this penis.

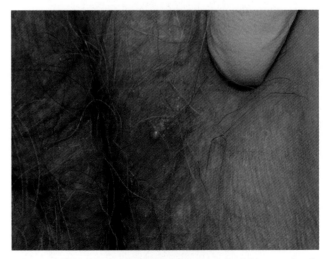

FIG. 8-31. This inflamed epidermal cyst of the labium majus is filled with purulent material, and it is of indistinguishable morphology from a furuncle: only the history of a longstanding preexisting nodule and a negative culture differentiate between these two diseases.

extend to surrounding skin. Multiple chronic or recurrently inflamed cysts represent hidradenitis suppurativa. Women with frequent inflammation of milia are easily misdiagnosed as having suppurative folliculitis.

Epidermal cysts do not require therapy except for cosmetic reasons or if there is inflammation. Inflamed cysts are best treated with 0.1 to 0.3 mL of triamcinolone acetonide, 3 to 5 mg/mL injected intralesionally before they become fluctuant. After they are fluctuant, incision and drainage can provide some comfort for the patient, but recurrence is common. Definitive therapy consists of excision, but cysts should not be excised while inflamed. When inflamed, cyst borders are indistinct and edematous, requiring a larger excision and more scarring than would occur in the absence of inflammation. Antibiotics are generally unhelpful acutely. However, patients with recurrently inflamed cyst nodules (hidradenitis suppurativa) or frequently inflamed milia benefit from the long-term administration of anti-inflammatory antibiotics such as twice-daily administered tetracycline or erythromycin 500 mg, doxycycline or minocycline 100 mg, clindamycin 150 mg, or double-strength trimethoprim-sulfamethoxazole.

Vestibular Cysts

Vestibular or mucous cysts of the vulva are relatively common cysts that arise from persistent urogenital sinus epithelium or from the obstruction of the minor vestibular glands (see also Chapter 9). Vestibular cysts are nodules, 2 mm to 2 cm, that can be skin-colored, yellow, or bluish (Fig. 8-32). Often, they are translucent, and, if

ruptured, these lesions emit clear mucus. These cysts are generally asymptomatic, although if large they can rarely cause dyspareunia or urinary tract obstruction. The diagnosis is usually made clinically, with the differential diagnosis primarily containing only other types of benign cysts. The differentiation of vestibular cysts from other local cysts is unimportant. Therapy is rarely necessary, but vestibular cysts can be surgically excised if they are symptomatic.

OTHER DISEASES THAT CAN APPEAR YELLOW OR PRODUCE CRUSTING

Any diseases that cause ulceration, erosion, or blistering can, when occurring on dry skin, cause crusting. These are generally the same diseases that produce erosions when occurring on more fragile mucous membrane epithelium, such as the vagina, or on modified mucous membrane, such as the glans penis and clinically nonhair-bearing skin of the vulva. Erosions on these epithelial surfaces often exhibit a yellow fibrin base.

HSV (see also Chapter 9) infections are usually classified as vesicular or erosive. However, like any vesicular eruption, this viral infection can exhibit a yellow morphology in several settings (Figs. 8-33 and 8-34). First, as vesicles on keratinized skin break, exudation and drying produce a yellow crust that can mimic impetigo. In addition, the vesicles of HSV infections often become secondarily cloudy when they occur on keratinized skin, where the skin is less fragile and vesicles do not quickly disintegrate. Finally, erosions on mucous membrane and modified mucous membrane skin frequently develop a yellowish coagulum at the base. Immunosuppressed patients are especially likely to acquire papular HSV infection, as adherent, coalescing papules of yellow fibrin form on erosions.

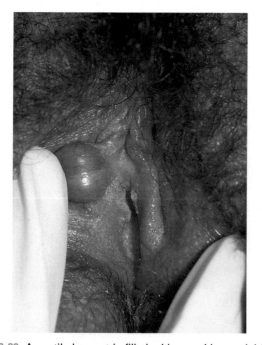

FIG. 8-32. A vestibular cyst is filled with mucoid material from vestibular glands and can appear yellow in some patients but skin-colored or bluish in others.

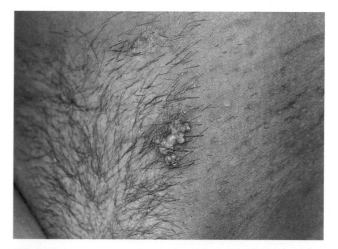

FIG. 8-33. Any blistering disease, including these vesicles from herpes simplex virus, appears pustular after they have been present for several days. However, piercing the blister reveals serous fluid rather than thick pus.

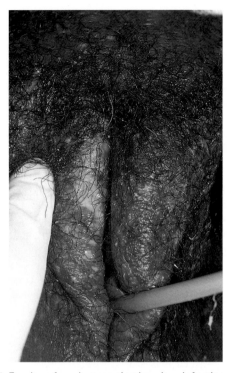

FIG. 8-34. Erosions from herpes simplex virus infection on a mucous membrane or modified mucous membrane typically leaves lesions with a nonspecific yellowish fibrin base that is indistinguishable from the appearance of erosions from any vesiculobullous disease.

The diagnosis of pustular HSV infection can usually be made by the small, uniform size of the pustules and by their grouped and fragile nature. The arcuate borders of erosions indicate the coalescing, blistering origins of the lesions and suggest a diagnosis of HSV infection. The diagnosis is confirmed by a viral culture. However, false-negative results are common, and polymerase chain reaction technique is not only the most sensitive diagnostic tool but now also cost effective. A biopsy from the edge of a lesion shows typical changes of a herpes blister, but HSV

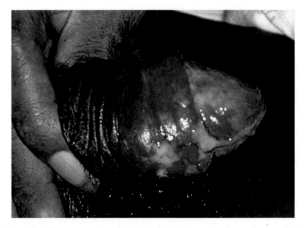

FIG. 8-35. The irregular and poorly demarcated erosions of this uncircumcised glans and prepuce are similar to the oral lesions of this patient with blistering erythema multiforme.

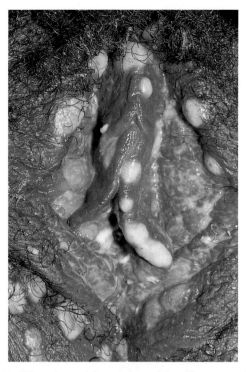

FIG. 8-36. Although condylomata lata of dry skin are manifested by flat-topped, skin-colored papules, these lesions of secondary syphilis on moist mucous membrane skin can leave thickened, yellow-white papules.

infection cannot be distinguished histologically from varicella-zoster virus infection.

Systemic courses of oral acyclovir, famciclovir, or valacyclovir are the mainstays of treatment for genital HSV infection.

Other common diseases that erode or blister in this area include bullous erythema multiforme, or Stevens–Johnson syndrome, a hypersensitivity reaction to either a medication or a recurrent HSV infection (Fig. 8-35). Aphthae frequently produce ulcers with a yellowish fibrin base. Blistering diseases such as impetigo, pemphigoid, and pemphigus vulgaris should sometimes be considered.

Condylomata lata (genital papules and plaques of secondary syphilis) can have a moist surface that appears yellowish white, although this condition is usually skin-colored when it occurs on dry skin (Fig. 8-36).

REFERENCES

1. Lorette G, Beaulieu P, Allaert FA, et al. Superficial community-acquired skin infections: prevalence of bacteria and antibiotic susceptibility in France. *J Eur Acad Dermatol Venereol.* 2009;23:1423–1426
2. Shapiro A, Raman S, Johnson M, et al. Community-acquired MRSA infections in North Carolina children: prevalence, antibiotic sensitivities, and risk factors. *N C Med J.* 2009; 70:102–107.

3. Stryjewski ME, Corey GR. New treatments for methicillin-resistant *Staphylococcus aureus*. *Curr Opin Crit Care*. 2009;15:403–412.

4. Sartorius K, Emtestam L, Jemec GB, et al. Objective scoring of hidradenitis suppurativa reflecting the role of tobacco smoking and obesity. *Br J Dermatol*. 2009;161:831–839.

5. Chandramohan K, Mathews A, Kurian A, et al. Squamous cell carcinoma rising from perineal lesion in a familial case of Hidradenitis suppurativa. *Int Wound J*. 2009;6:141–144.

6. Gener G, Canoui-Poitrine F, Revuz JE, et al. Combination therapy with clindamycin and rifampicin for hidradenitis suppurativa: a series of 116 consecutive patients. *Dermatology*. 2009;219:148–154.

7. van der Zee HH, Boer J, Prens EP, et al. The effect of combined treatment with oral clindamycin and oral rifampicin in patients with hidradenitis suppurativa. *Dermatology*. 2009;219:143–147.

8. Balik E, Eren T, Bulut T, et al. Surgical approach to extensive hidradenitis suppurativa in the perineal/perianal and gluteal regions. *World J Surg*. 2009;33:481–487.

9. Poulin Y. Successful treatment of hidradenitis suppurativa with infliximab in a patient who failed to respond to etanercept. *J Cutan Med Surg*. 2009;13:221–225.

10. Pelekanou A, Kanni T, Savva A, et al. Long-term efficacy of etanercept in hidradenitis suppurativa: results from an open-label phase II prospective trial. *Exp Dermatol*. 2009. Published on line September 16. [Epub ahead of print].

11. Lee RA, Dommasch E, Treat J, et al. A prospective clinical trial of open-label etanercept for the treatment of hidradenitis suppurativa. *J Am Acad Dermatol*. 2009;60:565–573.

12. Blanco R, Martínez-Taboada VM, Villa I, et al. Long-term successful adalimumab therapy in severe hidradenitis suppurativa. *Arch Dermatol*. 2009;145:580–584.

13. Soria A, Canoui-Poitrine F, Wolkenstein P, et al. Absence of efficacy of oral isotretinoin in hidradenitis suppurativa: a retrospective study based on patients' outcome assessment. *Dermatology*. 2009;218:134–135.

14. Sobel JD, Wiesenfeld HC, Martens M, et al. Maintenance fluconazole therapy for recurrent vulvovaginal candidiasis. *N Engl J Med*. 2004;351:876–883.

15. Witt A, Kaufmann U, Bitschnau M, et al. Monthly itraconazole versus classic homeopathy for the treatment of recurrent vulvovaginal candidiasis: a randomised trial. *BJOG*. 2009;116:1499–1505.

16. Singh N, Thappa DM. Circinate pustular psoriasis localized to glans penis mimicking 'circinate balanitis' and responsive to dapsone. *Indian J Dermatol Venereol Leprol*. 2008;74:388–389.

17. Ayala F. Clinical aspects and comorbidities of psoriasis. *J Rheumatol Suppl*. 2009;83:19–20.

18. Rallis E, Korfitis C, Stavropoulou E, et al. Clinical aspects and comorbidities of psoriasis. *J Rheumatol Suppl*. 2009;83:19–20.

19. Ko JM, Gottlieb AB, Kerbleski JF. Induction and exacerbation of psoriasis with TNF-blockade therapy: a review and analysis of 127 cases. *J Dermatolog Treat*. 2009;20:100–108.

20. Pang ML, Murase JE, Koo J. An updated review of acitretin—a systemic retinoid for the treatment of psoriasis. *Expert Opin Drug Metab Toxicol*. 2008;4:953–964.

21. Brenner M, Molin S, Ruebsam K, et al. Generalized pustular psoriasis induced by systemic glucocorticosteroids: four cases and recommendations for treatment. *Br J Dermatol*. 2009;161:964–966.

22. Sahlberg AS, Granfors K, Penttinen MA. HLA-B27 and host-pathogen interaction. *Adv Exp Med Biol*. 2009;649:235–244.

23. Berk DR, Hurt MA, Mann C, et al. Sneddon-Wilkinson disease treated with etanercept: report of two cases. *Clin Exp Dermatol*. 2009;34:347–351.

24. Voigtländer C, Lüftl M, Schuler G, et al. Infliximab (anti-tumor necrosis factor alpha antibody): a novel, highly effective treatment of recalcitrant subcorneal pustular dermatosis (Sneddon-Wilkinson disease). *Arch Dermatol*. 2001;137:1571–1574.

25. Al-Mutairi N, Al-Doukhi A, Al-Farag S, et al. Comparative study on the efficacy, safety, and acceptability of imiquimod 5% cream versus cryotherapy for molluscum contagiosum in children. *Pediatr Dermatol*. 2009. Published on line October 4. [Epub ahead of print].

26. Simonart T, De Maertelaer V. Curettage treatment for molluscum contagiosum: a follow-up survey study. *Br J Dermatol*. 2008;159:1144–1147.

27. Bard S, Shiman MI, Bellman B, et al. Treatment of facial molluscum contagiosum with trichloroacetic acid. *Pediatr Dermatol*. 2009;26:425–426.

28. Coloe J, Morrell DS. Cantharidin use among pediatric dermatologists in the treatment of molluscum contagiosum. *Pediatr Dermatol*. 2009;26:405–408.

29. Cathcart S, Coloe J, Morrell DS. Parental satisfaction, efficacy, and adverse events in 54 patients treated with cantharidin for molluscum contagiosum infection. *Clin Pediatr (Phila)*. 2009;48:161–165.

30. Hanna D, Hatami A, Powell J, et al. A prospective randomized trial comparing the efficacy and adverse effects of four recognized treatments of molluscum contagiosum in children. *Pediatr Dermatol*. 2006;23:574–579.

31. Binder B, Weger W, Komericki P, et al. Treatment of molluscum contagiosum with a pulsed dye laser: pilot study with 19 children. *J Dtsch Dermatol Ges*. 2008;6:121–125.

SUGGESTED READINGS

Alikhan A, Lynch PJ, Eisen DB. Hidradenitis suppurativa: a comprehensive review. *J Am Acad Dermatol*. 2009;60:539–561.

Buimer MG, Wobbes T, Klinkenbijl JH. Hidradenitis suppurativa. *Br J Surg*. 2009;96:350–360.

Chambers HF, Deleo FR. Waves of resistance: *Staphylococcus aureus* in the antibiotic era. *Nat Rev Microbiol*. 2009;7:629–641.

Cheng S, Edmonds E, Ben-Gashir M, et al. Subcorneal pustular dermatosis: 50 years on. *Clin Exp Dermatol*. 2008;33:229–233.

Revuz J. Hidradenitis suppurativa. *J Eur Acad Dermatol Venereol*. 2009;23:985–998.

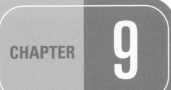

CHAPTER 9

Erosive and Vesiculobullous Diseases

LIBBY EDWARDS

The various erosive and blistering disorders are often morphologically indistinguishable when occurring on genital skin. Blisters are skin lesions that are filled with fluid. However, when blisters occur on fragile skin such as the genital area, the blister is unroofed quickly. This loss of epithelium results in a shallow area of denuded skin called an erosion, as distinguished from an ulcer, which is a deeper lesion, extending into or even through the dermis. Erosions can occur not only from ruptured blisters, but also from trauma, from epithelial necrosis produced by intense inflammation, or from necrosis resulting from tumor. Erosions resulting from a blister are usually well demarcated and round, or when blisters coalesce before eroding, arcuate erosions can result. Those resulting from trauma such as an excoriation are usually linear or angular. Erosive skin diseases can be infectious, immune-mediated, or malignant or can arise from excoriations from scratching, as in vulvar dermatoses. Ulcers are discussed in Chapter 10. There is overlap between erosive and ulcerative diseases, and many conditions may cause both together or sequentially.

NONINFECTIOUS INFLAMMATORY DERMATOSES THAT SOMETIMES ERODE

Erosive Lichen Planus

Lichen planus is a skin disease that exhibits variable morphologies on genital skin. Erosive lichen planus is the most common noninfectious erosive condition occurring on the vulva, although it is less common on the penis and almost nonexistent in circumcised men. Red papules (Chapter 3) are more common than erosions in men, and wet skin often exhibits white skin lesions (Chapter 11). Many patients exhibit more than one form of lichen planus.

Clinical Presentation

Erosive vulvovaginal lichen planus affects adults only, and women are far more often affected by the erosive form, particularly in the United States where circumcision is regularly performed on most newborn boys. Fewer than 25% of women with genital lichen planus have concurrent cutaneous involvement. Patients often report pruritus, but no pleasure with scratching, although the predominant complaint is that of burning, irritation, rawness, dysuria, dyspareunia, and postcoital bleeding. Many patients with erosive genital lichen planus also report mouth pain, especially with hard food such as chips, spicy foods, and acidic foods.

Although lichen planus manifests with many different morphologic appearances, classic lesions on keratinized skin are pruritic, violaceous, flat-topped papules (see Chapter 3). However, on mucous membranes, the most common morphologies are white lacy papules and plaques (see Chapter 11) or erosions. The white and eroded lesions can present separately or together. In 1982, Pelisse and associates described the vulvovaginal-gingival syndrome, introducing erosive lichen planus as a separate subgroup in women. Characteristically, these patients suffer erosions of the vulva, vagina, and oral mucosa at some stage of the disease, although not necessarily initially. Involvement of the modified mucous membranes of the vulva is usual, with bright red, thin epithelium and erosions most marked in the vestibule. These can be nonspecific, but often surrounding white epithelium and reticulate white lacy plaques reveal the diagnosis of lichen planus (Figs. 9-1 through 9-5). With chronic erosive lichen planus, scarring occurs (Fig. 9-6). Labial resorption and scarring of the clitoral hood over the clitoris are common. Narrowing of the introitus is also a frequent complication.

Vaginal erosions are usual with erosive vulvar lichen planus (Fig. 9-7). Even when vulvar lichen planus is papular rather than erosive, accompanying inflammatory vaginitis produced by lichen planus is common (see Chapter 15). Erosive vaginal lichen planus is tender and chronic and produces purulent vaginal secretions that incite an irritant contact dermatitis in the vestibule. Vaginal adhesions occur with severe disease, sometimes producing obliteration of the vaginal space that make sexual intercourse or the introduction of a speculum impossible.

Gingival lesions may be localized or generalized, primarily manifested by tender erosions and desquamative gingivitis, sometimes with surrounding solid or reticulate white papules (Fig. 9-8). Often, linear reticulate papules or erosions occur on the buccal mucosa (Fig. 9-9). Esophageal lichen planus is increasingly recognized and is more common than the literature suggests. Strictures

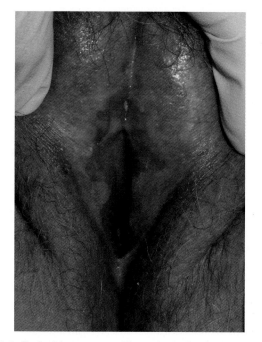

FIG. 9-1. Typical but nonspecific, red, shallow vestibular erosions with surrounding white epithelium are typical of erosive vulvar lichen planus. The characteristic resorption of vulvar architecture with loss of labia minora and scarring over the clitoris is present as well.

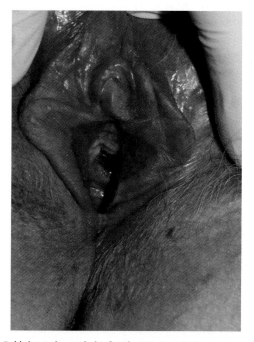

FIG. 9-2. Lichen planus is by far the most common cause of nonspecific chronic erosions, especially those that involve the vestibule.

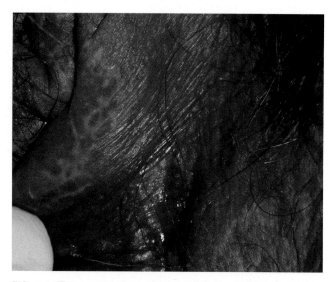

FIG. 9-3. This erosion is pathognomonic for lichen planus because of the surrounding white, interlacing papules.

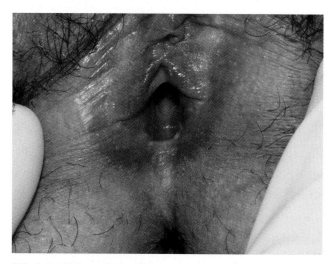

FIG. 9-4. Mild vestibular lichen planus can be confused with vestibulodynia (vulvar vestibulitis syndrome). However, the well-demarcated nature of the redness, the usual accompanying inflammatory vaginitis, and the frequent oral findings are simple methods for distinguishing the two conditions.

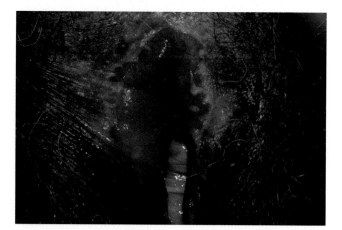

FIG. 9-5. Severe lichen planus is extremely painful and requires systemic as well as topical therapy.

producing dysphagia and weight loss are suggestive of this involvement, and squamous cell carcinoma of the esophagus is a serious complication (1).

Penile lichen planus is more commonly associated with lichen planus at other cutaneous sites than is vulvovaginal

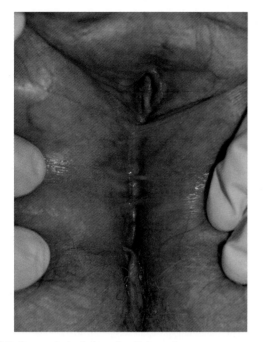

FIG. 9-6. Even relatively inactive lichen planus can eventuate in remarkable scarring, as has occurred in the patient with a 2 mm vaginal opening and urinary obstruction.

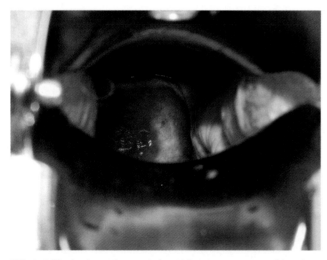

FIG. 9-7. Vaginal erosions are found in most women with vulvar lichen planus. Sometimes these are not seen on a speculum examination because of the difficulty of examining a painful vagina with a large speculum; however, purulent vaginal secretions that show parabasal cells and a lack of lactobacilli on wet mount are other signs of vaginal inflammation. Without treatment, the vagina can scar closed.

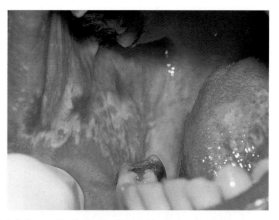

FIG. 9-8. Posterior buccal mucosal lesions regularly accompany genital lichen planus and occur often in any patient with any form of lichen planus on any skin surface.

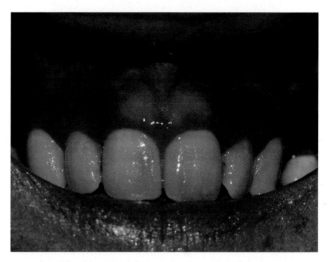

FIG. 9-9. Although gingival erosions are relatively uncommon in patients with lichen planus, patients with erosive genital lichen planus frequently exhibit this finding, producing the vulvovaginal-gingival and peno-gingival syndromes.

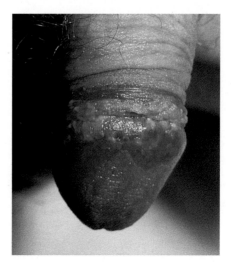

FIG. 9-10. The uncircumcised penis with erosive lichen planus, like the vulva, exhibits nonspecific erosions.

lichen planus. Lesions are less often eroded, but when erosions occur, they are very painful (Figs. 9-10 and 9-11). These erosions may be associated with oral lesions and run a similar prolonged clinical course to that seen in women (2). Men with erosive penile lichen planus also experience scarring, with phimosis if uncircumcised, or obliteration of the sharp distinction of the glans from the

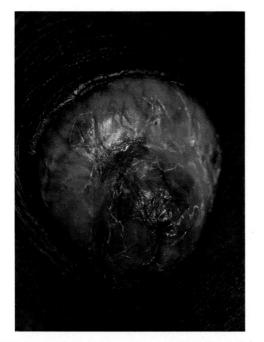

FIG. 9-11. Erosive lichen planus on an uncircumcised glans may appear crusted because of the dry environment.

shaft in the circumcised penis. Perianal lesions sometimes occur in both genders (Fig. 9-12).

There are rare reports of squamous cell carcinoma occurring in both vulvar and penile lichen planus. Indurated erosions and ulcers should be biopsied, as should chronic hyperkeratotic areas.

There have been reports of lichen planus occurring more often in patients with hepatitis C, and reports discounting this association. A recent meta-analysis reports that this association is real, at least in some geographic locations (3).

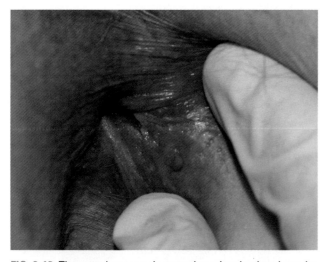

FIG. 9-12. The rectal mucosa is sometimes involved and can be subtle, requiring gentle eversion of that skin surface for detection. Again, a biopsy performed from the white, surrounding skin is most likely to yield the diagnosis.

Diagnosis

The diagnosis of lichen planus can be made with confidence when erosions are accompanied by white, lacy, reticulate, or fernlike papules of the genitalia or mouth. Otherwise, a biopsy is required, although most often the histology is returned as "lichenoid dermatitis" consistent with but not diagnostic of lichen planus. The biopsy should be taken from the edge rather than the center of an erosion, and it should be submitted for routine histology. If the biopsy is very nonspecific or is suggestive of an autoimmune blistering disease such as cicatricial pemphigoid or pemphigus vulgaris, an additional biopsy submitted for direct immunofluorescence will be necessary. This biopsy should be obtained from normal, perilesional skin and stored in transport media rather than formalin.

Histologic features of erosive lichen planus include a dense, lymphocytic, dermal bandlike infiltrate extending to and damaging the basal layer. A prominent granular cell layer, hyperkeratosis, and acanthosis are common, but erosive mucous membrane lichen planus often exhibits epithelial thinning and flattening. A biopsy of eroded skin that does not include epithelium cannot demonstrate a diagnosis of lichen planus, so biopsy sampling should include the epithelialized edge of an erosion. Colloid and Civatte bodies are frequently seen in the lower epidermis and upper dermis, and a direct immunofluorescent biopsy makes these more easily visualized.

Most chronic erosive skin diseases are in the differential diagnosis of erosive genital lichen planus. Pemphigus vulgaris and cicatricial pemphigoid are nearly indistinguishable, but less common and usually more easily diagnosed by routine and direct immunofluorescent biopsy. Often, surrounding white epithelium suggests the diagnosis of erosive lichen planus, but any chronic erosion can induce surrounding nonspecific white epithelium. Sometimes, this white epithelium can resemble lichen sclerosus, but lichen sclerosus never affects the vagina, and it shows a characteristic crinkled or occasionally waxy texture unlike that of lichen planus. Toxic epidermal necrolysis, severe erosive candidiasis, and an irritant contact dermatitis to an agent such as podophyllum resin can mimic erosive lichen planus, but these are acute rather than chronic in onset. Like erosive lichen planus, plasma cell mucositis also exhibits red, moist, glistening papules, and plaques that may appear erosive. The histology differentiates lichen planus from plasma cell vulvitis or balanitis and from the erosive genital lesions of graft versus host disease that may also be associated with lichenoid skin lesions.

Pathophysiology

Lichen planus is an inflammatory condition of unknown etiology. However, evidence suggests this disorder may be an autoimmune disease of cellular immunity. Injury of the basement membrane by cytotoxic T cells is central, and recent investigations report amplification of this injury by interferon alpha derived from plasmacytoid dendritic cells (4). Other autoimmune diseases cluster with lichen planus, including lichen sclerosus (5).

Management

The management of erosive lichen planus often is difficult. Mild disease is often adequately controlled by supportive measures and topical corticosteroids, whereas more severe disease requires the systemic use of systemic antimetabolites and immunosuppressive agents with variable success. Circumcision is sometimes curative in men (6).

Topical emollients such as petrolatum are soothing, as are measures such as air-drying rather than towel-drying. Because vulvovaginal lichen planus occurs primarily in the postmenopausal age group, topical or systemic estrogen replacement can be crucial, avoiding an additional and easily corrected cause for mucosal thinning.

First-line specific therapy for lichen planus is corticosteroid therapy. Potent topical steroid ointments (e.g., clobetasol propionate 0.05%) applied to vulvar or penile lesions twice daily can be beneficial. Creams, gels, lotions, and solutions are to be avoided because of the irritation induced by the alcohols regularly contained in these vehicles. This medication can also be inserted intravaginally at night, as can 25 mg hydrocortisone acetate rectal suppositories or hydrocortisone foam.

Systemic corticosteroids (prednisone 40 to 60 mg/day) effect significant and rapid improvement in most patients, but the condition recurs when the medication is stopped. The benefit is delayed in onset for all other treatments, and other therapies improve lichen planus less regularly. Methotrexate 25 mg weekly sometimes is beneficial for lichen planus (7). There are reports that oral retinoids such as isotretinoin 40 to 80 mg/day and acitretin at about 25 mg/day have been helpful, but side effects including teratogenicity and altered liver function require careful monitoring, and more evidence is needed from larger clinical trials as to their effectiveness. In addition, the long half-life of some retinoids is problematic. Other systemic treatments tried include oral griseofulvin at 500 mg twice daily, dapsone 100 to 150 mg daily, azathioprine, cyclophosphamide, mycophenylate mofetil, and hydroxychloroquine 200 mg twice daily, with anecdotal benefit in some patients; clinician familiarity with these medications for appropriate monitoring is important. Topical cyclosporine (using the oral liquid or solution intended for intravenous administration) four times a day has been useful for occasional patients, but the expense, local irritation, and minimal benefit render it impractical for most (8). Thalidomide at 100 to 150 mg/day is a theoretical potential therapy (9), as are topical tacrolimus (10) and pimecrolimus (11). More recently, topical rapamycin has been suggested as beneficial for refractory oral erosive lichen planus (12). Extracorporeal photochemotherapy has been reported beneficial in a

series of patients with refractory oral erosive lichen planus, an expensive therapy not available to most clinicians (13). No one therapy is ideal, and few produce consistent improvement without significant risks or side effects.

Lastly, surgery is occasionally needed to separate vaginal adhesions, reverse tightening of the introitus, or to uncover a buried clitoris. Skin disease should be controlled as well as possible before surgery is contemplated, and great care has to be taken postoperatively to prevent rapid scar reformation. Use of topical steroids and dilators is advisable.

Erosive anogenital lichen planus is chronic and painful, and there are no standard treatment measures that help all patients. Nor are there any controlled trials that evaluate therapy for anogenital lichen planus. However, experience suggests that there are various therapies that help some patients. Occasionally, erosive anogenital lichen planus remits, but this is the exception. Also, because of the risk of squamous cell carcinoma, patients should be checked regularly throughout the course of the disease.

Plasma Cell Balanitis and Vulvitis

The origin of Zoon balanitis or vulvitis (also called balanitis or vulvitis circumscripta plasmacellularis, inflammatory erythroplasia) is unknown, although some physicians believe that plasma cell vulvitis and balanitis are related to lichen planus (see also Chapter 3).

Clinical Features

Plasma cell vulvitis and balanitis present as a glistening, red, usually solitary plaque on the glans penis or vulva (Figs. 9-13 and 9-14). This may be asymptomatic or may present with mild pruritus. Erosive and vegetative types may occur, which are more painful. Lesions may

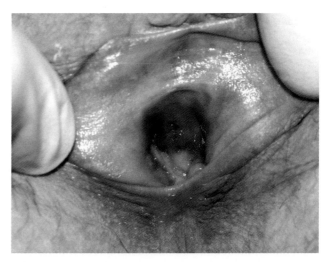

FIG. 9-13. This brown-red plaque around the urethral meatus is characteristic of plasma cell (Zoon) mucositis; this glistening plaque can be difficult to differentiate from an erosion at times.

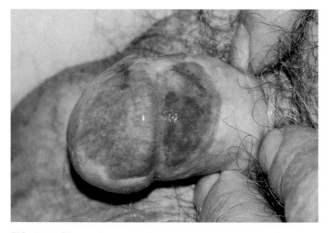

FIG. 9-14. The moist, eroded appearance is typical of plasma cell mucositis (Zoon balanitis) in male patients (Credit Errol Craig, MD).

persist for years, but they usually resolve slowly leaving a "rusty stain" resulting from microhemorrhage and hemosiderin deposition. The condition may recur.

Diagnosis

Plasma cell vulvitis and balanitis are diagnosed by the morphology of characteristic skin lesions, and it is confirmed on biopsy. Histology shows a thinned epidermis, sometimes with upper layers absent or detached from the dermis. Flattened keratinocytes separated by intercellular edema are distinctive. Red blood cells may be seen in the upper dermis and epidermis, and hemosiderin and vascular proliferation are common in the dermis. A dermal bandlike dense infiltrate with a predominance of plasma cells is characteristic.

Other diseases that can be confused with plasma cell vulvitis and balanitis include erosive lichen planus, intraepithelial neoplasia (also called Bowen disease, erythroplasia of Queyrat), and sometimes, Paget disease. Erosive candidiasis also can resemble Zoon vulvitis or balanitis.

Pathophysiology

The pathogenesis of plasma cell mucositis is unknown. Some believe that this may be related to lichen planus, and others suspect it is a nonspecific reaction pattern to an inflammatory process.

Treatment

In men, circumcision is curative. Otherwise, potent topical corticosteroids offer some symptomatic relief and improvement in appearance in many patients, but relapse is the rule on discontinuation of treatment. Topical tacrolimus, pimecrolimus, and masoprocol have been useful in some, but reported results of therapy are conflicting (14–16). Intralesional corticosteroids, imiquimod, and CO_2 laser have been reported beneficial at times (17–19).

There is one report of squamous cell carcinoma in situ (intraepithelial neoplasia) in a patient with plasma cell balanitis, so that ongoing surveillance is recommended (20).

Erosive Lichen Sclerosus (Lichen Sclerosus et Atrophicus, Hypoplastic Dystrophy)

Lichen sclerosus is a chronic fragile dermatosis characterized by atrophic white plaques, occurring most commonly on the genital skin of both sexes, although there is a female preponderance of 10:1 (see Chapter 11 for primary discussion).

The usual presenting symptom of lichen sclerosus is severe pruritus, often leading to painful erosions as this fragile skin is scratched (Fig. 9-15). These excoriations and other erosions resulting from fragility of the skin can be very painful and can predispose to secondary infection. The atrophic skin fissures more easily, so patients may present with pain on intercourse, and young girls often experience constipation resulting from pain of fissures with defecation (boys do not experience perianal lichen sclerosus). Lichen sclerosus is characterized by pallor and thin, crinkled skin; advanced disease is often associated with resorption of the labia minora, a clitoris covered by scar, and narrowing of the introitus. Purpura and hyperkeratosis are common, and lichen sclerosus may spread to perianal skin in women. Extragenital involvement occurs in about 6% of women of patients (unpublished data), and oral and vaginal mucosal involvement is rare.

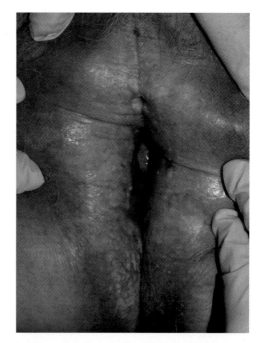

FIG. 9-15. Although lichen sclerosus is not primarily an erosive disease, intense itching with resulting rubbing of this fragile skin often produces erosions and purpura. There is fissuring of the anterior midline, as well as vestibular erosions following sexual activity.

Squamous cell carcinoma occurs in about 3% of patients with untreated vulvar lichen sclerosus, but erosive and hyperkeratotic lesions of lichen sclerosus in elderly patients are forms more likely to exhibit malignant change. In addition, lichen sclerosus is found in more than 50% of specimens from vulvectomies performed for squamous cell carcinoma.

Eroded lichen sclerosus is sometimes indistinguishable from erosive lichen planus, and these two diseases are known to coexist in some patients. Erosive and scarring lichen sclerosus can also mimic other chronic erosive or blistering diseases such as cicatricial pemphigoid and pemphigus vulgaris, so biopsy and examination of other mucous membranes and skin surfaces may be necessary to make the diagnosis of lichen sclerosus.

For men, circumcision is usually curative. Otherwise, the main treatment is potent topical corticosteroid ointment such as clobetasol propionate 0.05%, applied twice daily until improvement occurs, and then the frequency is reduced. Eroded lichen sclerosus is more likely than noneroded disease to present with bacterial or candidal superinfection, which should be addressed. In addition, these patients are more likely to develop superinfection after the initiation of an ultrapotent corticosteroid. Early detection and treatment, or even prophylaxis during the first week or so of therapy until the skin improves, can be extremely helpful.

This is a chronic skin disease that requires chronic corticosteroid therapy for ongoing control. Patients should undergo ongoing surveillance to assess the activity of the disease, side effects of medication, and any early signs of malignant transformation.

Lichen Simplex Chronicus (Eczema, Atopic Dermatitis, Neurodermatitis)

This excruciatingly pruritic condition exhibits erosions only secondarily, as a result of excoriation (see also Chapter 4). A genetic tendency to itch in the presence of local irritation initiates an itch–scratch cycle characterized by skin changes produced by rubbing (lichenification, scale, and erythema) and scratching (linear erosions of excoriation) (Figs. 9-16 and 9-17). The diagnosis is generally recognized by the history of scratching and the observation of irregular or linear erosions consistent with excoriations on the vulva or scrotum. Therapy includes topical corticosteroids, infection control, and nighttime sedation to minimize scratching during sleep.

Reiter Syndrome

The skin findings of Reiter syndrome classically include balanitis or cervicitis, often with erosions and crusting (see also Chapter 8). It is genetically determined and often runs a prolonged and relapsing course. This disease appears to be an abnormal host response to

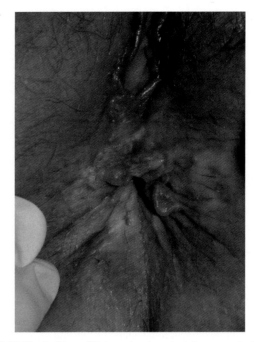

FIG. 9-16. The itching of lichen simplex chronicus results in rubbing that thickens the skin, producing the white color, and scratching that can produce erosions.

infection. Much more common in males, this response can occur either to a preceding enteric (gram-negative) infection or to a genitourinary, sexually transmitted *Chlamydia* infection.

One characteristic presentation consists of plaques of pustules that occur primarily on the glans penis, but these pustules erode quickly because of their fragile

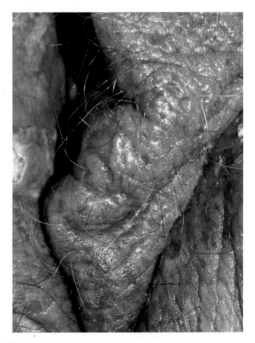

FIG. 9-17. Erosions with lichen simplex chronicus are most often linear and angular from scratching with fingernails.

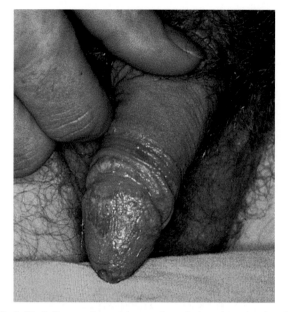

FIG. 9-18. Inflammation and pustules of the glans penis of a patient with Reiter syndrome often develop into erosions.

nature on thin skin. Crusting follows on the dry glans, but the uncircumcised glans exhibits erosions. Plaques with pustules and crusting occur on the vulva; palms and soles are often prominently involved (Fig. 9-18). On the palms and soles, these crusted plaques develop superimposed hyperkeratosis (keratoderma blennorrhagica). Other clinical features include acute oligoarthritis, usually of the knee or ankle, and problems with associated tendons and ligaments, conjunctivitis, mouth ulcers, urethritis or cervicitis, balanitis, and occasionally, cardiac problems.

The skin findings of Reiter syndrome are usually diagnosed by the clinical appearance and recognition of the constellation of symptoms. Unfortunately, there is no specific test for Reiter syndrome, but histologic confirmation of characteristic cutaneous abnormalities, which are identical to those of pustular psoriasis, is often helpful. Diseases that should be excluded include pustular psoriasis, gonococcal infection, and Behçet syndrome. Reiter syndrome is seen in human immunodeficiency virus (HIV)-positive patients.

Treatment is difficult because there is no one safe agent that dampens the host response overall. Antibiotics are used to shorten the initial infection, and otherwise each organ is treated symptomatically. Topical steroids may be helpful for the balanitis, but systemic steroids are reserved for severe complications such as cardiac involvement. Methotrexate and systemic retinoids such as acitretin are extremely useful for the skin abnormalities.

Necrolytic Migratory Erythema

This is a very rare condition that is caused by a glucagonoma, an α-cell tumor of the pancreas which is usually malignant. Serum levels of glucagon are elevated. Patients are usually ill with weight loss, diarrhea, malabsorption, and diabetes.

The rash begins as erythematous papules around orifices and flexures, including those of the genitalia. These papules coalesce into plaques, and central erosions occur and crust, eventually producing a circinate migratory erythema.

Histology of the skin shows superficial necrolysis and infiltration with lymphocytes. Treatment consists of removal of the tumor, if possible. Topical steroids may alleviate symptoms of the rash, but they do not clear it.

PRIMARY BLISTERING OR PUSTULAR INFECTIONS

Herpes Simplex Virus Infection

Herpes simplex virus (HSV) infection is a common sexually transmitted disease manifested by recurrent, painful, grouped vesicles that quickly erode into superficial coalescing erosions.

Clinical Presentation

Most common in younger individuals, herpes simplex virus infection is especially likely in those who have higher risks of contagion due to many lifetime sexual partners. HSV produces both primary and recurrent infections. Primary infection with HSV is often subclinical and unrecognized, but the classic primary infection by HSV is much more severe than recurrent episodes. Primary genital HSV infection follows exposure by 2 to 7 days and often exhibits associated fever, malaise, headache, and other constitutional symptoms. Regional lymphadenopathy is usual; pain and edema may cause urinary retention. The lesions initially occur as small (1- to 3-mm), scattered, and grouped vesicles occurring typically on the glans or shaft of the penis or the mucous membrane and modified mucous membrane portion of the vulva, sometimes extending to keratinized skin (Figs. 9-19 though 9-21). Because the vesicles are fragile and easily break, well-demarcated, discrete, round, and arcuate erosions (which indicate coalescing of the round erosions) often are seen rather than intact vesicles, especially on modified mucous membrane skin (Figs. 9-22 through 9-24). Healing may be complicated by secondary infection and irritation from overwashing or topical agents used empirically by an anxious patient.

After a primary infection, HSV remains latent in neuronal cells located in ganglia. Subsequently, the virus intermittently reactivates, thus producing recurrent disease that is usually milder and shorter in duration. Recurrent genital HSV infections are less painful, more localized, and less often associated with fever, arthralgias, and headache than primary disease. Many patients experience

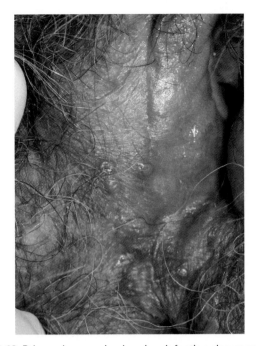

FIG. 9-19. Primary herpes simplex virus infection shows vesicles that are scattered and more generalized than that of recurrent disease. The vesicle with the central depression is specific for a herpes infection, either simplex or zoster.

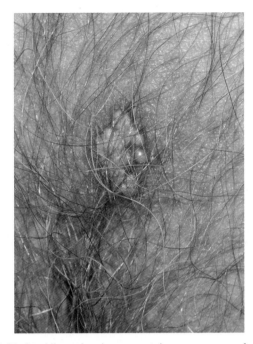

FIG. 9-21. Any blister develops a pustular appearance after several days; this does not signify bacterial infection, and the fluid remains clear when the blister is punctured.

a prodrome of tingling, burning, or dysesthesias before the onset of skin lesions. Recurrent HSV is most often located on the glans and shaft of the penis and the mucous membranes and modified mucous membrane portion of the vulva, but can occur on any epithelial surface, including the scrotum, perianal skin, and hair-bearing labia majora. Recurrent episodes are characterized by grouped vesicles that quickly develop into well-demarcated, round, and arcuate erosions. On dry, keratinized skin such as the shaft of the penis or the hair-bearing labia majora, round crusts may be the predominant lesion. Linear

fissures can appear as a manifestation of HSV infection, occurring most often in skin folds, such as the interlabial sulci of the vulva or within normal skin wrinkling of the penile shaft.

The primary episode of HSV infection for many patients is subclinical, so these people do not experience a classic primary episode of HSV infection and are thus unaware of their infection. Thus, their first clinical episode of infection exhibits the localized grouping of vesicles and

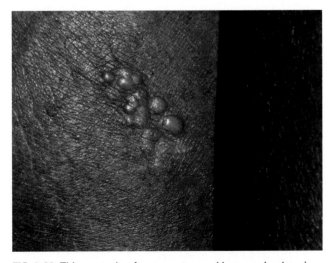

FIG. 9-20. This example of recurrent sacral herpes simplex virus infection shows the classic presentation of grouped vesicles occurring after a prodrome of burning or itching.

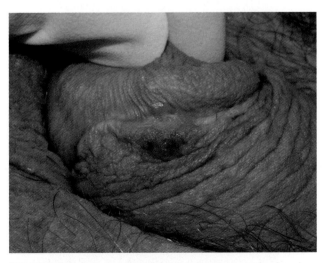

FIG. 9-22. On fragile, genital skin, blisters of herpes simplex virus infection rupture quickly, resulting in erosions or crusts. This penile erosion is nonspecific and is suspected by its recurrent nature and confirmed by culture or polymerase chain reaction technique.

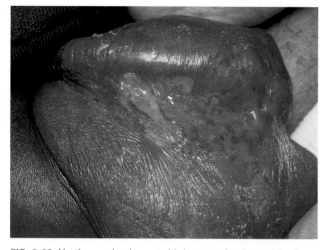

FIG. 9-23. Uncircumcised men with herpes simplex on the fragile glans generally never see clinical blisters, but only erosions.

erosions and milder clinical course of recurrent HSV infection. Because the appearance of this nonprimary but first clinical episode is delayed, the time and circumstances of transmission cannot be determined; on occasion, this delay is years long.

HSV infections often are associated with marked morbidity in immunosuppressed patients (see Chapter 16). Patients with altered cellular immunity, as occurs in those with HIV disease and patients receiving immunosuppressive agents, are at increased risk of ulcerative and chronic HSV infection (Fig. 9-25).

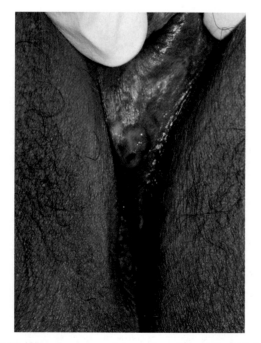

FIG. 9-24. When herpes vesicle rupture, the original blistering nature is recognized by the round, coalescing nature of the erosions.

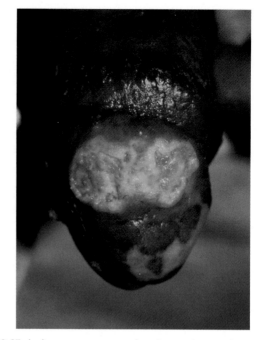

FIG. 9-25. In immunosuppressed patients, the erosions of herpes simplex virus infection enlarge into chronic ulcers.

Diagnosis

Although the diagnosis usually can be made on the appearance of skin lesions and history, laboratory confirmation of a genital HSV infection is desirable because of the psychologic impact of this disease on the patient and his or her partner. A viral culture from a swab of the base of a fresh erosion is the most common means of detecting HSV. However, false-negative results are a common occurrence in many laboratories, especially when delivery of the sample to the laboratory is delayed. Therefore, a negative culture should not convince a suspicious clinician to eliminate the diagnosis. Recently, the extremely sensitive polymerase chain reaction technique for detecting HSV has become widely available and reasonably priced, so this is now a test of choice (21). Although more uncomfortable, a shave skin biopsy from the edge of an erosion or of an intact vesicle is another very sensitive test to confirm the presence of a herpes virus infection, but a biopsy does not differentiate HSV from VZV. The Tzanck's preparation, although very quick, is less reliable, even in experienced hands. Direct immunofluorescent antibodies are available for HSV1 and 2 for more rapid diagnosis, although an adequate sample is of utmost importance. Scraping the base of the ulcer with a number 15 blade usually suffices for an adequate cell sample. Serology is not an adequate means of diagnosing an episode of HSV. Positive IgG for HSV varies very widely according to the country, occurring in up to 80% of adults; this denotes exposure, but not active or communicable disease (22). Negative serology indicates no past infection, but does not rule out a primary episode, since about 6 weeks is required for conversion.

The histologic appearance of HSV includes an intraepidermal vesicular dermatitis formed by acantholysis. Individual keratinocytes show intracellular edema (ballooning) and reticular degeneration (intracellular edema causing cell walls to burst). Eosinophilic intranuclear inclusion bodies may be present. Multinucleated keratinocytes are pathognomic for herpes virus infections but do not distinguish between HSV and varicella-zoster virus (VZV) infections.

HSV must be differentiated from several other vesicular and pustular diseases. Occasionally, the differentiation of genital HSV infection from VZV infection can be difficult, because both exhibit grouped vesicles or erosions. However, genital VZV infection usually occurs in the older patient and covers a dermatomal pattern, also affecting the medial thigh or buttock unilaterally. VZV infection occurs only once in the immunocompetent patient, rather than recurrently, as is usual with HSV infection. Another likely disease to confuse with genital HSV infection is candidiasis of the modified mucous membranes of the vulva or the uncircumcised glans penis, in which yeast can cause coalescing erosions when superficial pustules rupture. A fungal smear is positive in that case. Folliculitis, both irritant and staphylococcal, produces discrete red papules and pustules that can mimic HSV. Finally, blistering erythema multiforme both mimics and sometimes follows HSV infection. The most common cause of recurrent erythema multiforme is recurrent HSV infection in a patient with an enhanced immunologic response to this virus. These patients usually exhibit both intraoral and genital erosions that are less well demarcated, whereas HSV does not occur inside the mouth, except for the initial primary outbreak. In addition, the occurrence of red, nonscaling, flat-topped papules on the palms, soles, and sometimes other keratinized surfaces is common.

Pathophysiology

Herpes simplex virus (HSV) types 1 and 2 are double-stranded DNA viruses (*Herpesvirus hominis*) capable of producing vesicular and erosive mucocutaneous disease. Oral mucocutaneous and ocular disease is produced by HSV 1 in most cases, whereas genital HSV infection is caused by HSV 2 in the majority of affected patients. The proportion of HSV 1 occurring on the genital skin is increasing, presumably due to the increase in oral-genital sexual activity.

Management

The management of HSV infection begins with the sensitive and nonjudgmental education of the patient. The patient should be counseled regarding the infectious nature of the disease, its recurrent nature, and the importance of avoidance of sexual intercourse when open lesions are present. Circumcision and condoms have been shown to confer modest protection from infection (23,24). Patients should be aware that intermittent shedding of the virus occurs when there is no evidence of active HSV infection, and the infection can be transmitted even in the absence of blisters and erosions. In fact, most HSV infection is contracted during asymptomatic episodes. This shedding has also been documented in patients receiving long-term suppressive antiviral medication. Therefore, the use of a condom, even when there are no obvious lesions, is wise. The possibility of transmission of HSV to a newborn during delivery should be discussed to ensure the protection of future infants from maternal infection, although most neonatal HSV infections occur due to maternal primary infection.

Both primary and recurrent primary HSV infections are shortened by prompt treatment with specific oral antiviral agents, although some recurrent episodes are so mild that therapy is unwarranted. Three current choices for the treatment of recurrent HSV are as follows: 5 days of acyclovir 200 mg five times a day (or, for primary HSV infection, for 10 days), famciclovir 125 mg twice daily, and valacyclovir 500 mg twice daily (1 g twice daily for 10 days for primary HSV infection). These therapies exhibit equivalent efficacy, with choices made on the basis of cost and convenience of dosing. Side effects are minimal with each. Topical acyclovir exerts only minimal benefit. More recently, topical penciclovir has become available to shorten the course of HSV infection, but the benefit over placebo is minimal.

Intravenous acyclovir is occasionally needed if disease is severe, especially if the patient is immunosuppressed or if gastrointestinal absorption is a major problem, as can occur in the HIV-positive patient. Resistance of HSV to currently available oral medications occurs only occasionally and always in immunosuppressed patients. Foscarnet is an alternative treatment, although it is available only for intravenous use. Several other agents have been reported as beneficial in acyclovir-resistant HSV, including intravenous and topical cidofovir, topical trifluorothymidine, topical interferon-α in dimethyl sulfoxide, and imiquimod (25).

For patients experiencing frequent or severe episodes of HSV infection, chronic prophylactic acyclovir at a dose of 400 mg twice daily, famciclovir 250 mg twice daily, or valacyclovir 500 to 1000 mg/day is a safe, practical, and effective means of preventing most recurrences. Suppressive oral antiviral therapy also decreases asymptomatic shedding and, therefore, probably infectivity, but asymptomatic shedding of virus is not eliminated (26). Transmission of HSV infection still occurs in patients taking these medications and experiencing no clinical outbreaks.

Crucial to the management of anogenital HSV infection is counseling and psychological support. These patients exhibit marked anxiety, depression, fear, and self-esteem issues (27).

Some patients erroneously believe that HSV infection can be followed by postherpetic neuralgia. Fortunately, that is not a sequel to this infection; this only follows herpes zoster infection.

Herpes Zoster Infection (Shingles)

Varicella zoster virus (VZV) causes two diseases: herpes zoster, or shingles, and chicken pox. Both affect the genitalia but present very differently. The first episode of VZV (varicella, chicken pox) presents with generalized distribution of discrete red papules, vesicles, and crusts, but there is a predilection for the genital skin and vagina. Shingles, the second episode of VZV is localized, typically very painful, and with minimal constitutional symptoms. Hopefully, with the availability of the shingles vaccine, this condition will become uncommon.

Clinical Presentation

Herpes zoster occurs primarily in patients with immune deficiency by virtue of age, disease, or medications, but occasionally occurs in young and healthy individuals. The prevalence of this miserable condition should decrease as more older people receive the recently available vaccine.

Many patients experience a localized prodrome of pain, itching, burning, or aching, followed in one or a few days by pink, nonscaling plaques in a unilateral dermatomal distribution (Figs. 9-26 and 9-27) in the symptomatic area. Grouped vesicles overlying these red plaques quickly follow, then coalesce into larger blisters. Often, the blisters become purple or gray due to hemorrhage into the blister. Over the next 3 weeks, the blisters crust and heal. Blisters occurring on mucous membranes and modified mucous membranes of the genitalia are quickly unroofed due to friction on this moist and very thin skin, so that erosions usually predominate. Likewise, the friction from skin folds and clothing often tears blister roofs even on the more keratinized genital skin. Herpes zoster

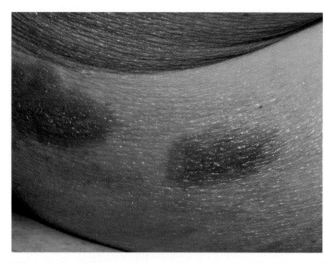

FIG. 9-27. In addition to the one-sided nature of the blisters of herpes zoster, patients with herpes zoster, unlike those with herpes simplex, do not experience recurrences.

can become ulcerative, chronic, or hyperkeratotic in immunosuppressed patients (see Chapter 16).

Sometimes, the eruption is accompanied by mild headache, malaise, and a low-grade fever. However, the primary complication of herpes zoster infection is the development of postherpetic neuralgia, in which chronic pain persists after the eruption resolves. This is more likely in individuals over 60 years of age and in immunosuppressed people. Some clinicians theorize that this may be responsible for some genital pain syndromes such as vulvodynia and scrotodynia, but preceding VZV infection affecting the genitalia is almost never identified in patients with genital pain syndromes. Unlike HSV, VZV does not recur in immunocompetent patients.

Diagnosis

The definitive diagnosis of herpes zoster is usually made on the basis of the presentation and morphology. When necessary, this can be confirmed by a positive culture or the identification of viral DNA with the PCR technique. The virus is rather fastidious, so cultures are sometimes falsely negative, but the PCR technique is very sensitive and now easily available. Tzanck's preparation from epithelial cells scraped from the base of a blister or erosion shows giant cells when examined microscopically, but the validity of this test is extremely dependent on the examiner, and the results are subjective. A biopsy is extremely sensitive but does not differentiate between HSV infection and herpes zoster, a distinction that can usually be made on clinical grounds. The histologic appearance of herpes zoster infection is identical to that of HSV infection. Keratinocytes swell and burst, and some epithelial cells form giant cells. Occasionally, leukocytoclastic vasculitis underlies these epithelial changes, but this does not indicate a primary or possibly systemic problem of vasculitis.

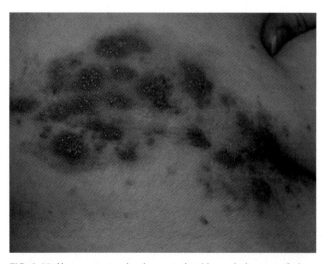

FIG. 9-26. Herpes zoster is characterized by red plaques of clustered vesicle that are unilateral and in a dermatomal distribution.

The differentiation of genital herpes zoster infection from HSV infection may be difficult. HSV is a recurrent disease, whereas herpes zoster is a one-time event, except in significantly immunosuppressed patients. Herpes zoster is unilateral, but vesicles may erode early in both diseases. Bullous impetigo and bullous pemphigoid can sometimes mimic herpes zoster, but these are usually bilateral and are not particularly painful. Bullous pemphigoid generally exhibits distant lesions that exclude the diagnosis of herpes zoster, and impetigo can be differentiated by culture.

Pathophysiology

Herpes zoster infection is a blistering disease that results from reactivation of VZV that has been latent in nerve ganglia since a remote episode of varicella. This condition occurs most often in older individuals whose immune system is less efficient or in immunocompromised patients.

Management

For most patients with herpes zoster, pain control is the most important aspect of care. Narcotic pain analgesia is usually needed for the first few weeks. The early diagnosis and treatment (within 72, but especially 48 hours) with oral antiviral therapy somewhat reduces the duration of an acute infection. This improvement is not striking, so therapy is optional in younger, healthy patients. However, immunosuppressed or very elderly people should be treated. Some studies have shown an arguably significant reduction of postherpetic neuralgia in patients treated early.

Choices include acyclovir 800 mg five times a day, famciclovir 500 mg three times daily, and valacyclovir 1 g every 8 hours. The advantage of the more expensive valacyclovir and famciclovir is the less frequent dosing schedule.

Those patients who experience postherpetic neuralgia deserve medication for neuropathic pain, including amitriptyline, gabapentin, pregabalin, venlafaxine, or duloxetine (see Chapter 5). Sometimes, referral to a pain clinic is necessary.

Otherwise, the best current management is prevention. A vaccine for the prevention of herpes zoster is now available, approved by the Food and Drug Administration for people over 60 years of age.

Candidiasis

Vaginal and vulvar infection with *Candida albicans* is common, but genital candidiasis in men is essentially confined to uncircumcised, incontinent, obese, or immunosuppressed men (see also Chapters 4, 8, 11, 14, and 15). Although genital *Candida albicans* infection is most often erythematous and scaling (see Chapter 3), severe disease sometimes produces erosions. Women present

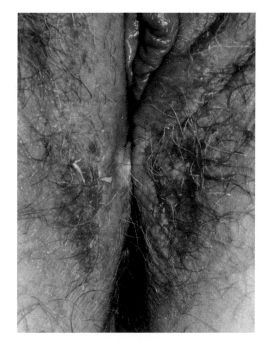

FIG. 9-28. Severe candidiasis produces pustules that rupture and coalesce into plaques with peripheral peeling.

with vaginal discharge, itching, and soreness of the vulva. Erythema, scale, and pustules that shed blister roofs and form coalescing superficial erosions are seen (Figs. 9-28 through 9-30). At the edge of eroded plaques are satellite pustules that erode into collarettes and round erosions. In addition, *Candida albicans* often produces linear erosions, or fissures, in the skin creases between the labia

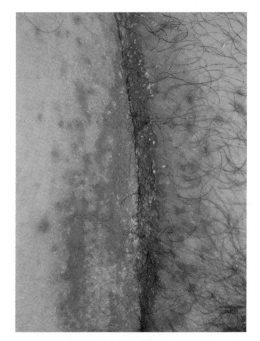

FIG. 9-29. As pustules of candidiasis lose their blister roofs, they are replaced with round, discrete erosions, often surrounding an intertriginous plaque, as in this elderly incontinent man.

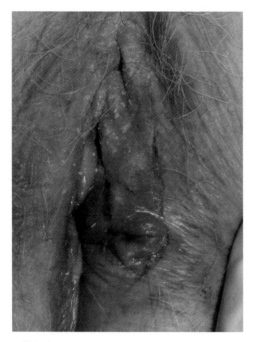

FIG. 9-30. Skin folds between the labia minora and labia majora and the gluteal cleft are areas that often fissure in a setting of inflammation, classically an infection with *Candida albicans.*

minora and labia majora. In men, candidal balanitis and intertrigo present with burning and itching, and with papules and pustules that merge to form eroded plaques. Predisposing factors for external and intertriginous genital candidiasis include diabetes mellitus, corticosteroid therapy, pregnancy, treatment with oral contraceptive pills or broad-spectrum antibiotics, an infected sexual partner, and immunosuppression. Local moisture and obesity also contribute.

HSV infection, Paget disease, Bowen disease (vulvar or penile intraepithelial neoplasia), eczema (lichen simplex chronicus), and irritant contact dermatitis can be mistaken for erosive candidiasis.

Histologically, epithelial edema is present, and a pustule is often seen just below the stratum corneum. Gram stain and periodic acid–Schiff stain reveal mycelia and occasional budding yeast in the stratum corneum. The diagnosis, however, is made most economically from fungal preparations of skin scrapings and wet mounts of vaginal secretions showing budding yeast forms and pseudohyphae. There are several adequate therapies for erosive candidiasis. Although topical azoles are effective, these medications are generally available only in creams, which sometimes irritate eroded skin. When possible, oral therapy with fluconazole at 100 to 200 mg/day or itraconazole 200 mg/day is a comfortable, safe, and effective alternative. Topical nystatin ointment applied four times daily is another soothing but messy alternative to creams in erosive candidiasis. When sufficiently healed, an azole cream can be used to complete healing, then either immediately with another episode, or daily as ongoing suppression for

patients with frequent recurrence. In women, topical vulvar therapy should be combined with vaginal treatment.

Impetigo

Impetigo is a bacterial infection of the superficial epidermis that can produce blisters and erosions (see Chapter 8). When caused by some phage types of *Staphylococcus aureus,* infection produces separation of the stratum corneum and rapid loss of this fragile blister roof. Well-demarcated, round erosions with collarettes are typical (Fig. 9-31). When produced by α-hemolytic *Streptococcus* infection, erosion and crusting are common. Impetigo is often associated with bacterial folliculitis, infection that has extended into nearby hair follicles, producing discrete red papules, pustules, and small erosions and crusts. The diagnosis is suspected by the morphology and is confirmed by a bacterial culture and response to therapy. Treatment consists of an antibiotic effective against both *S. aureus* and *Streptococcus* species, such as cephalexin, erythromycin, dicloxacillin, clindamycin, and trimethoprim–sulfamethoxazole. Unfortunately, resistant *S. aureus* has become common so that empiric therapy is often ineffective, and culture with sensitivities has become important. Despite prompt response to therapy, lesions sometimes recur after therapy. This occurs most often in patients who are nasal carriers of *S. aureus,* and

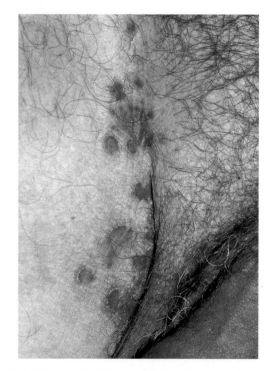

FIG. 9-31. The fragile blister roof of bullous impetigo erodes quickly, leaving very superficial round erosions with collarettes with an appearance similar to that of candidiasis. Often, however, individual erosions are larger than those caused by *Candida* and generally coalescence into a central plaque is less marked.

these patients benefit from the administration of intranasal mupirocin cream or ointment four times a day, for 1 week each month for several months to minimize this carrier state.

NONINFECTIOUS BLISTERING ERUPTIONS

Many of these diseases are autoimmune or hypersensitivity reactions. They cause blistering and erosions of skin and mucosal surfaces including the genitalia.

In autoimmune blistering diseases, autoantibodies are directed against target antigens that are involved in helping epithelial cells adhere to each other or in helping the epithelium adhere to the dermis. Such antibodies fix to the target antigen and trigger complement activation through the classical pathway, attracting eosinophils. Their subsequent degranulation releases proteolytic enzymes that lead to separation of epidermal cells, and a blister is formed. As with other blistering processes, lesions of mucous membranes and modified mucous membranes are so fragile that blisters are so transient as to be unnoticed, and the usual presentation is that of erosion. However, lesions on keratinized skin usually exhibit at least some clinical blisters.

Histology and immunofluorescent studies are essential for a correct diagnosis. Histologic samples are obtained from cutaneous and mucosal sites, from the edge of a blister or erosions for routine histology, and from nearby normal epithelium for direct immunofluorescent studies.

Pemphigus

Clinical Presentation

Pemphigus affects the skin and mucous membranes in people of middle and old age (mean age is the sixth decade). Childhood cases are rare.

Pemphigus vulgaris (common pemphigus) accounts for 80% of all patients with pemphigus. Of these, 60% present with oral lesions that may produce extensive erosion, and months may elapse before keratinized skin lesions form. More than 90% of patients with pemphigus vulgaris suffer mucosal involvement at some time during the course of the disease; genital involvement is common, and erosions are sometimes extensive. Mucosal sites reported include nose, pharynx, esophagus, conjunctiva, cervix, vagina, and rectum, and modified mucous membranes affected include the vulva. Blisters of pemphigus occurring on these areas quickly erode, so that the first recognized lesions usually are well-demarcated, bland, nonspecific, uniform erosions (Fig. 9-32). Although pemphigus is generally a nonscarring disease, the severely affected vulva exhibits resorption of the labia majora and the clitoris is covered by scar, and the uncircumcised penis may develop phimosis (Fig. 9-33).

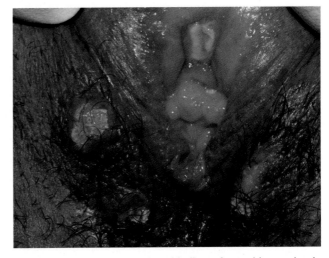

FIG. 9-32. The white, necrotic epithelium of pemphigus vulgaris quickly sloughs to nondescript form erosions.

Genital involvement in women occurs in over half of patients with pemphigus vulgaris. A series of 77 women showed that 92% of those affected experience erosions of the labia minora, 28% of the labia majora, 36% of the vagina, and 15% of the cervix (28). Papanicolaou smears in women with cervical pemphigus vulgaris show inflammation, acantholytic cells, and/or low-grade squamous intraepithelial neoplasia, which should not be confused with intraepithelial neoplasia requiring treatment.

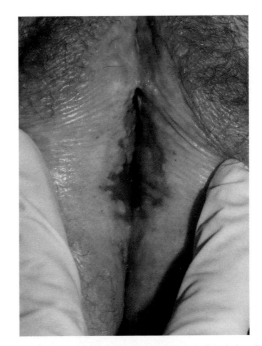

FIG. 9-33. Although a hallmark of pemphigus vulgaris is a lack of scarring, any chronic inflammatory condition on the vulva, including pemphigus vulgaris, can scar, with loss of labia minora. In addition, surrounding chronic inflammation creates nonspecific, white, variably thick skin.

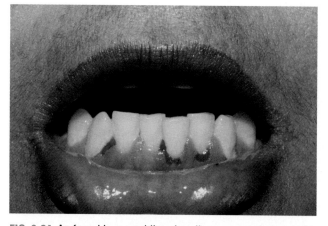

FIG. 9-34. As found in many blistering diseases, genital pemphigus vulgaris is generally accompanied by oral disease, manifested here by well-demarcated erosions of the gingivae.

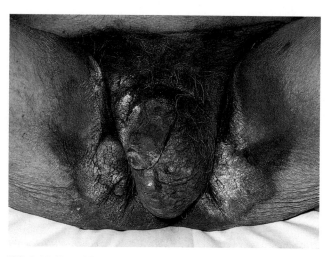

FIG. 9-36. Pemphigus vegetans produces thickened, hyperkeratotic plaques in areas of previous erosion and blistering.

Pemphigus vulgaris of the penis is less common than pemphigus of the vulva, and when present it occurs most often on the glans. The distal shaft and corona also are sites that are preferentially affected. The oral mucosa is usually affected in both men and women (Fig. 9-34).

Blisters on nonmucous membrane skin are superficial and flaccid and arise from noninflamed skin. With gentle traction on a blister, the tenuous adherence of the upper epidermis to underlying tissue allows the blister to extend (Nikolsky sign). Even on keratinized skin, these very superficial blisters rupture easily to leave large eroded areas,

but they normally heal without scarring (Fig. 9-35). However, the erosions of pemphigus vulgaris on the vulva produce resorption of the labia minora and clitoral hood, and pemphigus of the uncircumcised glans penis can cause phimosis.

Pemphigus vegetans is a variant characterized by erosions with peripheral pustules in the early phases of the disease. Later, large, vegetating, and almost verrucous plaques occur (Fig. 9-36).

Pemphigus foliaceus presents in older patients as superficial crusting plaques, often on the central trunk and in skin folds. The blistering nature can be identified by a careful observer by the well-demarcated and arcuate borders and by the realization that crusting is often a sign of blistering. This form of pemphigus generally spares mucous membranes, so the dry, keratinized skin of the genitalia is more likely than moist mucous membrane skin to be affected.

Diagnosis

The diagnosis is made from characteristic histologic changes on biopsies for routine microscopy and direct immunofluorescence. A skin biopsy shows an intraepidermal blister. Pemphigus vulgaris and early pemphigus vegetans exhibit a blister located just above the basal cell layer. The basal cells remain attached to the basement membrane, but not to each other or to overlying cells, thus producing a picture similar to that of a row of tombstones. In addition, within the blister cavity are epidermal cells that, with loss of cohesion to surrounding cells, appear round and are called acantholytic cells. Direct immunofluorescence biopsies obtained from normal-appearing skin near a blister or erosion show immunoglobulin G (IgG) deposition in the epidermal intercellular substance. In addition, indirect immunofluorescence of patients' serum showing antibodies that bind to the epidermal cell surface is characteristic of this disease. The patients' serum contains IgG

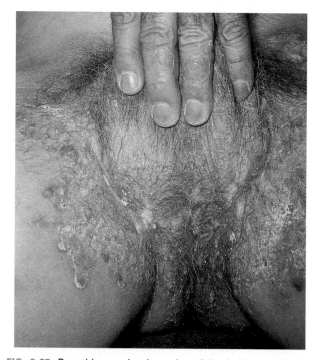

FIG. 9-35. Pemphigus vulgaris on keratinized skin appears as very superficial and flaccid blisters with frequent, superficial erosions but no tense blisters.

autoantibodies directed against the glycoproteins desmogleins and desmocollins in the desmosomes of stratified squamous epithelium.

Biopsies of pemphigus vegetans often show, in addition, neutrophilic inflammation producing intraepithelial abscesses. In its latter, hyperkeratotic form, pemphigus vegetans reveal squamous hyperplasia and pseudoepitheliomatous hyperplasia on biopsy, in addition to the characteristic suprabasilar blister. Pemphigus foliaceus shows a very superficial blister formed by acantholysis in the uppermost epidermis.

Pemphigus can be confused with most other blistering diseases. Pemphigus vulgaris often begins with mucosal erosions indistinguishable from erosive lichen planus. Routine biopsies usually differentiate the two diseases, and pemphigus vulgaris progresses to produce blisters and erosions on keratinized skin, unlike in lichen planus. Pemphigus vulgaris can mimic cicatricial pemphigoid, with both producing nonspecific mucosal erosions. The milder and intermittent occurrence of a fixed drug eruption and the explosive onset of blistering forms of erythema multiforme usually distinguish these diseases from pemphigus.

Pathophysiology

Pemphigus is a group of autoimmune intraepidermal bullous diseases produced by autoantibodies to the surface of epidermal cells. This ultimately produces a loss of adhesion of these cells that leads to a superficial blister within the epidermis. The most common and dangerous form of pemphigus, pemphigus vulgaris, is produced by loss of adhesion of the basal cells from the upper epidermis. Like pemphigus vulgaris, pemphigus vegetans is produced by a split in the epidermis just above the basal cell layer, but it is characterized by the later development of thickened, hyperkeratotic skin. Pemphigus foliaceus occurs when cells in the upper epidermis lose cohesion and form such a superficial blister that the blistering nature is often misdiagnosed clinically as scaling or crusting. Both drug-induced pemphigus (e.g., captopril, rifampicin) and paraneoplastic pemphigus are reported. One form of pemphigus, benign familial pemphigus (also called Hailey–Hailey disease), is of autosomal dominant rather than autoimmune origin, and it is discussed later in this chapter.

Management

Genital pemphigus is generally not controlled with topical therapy. This usually widespread disease is treated primarily systemically. The mainstay therapy of pemphigus is systemic corticosteroids, using prednisone or its equivalent at 60 to 150 mg/day. In addition, the steroid-sparing immunosuppressive medications cyclophosphamide or azathioprine are standard therapy for pemphigus; these begun as early as possible in the course of the disease because of the delay in the onset of benefit (29). Topical steroid treatment and measures to prevent secondary infection are also very important. Other treatments tried include gold, dapsone, antimalarials, cyclosporine, plasmapheresis, and intravenous immunoglobulins (29). Cyclophosphamide administered in intravenous pulses with steroid pulses (30) and oral mycophenolate have shown promise in the treatment of recalcitrant pemphigus (31). Rituximab has been examined in a series of 88 patients and was found to produce a complete response in 80.7%, partial response in 11.8%, no response in 5.7%, and death in 2.5% (32). Intravenous immunoglobulin, with and without rituximab, have been reported beneficial. Unlike most skin diseases in men, pemphigus is not cleared with circumcision and requires medical therapy.

The prognosis of pemphigus vulgaris has improved markedly since the use of corticosteroids. In the past, the disease itself or fulminant secondary infection led inexorably to death in the majority of cases. Current treatment has decreased mortality to 10%, and morbidity most often now results from adverse reactions to medication. Generally, after pemphigus is controlled, medications can be tapered to lower doses. Occasionally, medications can even be discontinued. However, recurrence is common and may occur after several years in remission.

Bullous Pemphigoid

Clinical Presentation

Bullous pemphigoid is the most common autoimmune blistering disease. It occurs at any age, but most commonly presents in adults older than 60 years. Men and women are affected equally. Genital involvement is relatively uncommon, occurring in about 10% of patients, with the keratinized epithelium more likely to be affected than the mucous membranes.

Pruritus is intense and may precede the blisters for months. In addition, before clinically obvious blisters occur, many patients exhibit pink plaques that mimic urticaria. Subsequently, small vesicles and then bullae arise from the inflamed plaques. Clinically, skin involvement may be minor or very extensive. The areas most likely to be involved are the hair-bearing areas of inner thighs, inguinal crease, and perineum. Blisters are tense and filled with straw-colored and, occasionally, hemorrhagic fluid (Figs. 9-37 and 9-38). Scarring does not occur in the absence of a complicating event such as secondary infection.

Diagnosis

A provisional diagnosis of bullous pemphigoid can be made on the basis of the morphology of the lesions and characteristic onset in elderly patients. However, confirmation by biopsy for routine histology and direct immunofluorescence is mandatory. Biopsy of an intact new blister shows characteristic histology; subepidermal blistering with a variable dermal inflammatory infiltrate including eosinophils is usual. Direct immunofluorescent

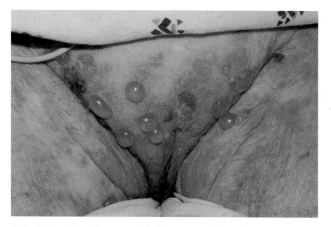

FIG. 9-37. The blisters of bullous pemphigoid occur from a deeper cleft in the skin, under the epidermis, resulting in tense, straw-colored blisters, rather than flaccid lesions. (Credit Errol Craig, MD.)

biopsy of perilesional skin shows in vivo deposition of IgG and complement components along the BMZ. A direct immunofluorescent examination of salt-split skin shows that the binding is epidermal, to the roof of the blister. This differentiates bullous pemphigoid from epidermolysis bullosa acquisita (EBA), in which the binding is to the base or dermal side of the blister. Indirect immunofluorescent studies of the sera of patients with bullous pemphigoid show the presence of IgG directed toward the pemphigoid target antigens in the lamina lucida of the BMZ.

Most other blistering diseases can be considered in the differential diagnosis of bullous pemphigoid. Blistering forms of erythema multiforme are sometimes difficult to distinguish, but erythema multiforme essentially always exhibits mucosal lesions, and the onset is generally more abrupt. Except for the absence of scarring, bullous

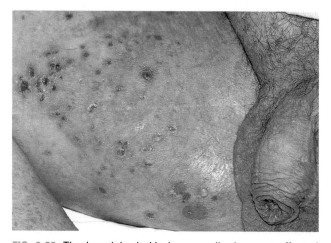

FIG. 9-38. The keratinized skin is generally the most affected area by bullous pemphigoid with relative sparing of the mucous membranes and modified mucous membranes.

pemphigoid is often indistinguishable from EBA, both clinically and histologically. A direct immunofluorescent study on salt-split skin is required for absolute differentiation of these two diseases. Pemphigus vulgaris, unlike bullous pemphigoid, generally affects mucous membranes prominently and is characterized by erosions and flaccid bullae, rather than by tense blisters. Less often, bullous impetigo can mimic bullous pemphigoid. However, blisters are usually few in number and flaccid, and of sudden and recent onset. Mucous membranes are spared.

Pathophysiology

This autoimmune blistering disease occurs when autoantibodies are directed at a portion of the basement membrane zone (BMZ), ultimately causing detachment of the epidermis from the dermis. Although usually occurring spontaneously and without an identifiable precipitating factor, bullous pemphigoid is sometimes associated with specific drugs, such as furosemide, penicillins, psoralens, ibuprofen, and some angiotensinconverting enzyme inhibitors. In addition, some systemic diseases appear to be linked, such as diabetes mellitus (perhaps by increased glycosylation of BMZ components), multiple sclerosis, and rheumatoid arthritis. Studies to establish such links are difficult because bullous pemphigoid is rare and affects the elderly in whom concomitant disease is more likely. Although an association of bullous pemphigoid with internal malignancy was reported in the past, more recent studies showed no or very little increase of malignancy compared with age- and sex-matched controls.

Management

For localized and prebullous disease, treatment with potent topical steroids is usually sufficient. For generalized bullous pemphigoid, systemic steroids are required in doses varying from 15 to 60 mg/day, tapered according to response. In the few patients who do not respond or whose response does not allow dose reduction, an immunosuppressive agent may be added, such as azathioprine, cyclophosphamide, or minocycline with nicotinamide. Methotrexate has also been used as a steroid-sparing agent (33). Supportive care and guarding against harmful side effects are important in these elderly patients.

In addition to this specific treatment for bullous pemphigoid, local care of the affected genitalia is important. Infection control and topical corticosteroids can minimize discomfort.

The lesions in bullous pemphigoid are nonscarring, and the course of bullous pemphigoid is self-limiting, with remission in treated patients occurring in 2 to 6 years. The condition may recur, but recurrences are usually milder than the initial bout. Treated patients have a mortality of 20%, little different to the natural course of the disease, but the treatment is suppressive and improves the pruritus and the quality of life.

Cicatricial Pemphigoid (Benign Mucous Membrane Pemphigoid)

Clinical Presentation

Cicatricial pemphigoid is much less common than bullous pemphigoid, but more likely to affect the mucous membrane of the genitalia than does bullous pemphigoid. The age of onset of cicatricial pemphigoid is middle to old age and is more common in women in a ratio of 1.5:1.

Cicatricial pemphigoid primarily affects the mucous membranes with resulting scarring. It affects keratinized skin only in about 30% of cases. Because the diagnosis is difficult in the absence of intact blisters on hair-bearing skin, it may be delayed or sometimes missed. Cicatricial pemphigoid usually starts with irritation, mild blisters, and erosions of the mouth, the eye, and the genitalia. Genital involvement is seen in 50% of cases of cicatricial pemphigoid. Men report penile lesions, dysuria, and difficulty retracting the foreskin. Women report pain, pruritus, and dysuria. Morphologically, genital cicatricial pemphigoid is characterized by painful erosions and scarring (Figs. 9-39 and 9-40). The preceding blisters are often short-lived, and the underlying blistering nature of the disease is missed. These mucous membrane erosions may progress rapidly to produce scarring with considerable morbidity. The initial, nonspecific, enlarging erosions produce scarring in more developed disease. Men may develop meatal stenosis and phimosis, and women may experience urethral

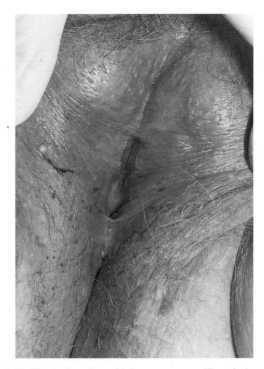

FIG. 9-40. The hallmarks, which are not specific, of cicatricial pemphigoid are its early and remarkable scarring and fragility; in this patient, active erosions are minimal but scarring is remarkable.

stenosis, fusion of the labia, clitoral burial, and introitus stenosis.

Painful erosion in the mouth is usual (Fig. 9-41). Erythema and erosions of the gingiva may lead to scarring and retraction with resulting secondary dental disease. Nasal mucosa, larynx, and pharynx may also be affected, and stridor or dysphagia may result. The eye,

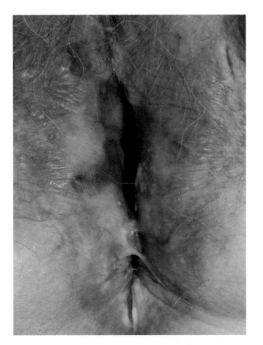

FIG. 9-39. Erosions and loss of vulvar architecture are typical of cicatricial pemphigoid, but these findings and the surrounding hypopigmented, thickened skin are nonspecific; both routine and direct immunofluorescent biopsies are required for diagnosis.

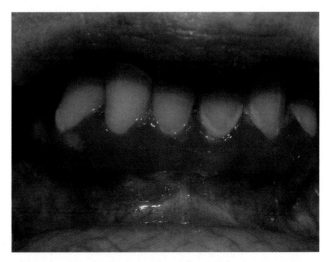

FIG. 9-41. Desquamative gingivitis indistinguishable from that of pemphigus vulgaris and, some cases, of erosive lichen planus, is usually seen in patients such as this with cicatricial pemphigoid.

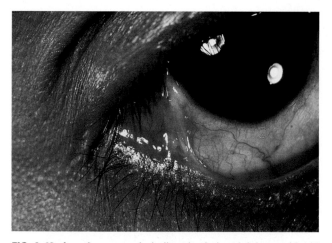

FIG. 9-42. A pathognomonic hallmark of cicatricial pemphigoid is scarring of the conjunctivae, with early synechiae between the palpebral and bulbar conjunctivae.

despite feeling dry and gritty, may appear normal initially, but an ophthalmologic examination detects early abnormalities: reduced lacrimation or adhesions of the bulbar and palpebral conjunctivae (Fig. 9-42). Later, more extensive scarring may cause severe adhesions, entropion, and corneal scarring with blindness.

Nonmucous membrane lesions, when present, are very helpful in suggesting the correct diagnosis by demonstrating the blistering nature of the process. Lesions are small, straw-colored blisters that may scar.

Patients with a more recently recognized form of cicatricial pemphigoid, antiepiligrin cicatricial pemphigoid, exhibit more recalcitrant disease, minor nonmucous membrane disease, and a relatively frequent association with solid tumors.

Diagnosis

The diagnosis is suspected by the constellation of ocular, oral, and genital irritation and erosions. The diagnosis is confirmed by typical routine histology of a blister or erosion that also shows no evidence of other diseases that clinically mimic cicatricial pemphigoid. The diagnosis can sometimes be definitively made by typical immunofluorescent studies. Histology shows a subepidermal blister, a mixed inflammatory infiltrate, and dermal scarring. Direct immunofluorescent biopsies may be negative but, when positive, are the same as in bullous pemphigoid. There is linear deposition of IgG, IgA, and C3 at the BMZ. Immunofluorescent studies of salt-split skin show the antibodies to be in the roof (epidermal) portion of the blister, although some are located in the floor (dermal) aspect of the blister. Multiple biopsies including oral and conjunctival specimens increase the positive yield.

All mucous membrane erosive diseases must be considered initially in patients with cicatricial pemphigoid. Blistering diseases that can mimic cicatricial pemphigoid include pemphigus vulgaris and epidermolyis bullosa

acquisita. Although the two diseases are clinically different, cicatricial pemphigoid and bullous pemphigoid appear identical histologically, and some target antigens in cicatricial pemphigoid (BP180 and BP230) are identical to those in bullous pemphigoid, although others involve laminin-5, the β_4-integrin, and other as yet unknown antigens. Because blisters are often not apparent in patients with cicatricial pemphigoid, other scarring diseases such as erosive lichen planus or erosive lichen sclerosus are in the differential diagnosis for genital cicatricial pemphigoid.

Pathophysiology

Cicatricial pemphigoid is a phenotype of a group of immunochemically distinct autoimmune subepidermal blistering diseases. As occurs with the closely related bullous pemphigoid, antibodies are directed against components of the basement membrane including laminin 5, resulting in a loss of adhesion of the epidermis to the dermis and subsequent blistering (34).

Management

Treatment is often difficult. Disease activity fluctuates naturally, and most treatment modifies disease activity but cannot suppress it. Systemic prednisone at 50 to 80 mg/day and reduced according to response may be helpful for the skin disease but is less helpful for mucosal disease. Steroid-sparing drugs may be needed (dapsone, oral or pulse cyclophosphamide, azathioprine). More recently, intravenous immunoglobulin has shown promise in the treatment of this disease. The anti-CD20 antibody rituximab may also provide benefit in some patients (35). Genital lesions may be improved by potent topical steroids, sometimes in combination with an anti-inflammatory antibiotic such as tetracycline. In addition, local care of the mucous membranes by multiple specialties and prevention of secondary infection are essential. Surgery and dilation may be needed to alleviate scarring when the skin disease is controlled.

Cicatricial pemphigoid is a chronic disease, although activity may fluctuate. Continuing care is necessary. There is no proven link with malignancy, but carcinoma has been reported, possibly from chronic erosion and immunosuppressive treatment.

Linear IgA Disease

Epidemiology and Clinical Morphology

Linear IgA disease (LAD) presents at any age, with the peak incidence at more than 60 years. It sometimes occurs in children, when it was formerly called "chronic bullous disease of childhood."

The initial presentation of LAD consists of annular, erythematous, nonscaling, red plaques with peripheral blistering (Fig. 9-43). These plaques gradually become more

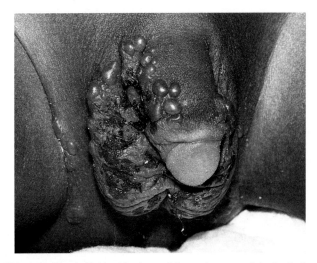

FIG. 9-43. The individual lesions of linear immunoglobulin A disease resemble those of bullous pemphigoid, with tense, straw-colored blisters.

generalized. Mucosal involvement with scarring may occur. Children present with genital and perioral blisters, suggesting the possibility of sexual abuse. Healing plaques may show postinflammatory pigmentation.

In the past, LAD was reported as associated with a number of autoimmune diseases, especially thyroid disease, vitiligo, rheumatoid arthritis, systemic lupus erythematosus, and pernicious anemia. However, studies on large numbers of adults with LAD showed a higher incidence of autoantibodies but no higher incidence of autoimmune disease. There is a definite increased incidence of lymphoproliferative disease in patients with LAD.

Diagnosis

This disease is suspected by the morphology of the skin lesions, and it is confirmed by routine biopsy as well as a biopsy for direct immunofluorescence and serum for indirect immunofluorescence. An extremely rapid response to dapsone therapy is a less-sophisticated diagnostic test. Histology shows a subepidermal blister with a neutrophilic infiltrate. Biopsies for direct immunofluorescence show a linear band of IgA deposition at the BMZ. Immunofluorescent studies of salt-split skin show the IgA deposition to be epidermal, and indirect immunofluorescent assays of serum show IgA antibodies in all children and most adults.

Initial, annular pink plaques can be confused with urticaria, and once blistering occurs, bullous pemphigoid and blistering erythema multiforme must be considered. However, the classic annular blistering plaques are unique to LAD.

Pathophysiology

Linear IgA disease (LAD) is an acquired autoimmune blistering disease (see also Chapter 14). The target antigens include collagen XVII (BP180) and its shed

ectodomain, leading to the production of plasminlike proteases and tissue damage (36). Amiodarone, antibiotics including vancomycin and amoxicillin/clavulinic acid, lithium, and nonsteroidal anti-inflammatory drugs have been shown to induce LAD (37,38), and although pregnancy improves the disease, a relapse is common 3 months postpartum. Such diseases, drugs, and hormonal changes may alter the ability of the IgA to bind antigen. Occasionally, localized LAD may occur at sites of cutaneous trauma such as a burn. There may be an increased incidence after infection or antibiotic administration, and in one series, a significantly higher number of patients with LAD had been exposed to building work in the 3 months before disease onset than in the general population.

Management

Systemic therapy is required for the control of LAD. Treatment with dapsone or sulfonamides produces improvement in patients with LAD within 48 hours. Systemic corticosteroids are necessary in some cases, and minocycline with nicotinamide, or azathioprine with dapsone, has been tried, sometimes successfully. Care of the mucous membranes, prevention of secondary infection, and use of topical steroids are also important in management.

Sixty percent of adults experience remission, usually within 3 years. The immune deposits are lost from the skin. The disease is self-limiting in children, with most experiencing remission before puberty. Mucous membrane lesions may be more recalcitrant.

Those patients with unusually severe disease may be more likely to have the antiepiligrin type of disease. This may be important because the immunosuppressive medications used for cicatricial pemphigoid may accelerate the activity of any underlying adenocarcinoma that is more likely to occur with this form of pemphigoid.

Epidermolysis Bullosa Acquisita

Clinical Presentation

Epidermolysis bullosa acquisita (EBA) is a rare disease that occurs most often in middle-aged and elderly patients. It is characterized by skin fragility, trauma-induced blisters, mucous membrane involvement in 50% of cases, and a tendency to heal with scarring. Early skin findings can be indistinguishable from bullous or cicatricial pemphigoid. Scarring of the skin leads to tapering of the fingers similar to that seen in scleroderma. In addition, cigarette paper texture of the skin is common, as is variegate cutaneous hyperpigmentation and hypopigmentation and milia.

On the genitalia, painful erosions are typical, and scarring may lead to phimosis in uncircumcised men and alteration of normal vulvar architecture and introital stenosis in women. Scarring of the conjunctivae, larynx, and esophagus also occurs.

Diagnosis

The diagnosis is suspected by it presentation, confirmed by a routine biopsy in association with direct and indirect immunofluorescent studies. Histology is similar to that of pemphigoid, showing a subepidermal blister with a mixed inflammatory infiltrate. A biopsy for direct immunofluorescence reveals IgG deposited along the basement membrane.

Bullous pemphigoid, cicatricial pemphigoid, porphyria cutanea tarda, and pemphigus vulgaris are the blistering/erosive diseases morphologically most similar to EBA. More advanced EBA with scarring of the fingers resembles scleroderma.

Pathophysiology

EBA is an acquired autoimmune blistering disease. The target antigen is collagen VII (the anchoring fibrils) in the dermis. This is shared as the target antigen in bullous systemic lupus erythematosus, but the latter is very different clinically, being a short-lived bullous disease in the setting of systemic lupus erythematosus. The same target antigen is found in congenital epidermolysis bullosa dystrophica, which presents in infancy with repeated blistering, scarring, and deformity.

Management

Treatment is difficult, and the course of EBA is prolonged, lacking the eventual remissions of some autoimmune blistering diseases. It may be unresponsive to steroids, both systemic and topical, or to immunosuppressive agents, dapsone, or tetracyclines. Data regarding therapy is limited to case reports and very small series. Colchicine (39), rituximab (40), and mycophenylate mofetil (41) have been reported useful in some. Supportive care is essential, especially if the disease is widespread, and careful attention to secondary infection of the genitalia may help to minimize scarring.

Pemphigoid Gestationis (Herpes Gestationis)

Pemphigoid gestationis is a dramatic autoimmune blistering disorder occurring in the second or third trimester of pregnancy, in the postpartum period, or in the setting of choriocarcinoma or hydatidiform mole. It may occur in any pregnancy but occurs earlier and more severely in subsequent pregnancies. Associated autoimmune disease has been reported, especially thyroid disease. It is rare; the incidence is reported from 1 in 3,000 to 1 in 60,000 pregnancies.

Clinically, in pemphigoid gestationis, intensely pruritic, pink, nonscaling plaques that resemble urticaria occur around the umbilicus and progress to a generalized bullous eruption. Vulvar involvement is not prominent, and mucosal involvement is mild. The disease often flares at delivery, and there is a tendency to premature delivery and low-birth-weight fetus. The neonate may be affected with mild cutaneous lesions in 10% of cases, but the condition resolves rapidly over a few weeks. The early onset of this disease in pregnancy and the presence of significant blistering may be associated with adverse outcomes, so that careful surveillance is important (42).

Direct immunofluorescence in pemphigoid gestationis shows C3 with or without IgG bound to the BMZ, and salt-split skin shows this to be epidermal. The target antigen is the BP180 in the hemidesmosomes. Indirect immunofluorescence shows that patients' sera can fix fresh C3 to skin BMZ.

Systemic steroids are the mainstay of treatment and can safely be used in pregnancy. Sometimes, topical steroids are sufficient. The dose can be tapered in the last trimester of pregnancy, but the dose may have to be increased to cope with the postpartum flare of disease. After delivery, the disease usually regresses spontaneously in weeks to months, although occasionally it remains active for years. It is hormone sensitive, and 30% of patients suffer an exacerbation with oral contraceptives.

Dermatitis Herpetiformis

Dermatitis herpetiformis is an autoimmune blistering disease that does not preferentially affect the genitalia. It is produced by IgA deposits in the upper dermis that ultimately produce a neutrophilic infiltrate and detachment of the epidermis from the dermis (43).

The hallmark of dermatitis herpetiformis is excruciating itching, accompanied by small, grouped vesicles that tend to occur on the elbows, knees, and lower back and buttocks. Because of rubbing and scratching that quickly break the vesicles, the blistering nature of the process is often obscured by excoriations. Dermatitis herpetiformis is associated with gluten-sensitive enteropathy that often is asymptomatic.

The diagnosis is made by the clinical picture, a characteristic routine biopsy of a blister or erosion, and a direct immunofluorescent biopsy that shows IgA in the dermal papillae. Dermatitis herpetiformis predictably responds quickly to oral dapsone. In addition, avoidance of all dietary gluten results in the alleviation of both enteropathy and skin disease, but the time to response is quite long.

Benign Familial Pemphigus (Hailey–Hailey Disease)

Clinical Presentation

Presenting in young adults, Hailey–Hailey is autosomal dominant, occurring in about half of family members in varying degrees of severity. The skin lesions of Hailey–Hailey disease are characterized by recurrent, small, usually subtle blisters and crusted erosions occurring on an erythematous base, largely in intertriginous zones and perianal skin (Figs. 9-44 through 9-46). These eventuate into thickened, macerated red plaques that exhibit

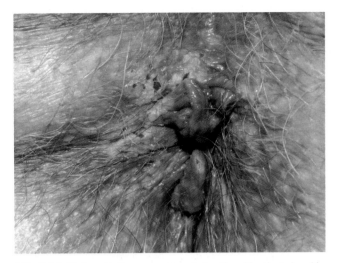

FIG. 9-44. Hailey–Hailey consists of fragile skin that, in skin folds, presents as thickened, white skin with angular, small fissures. Maceration is common.

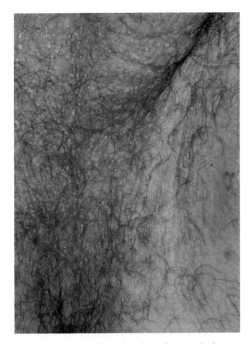

FIG. 9-46. Hailey–Hailey often develops into red plaques of redness and maceration that resemble eczema or lichen simplex chronicus, as seen on the scrotum and perineum of the son of the patient pictured in Fig. 9-45.

characteristic, short, irregular, linear fissures. Exudation is common, and vesicles may become pustules. There may be expanding erythematous plaques with peripheral scaling in the axillae, groin, and perineum that resemble a fungal infection. Mucous membrane lesions do not occur.

Diagnosis

The diagnosis is made on the basis of morphology, family history, and a routine biopsy. Histology reveals suprabasal blisters with acantholysis and areas of intraepidermal separation. Immunofluorescence is negative.

The most common morphology, that of exudative red, scaling plaques, can resemble tinea cruris, eczema, and psoriasis. When vesicles are pustular, candidiasis as a diagnosis or complicating factor should be considered. In addition, HSV can mimic the tiny erosions within the plaques. At times, HSV infection can secondarily infect Hailey–Hailey disease (Kaposi varicelliform eruption), so refractory disease should be evaluated for this possibility. However, the erosions of candidiasis and HSV are generally round or arcuate from coalescing blisters, whereas the small erosions from Hailey–Hailey disease are characteristically linear and angular.

Pathophysiology

Hailey–Hailey disease is an autosomal dominant disease resulting in a defect in normal adhesion between keratinocytes. This condition is associated with various mutations in the ATP2C1 gene, a gene responsible for controlling Ca2+ concentrations in the cytoplasm and Golgi apparatus of keratinocytes (44). Ca2+ in the cytoplasm is essential in keratinocyte differentiation (45).

The friction, heat, perspiration, bacterial and yeast colonization, and infection most marked in skin folds precipitate separation of the epidermis from the dermis and resulting erosions. HSV infection sometimes plays a role as well.

Management

There is no satisfactory, specific therapy for Hailey–Hailey disease. Supportive care is important, including the prompt treatment of secondary infection. Blistering can be minimized by the suppression of cutaneous bacteria by long-term administration of topical antibiotics such as clindamycin or erythromycin solutions, or oral medication such as doxycycline or clindamycin. In addition, an antiperspirant can reduce the friction that worsens with

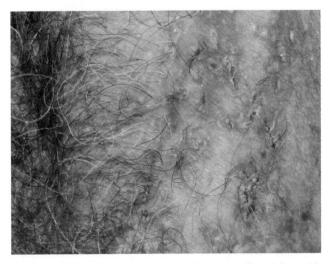

FIG. 9-45. Hailey–Hailey disease produces small vesicles with moist, white necrotic epithelium that leave linear erosions as they rupture.

sweating, and the subsequent blistering and maceration. However, antiperspirants can produce remarkable stinging and irritation when they are applied to very irritated, eroded, or macerated skin, so these agents should be used only as maintenance therapy on relatively well-controlled skin. If "clinical strength" over-the-counter potent antiperspirants up to 12% are not adequately effective, prescription-strength aluminum chloride can be used. Botulinum toxin type A has been reported as useful in some patients with Hailey–Hailey disease, presumably because of the antiperspirant activity (46).

Topical corticosteroids partially suppress the manifestations of Hailey–Hailey disease, but high-potency preparations are needed, and rebound of symptoms on reducing the dose is common. Tacrolimus has been beneficial for some but is irritating to most patients with active disease (47). Dapsone and methotrexate have been used successfully in some patients. Carbon dioxide laser therapy (48), photodynamic therapy (49), topical fluorouracil (50) and dermabrasion have been shown to produce benefit in some patients with recalcitrant disease, likely because of the surface damage and scarring that may disrupt sweat glands. These are all very uncomfortable therapies that should not be first-line. Retinoids such as acitretin may regulate differentiation and provide comfort to some patients (51). The course of the disease is one of spontaneous exacerbations and remissions. It is usually worse in hot summer months when sweating worsens the condition. There is no tendency to improve with age.

Bullous Erythema Multiforme (Stevens–Johnson Syndrome, Toxic Epidermal Necrolysis)

Clinical Presentation

Erythema multiforme is a self-limiting but sometimes recurrent hypersensitivity reaction. This presents with the sudden onset of erythematous flat papules that classically develop a darker, dusky erythema centrally due to more severe inflammation in that area; this produces a target contour (Fig. 9-47). With severe central inflammation and epidermal necrosis, the dermis and epidermis can separate, forming either a central blister, or necrotic epithelium simply sloughs, leaving erosions. When blisters on keratinized skin remain discrete and are associated with mucous membrane erosions, the condition is called Stevens–Johnson syndrome (Figs. 9-48 and 9-49). More severe disease that results in the coalescence of red skin and sheets of denuded epithelium is named toxic epidermal necrolysis (Figs. 9-50 through 9-53).

Usually, lesions appear abruptly and are generalized over the skin surface. However, blistering forms of erythema multiforme sometimes preferentially affect only the palms, soles, and mucous membranes. Blistering forms of erythema multiforme generally involve multiple

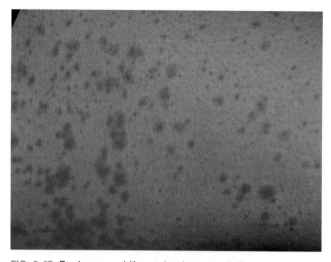

FIG. 9-47. Erythema multiforme begins as red, flat macules with dark centers that sometimes progress to necrosis and sloughing.

mucous membranes, and these blisters on fragile mucous membrane and modified mucous membrane rupture almost instantly, producing erosions rather than intact blisters. Usually, the blisters are never recognized clinically because of their short-lived nature.

Even though skin lesions generally heal quickly after the inciting agent is withdrawn or treated, scarring of the genitalia and eyes can be severe. Vaginal lesions occasionally result in synechiae, and uncircumcised men can experience phimosis and paraphimosis.

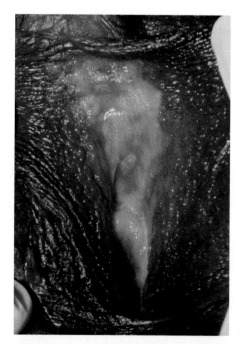

FIG. 9-48. Blisters of erythema multiforme on mucous membranes generally become immediate erosions that are indistinguishable from those of immunobullous diseases and lichen planus.

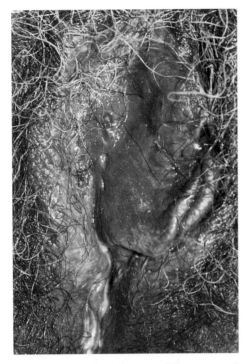

FIG. 9-49. Milder forms of erythema multiforme are characterized by scattered, discrete erosions of modified mucous membranes and mucous membranes, sometimes without blistering on keratinized skin.

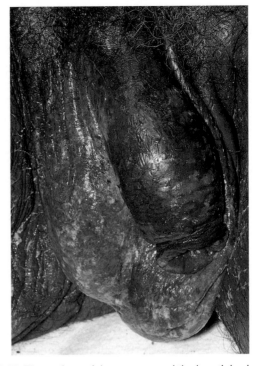

FIG. 9-51. The surface of the scrotum and the keratinized skin of the penis are preferentially affected over other keratinized surfaces in toxic epidermal necrolysis. This patient succumbed to his allergy to phenytoin.

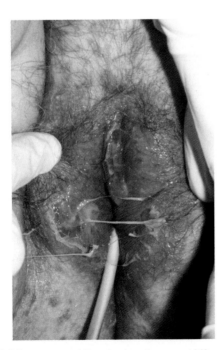

FIG. 9-50. More severe blistering erythema multiforme, called toxic epidermal necrolysis, is characterized by widespread erosion and flaccid blisters.

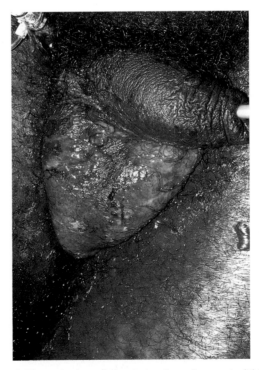

FIG. 9-52. The scrotal erosions were only a minor part of this patient's generalized blistering and erosive reaction to sulfonamide drugs.

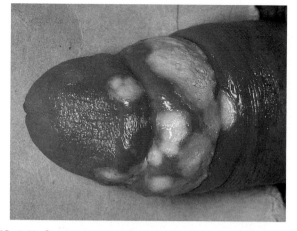

FIG. 9-53. Secondary infection can transform erosions of toxic epidermal necrolysis into ulcerations, as has occurred here. This underscores the importance of scrupulous local care and infection control.

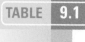

| TABLE 9.1 | Common medications causing blistering erythema multiforme (Stevens–Johnson syndrome and toxic epidermal necrolysis) |

Antibiotics
  Penicillins
  Cephalosporins
  Sulfonamides
Anticonvulsant medications
  Carbamazepine
  Barbiturates
  Phenytoin
  Lamotrigine
Cardiovascular medications
  Hydrochlorothiazide
  Furosemide
  Hydralazine
  Procainamide
Other
  Allopurinol
  All nonsteroidal anti-inflammatory medications
  Quinidine

From Roujeau JC, Stern RS. Severe adverse cutaneous reactions to drugs. *N Engl J Med.* 1994;331:1272, with permission.

Patients with widespread lesions are toxic, exhibit a marked risk of secondary infection and temperature instability, and generally experience the same complications as burn patients.

Diagnosis

The diagnosis of blistering erythema multiforme is made by the abrupt onset and clinical appearance in a person who is receiving a medication known to produce this reaction. The diagnosis should be confirmed by biopsy to rule out other diseases such as pemphigus vulgaris or cicatricial pemphigoid, which usually do not occur as quickly, but are treated very differently. The mortality of widespread disease is about 40%.

The most striking histologic abnormalities of blistering forms of erythema multiforme are epidermal. Early lesions show groups of necrotic keratinocytes, and more advanced disease shows liquefaction degeneration of the basal cell layer with extensive epidermal necrosis. Dermal chronic perivascular mononuclear inflammation is usual.

Pemphigus vulgaris can be almost indistinguishable from widespread toxic epidermal necrolysis, although it is usually slower in onset. Bullous pemphigoid can be similar, but usually spares mucous membranes, whereas cicatricial pemphigoid characteristically produces similar genital lesions. A fixed drug eruption can appear very similar, but the number of lesions is usually smaller.

Pathophysiology

Blistering erythema multiforme is an allergic reaction to either a medication or to recurrent HSV infection (Table 9-1). Although nearly every available medication has been reported to produce blistering erythema multiforme, sulfas, anticonvulsants, and lamotrigine are the medications most associated with this event (52). HLA genotype appears to have a significant association with the risk of blistering erythema multiforme (53). Although not yet available, rapid methods for evaluating increased risk by diagnosis of HLA status are in development (54).

Unlike other medication reactions, blistering of these diseases is preceded by the presence of increased levels of soluble Fas ligand levels in serum, which interacts with Fas on affected keratinocytes (55). The recent progress in elucidation of the pathogenesis of these diseases provides clues for the development of more effective therapies.

Management

Treatment includes stopping the offending drug. Those patients with recurrent HSV infection producing blistering erythema multiforme can be treated with chronic suppressive antiviral medication such as acyclovir 400 mg twice daily, famciclovir 250 mg twice daily, or valacyclovir 500 mg or 1 g/day, to prevent future recurrences. The acute treatment of HSV infection is not beneficial, because erythema multiforme follows the infection, and antivirals generally are useful for recurrent HSV infection only when they are begun immediately.

Supportive care is the second most important aspect of therapy. The aggressive identification and treatment of any secondary infection and fluid loss are essential. Referral to a burn unit for those with widespread disease is required in many people. Local care of the genitalia with generous lubrication and regular retraction of the glans in uncircumcised men can help to prevent scarring, as can the insertion of a vaginal dilator daily in women with vaginal involvement. Local yeast infections are especially common in this setting of frequent concomitant immunosuppressive and antibiotic use.

There are no controlled trials of therapy for erythema multiforme. Intravenous immunoglobulin therapy has been reported beneficial in the treatment of blistering forms of erythema multiforme (56). However, the use of systemic corticosteroids is very controversial and many consider corticosteroids to be contraindicated (57). Although some clinicians believe that the early institution of corticosteroids can limit blistering, prolonged use of systemic corticosteroids and their use after blistering has occurred do not improve the condition and can worsen the prognosis by increasing the risk of adverse reaction to the steroid. Intravenous immunoglobulins have been reported useful at times (58), but not all have had good results with this therapy. Cyclosporine, infliximab, and plasmapheresis have been used as well (59).

Fixed Drug Eruption

Clinical Presentation

A fixed drug eruption is a peculiar reaction to a medication consisting of a recurrent same-site skin lesion, occurring in any sensitized individual, independent of gender or age. Following exposure to the causative medication, the patient notes a single or a few lesions. On

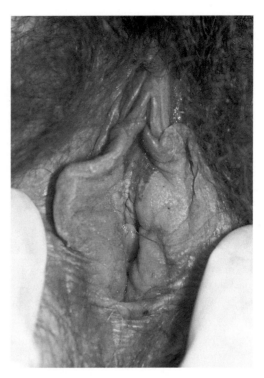

FIG. 9-55. The recurrent erosion of a fixed drug eruption occurs in the exact same spot, as in the anterior vestibule seen here, although new areas may appear with subsequent exposures as well.

keratinized skin, these present as well-demarcated, round, edematous, erythematous plaques that may blister. Lesions on mucous membranes such as the oral mucosa, the modified mucous membrane skin of the vulva, or the glans penis normally blister but quickly erode before the blister is recognized (Figs. 9-54 through 9-57). On this thinner, moist epithelium, the individual lesions are often more irregular in shape. These lesions are often accompanied by a burning sensation. Further exposures to the causative medication produce subsequent fixed drug reaction lesions at previously affected sites, although

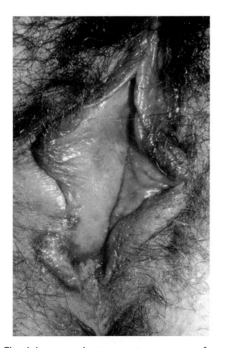

FIG. 9-54. Fixed drug eruption presents as one or a few erosions that occur with each exposure to medication and can be historically misdiagnosed as recurrent herpes simplex virus infection.

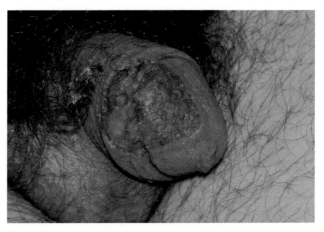

FIG. 9-56. This fixed drug reaction began as a fragile wheal that eroded and then crusted. (Credit Errol Craig, MD)

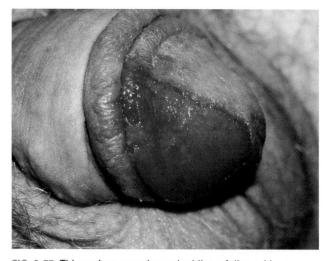

FIG. 9-57. This patient experienced a blister followed by an erosion representing a fixed drug eruption shortly after beginning doxycycline for acne.

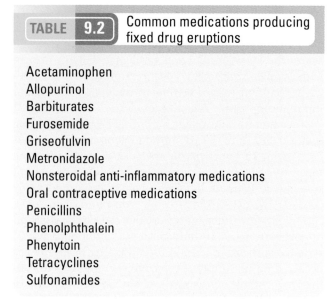

TABLE **9.2**	Common medications producing fixed drug eruptions

Acetaminophen
Allopurinol
Barbiturates
Furosemide
Griseofulvin
Metronidazole
Nonsteroidal anti-inflammatory medications
Oral contraceptive medications
Penicillins
Phenolphthalein
Phenytoin
Tetracyclines
Sulfonamides

each exposure may be associated with new lesions as well. The lesions disappear when the drug is withdrawn, although there may be some residual postinflammatory hyperpigmentation.

Diagnosis

The diagnosis of a fixed drug eruption is made by the abrupt onset of oral and/or genital erosions, often with blisters or edematous round plaques of keratinized skin, in the presence of a history of recent ingestion of a medication known to cause this skin eruption. Usually, the history also reveals that recurrent lesions in the same location have occurred in the past. Although mucous membrane erosions of a fixed drug eruption generally are nonspecific, keratinized skin lesions are often very helpful when present, and round, well-demarcated patches of deep postinflammatory hyperpigmentation from past episodes are pathognomonic. When needed, a biopsy is usually characteristic. Histologic findings include liquefaction degeneration of the basal cell layer, with upper dermal pigment incontinence. Dyskeratotic keratinocytes and separation of the epidermis from the dermis produce bullae. Epidermal necrosis with neutrophils is characteristic.

The history of recurrent genital and oral erosions in the same locations often suggests a diagnosis of recurrent HSV infection, but the morphology does not suggest a coalescence of small erosions of vesicles. The side of the lesions is more consistent with those of lichen planus, an immunobullous blistering disease, or trauma. Individual lesions are suggestive of blistering erythema multiforme, but the numbers of lesions is usually much fewer.

Pathophysiology

Fixed drug eruptions are uncommon, peculiar hypersensitivity reactions to any of several possible medications.

The eruption may occur as a result of activation of effector memory T cells within the epidermis of lesional skin (60). Causative drugs include tetracyclines, sulfonamides, analgesics, sedatives, oral contraceptives, metronidazole, as well as phenolphthalein "hidden" in some over-the-counter laxatives (Table 9-2) (61,62). Cross-reactivity of one drug with another to produce the rash can make the diagnosis more difficult. Occasionally, an offending medication cannot be identified.

Management

The most important aspects of treatment are the identification and elimination of the offending medication. Otherwise, therapy is supportive only. Soaks, infection control, and pain medication are mainstays.

Trauma and Iatrogenic and Artifactual Disorders

Clinical Presentation

The morphology of the erosions or blisters and the degree and timing of discomfort depend on the insult, with many producing immediate pain. Liquids often produce a drip pattern, and blisters produce a round erosion. Scratching, zipper, and bite trauma are manifested by irregular erosions.

Diagnosis

The diagnosis is usually made easily because the injury is immediately painful. In addition, the shape of the erosion is suggestive of the diagnosis.

Erosive lichen planus and autoimmune blistering diseases are occasionally mistaken for traumatic lesions. However, an examination of other areas usually shows evidence of these other diseases, and a biopsy can be helpful in difficult cases.

Pathophysiology

Erosions and blisters from trauma can occur from many different types of insults. A common cause of genital erosions is a chemical burn, particularly from wart therapies such as podophyllin, trichloroacetic and bichloroacetic acids, and fluorouracil. Less often, patient-applied podofilox or imiquimod produces erosions. Occasionally, alcohols and preservatives in creams, especially antifungal creams being used on irritated skin, can cause burning and erosions, as can an exaggerated reaction to gentian violet. Thermal burns can occur in this area, but these are uncommon, whereas blisters and erosions from cryotherapy for warts or dysplasia are usual reactions to treatment. Other traumas inflicted for medical purposes that cause erosions include laser surgery and electrocautery.

Nonmedical injuries include tearing of skin from a zipper, human bites, and injuries to the area designed to heighten sensation or to intensify orgasm, such as a rubber band applied around a penis and then inadvertently left in place, thus producing necrosis.

Management

Bland emollients, soaks, pain medication, and infection control are important. The prognosis depends upon the cause of the trauma.

Contact Dermatitis

Contact dermatitis can result from either an irritant or a specific allergen (see also Chapters 4 and 6). Irritant contact dermatitis is produced by a substance that directly and nonimmunologically damages the skin. An irritant

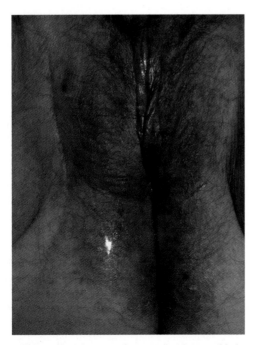

FIG. 9-58. This patient has erosions and redness of irritant contact dermatitis from compulsive scrubbing with antiseptic soap.

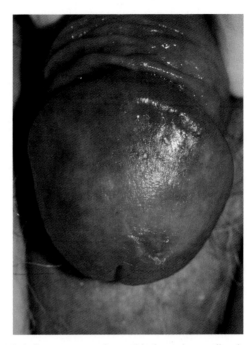

FIG. 9-59. Irritant contact dermatitis from the application of alcohol and hydrogen peroxide have caused redness, edema, and erosion of the glans.

reaction sufficient to produce erosions or blisters is generally called a burn (see the earlier discussion of trauma) (Figs. 9-58 and 9-59).

Allergic contact dermatitis is a cell-mediated type IV allergic reaction to a specific allergen, occurring at the point of contact. Common sensitizing allergens include topical creams containing the antibiotic neomycin, the preservative ethylenediamine, propylene glycol, the local anesthetics benzocaine and diphenhydramine, and some topical corticosteroids. The patient must be sensitized to the allergen. One or two days following subsequent exposure to the allergen, the rash develops. An acute, strong allergic contact dermatitis consists of confluent small, firm, and pruritic vesicles. This eruption may persist for 2 weeks. On the genitalia, this often presents as erosions and blisters on a background of erythema (Figs. 9-60 and 9-61). The diagnosis can be confirmed by patch testing normal skin with the suspected allergen. Treatment involves the elimination of responsible allergenic substances. Application of mild topical corticosteroids, use of ointment emollients, and cooling with ice packs cause rapid relief. Erosive allergic contact dermatitis often improves best with oral prednisone 40 to 60 mg each morning for 5 to 10 days.

PSEUDOVESICULAR CONDITIONS

Mollusca Contagiosa

Although mollusca contagiosa most often appear white or skin-colored and solid, these lesions are sometimes sufficiently shiny that they appear vesicular, leading to the

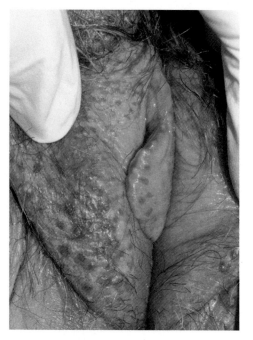

FIG. 9-60. The application of an over-the-counter anti-itch medication containing benzocaine and resorcinol eventuated into an allergic contact dermatitis characterized by blisters that eroded into small round erosions.

lay term "water warts" (Fig. 9-62). This condition is discussed primarily in Chapters 8, 11, and 12.

Hidradenoma Papilliferum

These small cystic tumors are classic on the vulva, and often appear vesicular with intermittent drainage of clear

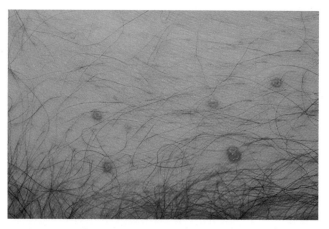

FIG. 9-62. These mollusca contagiosa resemble herpes vesicles, with the central depression that is characteristic of both mollusca and a herpes blister. However, these "water-warts" are firm to the touch and not fluid filled.

mucoid material from an overlying punctum (Figs. 9-63 and 12-34). However, these are most often solitary and solid to the touch. See also Chapters 11 and 12.

Lymphangiectasias and Lymphangioma Circumscriptum

Lymphangiectasias occur when firm edema obstructs lymphatic return, and dilated lymphatic vessels distend and are visible through the thinned epidermis (Figs. 9-64 and 12-47). Primary lymphangioma circumscriptum refers to a vascular malformation of the lymphatics that produces the same surface clinical appearance. Often, a deep

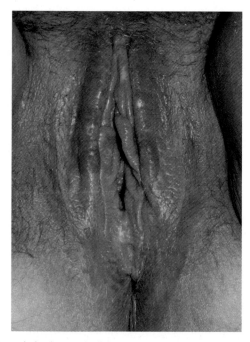

FIG. 9-61. Irritation and allergy to medications used for lichen simplex chronicus evolved into superimposed irritant and allergic contact dermatitis.

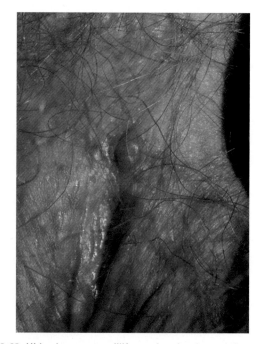

FIG. 9-63. Hidradenoma papilliferum is a benign cystic tumor of sweat glands that may appear vesicular. There is usually a central pit that can exude mucoid material.

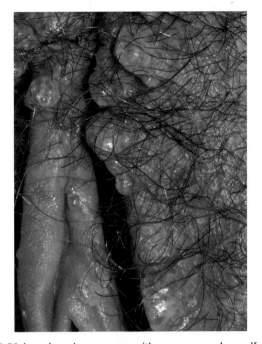

FIG. 9-64. Lymphangiomas occur either as a vascular malformation of lymphatics or, more often, as a result of chronic, firm edema that occludes lymphatic return, leading to dilated lymph vessels that protrude above the skin. This patient had chronic edema from Crohn disease.

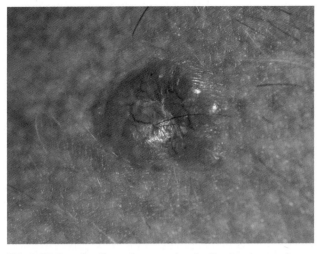

FIG. 9-65. Basal cell carcinomas classically show a pearly appearance that can mimic a blister; these can ulcerate as they enlarge.

component results in fairly widely scattered, grouped multiloculated bulging lymphatics protruding though the surface. These abnormalities not only mimic vesicles, but also can resemble raspberry-shaped genital warts.

MALIGNANCIES PRESENTING AS EROSIONS

Basal Cell Carcinoma

Basal cell cancers are associated, classically, with sites of sun exposure, but 10% occur on nonexposed sites and account for 5% of genital cancers (see Chapter 12). They occur more frequently in fair than dark-skinned men and women. Basal cell carcinomas are more common with increasing age and often present with itching but only minor pain or soreness. The lesions often display the typical pearly, rolled edge, with a central depression or necrotic erosion (Fig. 9-65), whence the term "rodent ulcer." They invade locally, but almost never metastasize. Still, local invasion and necrosis of untreated tumors cause significant tissue damage.

Diagnosis and treatment are affected by conservative local excision. Those in more difficult sites may be amenable to radiotherapy.

Invasive Squamous Cell Carcinoma

Squamous cell cancers account for more than 90% of genital cancers and often arise in the site of chronic scarring

or inflammation such as lichen sclerosus and lichen planus (see Chapter 12 for primary discussion) or some human papillomavirus infection. Squamous cell carcinomas occur most commonly in the older age group (the mean presenting age is older than 65 years), but it may present at any age from the 20s. The lesions present as red or skin-colored plaques or nodules that can erode or ulcerate as they enlarge (Fig. 9-66). There may be associated inguinal lymphadenopathy. Diagnosis is made by biopsy, and treatment is surgical.

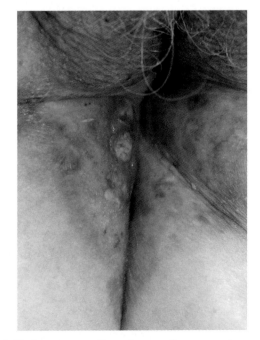

FIG. 9-66. Squamous cell carcinoma often presents as a red plaque, sometimes with erosions and ulcerations, and frequently with induration.

Intraepithelial Carcinoma (Vulvar Intraepithelial Neoplasia, Vaginal Intraepithelial Neoplasia, Penile Intraepithelial Neoplasia, Bowen Disease, Bowenoid Papulosis, Squamous Cell Carcinoma In Situ, Erythroplasia of Queyrat)

Intraepithelial neoplasia refers to dysplasia of the epidermis (see Chapter 12 for primary discussion). Genital intraepithelial neoplasia most often is related to human papillomavirus (HPV) infection, but it is also seen with longstanding lichen sclerosus and lichen planus. Patients experience itching, soreness, or no symptoms. Morphologically, cases of vulvar and penile intraepithelial neoplasia are often multifocal, and lesions may resemble viral warts, sometimes coalescing into plaques. Often, they are pigmented, erythematous, scaling, crusted, or eroded plaques (Fig. 9-67). Penile intraepithelial neoplasia occurs mainly in uncircumcised male patients and presents as a glazed red plaque of the glans and foreskin that may erode. It can cause phimosis and sometimes involves the distal urethra. The diagnosis is confirmed by biopsy, and treatment options include surgical excision, cryotherapy, CO_2 laser ablation, or topical fluorouracil. Imiquimod has been used as well. All patients should be followed up by careful observation for recurrence and possible evolution to invasive squamous cell carcinoma.

Extramammary Paget Disease
(see Chapter 6 for primary discussion)

Extramammary Paget disease is a rare neoplasm arising from dysplastic secretory glandular adenocarcinoma

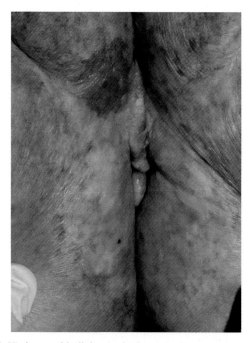

FIG. 9-67. Intraepithelial neoplasia can also appear red and eroded, but it is usually not associated with induration.

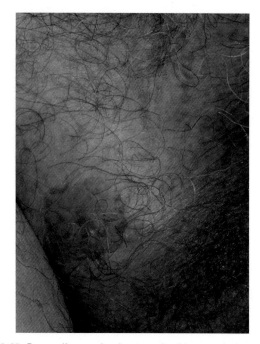

FIG. 9-68. Paget disease is characterized by a red plaque with erosions, and it may be mistaken for eczema or intraepithelial neoplasia.

cells occurring in the anogenital or axillary epidermis (see Chapter 6). Anogenital Paget disease most often is unassociated with malignancy, but there is an associated gastrointestinal or genitourinary malignancy in about 15% of patients.

Extramammary Paget disease generally presents as well-demarcated, slow-growing, eroded, itchy, red plaques (Fig. 9-68). When pruritus is a prominent feature, the area may become lichenified and may mimic benign dermatitis.

Diagnosis is by biopsy, and treatment is by surgical wide excision and should include investigations to find a local or distant tumor. Local recurrences requiring repeated excisions are usual.

GENITAL SKIN FOLD FISSURES

Genital skin fold fissures are not a disease, but a common clinical presentation of several genital diseases. Genital fissures, especially fissures of the vulva, produce stinging pain that patients often refer to as feeling like paper cuts. These erosions are often recurrent or chronic.

Clinical Presentation

Skin fold fissures consist of linear erosions within skin folds, especially the interlabial folds, edges of the clitoral hood in women, in the coronal sulcus and skin wrinkling of the penile shaft, and within the normal skin markings of the perineal body and perianal skin of both

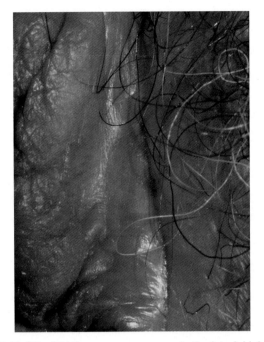

FIG. 9-69. Skin fold fissures are common in the interlabial folds and, in this case, are caused by candidiasis.

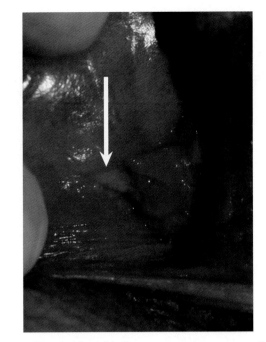

FIG. 9-71. Chronic idiopathic fissures sometimes occur adjacent to the hymeneal ring, generally requiring excision by a perineoplasty.

men and women (Figs. 9-69 through 9-73). These are so transient that the diagnosis is often made by the history in association with thin, red lines in the areas of fissuring or by having the patient return as soon as fissures recur. Sometimes, magnification is required for identification. At other times, the fissures are so deep as to actually represent ulcers.

Both skin fold fissures and posterior fourchette fissuring present with a tearing, stinging, burning sensation. The stinging often is accentuated when urine, semen, medicated creams, or even water touches the area. The

patient often reports prompt healing, but recurrence with sexual activity, rubbing, or scratching.

Diagnosis

The diagnosis of skin fold fissuring is made by its morphology. The diagnosis of the underlying cause is more difficult and requires the elimination or treatment of each individual cause. The diagnosis of the underlying cause provides the diagnostic dilemma in this condition.

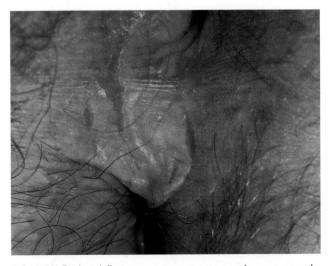

FIG. 9-70. Perineal fissures are most common in women; rubbing and scratching lichen simplex chronicus have produced these fissures.

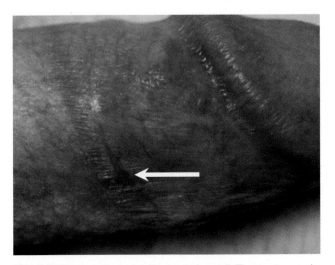

FIG. 9-72. Fissures occur on the penis as well. There was no obvious cause found for this fissure on the penile shaft.

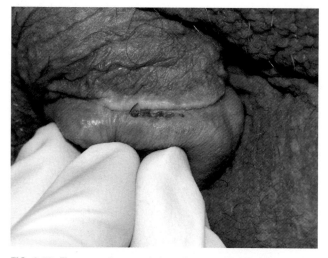

FIG. 9-73. Fissures also result from herpes simplex virus infection, as occurred in this patient who also has lichen sclerosus.

Pathophysiology

Skin fold fissures are nonspecific linear erosions with any irritation, often exacerbated by or precipitated by sexual activity. The most common underlying irritant to cause these is *Candida albicans* infection. When yeast is the primary cause, the gluteal cleft is often prominently involved.

Tinea cruris does not often produce fissures, because this is a disease of dry, keratinized skin rather than the vulva, penis, or perianal skin. Other infections that can cause fissuring are recurrent HSV infection, and vulvar or vaginal bacterial infection, most often *S. aureus* or *Streptococcus,* either α-hemolytic or group B *Streptococcus.* Although group B *Streptococcus* is nearly always an asymptomatic normal colonizer, occasionally it can contribute to vulvar irritation and fissuring.

Any itchy dermatosis, such as eczema (lichen simplex chronicus), lichen sclerosus, or psoriasis, can produce these skin fold fissures, which, in turn, increase itching, beginning or maintaining an itch–scratch cycle. Fissuring of the penis has been noted in association with penile intraepithelial neoplasia (Bowen disease).

Management

For skin fold fissures, the identification, treatment, and suppression of the underlying condition are crucial. When no underlying factors are identified, a trial of an antistaphylococcal or streptococcal antibiotic such as cephalexin, a topical corticosteroid ointment such as triamcinolone acetonide 0.1%, and an antifungal therapy such as fluconazole 150 mg every 4 to 7 days (or nystatin ointment, because creams may burn eroded skin) often produces significant control of fissures. After the skin has healed, the medications can be gradually discontinued, although recurrence is common.

In conclusion, erosive and bullous diseases affecting the genital areas are often painful and usually worrying for the patient. Diagnosis requires history, examination, and usually skin biopsies. Treatment needs to be combined with care and education of the patient and sometimes careful follow-up. Continuing research and advancement of knowledge increase the hope for more effective treatments and make this specialty an interesting area in which to work.

POSTERIOR FOURCHETTE VULVAR FISSURES

Clinical Presentation

Posterior fourchette fissures occur most often in premenopausal women and almost exclusively in sexually active individuals. The onset is usually sudden, without preceding trauma or infection; burning and splitting of the posterior fourchette occurs during sexual intercourse. Semen, water, and urine sting. The area usually heals quickly, but recurs with most acts of intercourse.

On clinical examination, there is a linear erosion at the midline posterior fourchette that may be thin and subtle, or relatively wide, obvious, and nearly ulcerative (Fig. 9-74). Some patients exhibit fairly long-lasting erythema of the area after healing. Posterior fourchette fissuring is easily seen when the patient presents within a day or two following sexual intercourse.

Some women report pain around the fissure but within the vestibule. Some clinicians postulate that fissuring occurs in association with vulvodynia, or vestibulodynia (Chapter 5).

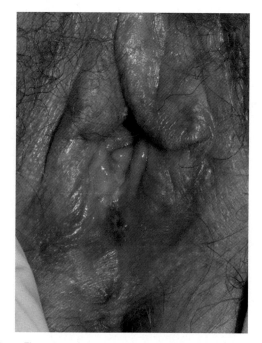

FIG. 9-74. Fissuring of the posterior fourchette during sexual activity is accompanied by a sensation of tearing and stinging.

Diagnosis

The diagnosis of a recurrent posterior fissure is easily made by the morphology and history. Diseases to consider in the differential include vestibulodynia (vulvar vestibulitis syndrome) because of the history of posterior vestibular pain with intercourse; examination of the patient the day following sexual activity reveals the presence of the fissure. Also to be considered is HSV infection, because HSV can present as recurrent fissures. The location and immediate occurrence with sexual activity usually suggest the correct diagnosis. PCR for HSV can be performed if necessary

Pathophysiology

Although some clinicians have implicated low estrogen levels as a cause of posterior fourchette fissuring, the addition of oral or topical estrogen replacement is not helpful. One report describes skin disease often detected on biopsy (62), but a biopsy of the posterior fourchette sometimes eventuates in poor healing, so sampling that avoids the midline is desirable. Some patients have tightness of the skin at the posterior fourchette, predisposing them to this condition. However, an additional factor is probably needed to allow splitting suddenly with intercourse, since many women exhibit this tight skin. Some believe that pelvic floor abnormalities may contribute to both vestibulodynia and posterior fourchette fissuring, helping to explain a possible association of these two conditions. Lichen sclerosus predisposes to posterior fourchette fissuring, and this fissuring resolves with treatment of the lichen sclerosus. Most women simply and relatively suddenly experience the onset of posterior fourchette fissuring with no known cause or accompanying abnormalities.

Management

The treatment of posterior fourchette fissuring can be difficult. Liberal lubrication during sexual activity, topical anesthetics such as lidocaine jelly 2%, and woman-on-top positioning is adequate therapy for some women. Simple lengthwise excision with suture closure of the fissuring area does not effect a cure and in fact often worsens the splitting as the caliber of the introitus is narrowed. However, a perineoplasty is usually curative. The skin surrounding the posterior fourchette is surgically excised, and vaginal epithelium is advanced to cover the defect. The success of the procedure depends largely on patient selection. Women should be evaluated for the likely presence of vestibulodynia before surgery, since their pain does not totally remit unless the entire vestibule is removed, or unless they receive medical treatment and/or physical therapy for vestibulodynia in addition to surgery.

REFERENCES

1. Chandan VS, Murray JA, Abraham SC. Esophageal lichen planus. *Arch Pathol Lab Med.* 2008;132:1026–1029.
2. Petruzzi M, DeBenedittis M, Pastore L, et al. Peno-gingival lichen planus. *Periodontology.* 2005;76:2293–2298.
3. Shengyuan L, Songpo Y, Wen W, et al. Hepatitis C virus and lichen planus: a reciprocal association determined by a meta analysis. *Arch Dermatol.* 2009;145:1040–1047.
4. Sontheimer RD. Lichenoid tissue reaction/interface: clinical and histological perspectives. *J Invest Dermatol.* 2009;129:1088–1099.
5. Cooper SM, Ali I, Baldo M, et al. The association of lichen sclerosus and erosive lichen planus of the vulva. *Arch Dermatol.* 2008;144:1502–1503.
6. Porter WM, Dinneen M, Hawkins DA, et al. Erosive penile lichen planus responding to circumcision. *J Eur Acad Dermatol Venereol.* 2001;15:266–268.
7. Jang N, Fischer G. Treatment of erosive vulvovaginal lichen planus with methotrexate. *Australas J Dematol.* 2008;49:216–219.
8. Conrotto D, Carbone M, Carrrozzo M, et al. Ciclosporin vs. clobetasol in the topical management of atrophic and erosive oral lichen planus: a double-blind, randomized controlled trial. *Br J Dermatol.* 2006;154:139–145.
9. Sharma NL, Sharma VC, Mahajan VK, et al. Thalidomide: an experience in therapeutic outcome and adverse reactions. *J Dermatolog Treat.* 2007;18:335–340.
10. Byrd JA, Davis MD, Rogers III RS. Recalcitrant symptomatic vulvar lichen planus: response to topical tacrolimus. *Arch Dermatol.* 2004;140:715–720.
11. Volz T, Caroli U, Ludtkele H, et al. Pimecrolimus cream 1% in erosive oral lichen planus—a prospective randomized double-blind vehicle study. *Br J Dermatol.* 2008;159:936–941.
12. Soria A, Agbo-Godeau S, Taïeb A, et al. Treatment of refractory oral erosive lichen planus with topical rapamycin: 7 cases. *Dermatology.* 2009;218:22–25.
13. Guyot AD, Farhi D, Ingen-Housz-Oro S, et al. Treatment of refractory erosive oral lichen planus with extracorporeal photochemotherapy: 12 cases. *Br J Dermatol.* 2007;156:553–556.
14. Virgili A, Mantovani L, Lauriola MM, et al. Tacrolimus 0. 1% ointment: is it really effective in plasma cell vulvitis? Report of four cases. *Dermatology.* 2008;216:243–246.
15. Stinco G, Piccirillo F, Patrone P. Discordant results with pimecrolimus 1% cream in the treatment of plasma cell balanitis. *Dermatology.* 2009;218:155–158.
16. Gunter J, Golitz L. Topical misoprostol therapy for plasma cell vulvitis: a case series. *J Low Genit Tract Dis.* 2005;9:176–180.
17. Tseng JT, Cheng CJ, Lee WR, et al. Plasma-cell cheilitis: successful treatment with intralesional injections of corticosteroids. *Clin Exp Dermatol.* 2009;34:174–177.
18. Frega A, Rech F, French D. Imiquimod treatment of vulvitis circumscripta plasmacellularis. *Int J Gynaecol Obstet.* 2006;95:161–162.
19. Retamar RA, Kien MC, Chouela EN. Zoon' balanitis: presentation of 15 patients, five treated with a carbon dioxide laser. *Int J Dermatol.* 2003;42:305–307.
20. Starritt E, Lee S. Erythroplasia of Queyrat of the glans penis on a background of Zoon plasma cell balanitis. *Australas J Dermatol.* 2008;49:103–105.
21. Ratnam S, Severini A, Zahariadis G, et al. The diagnosis of genital herpes beyond culture: an evidence-based guide for

the utilization of polymerase chain reaction and herpes simplex virus type-specific serology. *Can J Infect Dis Med Microbiol.* 2007;18:233–240.

22. Patnaik P, Herrero R, Morrow RA, et al. Type-specific sero-prevalence of herpes simplex virus type 2 and associated risk factors in middle-aged women from 6 countries: the IARC multicentric study. *Sex Transm Dis.* 2007;34:1019–1024.

23. Tobian AA, Serwadda D, Quinn TC, et al. Male circumcision for the prevention of HSV-2 and HPV infections and syphilis. *N Engl J Med.* 2009;360:1298–1309.

24. Martin ET, Krantz E, Gottlieb SL, et al. A pooled analysis of the effect of condoms in preventing HSV-2 acquisition. *Arch Intern Med.* 2009;169:1233–1240.

25. Lolis MS, González L, Cohen PJ, et al. Drug-resistant herpes simplex virus in HIV infected patients. *Acta Dermatovenerol Croat.* 2008;16:204–208.

26. Martens MG, Fife KH, Leone PA, et al. Once daily valacyclovir for reducing viral shedding in subjects newly diagnosed with genital herpes. *Infect Dis Obstet Gynecol.* 2009;105376. [Epub Aug 10].

27. Mark H, Gilbert L, Nanda J. Psychosocial well-being and quality of life among women newly diagnosed with genital herpes. *J Obstet Gynecol Neonatal Nurs.* 2009;38:320–326.

28. Akhyani M, Chams-Davatchi C, Naraghi Z, et al. Cervicovaginal involvement in pemphigus vulgaris: a clinical study of 77 cases. *Br J Dermatol.* 2008;158:478–482.

29. Roujeau JC, Ingen-Housz-Oro S, Leroux C, et al. Treatment of bullous pemphigoid and pemphigus. The French experience, 2009 update. *G Ital Dermatol Venereol.* 2009;144:333–338.

30. Kandan S, Thappa DM. Outcome of dexamethasone-cyclophosphamide pulse therapy in pemphigus: a case series. *Indian J Dematol Venereol Leprol.* 2009;75:373–378.

31. Baskan EB, Yilmaz M, Tunali S, et al. Efficacy and safety of long-term mycophenolate sodium therapy in pemphigus vulgaris. *J Eur Acad Dermatol Venereol.* 2009. [Epub ahead of print].

32. Leuci S, Levine D, Zhang J, et al. Response in patients with pemphigus vulgaris to rituximab therapy. Basis of the biology of B cells. *G Ital Dermatol Venereol.* 2009;144:379–409.

33. Gürcan HM, Ahmed AR. Analysis of current data on the use of methotrexate in the treatment of pemphigus and pemphigoid. *Br J Dermatol.* 2009;161:723–731.

34. Rose C, Schmidt E, Kerstan A, et al. Histopathology of anti-laminin 5 mucous membrane pemphigoid. *J Am Acad Dermatol.* 2009;61:433–440.

35. Taverna JA, Lerner A, Bhawan J, Demierre MF. Successful adjuvant treatment of recalcitrant mucous membrane pemphigoid with anti-CD20 antibody rituximab. *J Drugs Dermatol.* 2007;6: 731–732.

36. Hoffman SC, Voith U, Schonau V, et al. Plasmin plays a role in the in vitro generation of the linear IgA dermatosis antigen LADB97. *J Invest Dermatol.* 2009;129:1730–1732.

37. Panasiti V, Rossi M, Devirgiliis V, et al. Amoxicillin-clavulanic acid-induced linear immunoglobulin. A bullous dermatosis: case report and review of the literature. *Int J Dermatol.* 2009; 48:1006–1010.

38. Khan I, Hughes R, Curran S, et al. Drug-associated linear IgA disease mimicking toxic epidermal necrolysis. *Clin Exp Dermatol.* 2009;34:715–717.

39. Tanaka N, Dainichi T, Ohyama B, et al. A case of epidermolysis bullosa acquisita with clinical features of Brunsting-Perry

40. pemphigoid showing an excellent response to colchicine. *J Am Acad Dermatol.* 2009;61:715–719.

40. Schmidt E, Broker EB, Goebeler M. Rituximab in treatment-resistant autoimmune blistering skin disorders. *Clin Rev Allergy Immunol.* 2008;34:56–64.

41. Marzano AV, Ramoni S, Spinelli D, et al. Refractory linear, IgA bullous dermatosis successfully treated with mycophenolate sodium. *J Dermatology Treat.* 2008;19:364–367.

42. Chi CC, Wang SH, Charles-Holmes R, et al. Pemphigoid gestationis: early onset and blister formation are associated with adverse pregnancy outcomes. *Br J Dermatol.* 2009;160: 1222–1228.

43. Caproni M, Antiga E, Melani L, et al; Italian Group for Cutaneous Immunopathology. Guidelines for the diagnosis and treatment of dermatitis herpetiformis. *J Eur Acad Dermatol Venereol.* 2009;23:633–638.

44. Hamada T, Fukuda S, Sakaguchi S, et al. Molecular and clinical characterization in Japanese and Korean patients with Hailey–Hailey disease: six new mutations in the ATP2C1 gene. *J Dermatol Sci.* 2008;51:31–36.

45. Aberg KM, Racz E, Behne MJ, et al. Involucrin expression is decreased in Hailey–Hailey keratinocytes owing to increased involucrin mRNA degradation. *J Invest Dermatol.* 2007;127: 1973–1979.

46. Koeyers WJ, Van Der Geer S, Krekels G. Botulinum toxin type A as an adjuvant treatment modality for extensive Hailey–Hailey disease. *J Dermatolog Treat.* 2008;19:251–254.

47. Rocha Paris F, Fidalgo A, Baptista J, et al. Topical tacrolimus in Hailey–Hailey disease. *Int J Tissue React.* 2005;27:151–154.

48. Collet Villette AM, Richard MA, Fourquet F, et al. Treatment of Hailey–Hailey disease with carbon dioxide laser vaporization. *Ann Dermatol Venereol.* 2005;132:637–640.

49. Fernandez Guarino M, Ryan AM, Harto A, et al. Experience with photodynamic therapy in Hailey–Hailey disease. *J Dermatolog Treat.* 2008;19:288–289.

50. Dammak A, Camus M, Anyfantakis V, et al. Successful treatment of Hailey–Hailey disease with topical 5-fluorouracil. *Br J Dermatol.* 2009;161:967–968.

51. Berger EM, Galadari HI, Gottlieb AB. Successful treatment of Hailey–Hailey disease with acitretin. *J Drugs Dermatol.* 2007;6: 734–736.

52. Levi N, Bastuji-Garin S, Mockenhaupt M, et al. Medications as risk factors of Stevens–Johnson syndrome and toxic epidermal necrolysis in children: a pooled analysis. *Pediatrics.* 2009;123: 297–304.

53. Phillips EJ, Mallal SA. HLA and drug-induced toxicity. *Curr Opin Mol Ther.* 2009;11:231–242.

54. Cheng SH, Kwan P, Ng HK, et al. New testing approach in HLA genotyping helps overcome barriers in effective clinical practice. *Clin Chem.* 2009;55:1568–1572.

55. Abe R. Toxic epidermal necrolysis and Stevens–Johnson syndrome: soluble Fas ligand involvement in the pathomechanisms of these diseases. *J Dermatol Sci.* 2008;52:151–159.

56. Hanken I, Schimmer M, Sander CA. Basic measures and systemic medical treatment of patients with toxic epidermal necrolysis. *J Dtsch Dermatol Ges.* 2009. [Epub ahead of print].

57. Lissia M, Mulas P, Bulla A, et al. Toxic epidermal necrolysis (Lyell's disease). *Burns.* 2009. [Epub ahead of print].

58. Molgó M, Carreño N, Hoyos-Bachiloglu R, et al. [Use of intravenous immunoglobulin for the treatment of toxic epidermal necrolysis and Stevens–Johnson/toxic epidermal necrolysis

overlap syndrome. Review of 15 cases]. *Rev Med Chil.* 2009; 137:383–389.

59. Koh MJ, Tay YK. An update on Stevens–Johnson syndrome and toxic epidermal necrolysis in children. *Curr Opin Pediatr.* 2009;21:505–510.

60. Mizukawa Y, Shiohara T. Fixed drug eruption: a prototypic disorder mediated by effector memory T cells. *Curr Allergy Asthma Rep.* 2009;9:71–77.

61. Patel RM, Marfatia YS. Clinical study of cutaneous drug eruptions in 200 patients. *Indian J Dermatol Venereol Leprol.* 2008;74:430.

62. Sehgal VN, Srivastava G. Fixed drug eruption (FDE): changing scenario of incriminating drugs. *Int J Dermatol.* 2006;45: 897–908.

SUGGESTED READINGS

Alessi E, Coggi A, Gianotti R. Review of 120 biopsies performed on the balanopreputial sac. from zoon's balanitis to the concept of a wider spectrum of inflammatory non-cicatricial balanoposthitis. *Dermatology.* 2004;208:120–124.

Alexandroff AB, Harman KE. Blistering skin disorders: an evidence-based update. Conference report. *Br J Dermatol.* 2009;160:502–504.

Daniel E, Thorne JE. Recent advances in mucous membrane pemphigoid. *Curr Opin Ophthalmol.* 2008;19:292–297.

Edwards L. Vulvar fissures: causes and therapy. *Dermatol Ther.* 2004; 17:111–116.

Fromowitz JS, Ramos-Caro FA, Flowers FP. Practical guidelines for the management of toxic epidermal necrolysis and Stevens-Johnson syndrome. *Int J Dermatol.* 2007;46:1092–1094.

Kennedy CM, Galask RP. Erosive vulvar lichen planus: retrospective review of characteristics and outcomes in 113 patients seen in a vulvar specialty clinic. *J Reprod Med.* 2007;52:43–47.

Khalili B, Bahna SL. Pathogenesis and recent therapeutic trends in Stevens–Johnson syndrome and toxic epidermal necrolysis. *Ann Allergy Asthma Immunol.* 2006;97:272–280.

Malik M, Ahmed AR. Involvement of the female genital tract in pemphigus vulgaris. *Obstet Gynecol.* 2005;106:1005–1012.

Money D, Steben M; Society of Obstetricians and Gynaecologists of Canada. SOGC clinical practice guidelines: genital herpes: gynaecological aspects. Number 207, April 2008. *Int J Gynaecol Obstet.* 2009;104:162–166.

Moyal-Barracco M, Edwards L. Diagnosis and therapy of anogenital lichen planus. *Dermatol Ther.* 2004;17:38–46.

Patrício P, Ferreira C, Gomes MM, et al. Autoimmune bullous dermatoses: a review. *Ann N Y Acad Sci.* 2009;1173:203–210.

Retamar RA, Kien MC, Chouela EN. Zoon's balanitis: presentation of 15 patients, five treated with a carbon dioxide laser. *Int J Dermatol.* 2003;42:305–307.

Smith PD, Roberts CM. American college health association annual Pap test and sexually transmitted infection survey: 2006. *J Am Coll Health.* 2009;57:389–394.

Virgili A, Levratti A, Marzola A, et al. Retrospective histopathologic reevaluation of 18 cases of plasma cell vulvitis. *J Reprod Med.* 2005;50:3–7.

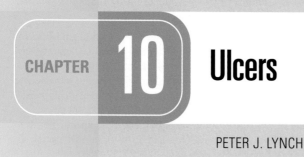

CHAPTER 10 Ulcers

PETER J. LYNCH

Erosions and ulcers occur when tissue is lost from the surface of the skin. They are differentiated on the basis of depth. Tissue loss limited to the epithelium produces erosions, whereas tissue loss that extends into, or through, the dermis is termed an ulcer. The base of an erosion either may be red or may be covered with a loosely adherent yellow crust. The base of an ulcer, on the other hand, may be red or may be covered with a crust that has red, blue, or black heme pigment due to the destruction of blood vessels within the dermis. The crusts covering ulcers may also have considerable fibrin in them and for this reason are adherent and tenacious; this is sometimes termed eschar formation (see Chapter 9 for the coverage of erosions). Ulcers due to infection are discussed in the first portion of this chapter and those that are noninfectious in etiology are discussed in the latter half.

SYPHILIS

Syphilis is a sexually transmitted infection that is characterized by asymptomatic periods of varying duration, interrupted by three stages of clinical disease. In primary syphilis, a painless and nontender ulcer ("chancre") develops, most often in or around the genitalia. The major discussion of syphilis will be found in this chapter with brief mention made of secondary syphilis in Chapter 12. Although syphilis is a global problem, the data in this chapter refer primarily to syphilis in Western countries.

Clinical Presentation

According to the 2007 Centers for Disease Control (CDC) report, the rate of primary and secondary syphilis in the United States declined 90% from 1990 to 2000 at which point it reached its nadir (1). Since then the rate has been steadily increasing. Most of this increase has been in men, primarily among men who have sex with men (MSM) (1). This population now accounts for about 65% of all of the cases of early syphilis. In 2007, the incidence of syphilis was 6.6 per 100,000 for men and 1.1 per 100,000 for women. The rate is appreciably higher in Hispanic and African American men than that in non-Hispanic white men. Syphilis occurs most frequently between the ages of 20 and 24 in women and 20 and 30 in men. The data for Australia and European countries is quite similar to that

found in the United States (2,3). Coinfection with human immunodeficiency virus (HIV) is encountered frequently.

After an incubation period of 9 to 90 days (average of 3 weeks), the primary lesion occurs at the original site of inoculation. It begins as a small red papule that quickly enlarges and ulcerates to form a painless ulcer ("chancre") that may be up to 2 cm in diameter. A chancre has a clean, red, glistening base (Figs. 10-1 and 10-2). A small amount of nonpurulent, watery exudate may be present. The ulcer borders are sharply demarcated and are characteristically raised and indurated. The chancre is painless and usually nontender. The base feels firm on palpation. Most patients present with a solitary ulcer, but two or even multiple lesions are possible. Chancres are located most often at the distal tip of the penis in men and on the labia majora or vestibule in women. However, it is likely that many chancres in women are never observed due to a location within the vagina or on the cervix. For this reason, the first clinical presentation of syphilis in women is more likely to be at the secondary stage than is true for men. Individuals who have receptive anal intercourse may develop chancres within or around the anus. Secondary bacterial infection of ulcerative lesions may distort the clinical presentation, causing tenderness and purulent discharge. Within about 1 week of chancre formation in the anogenital area, unilateral or bilateral inguinal regional lymphadenopathy develops as nontender, firm, rubbery, mobile lymph nodes.

Diagnosis

The presence of a solitary, nontender ulcer with a clean, firm base is highly likely to represent primary syphilis. Nevertheless, a clinical diagnosis must be confirmed by laboratory means. In years past, the quickest confirmation could be obtained by a dark-field examination carried out on site by the clinician. Unfortunately, this test has almost completely disappeared due to the lack of dark field microscopes in clinicians' offices and the declining skills in carrying out this test. For this reason, a serologic test for syphilis needs to be obtained. The most commonly used nontreponemal serologic tests are the Venereal Disease Research Laboratory (VDRL) and the rapid plasma regain (RPR) tests, both of which detect antibodies to cardiolipin. These are readily available, cheap, and reliable. In addition, positive results can be titrated providing a valuable tool for determining response to

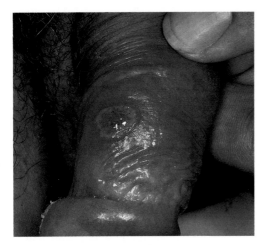

FIG. 10-1. This is a classical indurated, well-demarcated chancre with a glistening red base.

therapy. Unfortunately, there are several drawbacks to these tests: (1) the test may not become positive until 1 or 2 weeks after the chancre has appeared; (2) false-positive tests occur with some frequency; and (3) false-negative tests may occur due to the prozone phenomenon especially in those patients who are coinfected with HIV.

Because of these drawbacks, treponemal-specific tests such as the fluorescent treponemal antibody absorbed test (FTA-ABS), the *Treponemal pallidum* particle agglutination test (TP-PA), the *T. pallidum* hemagglutination assay (TP-HA), and Western blots are available. These tests offer nearly 99% sensitivity and 99% specificity. Interestingly, some large laboratories are reversing the algorithm and are using automated enzyme immunoassays (EIAs) for initial screening followed by a VDRL or RPR if positive results are obtained. This latter approach may offer some cost savings but can cause difficulties due to both occasional false-positive results with EIAs and the fact that unlike the nontreponemal tests, they may remain positive after previous effective treatment

and thus cannot be used for determining a response to therapy (4).

Both the nonspecific and the specific serologic tests can remain negative for 7 to 14 days after a chancre appears. In this situation, biopsy should be considered for any lesion that is clinically suspicious for syphilis. The histologic presence of numerous plasma cells would then be followed by the use of a silver stain (e.g., Warthin–Starry stain) to identify the presence of spirochetes. Patients with syphilis are likely to have been exposed to other sexually transmitted diseases. For this reason, patients should be examined and tested for other infections when a diagnosis of syphilis has been established.

The two main considerations in the list of differential diagnoses are aphthous ulcers and genital herpes (HSV) infection, especially when the latter occurs in an immunosuppressed individual. Genital herpes occurring in those who are immunosuppressed may present with fairly deep, persistent, and relatively less painful ulcers rather than the more typical, transient, painful erosions seen in immunocompetent persons. Individual aphthous ulcers (as occur in complex aphthosis and Behçet disease) are similar in appearance to a chancre but, in contrast, several ulcers are usually present, they are extremely painful, and they tend to occur mostly in adolescent women. Chancroid is vanishingly rare in Western countries and is associated with a crusted base along with considerable pain and tenderness. Anogenital ulcers occur with Crohn disease, hidradenitis suppurativa, and granuloma inguinale, but the morphology is different as is the histopathology.

PRIMARY SYPHILIS:	**Diagnosis**

- One or two relatively painless genital ulcers
- Ulcer base is clean without crust or eschar
- Base of the ulcer is firm and nontender on palpation
- Positive RPR or VDRL; confirmed by positive FTA-ABS
- If serology is negative, repeat tests in 1 week or biopsy

Pathophysiology

Syphilis is caused by the spirochete, *Treponema pallidum*. The level of contagion for syphilis is very high; it has been estimated that about one third of individuals having direct contact with a chancre will develop syphilis. The likelihood of infection is further enhanced in the presence of even minor breaks in the skin as well as in a setting of immunosuppression such as occurs with HIV infection (5). The reverse is also true. There is an increased risk for the acquisition of HIV in patients with chancres. Many (6), but not all (7), studies suggest that circumcision in males reduces the likelihood of acquiring

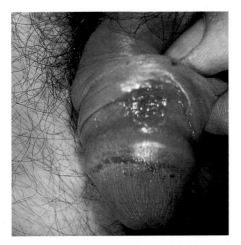

FIG. 10-2. Clean, firm borders and a base with slight nonpurulent exudate are typical of a chancre.

syphilis. The incubation period after exposure to *T. pallidum* is quite variable but averages about 3 weeks. Unfortunately, before the end of the incubation period and therefore before the development of a chancre, spirochetes have already gained access to the regional lymph nodes. For this reason, syphilis can be viewed as a systemic infection from its earliest inception.

Management

If untreated, a chancre undergoes spontaneous, non-scarring resolution within about 1 to 2 months. This leads the patient to the misconception that the process has healed and that it is not necessary to seek medical attention. However, as indicated above, syphilis becomes a systemic infection soon after the initial inoculation with the result that after a short latent period the generalized lesions of secondary syphilis are highly likely to appear. Rarely, secondary lesions may appear, without a latent period, while the chancre is still present. If the symptoms and signs of secondary syphilis are unrecognized and the patient remains untreated, the patient enters another latent period, leading some years later to the possibility of tertiary syphilis.

Most clinicians in the United States follow the treatment guidelines published by the CDC. The most recent update is from 2006 where benzathine penicillin G 2.4 million units, administered intramuscularly in a single dose, is the recommended therapy for primary and secondary syphilis (8). Note that Bicillin L-A (containing only benzathine penicillin) is to be used rather than Bicillin C-R that contains a combination of benzathine penicillin and the short-acting procaine penicillin. No penicillin resistance has yet been noted. Guidelines that are somewhat similar to those of the CDC have been developed for the United Kingdom and Europe (9,10). Because of their similarity, they will not be reviewed here.

For those who are allergic to penicillin, the CDC recommends desensitization rather than use of a second-line treatment with a nonpenicillin product. However, where desensitization is not feasible, it is appropriate to use alternative antibiotics such as doxycycline (100 mg orally twice daily for 14 days), ceftriaxone (1 g IM daily for 10 days), or azithromycin (2 g in a single oral dose) (8). The CDC recommendation for desensitization stems from a relative lack of published experience with all three of these agents together with some reports of azithromycin resistance. Patients who are pregnant should be treated with penicillin. Limited evidence suggests that in HIV infected persons, the response to therapy may be somewhat diminished. For this reason, some clinicians choose to repeat the 2.4 million units of benzathine penicillin weekly for 3 weeks.

The Jarisch–Herxheimer reaction is an acute febrile reaction that may occur within 24 hours of treatment for syphilis, regardless of the treatment regimen used. Symptoms include headache, malaise, myalgia, arthralgia, and fever. This transient reaction occurs most commonly after treatment for early syphilis and requires only reassurance, bed rest, and antipyretics for management.

Patients who are treated for primary or secondary syphilis require follow-up documentation of response. This is done by determining the titer of the RPR or VDRL antibodies at periodic intervals until at least a fourfold drop in titer has been obtained. Note that although either the RPR or the VDRL can be used, the same test must be used consistently as the titer levels differ between the two tests. Nearly all patients with early syphilis will eventually develop a negative RPR or VDRL test. However, this is not true for the treponemal specific tests (see above) where lifelong positivity usually continues.

PRIMARY SYPHILIS: **Management**

- Benzathine penicillin (Bicillin L-A) single dose 2.4 million units IM
- Consider repeating the dose if the patient is HIV positive
- Desensitize if the patient is allergic to penicillin
- Or, doxycycline 100 mg b.i.d. × 14 days, azithromycin 2 g as single dose
- Follow RPR or VDRL titer until negative

CHANCROID

Clinical Presentation

Chancroid is seldom encountered in Western societies. In the United States, fewer than 50 cases per year are reported to the CDC. However, within the last decade, the disease has occurred in clusters in several large cities of America. These mini-epidemics are usually associated with exposure to a single infected prostitute. Chancroid predisposes to the development of HIV infection and persons with chancroid are quite likely to have other sexually transmitted diseases as well.

After a short incubation period of 3 to 7 days, a small red papule or pustule appears at the site of inoculation. This inflammatory lesion may be either asymptomatic or tender. The area then quickly evolves into an extremely painful, deep, shaggy ulcer with ragged, soft, undermined margins (Figs. 10-3 and 10-4). In contrast to the chancre of syphilis, induration is not typically present. The base of the ulcer is friable and is often covered with a yellow-gray, foul-smelling, necrotic exudate. Most patients present with one or two ulcers, but multiple or giant ulcer formation is not uncommon. Fifty percent of patients develop painful, most often unilateral, inguinal lymphadenitis. Massively enlarged nodes (bubo formation) develop in 25% of cases and when untreated may become fluctuant with spontaneous rupture and chronic drainage.

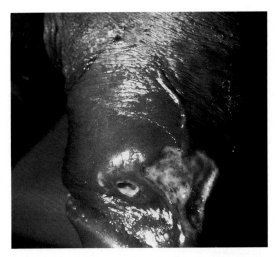

FIG. 10-3. The ulcer of chancroid typically exhibits a shaggy border with a somewhat purulent red base. (Courtesy of Jack Mosley.)

Diagnosis

There are no easily available diagnostic tests for chancroid. The causative bacterium, *Haemophilus ducreyi*, is difficult to identify on smears taken from the ulcer even when special stains such as the Giemsa stain are used. *H. ducreyi* can only be cultured on special media and unfortunately this media is not available commercially. As a result, most laboratories do not offer the ability to culture this bacterium. Biopsy does reveal a fairly characteristic pattern consisting of three separate horizontal zones with distinctive vascular changes. The floor of the ulcer shows necrosis, red blood cells, neutrophils, and fibrin. Underlying this is a wide area of new vessel formation with proliferating endothelial cells that sometimes

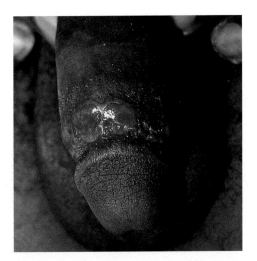

FIG. 10-4. These well-demarcated round ulcerations of chancroid on the distal shaft are uniform and atypical, demonstrating that diagnosis often cannot be made on the basis of morphology.

obstruct the lumina. The deepest portion of the histologic changes shows an inflammatory infiltrate of plasma cells and lymphoid cells.

The CDC indicates that a presumptive clinical diagnosis can be made if all of the following criteria are met: (1) the ulcers are painful and tender; (2) a serologic test for syphilis, taken at least 7 days after the ulcer has appeared, is negative; (3) the clinical presentation, including lymphadenopathy, is typical for chancroid; and (4) a test for HSV performed on the ulcer is negative (8). Primary syphilis, genital HSV infection, lymphogranuloma venereum, granuloma inguinale, ulcerated carcinoma, or secondarily infected traumatic lesions may all mimic chancroid.

CHANCROID:	Diagnosis

- Single, sometimes two or three, painful ulcers
- Base of ulcer is covered with purulent crust
- Base is soft and very tender on palpation
- Inguinal lymphadenopathy is usually present
- Biopsy if confirmation of the diagnosis is needed

Pathophysiology

Chancroid is caused by the fastidious, gram-negative, aerobic or facultative anaerobic bacterium, *H. ducreyi*. It is highly contagious and experimental transfer from human to human is fairly easily carried out (11).

Management

Untreated, the ulcer of chancroid lasts about 2 months before spontaneous healing, generally with scarring, takes place. Ulceration and drainage from the enlarged nodes, if present, can last even longer. The CDC indicates that all of the following can be used for treatment: azithromycin (1 g orally in a single dose), ceftriaxone (250 mg IM in a single dose), ciprofloxacin (500 mg orally twice a day for 3 days), and erythromycin base (500 mg orally three times a day for 7 days) (8). With any of these treatments, healing of the ulcer occurs in about 1 week with lymph node response occurring much more slowly. Greatly enlarged, fluctuant nodes may require needle aspiration or incision and drainage.

CHANCROID:	Management

- Azithromycin 1 g orally in a single dose or
- Ceftriaxone 250 mg IM as a single dose
- Incise and drain if lymph node is fluctuant
- Follow to ensure complete healing

GENITAL HERPES IN IMMUNOSUPPRESSED INDIVIDUALS

HSV infection causes shallow, self-healing genital *erosions* in persons with normal immune status. This presentation of genital herpes is covered in Chapter 9. However, in those who are immunosuppressed, HSV infection becomes locally more severe as reflected by the development of chronic *ulcers* rather than transient erosions.

Clinical Presentation

In normal circumstances, control of HSV infection depends in large part on the presence of an intact cell-mediated immune system. For this reason, it is not surprising that evidence of genital HSV infection becomes prolonged and more severe in patients who are chronically immunosuppressed due to such disorders as HIV infection, malignancy (especially of hematopoietic origin), and those receiving long-term immunosuppressant medications for any reason. HSV infection, usually due to HSV type 2, then transforms from an erosive to an ulcerative disease.

In immunosuppressed patients, the lesions of HSV most often arise from reactivation of preexisting disease rather than from a primary infection. As is true for HSV infection occurring in immunocompetent patients, immunosuppressed patients describe accompanying pain (though frequently less severe) and careful questioning usually reveals prior, more typical recurrent episodes of genital herpes.

HSV outbreaks in immunosuppressed patients start as grouped vesicles on an erythematous base. The roofs of these vesicles disintegrate almost immediately leaving well-demarcated, discrete erosions. However, unlike the situation in immunocompetent patients, the erosions may not heal, but rather coalesce and deepen to form large, well-demarcated ("punched out"), somewhat painful, nonhealing ulcers (Figs. 10-5 through 10-9). These ulcers may be superficial initially but often become deeper (Fig. 10-10). Secondary bacterial infection is possible but does not occur frequently. The configuration of the ulcers may be round but arcuate shapes are common due to coalescence of centrifugally expanding ulcers (Fig. 10-11). In men, chronic HSV ulcers are commonly found in a perianal distribution but also occur on the penis, scrotum, or in the groin. In women, ulcers may involve the mucosal portion of the vulva but also may extend to the labia majora and minora and even to the groin or inner thighs. As for men, HSV infection may also occur in a perianal location. In a small percentage of cases, HSV lesions in immunocompromised individuals may appear as eroded or ulcerated papules or nodules.

Diagnosis

A high index of suspicion should be present for HSV infection in any chronic, nonhealing ulcer in an

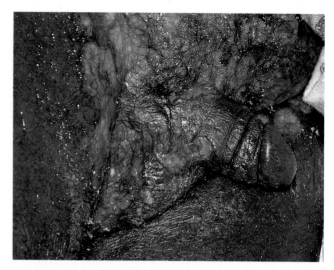

FIG. 10-5. Herpes simplex virus infection in an immunosuppressed patient, such as this man with HIV, becomes chronic with relentless extension and ulceration.

immunosuppressed patient. A viral culture will usually confirm a clinically suspected diagnosis but viral growth may be slow and results may be delayed for a week or more (8). Examination of a stained smear taken from the base of the lesion (A Tzanck preparation) is less reliable for the diagnosis of a chronic ulcerative herpetic infection than is true for HSV infection in immunocompetent patients (8). Direct immunofluorescent antibody testing is available in most labs and offers a rapid diagnosis. This is accomplished by scraping the base of the ulcer with a number 15 blade and smearing the material collected on a microscope slide. The slide is then submitted to the laboratory and the results may be available within an hour or two.

The characteristic histologic features in HSV infection include ballooning degeneration of keratinocytes, reticular degeneration, and formation of multinucleated keratinocytic giant cells. Multinucleated keratinocytes are

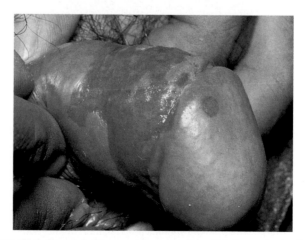

FIG. 10-6. Although this man has extension of his herpetic penile erosion, it has lost the classic arcuate borders from coalescing vesicles and now is only a nonspecific erosion.

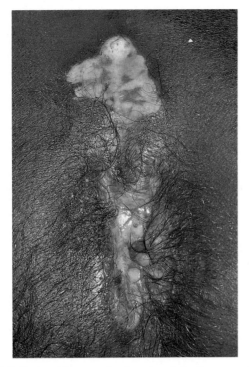

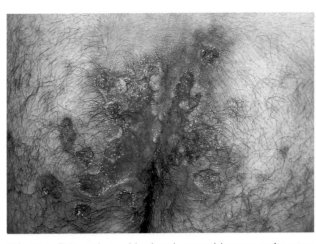

FIG. 10-9. This patient with chronic sacral herpes resistant to antiviral medication exhibits both extension and healing simultaneously.

FIG. 10-7. Perianal herpes simplex virus infection can also extend peripherally and deeply, producing a yellow fibrin base characteristic of ulceration of any cause.

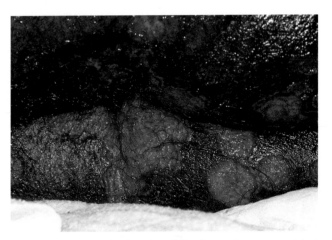

FIG. 10-10. Herpes simplex virus infection resistant to antiviral agents in this man with AIDS has produced a peripherally enlarging perianal ulcer despite appropriate antiviral therapy.

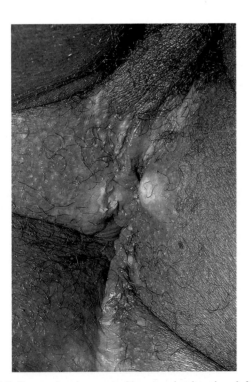

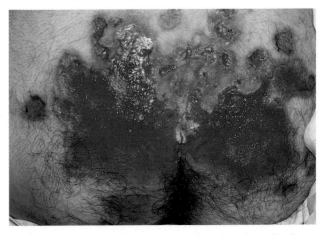

FIG. 10-8. Deeper involvement of herpes simplex virus infection in an immunosuppressed patient such as this woman with chronic lymphocytic leukemia sometimes produces indurated lesions.

FIG. 10-11. The most common cause of genital ulceration in an immunosuppressed patient is herpes simplex virus infection.

pathognomonic for herpes virus infections, but they do not distinguish between HSV and varicella-zoster virus infection. Polymerase chain reaction (PCR) techniques, which are exquisitely sensitive, can be used in instances where the clinical picture highly suggests HSV infection but where other diagnostic tests are negative (8).

Although the presence of multiple well-demarcated, painful, chronic ulcers is highly suggestive of HSV infection, several other ulcerating infections must be considered in the list of differential diagnoses. Syphilis produces one or more relatively short-lived, firm, painless, noncrusted ulcers. Chancroid causes a painful, ragged crusted ulcer and may cause massive painful inguinal adenitis. Granuloma inguinale consists of one or more genital ulcers, often linear in configuration, containing exuberant granulation tissue. Rarely cytomegalovirus (CMV) has been reported to cause large, deep, necrotic ulcers in immunosuppressed patients, particularly those with acquired immunodeficiency syndrome (HIV/AIDS). Biopsy confirmation for CMV infection may be needed because HSV infection can occur concomitantly with CMV and may overgrow CMV in viral culture. Noninfectious causes such as aphthous ulcers and Crohn disease should also be considered.

HSV IN IMMUNOSUPPRESSED: **Diagnosis**

- Patient is significantly immunosuppressed
- Punched out ulcers or ulcerated nodules
- Arcuate configuration when confluence of ulcers occurs
- Lesions are variable in terms of pain
- HSV culture, immunofluorescent smear, or biopsy to confirm

Management

Left untreated, HSV ulcers in immunosuppressed patients may persist indefinitely. However, complete response to medical therapy is usually prompt. The CDC recommends acyclovir 400 mg orally three to five times daily until clinical resolution is attained (8). Famciclovir (500 mg orally twice daily) or valacyclovir (1.0 g orally twice daily) administered for 5 to 10 days is also effective (8). Rarely, intravenous acyclovir may be necessary if there is inadequate response to oral therapy (8). It is given as 5 to 10 mg/kg every 8 hours for 2 to 7 days or until clinical resolution is achieved.

Resistance to acyclovir has been reported to occur in up to 10% of immunocompromised individuals receiving long-term therapy to suppress outbreaks of HSV. All acyclovir-resistant strains are resistant to valacyclovir and most are resistant to famciclovir as well. The currently recommended treatment for acyclovir-resistant anogenital herpes is intravenous foscarnet in a dosage of 40 mg/kg every 8 hours until clinical resolution occurs. For HIV/AIDS patient not already receiving highly active retroviral therapy (HAART), starting such a regimen can lead to improvement though there is also some risk of exacerbation of latent HSV infection as part of the immune reconstitution inflammatory syndrome when this is done (12). Additional, new medications that are potentially usable are described in a recent review article on HSV therapy (13).

HSV IN IMMUNOSUPPRESSED: **Management**

- Start HAART therapy if not already underway
- Acyclovir 400 mg orally 5 × per day until ulcers are healed or
- Famciclovir 500 mg b.i.d. or
- Valacyclovir 1.0 g b.i.d.
- Foscarnet 40 mg/kg t.i.d. if the ulcer is acyclovir resistant

---

GRANULOMA INGUINALE (DONOVANOSIS)

Granuloma inguinale is a chronic, mildly contagious bacterial infection with a slowly progressive and destructive course. Four different clinical variants of the disease exist and this variability can result in a vast array of difficult-to-diagnose clinical presentations. These include ulcerovegetative (the most common), nodular, hypertrophic, and cicatricial forms of the disease.

Clinical Presentation

Granuloma inguinale is rarely encountered in North America and Europe, but it is endemic in some tropical and subtropical areas such as the Caribbean, Africa, Australia, southern India, South America, and Southeast Asia. It occurs most commonly in those of lower socioeconomic class. The majority of cases are found in adults where the transmission is sexually transmitted but nonvenereal transmission is possible and may account for most of the cases reported in babies and children.

The incubation period is typically less than 2 weeks but it can be up to 3 months in duration. The ulcerovegetative form of the disease is by far the most common clinical presentation. In this type of granuloma inguinale, the onset is insidious with formation of solitary or multiple, painless, firm papules or nodules at the site of inoculation. These lesions then erode to form soft, friable, painless ulcers that often involve skin folds (Figs. 10-12 and 10-13). In these sites, the ulcers characteristically have a linear, "knife cut," morphology. The base of the ulcers is usually clean (noncrusted) with beefy-red granulation tissue. The margins are sharp and rolled borders are usually present. There is often progressive enlargement of some portion of

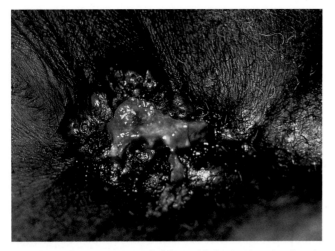

FIG. 10-12. This perianal ulceration with heaped-up borders is typical of granuloma inguinale (Donovanosis). (Courtesy of Jack Mosley.)

the ulcers while other portions are undergoing healing with fibrosis and scarring. In the less often encountered nodular variant of the disease, soft red papules and/or nodules develop and subsequently ulcerate. The ulcers on the surface of these lesions also contain appreciable amounts of granulation tissue. The hypertrophic form of granuloma inguinale consists of large vegetating masses, whereas the cicatricial variant is associated with expanding plaques of scar tissue.

Lesions in men most often occur in the anal and perianal area but also can be found in the coronal sulcus or on the inner aspect of the foreskin in uncircumcised individuals. In women, the vulva is most often involved but rarely lesions occur on the cervix. In both sexes, lesions may be found in the intertriginous folds of the

perigenital skin. Typically, lymphadenopathy does not occur but spread of the infection to areas around the inguinal lymph nodes may cause swelling and ulceration. This process is termed pseudobubo. This lack of lymph node enlargement is characteristic enough to be a helpful in clinical diagnosis.

Complications of chronic disease include architectural distortion and destruction of the genitalia as well as phimosis, lymphedema, and elephantiasis-like swelling of the vulva.

Diagnosis

Clinically suspicious lesions can be confirmed by a histologic demonstration of clustered bacteria (Donovan bodies) located within macrophages. This can be carried out using a snip of granulation tissue taken from the base of the ulcers. This tissue is crushed between two glass slides. The material is then fixed and stained with Wright or Giemsa stain after which the characteristic Donovan bodies can usually be identified located within the cytoplasm of mononuclear inflammatory cells.

The causative bacterium is very hard to culture. For this reason, biopsy is appropriate if tissue smears are negative in a patient with clinically suspicious lesions. Histology of the lesion shows acanthosis and an extensive dermal infiltrate composed of plasma cells and histiocytes. Warthin–Starry or Giemsa stain usually reveals large macrophages with cytoplasmic vacuoles containing bacteria (Donovan bodies). Ultrathin plastic-embedded sections may be superior to routinely processed paraffin-embedded sections for the demonstration of this organism in tissue.

Syphilis, chancroid, genital herpes in the immunosuppressed, amebiasis, and lymphogranuloma venereum are infections that may be confused with granuloma inguinale. Noninfectious conditions to be considered are cutaneous Crohn disease, hidradenitis suppurativa, and Langerhans cell histiocytosis. Occasionally the marked epithelial hyperplasia seen on histopathologic examination has been misinterpreted as suggesting squamous cell carcinoma.

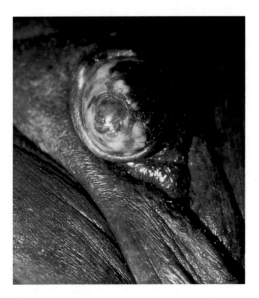

FIG. 10-13. Granuloma inguinale can produce a keratotic ulceration as seen on the glans penis. (Courtesy of Jack Mosley.)

GRANULOMA INGUINALE:	Diagnosis

- One or more very slowly enlarging ulcers
- Configuration may be arcuate or linear
- Linear "knife cut" ulcers in skin folds are characteristic
- Ulcer borders are rolled; base has granulomatous appearance
- Confirm by the presence of bacteria in macrophages on crushed smear or biopsy

Pathogenesis

The cause of granuloma inguinale is the bacterium *Klebsiella granulomatosis* which was previously termed *Calymmatobacterium granulomatosis*. This is a gram-negative, short, intracellular bacterium. As indicated above, it is not a particularly contagious process, but the likelihood of infection appears to be enhanced in the presence of poor hygiene and/or breaks in the skin.

Management

Left untreated, the ulcers of granuloma inguinale slowly heal over months to years leaving residual scar formation and genital architectural distortion or destruction. Chronic massive edema (elephantiasis) of the genitalia frequently develops. This is particularly like to happen with the vulva. The 2006 CDC treatment guidelines suggest treatment with one of several types of antibiotics such as doxycycline (100 mg orally twice daily), azithromycin (1.0 g orally once weekly), ciprofloxacin (750 mg orally twice daily), erythromycin base (500 mg orally four times a day), or trimethoprim–sulfamethoxazole (160/800 mg orally twice daily) (8). All of these antibiotics should be administered for a minimum of 3 weeks. If the healing is not complete by then, treatment should continue until this occurs.

GRANULOMA INGUINALE:	Management

- Doxycycline 100 b.i.d. or
- Azithromycin 1.0 g weekly or
- Ciprofloxacin 750 mg b.i.d.
- Treat until the ulcers are healed but for at least 3 weeks

LYMPHOGRANULOMA VENEREUM

Lymphogranuloma venereum is a sexually transmitted disease that is caused *Chlamydia trachomatis*. The initial lesion may be a papule or an ulcer but these lesions quickly heal spontaneously and patients present with impressive lymphadenopathy rather than an ulcer. For this reason, the primary discussion of this disease will be found in Chapter 12.

EPSTEIN–BARR VIRUS AND CYTOMEGALOVIRUS-ASSOCIATED ULCERS

Even though these ulcers are associated with infectious disease, they are discussed in the next section because their clinical appearance is identical to that of aphthous ulcers and it is likely these viral infections simply trigger the development of aphthae rather than causing the ulcers by direct infection of the skin.

APHTHOUS ULCER AND COMPLEX APHTHOSIS

Aphthous ulcers (synonyms: aphthae, aphthous stomatitis, "canker sores") are extremely common in the oral cavity but are encountered infrequently on the genitalia. The adjectives "minor" (<1 cm; heal without scarring), "major" (>1 cm; may heal with scarring), and "herpetiform" (10 or more, very small clustered) are used for the morphologic description of aphthous ulcers. The term "complex aphthosis" was coined by Jorizzo et al. and this term is used for either of two groups of patients: (1) individuals with three or more, almost constantly present, oral aphthae and (2) those with recurrent oral and genital aphthae. Aphthous ulcers may be "primary" (idiopathic and not occurring in direct association with other conditions) or "secondary" (associated with some other medical disorder more often than would be expected by chance). There is no difference in clinical or histologic appearance between primary and secondary form of aphthous ulcers. On the basis of the similarity of clinical morphology and course of disease, I, along with others, believe that "Lipschutz ulcer" and "ulcus vulvae acutum" are synonyms for primary aphthous ulcers of the vulva (Fig. 10-14) (14,15).

Clinical Presentation

The lifetime incidence of primary *oral* aphthae is usually given as about 30% but some estimates are as high as 60%. Data regarding the incidence of primary *genital* aphthous ulcers are not available but it must be much less than 1% given the relatively few published studies of this disorder. Two reports of 54 and 55 patients with complex aphthosis are available but, unfortunately, the authors of

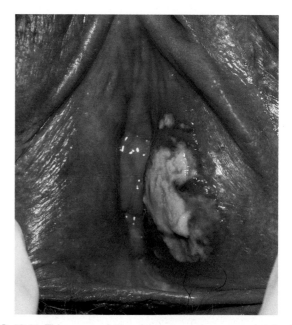

FIG. 10-14. This young girl has large, irregular, very painful aphthous ulceration of the vulvar vestibule. Such lesions are sometimes termed ulcus vulvae acutum.

these studies did not separately provide data for the two groups of patients included under the rubric of complex aphthosis: those with both genital and oral ulcers as compared to those with nearly constant oral ulcers, only (16,17). On the basis of my experience, I believe that *primary* aphthous ulcers of the genitalia occur almost only in females and almost only in girls and women up to the age of 25. The few genital aphthous ulcers that I have seen in men were *secondary* and occurred in the setting of Behçet disease. My experience is supported by the almost total lack of published reports of primary aphthous ulcers involving male genitalia and by the fairly large series of primary aphthous ulcers reported in young women by Huppert et al. (18). Since this is the largest published series of primary genital aphthae, much of the material below is based on information from that manuscript.

Most but not all patients with genital aphthous ulcers also have a history of oral aphthae. These patients, then, can be said to have complex aphthosis. Ulcers at these two sites may or may not occur synchronously. Aphthous ulcers of the vulva primarily occur within the vulvar vestibule, but lesions can also develop on the outer labia minora, the labia majora, the perineum, and at the vaginal introitus. The diameter (up to 2 cm) and depth (up to 1 cm) of the genital ulcers tend to be greater than those occurring in the mouth. Intravaginal, especially introital, ulcers are also possible though the frequency and appearance of such lesions is not clearly described in the medical literature. Interestingly, and in complete contrast to oral aphthae, those developing on the genitalia often occur on keratinizing, as well as mucosal, epithelium.

The majority of patients have two or more ulcers and, when multiple, confluence may occur leading to very large ulcers with gyrate borders (Fig. 10-15). The base of the

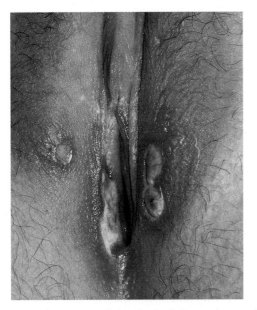

FIG. 10-15. Coalescing, well-demarcated, large, deep aphthae on the vulva and perivulvar tissue of a young girl.

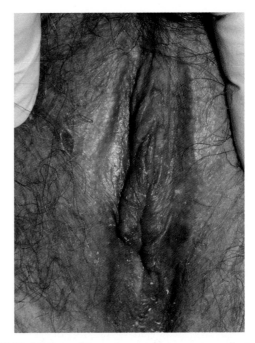

FIG. 10-16. Aphthae of the vulva can be large or small, single or multiple, and occur on either keratinized hair-bearing skin as on this right labium majus, the modified mucous membranes as seen on the left interlabial sulcus, or on the true mucous membranes of the vestibule or vagina.

ulcers can be bright red or may be covered with either gray, necrotic material or heme-colored eschar (Fig. 10-16). Genital ulcers are extremely painful and their appearance is sometimes preceded by, or accompanied by, low-grade fever, malaise, gastrointestinal, and/or respiratory symptoms. Larger genital lesions may heal with scarring. Genital aphthous ulcers in men tend to occur more often on the scrotum than on the penis but are otherwise similar to those that occur in women.

Just as is true for oral lesions, genital ulcers can recur at periodic intervals though the recurrence rate seems to be less frequent than for oral ulcers. In the study by Huppert et al., 35% of patients with genital aphthae either provided a history of preceding genital ulcers or developed recurrent ulcers during a year of follow-up (18). This rate of multiple episodes fits with my experience as well.

Diagnosis

The diagnosis is made on a clinical basis as there are no characteristic histologic or laboratory abnormalities. Some patients do have antibodies to Epstein–Barr virus (EBV) and/or CMV but what, if any, role these viruses play in the direct cause of these genital ulcers is controversial (see below). Biopsy reveals only nondiagnostic acute and chronic inflammation but may be desirable, or even necessary, to rule out other causes of genital ulceration.

Most clinicians initially, and incorrectly, believe that patients with genital aphthous ulcers have HSV infection.

However, HSV infection in *immunocompetent* patients leads only to erosions, not the deeper ulcers found in complex aphthosis. Nevertheless, it is appropriate to obtain HSV cultures or immunofluorescent antibody studies so as not to miss this common and easily treatable infection. Primary syphilis and chancroid cause ulcers but these are unlikely to be confused with aphthae because of lack of pain in the former and impressive lymphadenopathy in the latter.

It may be hard to distinguish primary from secondary aphthous ulcers because the occurrence of aphthae may precede evidence for the development of an associated disease by months or even years. The disease that most often needs to be considered in a list of potentially linked secondary disorders is Behçet disease. Oral and genital ulcers are the two most common findings in both complex aphthosis and Behçet disease and they have an identical clinical appearance in both of these settings. Unfortunately, there are no laboratory tests that definitively identify Behçet disease, with the result that making this diagnosis generally depends on the patient meeting the clinical diagnostic criteria established by the International Study Group (ISG) in 1990. Unfortunately, these criteria are rather broad and some of us believe that their use leads to overdiagnosis of Behçet disease (16). For this reason, other diagnostic criteria have been proposed. The criteria of the Behçet's Research Committee of Japan in 2003 are notable but they were primarily developed to be used for research purposes rather than for use as a clinical diagnostic tool (see Behçet disease). Moreover, since the symptoms and signs of Behçet disease usually evolve over a considerable period of time, patients with complex aphthosis need to be followed on a regular basis as a few such individuals may eventually develop Behçet disease. But in my experience, and in the experience of others, this happens only rarely in Western countries (16).

Secondary aphthous ulcers occur with several other conditions, most commonly inflammatory bowel disease and HIV/AIDS. Rare disorders that are accompanied by aphthae include cyclic neutropenia, lupus erythematosus, and the MAGIC (mouth and genital ulcers with inflamed cartilage) and PFAPA (periodic fever, aphthae, pharyngitis, and adenitis) syndromes.

APHTHOUS ULCERS:　　　　　　**Diagnosis**

- Occurrence primarily in girls and young women
- Several, punched out, very painful ulcers
- Flulike prodrome may precede or accompany ulcers
- Arcuate configuration when ulcers become confluent
- Rule out HSV, syphilis, and chancroid
- Look for associated systemic disease, especially Behçet disease and inflammatory bowel disease

---

Pathophysiology

The cause of oral and genital aphthous ulcers is unknown. Familial cases of oral, but not genital, aphthae occur with some frequency suggesting the possibility of a genetic predisposition. Other etiologic possibilities include the development of a brisk autoimmune, cell-mediated response to one or more antigens. The antigens most often considered are those relating to microbial proteins. A reaction to such antigens might cause crossover reactivity to self-antigens through the process of molecular mimicry. A somewhat similar hypothesis is based on the frequent association of aphthous ulcers with Crohn disease. In Crohn disease, there are mutations in several genes having to do with the processing of bacteria, suggesting that immunodeficiency rather than autoimmunity may be the critical pathway through which this inflammatory bowel disease develops (19). Thus it might be speculated that, because of the frequent association of aphthous ulcers with several viral infections, a somewhat similar mechanism might play a role in the development of aphthae. In addition, at least two well-recognized triggering factors include the development of aphthous ulcers at sites of trauma (pathergy) and at times of increased psychological stress.

No matter what the initiating events are, the end result is the development of a brisk influx of inflammatory cells with elaboration of inflammatory cytokines such as interleukin 2 and tumor necrosis factor alpha. The resultant severe inflammation leads to vascular destruction, induction of localized tissue necrosis, and subsequently ulcer formation.

Management

With the obvious exception of "swish and swallow" approaches, the treatment of genital aphthae is similar to that employed for oral aphthous ulcers. Symptomatic treatment is possible with topically applied anesthetics such as 5% lidocaine ointment applied several times per day. If pain is not controlled with this approach, the nerve ending in the ulcer can be destroyed chemically using the application of a standard silver nitrate stick (20). Topically applied steroids such as 0.05% clobetasol ointment may be somewhat helpful in mild cases, but depending on a patient's tolerance, intralesional injections of triamcinalone (Kenalog) 10 mg/mL directly into each ulcer base are appreciably more effective.

A topical approach used alone genital ulcers is seldom successful. For this reason, I usually initiate oral prednisone therapy (40 mg each morning for 7 to 10 days) at the first visit. This leads to satisfactory healing in most patients and can be repeated as necessary with recurrent episodes of ulceration. As an alternative to oral prednisone, nonsteroidal anti-inflammatory therapy can be offered with oral antibiotics (either doxycycline or minocycline 100 mg twice daily), pentoxyfylline (400 mg t.i.d.), colchicine

(0.6 mg b.i.d. to t.i.d.), or dapsone (100 to 150 mg/day) (21,22). The latter two agents used alone or together are quite effective especially when used on a long-term basis where they may decrease the frequency of recurrences as well as leading to healing of already existent ulcers (17). A complete review of these and other medications is available in a recent publication (23). For the minority of patients who fail to respond to these relatively safe approaches, the therapies described in the next section on Behçet disease can be considered.

With or without treatment, patients in Western countries with complex aphthosis have an excellent prognosis. When those patients with recognized associated disease are excluded, it can be said that patients with primary complex aphthosis have an excellent prognosis. It is certainly true that a few patients with primary complex aphthosis might go on to develop associated illness, especially Behçet disease, but this appears to happen only rarely in Western countries. This observation is supported by data from the series of Letsinger et al. and that of Huppert et al., where no patients with primary complex aphthosis went on to develop Behçet disease over limited periods of follow-up (16,18). For this reason, I believe that it is undesirable, and even inappropriate, to indicate that patients of American and European ancestry who fail to meet rigorous diagnostic criteria for Behçet disease at the time of first evaluation have, or are likely to develop, this disorder in the future.

APHTHOUS ULCERS:	Management

- Topical 5% lidocaine ointment
- Light application of silver nitrate sticks
- Prednisone 40 mg orally for 7 to 10 days
- Colchicine 0.6 mg b.i.d. or t.i.d. and/or
- Dapsone 100 to 150 mg/day

BEHÇET DISEASE

Behçet disease is a rare disorder first described as a triad of oral aphthous ulcers, genital aphthous ulcers, and uveitis. It is now considered a multisystem disease with potential development of problems in many organs such as the skin, joints, cardiovascular system, central nervous system, and gastrointestinal tract. Since it is a disease that will rarely be encountered by the audience for whom this book is intended, only a brief discussion emphasizing the presence of oral and genital aphthae is included in this section.

The prevalence of this disease is quite high in the Mediterranean, Middle East, and Japan. Turkey has the highest prevalence with a rate of 100 to 400/100,000 individuals. In Western countries, Behçet disease is quite rare and has a prevalence of less than 1/100,000. In all countries, the disease occurs more frequently, and with greater severity, in men. In both sexes, the usual age of onset is

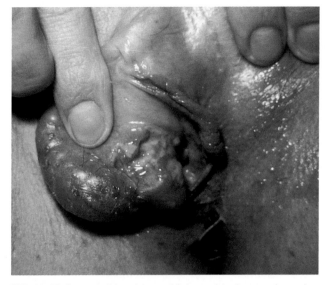

FIG. 10-17. Remarkable edema with irregular shaggy ulceration and white fibrin base in this woman with Behçet disease. (Courtesy of Fenella Wojnarowska.)

between 20 and 40 and it uncommonly develops after mid-adult life.

Recurrent oral and genital aphthous ulcers are the most common clinical signs in patients with Behçet disease. They are identical with those seen in complex aphthosis though they may be larger, more painful, and more frequently recurrent than in primary complex aphthosis (Figs. 10-17 and 10-18). Because of these similarities and the

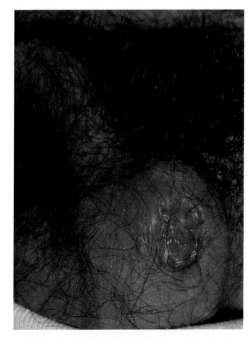

FIG. 10-18. Ulcers associated with Behçet disease in men can affect any area, including the scrotum; the differentiation between aphthae and Behçet disease cannot be made on clinical morphology, but only after evaluation and the identification of systemic involvement.

lack of pathognomonic laboratory findings, it is difficult, and sometimes impossible, to determine with certainty whether the correct diagnosis is that of complex aphthosis or Behçet disease.

The majority of clinicians use the 1990 ISG criteria for the diagnosis of Behçet disease (24). These criteria require recurrent oral ulcerations plus any two of the following: recurrent genital ulceration, uveitis (or other listed orbital abnormalities), evidence of pathergy, or certain skin disorders. Unfortunately, several of the listed skin conditions (erythema nodosum, pseudofolliculitis, papulopustular lesions, and acneiform nodules) are very common and are quite nonspecific. Western patients with genital aphthous ulcers regularly meet two of the criteria (the recurrent oral and genital ulcers) and, because of their age, most also have, or will develop, papulopustular lesions or acneiform nodules. Thus, strictly speaking, they meet the ISG criteria for a diagnosis of Behçet disease even though almost all of them neither have nor will develop the classical findings of this severe life-threatening disorder. Labeling these patients as having Behçet disease is clearly a disservice to the patients and their families. It seems most appropriate to instead work with a diagnosis of complex aphthosis until, and if, a diagnosis of Behçet disease can be subsequently established indisputably.

Other somewhat more specific sets of diagnostic criteria (notably those of O'Duffy in 1974 and those of the Behçet's Disease Research Committee of Japan in 2003) have been proposed (24). But, in my opinion, the former does not add sufficient specificity and the latter is too complicated and cumbersome to use in a clinical setting.

Material covering the extracutaneous clinical manifestations, list of differential diagnoses, and pathogenesis of Behçet disease can be found in two recent review articles (21,25). The treatment of the mucocutaneous ulcers is the same as is described in the section on complex aphthosis above. Additional systemic therapy is available for those patients with more severe or treatment-resistant disease. These agents include azathioprine, cyclophosphamide, cyclosporine, methotrexate, and the tumor necrosis factor alpha inhibitors, etanercept, and infliximab (23,25).

APHTHOUS-LIKE ULCERS ASSOCIATED WITH VIRAL INFECTIONS

Ulcers that are identical in every way to aphthous ulcers have been reported to arise in association with several viral diseases. In most of these instances, the genital aphthae have developed in young women with EBV infection. About 20 such patients have been reported (18,26). These patients developed their vulvar lesions after a short prodrome of fever, malaise, and fatigue. With rare exceptions, no EBV virus was found on viral culture or PCR on ulcer tissue and the diagnosis was made on the basis of

positive IgM antibodies to viral capsid antigen. These ulcers resolve in the same manner as do conventional aphthous ulcers and no specific treatment was found to be necessary. There are no reports of these EBV-associated aphthous-like ulcers occurring in boys or men.

Aphthous-like ulcers have also been reported in a few *immunocompetent* patients with CMV infection (18,27). These patients also were young women presenting with vulvar ulcers that developed after a short flu-like prodrome. Here too, the diagnosis was made on the basis of serology demonstrating IgM antibodies to CMV, though in one case, CMV was cultured from the ulcer. No genital ulcers in immunocompetent men appear to have been reported, but the situation in those patients who are *immunocompromised* may be somewhat different. Most of these patients have been men who developed aphthous-like perianal ulcers. Coinfection with HSV was noted in some of the ulcers (28). It is possible that, in these immunosuppressed patients, the CMV was caused directly by inoculation as a sexually transmitted disease. Aphthous-like ulcers, most often in the mouth, occur in some men with HIV infection and at least one young girl was reported to have developed vulvar ulcers in association with influenza A infection (15).

The relationship of these viral infections to the development of genital aphthous-like ulcers is controversial. The relative lack of evidence indicating the presence of viruses in the ulcers and the fact that almost all of the patients are young women lead me to think that these infections simply triggered the development of conventional aphthous ulcers rather than that the ulcers were caused by way of local infection. This explanation would be analogous to the triggering of erythema multiforme in some patients with HSV infection or the development of Gianotti–Crosti syndrome with any one of several viral diseases.

APHTHOUS-LIKE ULCERS ASSOCIATED WITH MEDICATIONS

Nicorandil is a medication widely used in European countries for the treatment of angina. It is not approved for use in the United States. It has a vasodilator effect that occurs as a result of its action on potassium channels. Oral aphthous-like ulcers occur with some frequency in patients taking nicorandil. Anal and perianal ulcers occur with somewhat less frequency (29). Only a handful of patients with penile (30) and vulvar (31) ulcers have been reported. The morphology of the ulcers is similar to the large deep ulcers seen in major aphthous ulcers. The pathophysiology for the development of the ulcers is unknown though a "vascular steal" phenomenon is the leading hypothesis. The ulcers tend to occur in patients taking higher doses of the nicorandil but not all cases seem to be dose related. Discontinuation of the drug is necessary to obtain healing, but once this is accomplished the ulcers heal spontaneously in 2 to 10 weeks.

Foscarnet is an antiviral agent administered intravenously to patients with drug-resistant HSV and CMV infections. Penile aphthous-like ulcers occur quite frequently though almost all of the reports are in the older medical publications and do not give incidence data. Vulvar ulcers are extremely rare. The reason for this difference is not known. The pathophysiology for the development of these ulcers is also unknown. They resolve spontaneously if foscarnet is discontinued. Genital aphthous-like ulcers have also been reported to have occurred in a few patients receiving *anti-retroviral therapy* for HIV infection.

CROHN DISEASE

Crohn disease is a chronic granulomatous inflammatory process that may affect any region of the intestinal tract. It is associated with a variety of extraintestinal manifestations, such as cutaneous lesions, joint involvement, and ophthalmic disease. Extension of bowel disease to perianal or peristomal skin is quite common. "Metastatic" Crohn disease (cutaneous granulomatous lesions that are separated from affected bowel by normal skin) occurs much less often.

Clinical Presentation

Crohn disease occurs fairly frequently in Western countries. The prevalence is approximately 100 to 200 per 100,000 persons. Perianal cutaneous Crohn disease occurs in a significant proportion of these patients, and while it usually develops as a direct extension from adjacent rectal Crohn disease, it can exist at considerable distance from foci of Crohn disease occurring elsewhere in the intestinal tract. Rarely, perianal disease precedes the development of recognized Crohn disease in the intestine.

If one excludes perianal Crohn disease contiguous with intestinal disease and also excludes genital edema due to Crohn disease, true "metastatic" Crohn disease involving the vulva, penis, and scrotum appears to occur only rarely. In fact, there are fewer than 100 reported cases with vulvar involvement and fewer than 50 with penile or scrotal involvement. However, my experience and that of others suggests that, at least for the vulva, this is a considerable underestimate of its real incidence. As is true for perianal Crohn disease, "metastatic" involvement of the genitalia precedes the development of Crohn disease in only a relatively small percentage of cases. However, this is probably an underestimation due both to a reluctance to accept the possibility that Crohn disease can arise as "primary" in the skin and to an unwillingness to carry out imaging and/or visualization of intestinal tract in otherwise asymptomatic patients. In any event, there appears to be

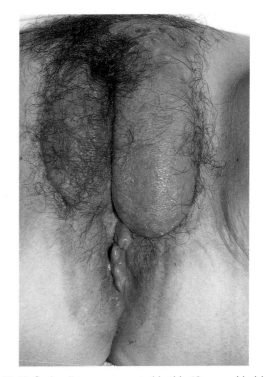

FIG. 10-19. Crohn disease presented in this 13-year-old girl as a painless, enlarged, and indurated left labium majus, followed over the next several years by perianal, fibrotic skin tags and a perianal fistula.

little relationship between the activity and/or severity of intestinal Crohn disease and the development of cutaneous lesions.

Edema, with or without granulomatous change on biopsy, is the most common clinical finding in both men and women (Figs. 10-19, 10-20, and 12-49). It may precede,

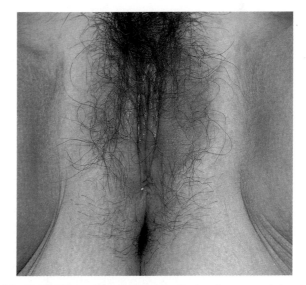

FIG. 10-20. This patient had known Crohn disease and developed mild asymptomatic edema of the left labium majus that showed changes consistent with cutaneous Crohn disease on biopsy.

occur concomitantly with, or follow a diagnosis of intestinal disease. In women, the edema may be unilateral or bilateral and in some instances small areas of edematous outpouching may give the labia minora a somewhat characteristic "multinodular" shape. Biopsy of this edematous tissue is rarely performed and for this reason it is not possible to state the frequency with which the edema is simply passively present versus its association with granulomatous inflammation. It should be noted, however, that nonspecific granulomatous changes are generally present in the edematous vulvae of women with the condition known as Melkersson–Rosenthal disease (Chapter 12), and it has been hypothesized that this condition represents a forme fruste of Crohn disease (32).

Perianal Crohn disease occurs in both sexes and includes the nonspecific findings of edematous skin tags and anal fissures as well as the much more characteristic fistulas and abscesses (33,34). Abscess formation typically begins with localized erythematous or violaceous nodular swelling. Progression to ulceration is common. While it is most common for these fistulae and abscesses to be found in a perianal location, they may also occur throughout the entire anogenital area. Linear fissures and deeper linear ulcers, most often occurring in the skin folds, represent the most characteristic lesions in anogenital Crohn disease (Fig. 10-21). Indeed in Western countries such lesions are nearly pathognomonic of the disease. These linear ulcers have been described frequently in women (34) but less often in men.

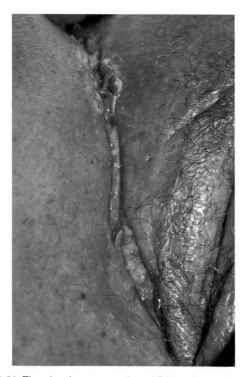

FIG. 10-21. The classic presentation of Crohn disease is a linear, "knifelike," ulceration.

Diagnosis

In the setting of previously diagnosed intestinal Crohn disease, it is often possible to make a clinical diagnosis of cutaneous Crohn disease when anogenital fistulae and/or linear skin fold ulcers are present. With less characteristic clinical lesions, or in the absence of recognized intestinal Crohn disease, a biopsy is necessary. Unfortunately, the granulomatous inflammation in cutaneous Crohn disease seems to be less characteristic than the microscopic changes that occur within the intestinal lesions. This often results in a hedged pathology report that simply indicates the presence of "granulomatous inflammation." In this situation, the diagnosis is established by clinical–pathologic correlation. Alternatively, when no established diagnosis of intestinal Crohn disease is present, radiologic and/or endoscopic examination should be strongly considered as intestinal Crohn disease may be present in some, otherwise asymptomatic, patients (32,34).

Several disorders need to be considered in the differential diagnosis of Crohn disease. As indicated above, genital edema with histologic evidence of granulomatous inflammation similar to that of Crohn disease occurs in the condition termed Melkersson–Rosenthal disease. It is not clear whether or not this disease is a distinct entity or is a forme fruste of Crohn disease (32,35).

Hidradenitis suppurativa is the disease most often confused with cutaneous Crohn disease. Patients with anogenital hidradenitis suppurativa may present with abscesses and fistulas that are very similar to those found in Crohn disease. On biopsy, these lesions of hidradenitis suppurativa generally show nonspecific granulomatous inflammation making differentiation between the two disorders very difficult. The presence of abscesses in the axillae, or anywhere along the milk line, together with the presence of atypical comedones in any of these locations, will correctly identify hidradenitis suppurativa. However, it should be noted that these two diseases have been reported to occur concomitantly more often than chance alone would suggest (36).

Linear ulcers like those in Crohn disease also occur in granuloma inguinale and Langerhans cell histiocytosis. Biopsy will allow for correct identification of these two diseases. Behçet disease, herpes genitalis in an immunosuppressed patient, syphilis, granuloma inguinale, chancroid, traumatic ulcerations, and ulcerated carcinoma cause anogenital ulcers but these disorders are less likely to be confused with Crohn disease.

CROHN DISEASE:	**Diagnosis**

- History of intestinal symptoms and signs
- Perianal tags and/or genital edema
- Abscesses and/or fistulas
- Linear "knife cut" ulcers in skin folds
- Biopsy to confirm

Pathophysiology

The cause of Crohn disease is unknown. Mutations in the *NOD 2*, *ATG16L1*, and *IRGM* genes are generally present in patients with Crohn disease (19). These genes play a role in the processing of bacteria present both in the intestinal wall and in the lumen. When mutated, abnormal processing occurs and this leads to a delay, or even lack, of bacterial clearance. In this situation, the bacteria are sequestered in areas of granulomatous inflammation (37). At this point it is uncertain whether the inflammation represents an autoimmune reaction or a primary immunodeficiency (19). While either or both of these hypothesis might explain the development of intestinal disease, it is not at all clear how either explanation might lead to cutaneous lesions that are not in contiguity with areas of intestinal disease.

Management

Therapy directed toward intestinal disease should be instituted for untreated patients with active bowel symptoms and signs. However, effective control of the bowel disease may or may not result in resolution of the cutaneous Crohn disease. Such treatment generally requires the use of systemic corticosteroids, methotrexate, sulfasalazine, or metronidazole administered either individually or in combination. The indications and dosing for these agents is beyond the scope of this book, but this information can be found in medical textbooks and in recent review (38). Special mention should be made of the relatively new biologic agents. Most of the products used for Crohn disease are inhibitors of the inflammatory cytokine, tumor necrosis factor alpha, but other biologics, directed toward different aspects of immune response, are in clinical trials (39,40). These biologic agents are very effective but their use is associated with considerable potential for adverse events, and as a result they are generally considered as second-line drugs.

When intestinal disease is inactive or not present, local therapy can be implemented. Fluctuant abscesses should be incised and drained. Smaller, solid inflammatory lesions can be intralesionally injected with triamcinalone acetonide (Kenalog) in a concentration of 10 to 20 mg/mL. Localized areas of persistent edema can be similarly treated with intralesional triamcinalone injections. Surgery, which is beyond the scope of this book, will be required for fistulas.

In terms of prognosis, the genital edema ("elephantiasis") that occurs with Crohn disease is extremely persistent and disfiguring. Likewise, the ulcers, abscesses, and fistulas are very destructive and cause appreciable scarring and architectural distortion. As is true for several other genital chronic inflammatory diseases, such as lichen sclerosus, lichen planus, and hidradenitis suppurativa, a possibility exists that squamous cell carcinoma may develop in nonhealing lesions (41).

CROHN DISEASE: **Management**

- Control associated bowel disease; refer if necessary
- Intralesional triamcinalone 10 mg/mL for solid lesions
- Incise and drain fluctuant lesions
- Consider oral prednisone or tumor necrosis factor alpha inhibitors
- Observe for the possible development of squamous cell carcinoma

---

PYODERMA GANGRENOSUM

Pyoderma gangrenosum belongs to the group of diseases known as the neutrophilic dermatoses. It is the most commonly encountered member of this family but it is rarely reported to involve the anogenital area. Nevertheless, because pyoderma gangrenosum can be associated with serious, even life-threatening, problems it is discussed in this chapter.

Clinical Presentation

The overall annual incidence of pyoderma gangrenosum is about 1 per 100,000 persons. Most often it develops in early and mid-adult life. It is equally common in men and women. The ulcers of pyoderma gangrenosum usually occur on the lower legs but lesions in other sites, such as the perianal area, occasionally develop. Fewer than 20 cases of vulvar pyoderma gangrenosum and about a dozen cases involving the penis and/or scrotum have been reported (42,43).

Pyoderma gangrenosum usually starts with one or more inflammatory pustules, papules, or nodules. The initial lesion becomes violaceous and then breaks down to form an ulcer. Less often pyoderma starts a hemorrhagic bulla or plaque that then also breaks down to form an ulcer. Classically, the ulcers of pyoderma gangrenosum are deep with overhanging, undermined violaceous borders. However, those lesions that begin as hemorrhagic bullae and plaques may present with more shallow ulcers (Fig. 10-22). Most often only a solitary ulcer is present but occasionally multiple lesions can be found. Pathergy, the development of a lesion at a site of trauma, is often noted to account for the site of lesion formation.

An underlying, associated systemic disorder is found in about half of the patients. Most commonly this is inflammatory bowel disease, especially Crohn disease. Other related conditions include rheumatoid arthritis, lupus erythematosus, hematopoietic malignancy, and various gammopathies.

Diagnosis

If the lesion is classical in appearance, a clinical diagnosis is possible. There are no characteristic laboratory

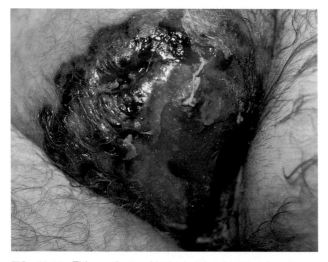

FIG. 10-22. This patient with leukemia developed a large, necrotic, and hemorrhagic bullous plaque that proceeded to ulcerate and proved to be bullous pyoderma gangrenosum. After necrotizing fasciitis was ruled out, he was treated successfully with systemic corticosteroids.

abnormalities. Biopsy should be carried out from tissue located 5 to 10 mm from the edge of the ulcer. If a dense infiltrate of neutrophils is present, clinicopathologic correlation can lead to the correct diagnosis. However, often in older ulcers, only nonspecific inflammation may be found in which case a diagnosis can only be established by ruling out other diseases described on the list of differential diagnoses. Such conditions include aphthous ulceration, Behçet disease, and cutaneous Crohn disease. Necrotizing fasciitis, termed Fournier gangrene when the anogenital area is involved, mimics the appearance of the bullous form of hemorrhagic pyoderma gangrenosum and is a strong consideration if fever, malaise, and an elevated white blood cell count are present.

PYODERMA GANGRENOSUM: **Diagnosis**

- Rapid development of painful ulcer with purpuric borders
- Classical ulcer is deep with undermined margins
- Bullous hemorrhagic form is shallow with purpuric blister roof over part or all of the ulcer
- Biopsy to confirm
- Look for associated disease, especially Crohn disease, lupus erythematosus, rheumatoid arthritis, and hematopoietic malignancy

---

Pathogenesis

The cause of pyoderma gangrenosum is unknown. It appears to be a reactive neutrophilic inflammatory reaction that appears to be preferentially directed toward the

dermal, rather than epidermal, tissue. Tissue breakdown occurs both as a result of the inflammation and as a result of anoxia when the blood vessels are destroyed. The vascular involvement seems not to be a form of conventional vasculitis.

Management

Pyoderma gangrenosum is a chronic condition in which spontaneous healing is unlikely or, at least, is significantly delayed. Therapy is difficult as might be supposed given the numerous agents that have been recommended (44). Systemic corticosteroids represent the first line of treatment. Prednisone is administered in a dose of 60 mg/day until healing begins. At that time, the dose can be tapered but it is likely that even for relatively mild disease, 2 months of steroid therapy will be necessary. Intralesional triamcinalone acetonide (Kenalog) in a concentration of 10 to 20 mg/mL can be used alone, for small ulcers, or as adjunctive therapy for larger ones. Other oral nonsteroidal anti-inflammatory agents such as doxycycline, minocycline, colchicine, dapsone, and thalidomide can be used either alone or in combination. These medications can be very helpful in minimizing the dose and/or duration of corticosteroid therapy. Cytotoxic agents, cyclosporine, and the biologic inhibitors of the inflammatory cytokine tumor necrosis factor alpha may be required for severe and recalcitrant disease. Treatment of any underlying, associated disease is useful but does not necessarily lead to resolution of the ulcers.

Healing occurs with or without scarring depending on the depth, diameter, and duration of the original ulcer. Otherwise, the prognosis is that for any underlying systemic disease that might be present in association with the pyoderma gangrenosum.

PYODERMA GANGRENOSUM: **Management**

- Prednisone 60 mg orally qAM; taper as healing occurs
- Intralesional triamcinalone 10 mg/mL as adjuvant therapy
- Oral antibiotics and dapsone for their anti-inflammatory effect
- Cyclosporine and/or tumor necrosis factor alpha inhibitors if necessary
- Treat any underlying disease that is present

ULCERS DUE TO EXTERNAL TRAUMA

External trauma can lead to the development of ulcers. A clue suggesting a traumatic etiology often comes from the presence of a linear or angular ulcer configuration. Traumatic ulcers arise in several contexts: (1) deep excoriation ("gouging"), (2) unintentional induction by the patient or the clinician, and (3) intentional, but usually unacknowledged, self-induction by the patient.

Deep Excoriation

Chronic scratching, most often in the setting of lichen simplex chronicus (see Chapter 4), represents the most common cause of traumatic genital ulcers. These ulcers are usually located on the scrotum in men and on the labia majora and pubic region in women. Patients may acknowledge that their scratching is causing ulcers, but in some instances (when the scratching occurs at a subconscious level or while the patient is asleep) the patient may be unaware of the role he or she is playing in the ulcer etiology. Whether aware of the scratching or not, patients are unable to discontinue the scratching of their own volition. For this reason, admonition by the clinician to stop scratching cannot be complied with and is usually counterproductive. Though not usually defined as such in psychiatric terms, this chronic scratching can be viewed as an obsessive–compulsive disorder (OCD) and thus will often require the use of psychotropic medication to interrupt the process (45).

In addition to the standard therapy for pruritus (see Chapters 2 and 4), use of a selective serotonin reuptake inhibitor (SSRI) is usually warranted. Most of these agents are approved for treatment of OCD and for this reason can reasonably be used in the setting of habitual, destructive excoriation (45). The normal stating dose should be used but often double or even triple that amount will be required. These medications can be taken in the morning or in the evening. I prefer the former as in almost all cases hydroxyzine 25 to 75 mg or doxepin 25 to 75 mg should be administered 2 hours before bedtime (see Chapters 2 and 4). There is some potential for drug–drug interaction between the SSRIs and the tricyclics, so care should be taken when maximizing the dose of either agent. Onset of action may be slow and a period of 4 to 6 weeks must be allowed to determine the level of effectiveness. If the patient is still gouging at that time, the use of an antipsychotic agents should be considered, as these medications are quite valuable for the therapy of SSRI-resistant OCD, including that of chronic excoriation (46).

Acknowledged External Trauma

Clinicians may prescribe, or apply, medications that potentially can cause either erosions or ulcers. The three medications most often responsible are clinician-applied trichloroacetic acid and patient-applied fluorouracil or imiquimod. The caustic reaction to these agents is not immediate and tissue destruction may not occur for days or even a week or so. When patients are given prescriptions for imiquimod or fluorouracil, they should be warned to stop the applications if inflammation becomes

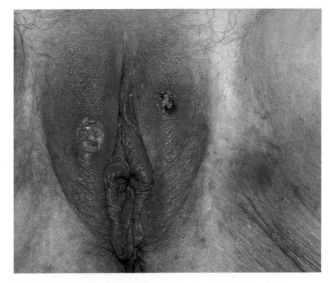

FIG. 10-23. These round ulcers in a background of deep erythema and edema of the labia majora resulted from compulsive, frequent scrubbing with antiseptic solutions.

more than moderately severe. Similarly, and not unexpectedly, ulcers can also occur following the use of liquid nitrogen and ablative electrosurgical and laser therapy.

Patients, especially women, sometimes have the perception that the anogenital area is "dirty," and for this reason, extraordinary approaches to hygiene may be used. They might then scrub with a stiff brush, apply bleach, or overuse cleansers that were never designed for application to the skin (Fig. 10-23). Patients who are incontinent or have chronic vaginal discharge may persistently occlude the anogenital area with diapers or panty liners, respectively. The chronic presence of moisture can then lead to breakdown of the skin and the formation of erosions and ulcers (see Chapter 2).

Genital ulcers may develop as a result of ritualistic female mutilation used for proof of virginity or circumcision to reduce libido. This is still practiced in some African societies but can also occasionally be encountered in Western countries (47).

Unacknowledged External Trauma

Patients with psychiatric disorders may mutilate the skin by way of burning, cutting, gouging, or other forms of self-mutilation. This may occur because they fear that something is abnormally present in the skin (delusions of parasitosis, morgellon disease) and they then feel compelled to physically remove these perceived bugs or fibers. They often deny that any behavior on their part is responsible for the repeated and persistent ulceration. Alternatively, traumatic self-abuse can represent a psychiatrically abnormal behavior pattern in adolescents, particularly young women (48). This frequently involves genital cutting as was vividly

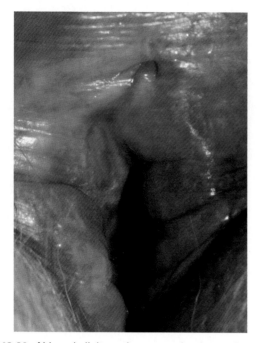

FIG. 10-24. Although lichen planus nearly always is erosive rather than ulcerative, this patient with the fragile skin of lichen planus shows a discrete ulceration.

portrayed in the recent movie *The Piano Teacher*. In men, penile implantations and other forms of penile manipulation up to, and including, penile amputation may be carried out (49). Patients who self-mutilate have extremely serious psychological problems requiring referral to psychiatrists rather than treatment by dermatologists and gynecologists.

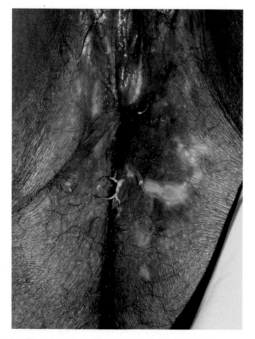

FIG. 10-25. The draining sinus tracts of hidradenitis suppurativa often develop into nonhealing ulcers.

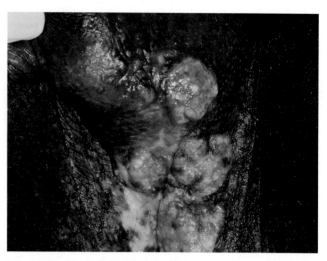

FIG. 10-26. Ulcerated exophytic lesions are generally tumors, such as this squamous cell carcinoma of the penis and scrotum.

MISCELLANEOUS ULCERS

Ulcers can arise at the site of what originally were erosions. Thus ulcers may sometimes occur in erosive lesions of lichen sclerosus and lichen planus (Fig. 10-24). Hidradenitis suppurativa generally presents with abscesses and fistulas but either of these may result in chronic ulceration (Fig. 10-25). When tumor growth outstrips its blood supply, the surface may undergo necrosis resulting in the development of an ulcer (Fig. 10-26).

REFERENCES

1. Center for Disease Control and Prevention. Sexually transmitted diseases surveillance, 2007. Syphilis. Available at: http://www.cdc.gov/std/stats07/syphilis.htm. Accessed August 8, 2009.
2. Bourke S, Schmidt T. Sexually transmissible infections—old enemies and a new friend. *Aust Fam Physician*. 2009; 38:373.
3. Viñals-Iglesias H, Chimeros-Küstner E. The reappearance of a forgotten disease in the oral cavity: syphilis. *Med Oral Patol Oral Cir Bucal*. 2009;14:e416–e420.
4. Marangoni A, Moroni A, Accardo S, et al. Laboratory diagnosis of syphilis with automated immunoassays. *J Clin Lab Anal*. 2009;23:1–6.
5. Phipps W, Kent CK, Kohn R, et al. Risk factors for repeat syphilis in men who have sex with men, San Francisco. *Sex Transm Dis*. 2009;36:331–335.
6. Weiss HA, Thomas SL, Munabi SK, et al. Male circumcision and risk of syphilis, chancroid, and genital herpes: a systematic review and meta-analysis. *Sex Transm Infect*. 2006;82: 101–109.
7. Tobian AA, Serwadda D, Quinn TC, et al. Male circumcision for the prevention of HSV-2 and HPV infection and syphilis. *N Engl J Med*. 2009;360:1298–1209.
8. Workowski KA, Berman SM. Sexually transmitted diseases treatment guidelines, 2006. *MMWR*. 2006;55(RR11):1–94.

9. Kingston M, French P, Goh B, et al. UK national guidelines on the management of syphilis 2008. *Int J STD AIDS*. 2008;19:729–740.

10. French P, Gomberg M, Janier M, et al. IUSTI: 2008 European guidelines on the management of syphilis. *Int J STD AIDS*. 2009;20:300–309.

11. Janowicz DM, Ofner S, Katz BP, et al. Experimental infection of human volunteers with *Haemophilus ducreyi*: fifteen years of clinical data and experience. *J Infect Dis*. 2009;199:1671–1679.

12. Marais S, Wilkinson RJ, Pepper DJ, et al. Management of patients with the immune reconstitution inflammatory syndrome. *Curr HIV/AIDS Rep*. 2009;6:162–171.

13. Superti F, Ammendolia MG, Marchetti M. New advances in anti-HSV chemotherapy. *Curr Med Chem*. 2008;15:900–911.

14. Hernández-Nuñez A, Cordoba S, Romero-Maté A, et al. Lipchütz ulcers—four cases. *Pediatr Dermatol*. 2008;25:364–367.

15. Wetter DA, Bruce AJ, MacLaughlin KL, et al. Ulcus vulvae acutum in a 13-year-old girl after influenza A infection. *Skinmed*. 2008;7:95–98.

16. Letsinger JA, McCarty M, Jorizzo JL. Complex aphthosis: a large case series with evaluation algorithm and therapeutic ladder from topicals to thalidomide. *J Am Acad Dermatol*. 2005;52:500–508.

17. Lynde CB, Bruce AJ, Rogers RS III. Successful treatment of complex aphthosis with colchicine and dapsone. *Arch Dermatol*. 2009;145:273–276.

18. Huppert JS, Gerber MA, Deitch HR, et al. Vulvar ulcers in young females: a manifestation of aphthosis. *J Pediatr Adolesc Gynecol*. 2006;19:195–204.

19. Coulombe F, Behr MA. Crohn's disease as an immune deficiency? *Lancet*. 2009;374:769–770.

20. Alidaee MR, Taheri A, Mansoori P, et al. Silver nitrate cautery in aphthous stomatitis: a randomized controlled trial. *Br J Dermatol*. 2005;153:521–525.

21. Keogan MT. Clinical immunology review series: an approach to the patient with recurrent orogenital ulceration including Behçet's syndrome. *Clin Exp Immunol*. 2009;156:1–11.

22. Mimura MA, Hirota SK, Sugaya NN, et al. Systemic treatment in severe cases of recurrent aphthous stomatitis: an open trial. *Clinics*. 2009;64:193–198.

23. Hatemi G, Silman A, Bang D, et al. EULAR recommendations for the management of Behçet's disease. *Ann Rheum Dis*. 2008;67:1656–1662.

24. Dervis E, Geyik N. Sennsitivity and specificity of different diagnostic criteria for Behçet's disease in a group of Turkish patients. *J Dermatol*. 2005;32:266–272.

25. Mendes D, Correia M, Barbedo M, et al. Behçet's disease—a contemporary review. *J Autoimmun*. 2009;32:178–188.

26. Barnes CJ, Alió AB, Cunningham BB, et al. Epstein–Barr virus associated genital ulcers: an under recognized disorder. *Pediatr Dermatol*. 2007;24:130–134.

27. Martin JM, Godoy R, Calduch L, et al. Lipschütz acute viral ulcers associated with primary cytomegalovirus infection. *Pediatr Dermatol*. 2008;25:113–115.

28. Abe M, Sawamura D, Ito S, et al. Perianal cytomegalovirus ulcer following herpes simplex virus in a patient with idiopathic thrombocytopenic purpura treated with immunosuppressants. *Clin Exp Dermatol*. 2005;30:596–598.

29. Akbar F, Maw A, Bhowmick A. Anal ulceration induced by nicorandil. *BMJ*. 2007;335:936–937.

30. Birnie A, Dearing N, Littlewood S, et al. Nicorandil-induced ulceration of the penis. *Clin Exp Dermatol*. 2008;33:215–216.

31. Claeys A, Weber-Muller F, Trechot P, et al. Cutaneous, perivulvar and perianal ulcerations induced by nicorandil. *Br J Dermatol*. 2006;155:477–500.

32. Saha M, Edmonds E, Martin J, et al. Penile lymphedema in association with asymptomatic Crohn's disease. *Clin Exp Dermatol*. 2009;34:88–90.

33. Vermeire S, Van Assche G, Rutgeerts P. Perianal Crohn's disease: classification and clinical evaluation. *Dig Liver Dis*. 2007;39:959–962.

34. Andreani SM, Ratnasingham K, Dang HH, et al. Crohn's disease of the vulva. *Int J Surg*. 2010;8:2–5.

35. Tonkovic-Capin V, Galbraith SS, Rogers RS III, et al. Cutaneous Crohn's disease mimicking Melkersson–Rosenthal syndrome: treatment with methotrexate. *J Eur Acad Dermatol Venereol*. 2006;20:449–452.

36. van der Zee HH, van der Woude CJ, Florencia EF, et al. Hidradenitis suppurativa and inflammatory bowel disease: are they associated? Results of a pilot study. *Br J Dermatol*. 2009;162:195–197. [Epub ahead of print].

37. Xavier RJ, Podolsky DK. Unraveling the pathogenesis of inflammatory bowel disease. *Nature*. 2007;448:427–434.

38. Baumgart DC, Sandborn WJ. Inflammatory bowel disease: clinical aspects and established and evolving therapies. *Lancet*. 2007;369:1641–1657.

39. Rutgeerts P, Vermeire S, Van Assche G. Biological therapies for inflammatory bowel disease. *Gastroenterology*. 2009;136:1182–1197.

40. Peyrin-Biroulet L, Desreumaux O, Sandborn WJ, et al. Crohn's disease: beyond antagonists of tumor necrosis factor. *Lancet*. 2008;372:67–82.

41. Kesteson JP, South S, Lele S. Squamous cell carcinoma of the vulva in a young woman with Crohn's disease. *Eur J Gynaecol Oncol*. 2008;29:651–652.

42. Sau M, Hill NCW. Pyoderma gangrenosum of the vulva. *Br J Obstet Gynaecol*. 2001;108:1197–1198.

43. Parren LJ, Nellen RG, van Marion AM, et al. Penile pyoderma gangrenosum: successful treatment with colchicine. *Int J Dermatol*. 2008;47(suppl 1):7–9.

44. Cohen PR. Neutrophilic dermatoses: a review of current treatment options. *Am J Clin Dermatol*. 2009;10:301–312.

45. Ravindran AV, da Silva TL, Ravindran LN, et al. Obsessive-compulsive spectrum disorders: a review of the evidence-based treatments. *Can J Psychiatry*. 2009;54:331–343.

46. Bloch MH, Landeros-Weisenberger A, Kelmendi B, et al. A systematic review: antipsychotic augmentation with treatment refractory obsessive-compulsive disorder. *Mol Psychiatry*. 2006;11:622–632.

47. Shah G, Susan L, Furcroy J. Female circumcision: history, medical and psychological complications, and initiatives to eradicate this practice. *Can J Urol*. 2009;16:4576–4579.

48. Laukkanen E, Rissanen ML, Honkalampi K, et al. The prevalence of self-cutting and other self-harm among 13- to 18-year-old Finnish adolescents. *Soc Psychiatry Psychiatr Epidemiol*. 2009;44:23–28.

49. Ristić DI, Petrović D, Cirić Z. Penle self-mutilation—two cases in one family. *Psychiatr Danub*. 2008;20:332–335.

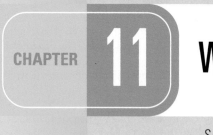
White Lesions

SALLIE M. NEILL

Skin pigmentation depends on melanin-containing melanosomes produced by melanocytes. Variation in pigmentation is due to differences in melanocyte numbers and to the numbers and size of melanosomes. White lesions may arise from damage to melanocytes, causing a temporary decrease in melanin production (hypopigmentation), or from total destruction of melanocytes, resulting in absent pigmentation (depigmentation). Loss of color of the skin is not always the result of melanocyte number or melanogenic activity and is seen in:

maceration of the skin due to hydration of top layer of the epidermis, produced when the stratum corneum is thickened by inflammation or friction.
scarring where the white appearance is due to a combination of both vascular and optical effects that are caused by changes of the dermis and epidermis.

WHITE PATCHES AND PLAQUES

Vitiligo

Vitiligo is a depigmenting condition of the skin and hair affecting approximately 1% to 2% of the population worldwide. Autoimmune, genetic, autocytotoxic, neural, environmental, and genetic factors have all been implicated (1). There is a strong genetic link as up to 30% of the affected individuals have a family history of the disorder and it seems that genetically predisposed individuals have melanocytes that are prone to damage which then undergo responses that lead to depigmentation. There are two forms of vitiligo, *segmental* which is unilateral occurring at a young age and *nonsegmental* which is generalized, bilateral running a chronic and unpredictable course. Patients with generalized vitiligo exhibit an increase in other autoimmune diseases, especially thyroid disease and have more circulating autoantibodies in general. Occupational vitiligo can occur in the genital area in men as a result of destruction of melanocytes by exposure to *para*-tertiary-butylphenol, a substance found in resins for adhesives in the car industry (2).

Clinical Presentation

Vitiligo is characterized by a total loss of pigmentation with no evidence of any textural change to the skin, that is, there is no scaling, crusting, or induration (Figs. 11-1 through 11-3). There may be an accentuation of the pigment in the skin bordering the depigmented lesions. Wood's light can be used to distinguish the depigmentation seen in vitiligo which appears brilliantly white rather than the hypopigmentation of other disorders where the lightening is more subtle. Patients usually present with extragenital lesions in the summer months when the areas burn or become more noticeable because of tanning of surrounding unaffected skin. There is a predilection for body sites that are normally hyperpigmented including the face, flexures, areola of the nipples, and the external genitalia. The pigment loss can be patchy or extensive and confluent. Vitiligo can exhibit the Köebner phenomenon, the occurrence of a skin disease in an area of injury or inflammation. The hairs in affected areas may lose their pigment and remain white even after spontaneous recovery of the skin. Spontaneous remission does occur, particularly in young children, but this is rarer in adults. Perifollicular hyperpigmentation is the first sign of recovery.

Diagnosis

The diagnosis of vitiligo is usually made clinically by the distribution of the depigmentation, absence of textural change, and the presence of a hyperpigmented border. Illumination of the skin with Wood's light helps to delineate the extent of the vitiliginous areas, as it accentuates and highlights areas that may not be seen easily in visible light and furthermore helps in the differentiation of disorders characterized by hypopigmentation. A biopsy may be necessary in some cases.

Histopathologically, there is an absence of melanocytes and melanin in the epidermis. This can be difficult to discern on routine hematoxylin and eosin stains, but incubation with 0.01% 3,4-dihydroxyphenylalanine (also called dopa) stains enzymatically active melanocytes black in the basal layer, and electron microscopy can demonstrate the loss of the melanocytes. There is also a mild to moderate dermal lymphocytic infiltrate at the borders of some lesions, and melanocytes in this area often appear large with long dendrites containing melanin.

Confusion of vitiligo with postinflammatory hypopigmentation can arise, particularly in the early lesions of vitiligo. This can be an especially difficult

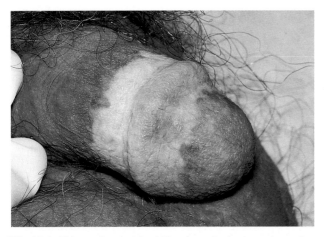

FIG. 11-1. This patient with vitiligo has depigmented patches without surface texture change and associated patchy peripheral hyperpigmentation.

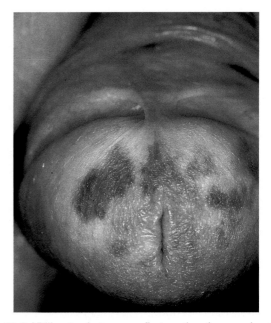

FIG. 11-2. Vitiligo tends to occur first on the glans, and patchy hyperpigmentation may or may not occur.

differentiation in black patients with hypopigmentation as a postinflammatory sequelae of the original inflammatory condition, for example, eczema or psoriasis. Pityriaisis versicolor enters the differential diagnosis at extragenital sites. The main diffential diagnosis in the anogenital area is lichen sclerosus. This has a similar marble white color, but the crinkled, rough textural changes in the skin help to differentiate this condition. A confusing picture arises with the relatively common coexistence of both vitiligo and lichen sclerosus. The anesthetic, hypopigmented patches of leprosy may also mimic vitiligo, but testing for sensation within the white skin is normal in vitiligo. Vitiligo-like change can be induced by the topical immunonmodulatory cream, imiquimod, used for treating genital warts (3).

inhibitor pimecrolimus can be used if a topical steroid is ineffective. Depigme-ntation of normal skin should be reserved for those patients with more than 50% skin involvement. Phototherapy can be used for extragenital vitiligo. Surgical treatment involves split skin grafting or minigrafting. However, most of these treatments are unsuitable for genital skin, particularly phototherapy because of the increased risk of cutaneous malignancy. Reassurance and support should be offered.

VITILIGO: **Diagnosis**

- White, depigmented patches
- No scale, surface change, or texture change of any kind
- Biopsy generally not necessary, and routine histology is often normal; may require dopa stains to confirm absence of melanocytes

---

Management

Treatment to encourage repigmentation in vitiligo includes medical and surgical therapies (4). Medical treatment includes a trial of a potent topical corticosteroid (i.e., clobetasol propionate) for no longer than 8 weeks. Care must be taken, particularly in the genitocrural folds, inner upper thighs, and scrotum as these areas are susceptible to steroid atrophy. Topical calcipotriol, a vitamin D analog (5), or the calcineurin

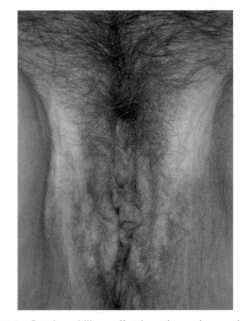

FIG. 11-3. Patchy vitiligo affecting the vulva and genito crural folds.

VITILIGO: Management

- No satisfactory therapy for repigmenting the genital area, but the following are occasionally useful, alone or in combination
  - Topical ultrapotent corticosteroid ointment applied b.i.d. in 6- to 8-week pulses
  - Tacrolimus or pimecrolimus applied b.i.d. ongoing
  - Calcipotriol (calcipotriene) cream applied b.i.d.
  - Ultraviolet light not practical, and confers risk of malignancy
- When large areas of the body are affected, remaining normal skin can be depigmented permanently with 20% monobenzylether of hydroquinone applied twice a day to even the skin color

POSTINFLAMMATORY HYPOPIGMENTATION: Diagnosis

- Usually, history of preceding inflammatory process; diaper dermatitis, lichen simplex chronicus, trauma of wart therapy, etc.
- Pale, hypopigmented patches
- No scale or surface change, except for that associated with any ongoing underlying etiologic inflammatory process
- Distribution correlates with previous inflammatory process
- Biopsy generally not necessary for diagnosis; stains show presence of melanocytes

Postinflammatory Hypopigmentation and Depigmentation

Clinical Presentation

The loss of pigment is often very subtle, and usually there is no associated surrounding hyperpigmentation. Under Wood's light examination, there is no enhancement of the hypopigmentation. However, patients with a dark complexion, and those who had past or present lesions of eczema or psoriasis, sometimes exhibit striking postinflammatory pigment loss that is accentuated by Wood's light, almost indistinguishable from vitiligo. It is possible that these are examples of the Köebner phenomenon localized to the sites of the inflammatory disease.

Diagnosis

The diagnosis can usually be determined by the pattern of hypopigmentation in association with the past or present existence of skin disease or injury. A biopsy is only occasionally required and shows a decreased amount of melanin in the basal keratinocytes, but melanocytes are present. Pigment-ladened macrophages may be present in the underlying dermis.

The pallor of lichen sclerosus, lichen planus, and lichen simplex may be similar to postinflammatory hypopigmentation but the textural changes and scarring help to distinguish these disorders. Vitiligo due to depigmentation can mimic postinflammatory hypopigmentation and Wood's lamp examination can usually differentiate between the two.

Pathophysiology

Any inflammatory dermatosis or injury can leave residual hypopigmentation or hyperpigmentation in the affected areas (Fig. 11-4). Postinflammatory hypopigmentation is more common in conditions that disrupt the integrity of the basement membrane zone, resulting in damage to the melanocytes and their function. In tinea versicolor, oxidation products are produced which are able to inhibit the tyrosinase activity of the melanocytes. Finally, permanent hypopigmentation may be a sequelae of destructive treatments in which the melanocytes may be more susceptible to damage, as seen after cryotherapy or radiotherapy.

Management

There is no treatment for postinflammatory hypopigmentation but the normal skin pigmentation returns spontaneously with time. If the underlying dermatosis

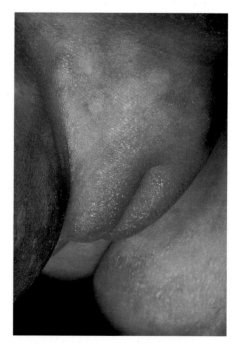

FIG. 11-4. This child still shows remaining erythema and roughness from her diaper rash; the area of pigment lightening is characteristic of postinflammatory hypopigmentation.

that caused the problem is still present, this should be treated to prevent further hypopigmentation.

POSTINFLAMMATORY HYPOPIGMENTATION:	Management

- Control of any ongoing underlying inflammatory process
- Otherwise, self-resolving; no therapies hasten repigmentation

Lichen Sclerosus

Lichen sclerosus is a relatively common disease with a predilection for the anogenital skin. The terms leukoplakia, kraurosis vulvae, and balanitis xerotica used to describe genital atrophy and pallor in the past are now recognized as probable examples of lichen sclerosus. It is commoner in women with an estimated prevalence of between 1 in 300 and 1 in 1000 of the population.

Clinical Presentation

The peak times of presentation of lichen sclerosus are childhood and later life, particularly after menopause. In young boys, lichen sclerosus presents with phimosis and is probably the main reason why a medical circumcision is required around the age of 6 or 7 years. The lichen sclerosus often goes unrecognized, particularly if there is no histologic examination of the tissue removed at the time of surgery. Constipation is often the presenting symptom in young girls because lichen sclerosus around the rectal canal causes fissuring and painful defecation with consequent anal retention. Perianal involvement does not seem to occur in male patients. An intense itch is the primary symptom of anogenital lichen sclerosus with pain as a secondary symptom when there is ulceration and erosions.

The classic findings of early lichen sclerosus consist of pearly white papules and plaques. In the male these occur on the glans and prepuce of the penis and less commonly the shaft, whereas in the female the labia minora, clitoris, and interlabial sulci are the most frequent sites affected (Figs. 11-5 through 11-12). The lesions can become confluent and can spread out to involve the skin of the genitocrural folds and down to the perianal area in a figure-of-eight configuration. The epidermal atrophy when present gives the skin surface the texture of wrinkled cigarette paper and a shiny appearance. Ecchymosis when seen is pathognomonic for this disorder as the upper dermal vessels in the area of hyalinization are easily damaged. These ecchymoses can be mistaken for evidence of abuse in young girls. Additional signs include erosions, ulceration, and areas of hyperkeratosis.

The scarring that accompanies lichen sclerosus typically results in sealing of the clitoral hood concealing

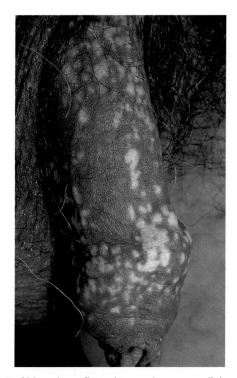

FIG. 11-5. Although at first glance, these very light papules mimic vitiligo, the crinkled texture change is pathognomonic for lichen sclerosus rather than vitiligo.

the glans clitoris underneath, shrinkage or loss of the labia minora, and more rarely some narrowing of the anterior and/or posterior aspects of the introitus (Fig. 11-13). Introital narrowing is unusual in women because lichen sclerosus appears to spare mucosal, non-

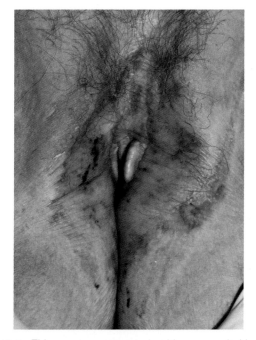

FIG. 11-6. This woman presented with severe itching, so scratching in the setting of the fragility typical of lichen sclerosus resulted in the classic finding of purpura.

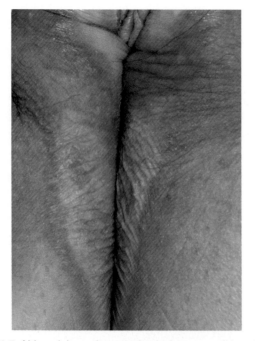

FIG. 11-7. Although hypopigmentation is the most striking abnormality in lichen sclerosus, the texture change is the key to diagnosis; the crinkled appearance seen here, and the distribution on the vulva and perianal skin are characteristic.

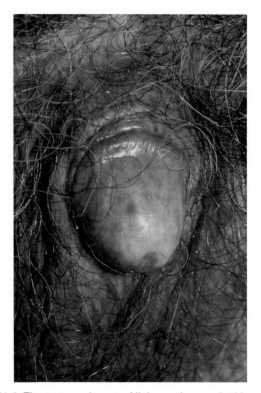

FIG. 11-9. The texture change of lichen sclerosus in this patient is manifested by shininess. The glans and inner prepuce are the most commonly affected areas.

cornified stratified epithelium. There can be involvement of the modified mucous membrane at junctional zones such as the vestibule, but the vagina is never involved. Perianal involvement appears to occur exclusively in female patients.

Since lichen sclerosus is more likely to affect uncircumcised men, the scarring leads to a gradual tightening of the prepuce and eventually phimosis (Fig. 11-14). The coronal sulcus can also become obliterated with adhesions (Fig. 11-15). Lichen sclerosus sometimes involves the

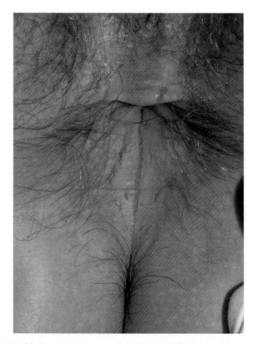

FIG. 11-8. Lichen sclerosus of perianal skin is very common in female patients, although it is not seen in male patients. Fissuring that produces pain with defecation contributes to constipation, a common presenting symptom in girls.

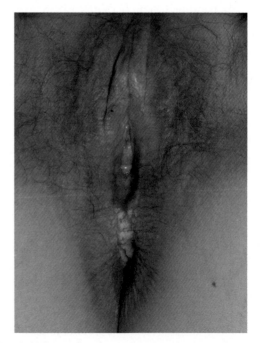

FIG. 11-10. Lichen sclerosus eventuates in resorption of architecture; the left labium minus has disappeared, and there is edema and midline scarring of the clitoral hood, an area of early and prominent involvement.

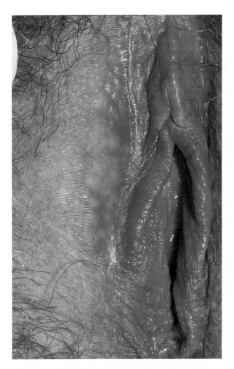

FIG. 11-11. Very early lichen sclerosus can be quite subtle, with mild hypopigmentation, poorly demarcated borders, and even a more waxy texture as pictured here in the anterior, interlabial fold.

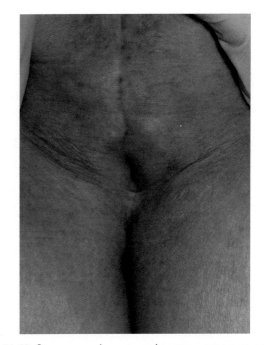

FIG. 11-13. Severe scarring occurs in some women as well as men; all vulvar architecture has been obliterated in this elderly woman with longstanding disease. Urinary obstruction occasionally occurs.

cornified epithelium surrounding the urethral meatus and lower part of the urethra (Fig. 11-16).

Extragenital lichen sclerosus in men is rare but occurs in up to a third of women. Extragenital sites occur on the upper back, axillae, volar aspects of the wrists, and in areas exposed to friction such as the shoulders and inframammary areas. The distribution of lesions in the friction zones can be partly explained by the Köebner phenomenon. Very rare instances of face, scalp nails, and mouth have all been reported. Oral lesions of lichen

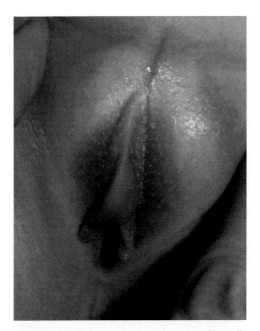

FIG. 11-12. Although lichen sclerosus is generally a disease of adults, its occurrence is well recognized in children, especially prepubertal girls, who are at risk of significant scarring of the vulva. Hypopigmentation, shiny texture, and purpura of the right labium minus are pathognomonic for lichen sclerosus. Edema of the clitoral hood is common as well.

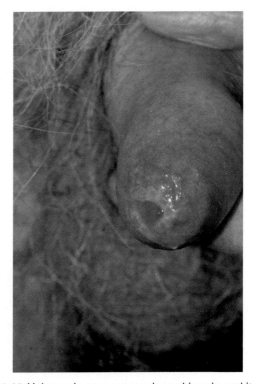

FIG. 11-14. Lichen sclerosus can produce phimosis, and it is the most common cause of phimosis in boys. (Courtesy of Errol Craig, MD.)

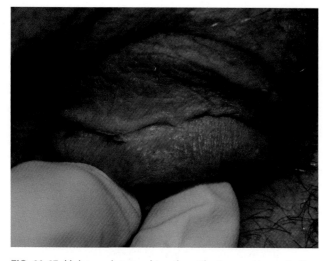

FIG. 11-15. Lichen sclerosus in male patients occurs most often on the glans, corona, and inner prepuce; scarring of the corona to the shaft has begun in this man.

sclerosus are extremely uncommon, and most of the lesions seen involve the frictional sites which can become cornified, on the buccal mucosae, dorsal aspect of the tongue, and attached gingivae (6).

There is an association with the other lymphocyte-mediated disorders such as lichen planus and morphoea and some patients can develop all three conditions. Vitiligo may also accompany lichen sclerosus.

There is a small risk, 4% or less, of neoplastic change and the development of a squamous cell carcinoma in long-standing untreated lichen sclerosus (Fig. 11-17). Verrucous carcinoma also has been associated with lichen sclerosus (Fig. 11-18).

Diagnosis

Although a diagnosis of lichen sclerosus can be made clinically in typical cases, histologic confirmation is ideal

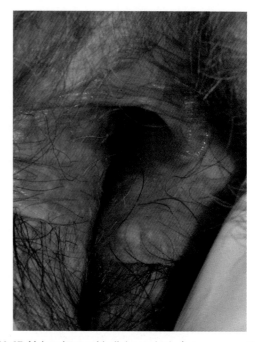

FIG. 11-17. Vulvar intraepithelial neoplasia (squamous cell carcinoma in situ) can present as red plaques within lichen sclerosus.

to differentiate lichen sclerosus from lichen planus and to detect if there is a thickened epidermis. However, the hyalinization of lichen sclerosus is lost if a potent topical steroid has been used. The skin that exhibits fine crinkling or ecchymosis is the ideal site for biopsy.

In uncomplicated lichen sclerosus, a biopsy shows an epidermis that is hyperkeratotic, thinned, and effaced. The epi-

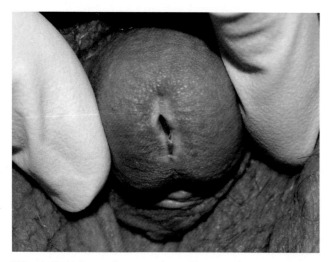

FIG. 11-16. Lichen sclerosus often affects urethral meatus and can cause strictures.

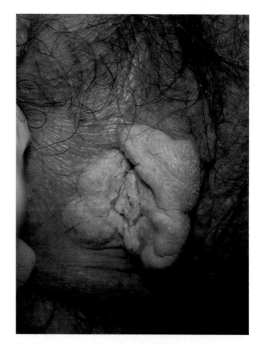

FIG. 11-18. This warty growth represents a verrucous carcinoma arising on a background of lichen sclerosus. Even clinically unimpressive thickened white areas of lichen sclerosus that do not promptly respond to therapy should be biopsied.

dermis overlies a band of hyalinization in the upper dermis with a mixed lymphocytic infiltrate immediately below it. In some areas, small foci of lichenoid change are found where the infiltrate abuts the dermoepidermal junction. Rarely, the epidermis exhibits the histologic features of squamous cell hyperplasia, that is, it is thickened (acanthotic). This is important as there seems to be an association with this kind of change and development of squamous cell carcinoma.

The pallor, atrophy, and loss of the normal anatomic features associated with well-established lichen sclerosus can be seen as a common end-stage picture of other inflammatory, scarring dermatoses, most notably lichen planus, cicatricial pemphigoid, and morphoea. Perianal itching with lichen simplex in children also raises the possibility of pinworm infestation.

LICHEN SCLEROSUS: **Diagnosis**

- White, crinkled, or shiny plaques
- Cornified epithelium of the vulva, perineal body, and perianal skin of women; primarily of the glans and prepuce of men
- Scarring often prominent
- Confirmed by biopsy that shows upper dermal chronic inflammatory infiltrate, hyalinization of the upper dermis, and disruption of basement membrane

---

Pathophysiology

It is a chronic lymphocyte-mediated inflammatory dermatosis with increasing evidence that it is an autoimmune-mediated disorder. There is a strong association with other autoimmune diseases particularly thyroid disease in women and circulating autoantibodies (7). The etiologic role of the infective agent *Borrelia burgdoferi* in extragenital disease is debated. However, it appears not to be implicated in genital lichen sclerosus (8).

Management

Treatment of choice in women and girls is an ultrapotent topical corticosteroid ointment (i.e., clobetasol propionate 0.05%) (Figs. 11-19A and B) (9,10). Randomized, controlled trials to support one ultrapotent steroid over another or for the length of time for the initial treatment are lacking. An ointment is preferred as it is well tolerated if there are painful fissures and erosions. Initially, this medication is applied once at night and then is gradually reduced in frequency as the symptoms and signs resolve. Generally, application can be reduced to as when required for long-term maintenance therapy after 3 or 4 months. Although superpotent corticosteroids have traditionally been avoided on genital skin, long-term studies have confirmed that these medications are safe (11). Thirty grams of the ointment should last 3 months for initial treatment and then 30 g can be used safely in 6 to 12 months for maintenance therapy. Patients should be reevaluated monthly for corticosteroid atrophy, improvement, and secondary infections while they are receiving daily therapy. Patients who fail to improve and who are using the treatment correctly should be reevaluated to ensure the correct primary diagnosis has been made or to detect the presence of an additional cutaneous diagnosis, for example, an irritant contact dermatitis (urinary incontinence), preneoplastic, or neoplastic change. Men with lichen

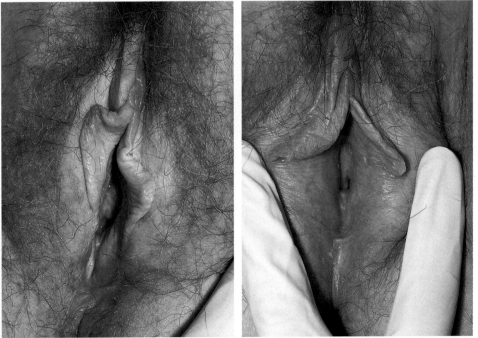

A   B

FIG. 11-19. **(A)** This patient with classic lichen sclerosus presented with severe itching and dyspareunia and was treated with clobetasol propionate 0.05% twice daily. **(B)** The same patient after 4 months of daily clobetasol showing a return to normal skin color and texture.

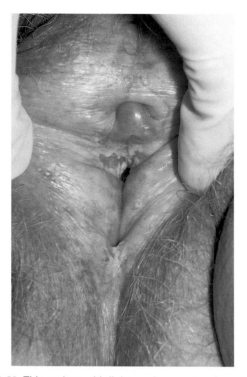

FIG. 11-20. This patient with lichen sclerosus has been treated unsuccessfully with testosterone, with resulting enlargement of the clitoris in a setting of progressive erosions, hyperkeratosis of the anterior fourchette, and agglutination of the labia minora.

sclerosus are nearly always uncircumcised and the use of a topical ultrapotent steroid may help but many will require circumcision (12). A soap substitute is useful and topical barriers should be added in if there is urinary or fecal incontinence.

Other medical treatments: Topical testosterone propionate is no longer used for the treatment of lichen sclerosus (Fig. 11-20). The topical calcineurin inhibitors tacrolimus and pimecrolimus have been used for lichen sclerosus that is resistant to topical corticosteroids or in cases where there have been steroid side effects (13–15), but these should be used with caution (16). Topical retinoids and vitamin D analogs are helpful particularly if there are areas of hyperkeratosis but their irritant effect limits their use. Phototherapy with UVA1 and photodynamic therapy have also been tried (17,18).

Surgery is indicated only if there is severe phimosis in men, or marked introital narrowing in women that interferes with sexual function, symptomatic clitoral pseudocyst, or in the development of squamous cell carcinoma or intraepithelial neoplasia.

The majority of lichen sclerosus cases experience an improvement or remission at puberty, but in some studies this has not always been the case (19). The symptoms often improve as estrogen produces more resilient epithelium, but ongoing scarring can occur in the absence of symptoms in untreated skin. Long-term follow-up two or three times a year is required if there is continuing active disease to monitor the skin for side effects from the topical corticosteroid or changes that might suggest neoplastic change. Lifelong monitoring of patients who have had a preneoplastic or neoplastic change is advised particularly as many are elderly and unlikely to notice suspicious change themselves.

LICHEN SCLEROSUS:	**Management**

- Correction of infection, local estrogen deficiency, irritant contact dermatitis, etc.
- Circumcision for men is usually curative, otherwise, as below for women
- Topical ultrapotent corticosteroid ointment (clobetasol propionate 0.05%, etc.)
  - once or twice a day until normal texture
  - then once three times a week ongoing, or midpotency corticosteroid (trimacinolone 0.1%, etc.) daily to maintain control
- Tacrolimus or pimecrolimus applied b.i.d. is second-line therapy
- Careful follow-up, monthly until disease is controlled, then twice yearly, to evaluate for side effects of medication, for control of disease, for changes of malignancy

Lichen Planus

Lichen planus is discussed primarily in Chapter 9, also in Chapters 6 and 15; only the white morphology is discussed here. Lichen planus is an inflammatory, autoimmune lymphocyte-mediated disease with variable morphology. Mucous membrane disease consists classically of either erosions or white, reticulate striae, although the white changes are sometimes those of more uniform white epithelium.

Clinical Presentation

The morphology of white lesions of lichen planus includes papules, lacy striae, annular lesions, plaques as well as hyperkeratotic papules and plaques (Figs. 11-21 through 11-28). Typical white, fine Wickham striae are seen so commonly in the mouth but are a less frequent finding on the anogenital skin. A confluent uniform, whitened epithelium that mimics lichen sclerosus can occur, although crinkling and ecchymosis are absent. Scarring is frequently absent or minimal, but in some cases it may be extensive.

The erosive form, discussed in Chapter 9, affects predominantly the mucosal surfaces and is often associated with adjacent white lesions. In the syndrome of Hewitt and Pelisse, also known as the vulvovaginal gingival syndrome, the affected areas are the gingivae, the vagina, and the vulvar vestibule (20) (Figs. 11-24 and 11-25). The areas involved have a characteristic glazed erythema or are frankly eroded

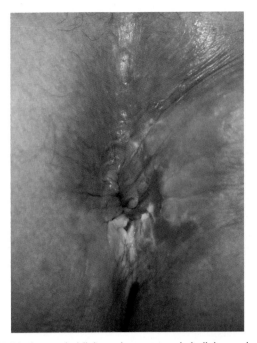

FIG. 11-21. Anogenital lichen planus can mimic lichen sclerosus; lichen planus should be considered in areas of white epithelium, especially when erosions are striking, or, in women, if accompanied by vaginal erosions. Usually, this white epithelium of lichen planus does not have the crinkled or shiny texture of lichen sclerosus.

and bordered by an edge of whitened hyperkeratotic epithelium. This edge is the best site for biopsy, as often the areas of glazed erythema, particularly in the vestibule, do not show the characteristic features of lichen planus and many are reported as a plasma cell mucositis (21).

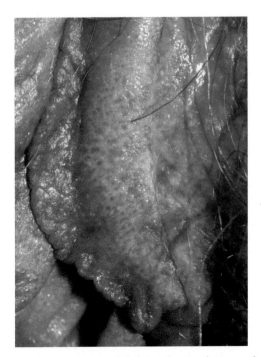

FIG. 11-22. Classic mucosal lichen planus shows reticulate white striae producing a fernlike or lacy pattern as seen here on the left lateral labium minus.

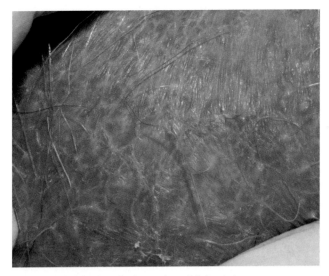

FIG. 11-23. White interlacing striae of lichen planus are seen on this man's scrotum.

Anogenital lichen planus may be asymptomatic, but patients usually complain of dyspareunia, pain, and itching.

Diagnosis

The diagnosis is usually confirmed by biopsy with substantiating evidence of typical oral lesions or lichen planus at extragenital sites. In the classic form of lichen planus, there is thinning and irregular acanthosis of the epidermis with a "saw-tooth" pattern of the rete ridges.

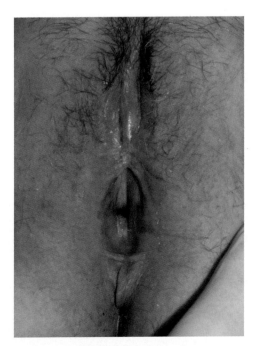

FIG. 11-24. This patient with erosive lichen planus presented with severe pain and dyspareunia. The vestibular location of her erosions is characteristic, but the surrounding white epithelium is suggestive of lichen sclerosus. Agglutination of the labia minora and clitoral hood are consistent with both diagnoses, and a biopsy of white epithelium is needed to definitively diagnose lichen planus.

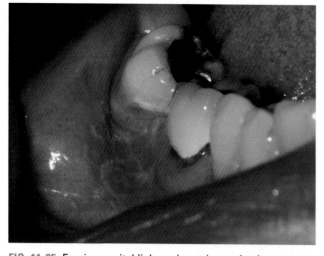

FIG. 11-25. Erosive genital lichen planus is nearly always associated with oral disease, seen here in its classic form. There are white striae on the mandibular gingiva.

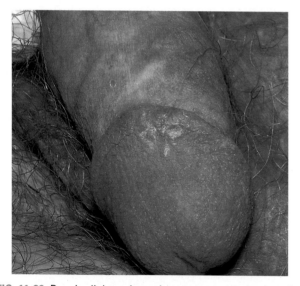

FIG. 11-26. Papular lichen planus is more common than erosive lichen planus in men, and a usual presentation is that of irregular white papules, most often on the glans.

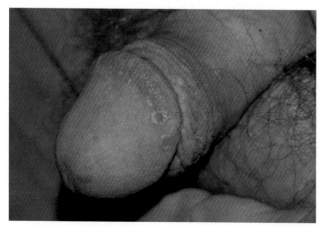

FIG. 11-27. Lichen planus on the glans is often annular. (Courtesy of Errol Craig, MD.)

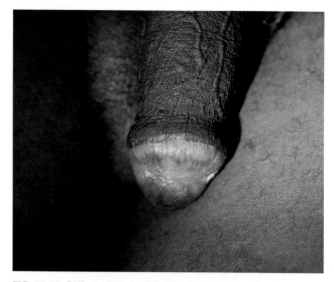

FIG. 11-28. Diffuse white epithelium is most often lichen sclerosus, but can occur with lichen planus as well. A biopsy to confirm lichen sclerosus of the glans in this man instead revealed lichen planus.

The granular layer is prominent, and there is a dense lymphocytic infiltrate along the dermoepidermal junction attacking the basal layer. The basement membrane zone becomes vacuolated with the formation of dyskeratotic cells known as colloid bodies found in the lower epidermis and occasionally upper dermis. There may also be a degree of pigmentary incontinence into the underlying dermis. The chronic hypertrophic forms and mucous membrane lesions often lack characteristic histologic features, thus making the diagnosis very difficult.

The typical fernlike, reticulate, white lesions of lichen planus are characteristic for this disease, but the white

LICHEN PLANUS (WHITE MORPHOLOGY):   **Diagnosis**

- Women: white, reticulate striae, or white epithelium surrounding erosions of the vulva and vestibule; vaginal erosions and inflammatory vaginal secretions common
- Men: white reticulate or annular striae, flat-topped white papules most common on glans. Less often, erosions with surrounding white epithelium
- Both women and men, oral lichen planus with white striae common, +/– buccal mucosal or gingival erosions
- Scarring often prominent
- Confirmed by biopsy that shows upper dermal chronic inflammatory infiltrate abutting and disrupting the basement membrane, dyskeratotic cells. Often, biopsy is interpreted as nonspecific "lichenoid dermatitis" so that diagnosis is made by clinical correlation

color sometimes raises the possibility of candidosis or the white papules seen on modified mucous membranes in Reiter disease. Lupus erythematosus is rare on the anogenital skins but the lesions are very similar to lichen planus. Immunofluorescent studies should help in the differentiation. When lichen planus presents as papules or plaques of uniform, white epithelium, a differentiation of lichen planus from lichen simplex, lichen sclerosus, macerated, psoriasis or eczema, Hailey–Hailey disease, fungal infection, and vitiligo must be made. In longstanding disease, particularly the hypertrophic form in which there is complete loss of the vulvar architecture, lichen planus is indistinguishable from end-stage lichen sclerosus, morphoea, or cicatricial pemphigoid.

Management

First-line treatment of lichen planus consists of topical corticosteroids, usually a superpotent medication such as clobetasol propionate 0.05%. On occasion, the addition of tetracycline in the formulation helps. Vaginal involvement requires the use of a steroid foam preparation or suppository. Although mucoerosive disease and hypertrophic lesions are often unresponsive to this therapy, epithelium whitened by lichen planus usually responds well to topical treatment. Topical tacrolimus can be used in steroid unresponsive cases (22) and is most effective in deeply fissured disease. It should be used for a limited time because of the unknown risk of the effect of this immunosuppressant medication. The other possible treatments include oral or topical cyclosporine, oral hydroxychloroquine, synthetic retinoids, azathioprine, and methotrexate. Those patients with resistant, destructive disease should ideally be seen and managed in specialized units run by multidisciplinary teams.

LICHEN PLANUS (WHITE MORPHOLOGY):	Management

- Correction of infection, local estrogen deficiency
- Men: circumcision if sufficiently severe, otherwise as for women
- Women: topical ultrapotent corticosteroid ointment (clobetasol propionate 0.05%, etc.) once or twice a day until normal texture, then decrease frequency as possible to maintain control
- Tacrolimus or pimecrolimus applied b.i.d. is second-line therapy; may be used with a corticosteroid for added benefit when required
- When required, systemic antimetabolites (methotrexate, azathioprine, etc.), immunosuppressives (mycophenylate mofetil, etanercept adalimumab, etc.), retinoids
- Careful follow-up, monthly at first to evaluate for side effects of medication, for control of disease, for changes of malignancy

Lichen Simplex Chronicus

Lichen simplex chronicus (histologically reported as squamous cell hyperplasia) was also termed neurodermatitis and refers to the lichenification seen on an area of skin secondary to scratching or rubbing when there is no identifiable underlying dermatosis. Lichen simplex chronicus is discussed primarily in Chapter 4, and only the white morphology is presented here.

Lichen simplex chronicus occurring on keratinized skin generally presents as red or hyperpigmented, lichenified plaques, often with excoriations. The anogenital skin is damp as it is an occluded site trapping moisture which in turn will whiten hyperkeratotic lichenified skin (Figs. 11-29 and 11-30). An obese patient is more prone to this white coloration of intertriginous lichen simplex chronicus than a leaner person.

The diagnosis can usually be made on the basis of lesional morphology, site, and asymmetry with a lack of genital scarring. Nevertheless, severe superimposed lichen simplex chronicus can obscure underlying lichen sclerosus and, less often, lichen planus. In these cases, a biopsy should be performed. The histologic picture is characterized by marked hyperkeratosis overlying a psoriasiform, hyperplastic epithelium with a prominent granular cell layer. The rete ridges are irregularly elongated, and there is a perivascular infiltrate of lymphocytes and eosinophils. There is lamellar fibrosis of the papillary dermis and, sometimes, perineural fibrosis. Spongiosis is present.

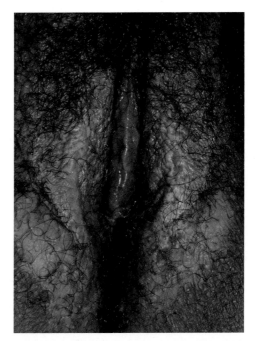

FIG. 11-29. Lichen simplex chronicus is characterized by very itchy skin that thickens as a result of rubbing and scratching. The thick skin is white because it is moist; the surrounding skin is hypopigmented due to postinflammatory hypopigmentation. These changes are especially common in patients who have naturally dark complexions, such as patients of African background.

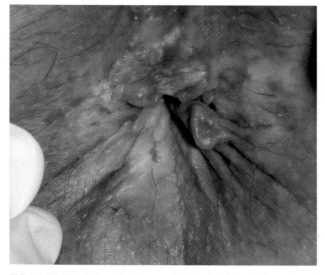

FIG. 11-30. The lichenification and excoriations of this perianal skin suggests lichen simplex chronicus, but lichen sclerosus and lichen planus can sometimes present similarly.

Hailey–Hailey disease (benign familial pemphigus), psoriasis, extramammary Paget disease, and the hypertrophic forms of lichen planus and lichen sclerosus can all resemble lichen simplex chronicus. A biopsy is indicated if there is poor response to therapy with a potent topical corticosteroid.

Therapy is discussed in detail in Chapter 4. The important aim of treatment is to break the itch–scratch cycle. A potent topical steroid (i.e., clobetasol propionate 0.05% applied once or twice daily) is the first-line treatment. However, care must be taken to avoid the risk of local adverse reactions. A lower-potency topical corticosteroid can be substituted as the patient improves. The identification and elimination of infection are essential, and a sedating antihistamine administered orally at night minimizes nighttime scratching. Topical doxepin, which is an antihistamine cream, can be used in resistant cases.

Candidosis

Although the primary lesions of candidosis are red plaques and erosions, mucous membrane candidosis, especially when severe, can exhibit white epithelium or a surface covered in a white adherent exudate which can be removed by scraping the area (Figs. 11-31 and 11-32). *Candida* infection is more completely discussed in Chapters 6 and 15. The causative organism of candidosis characterized by white lesions is usually *Candida albicans* or, less often, *C. tropicalis*. Although other strains such as *C. (Torulopsis) glabrata* and *C. parapsilosis* can also cause vulvovaginal symptoms, these forms of *Candida* generally produce only irritation of the mucous membrane skin of the vagina and introitus, rather than white lesions of keratinized, exterior skin.

The white lesions of vulvar or penile candidosis are seen most often in patients who are obese, diabetic, or

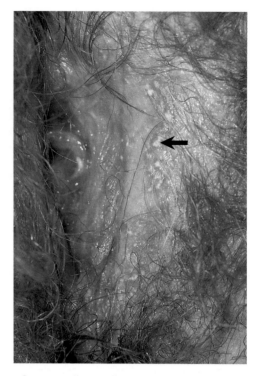

FIG. 11-31. Occasionally, candidiasis can appear white *(arrow)*, either because of white, clumped "cottage cheese" discharge or, as is seen here, because of superficial pustules and white epithelium of ruptured blister roofs.

immunosuppressed. Other patients exhibit coalescing white papules that represent fragile pustules with macerated blister roofs (Figs. 11-31 and 11-32).

Most candidal vulvitis is found in conjunction with vaginal candidosis and the term vulvovaginitis would be a more accurate description of the problem. However, more commonly, the *Candida* is a superimposed problem on eczema or psoriasis when there is bowel carriage of *Candida*. This overgrowth of the *Candida* on a background dermatitis exacerbates the underlying dermatosis, so both conditions should be treated simultaneously.

Men without evidence of impaired immunity can acquire genital candidosis through contact with affected sexual partners or, from *Candida* colonizing the bowel, especially when there is an underlying dermatosis, obesity, or incontinence. The favored sites are the inner surface of the prepuce or the glans penis. Although the patches are usually erythematous and eroded, the initial lesion can be pustular or can exhibit white, macerated epithelium similar to that seen in some women. The diagnosis is generally made by the identification of candidal pseudohyphae and hyphae on direct microscopy or by a swap culture on Sabouraud agar.

Diagnosis

The diagnosis is made by the appearance and confirmed by a microscopic fungal examination of secretions or skin, or a culture.

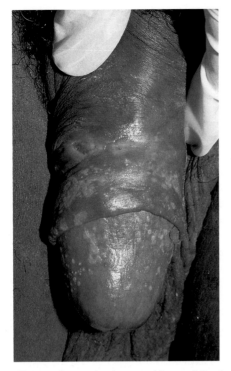

FIG. 11-32. This uncircumcised man with candidiasis also exhibits white papules.

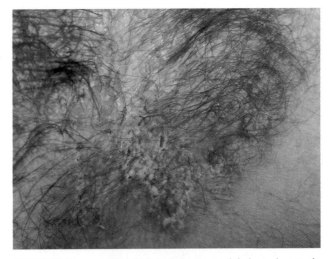

FIG. 11-33. Any superficial blistering can result in hyperkeratosis and maceration that appears white when moist, as seen in this patient with Hailey–Hailey disease (benign familial pemphigus).

Many dermatoses can be mistaken for candidal vulvitis and include eczema, psoriasis, Hailey–Hailey (benign familial pemphigus) (Fig. 11-33). The soft, hydrated epithelium of blisters and hyperkeratotic skin affected by pemphigus vegetans can resemble *Candida* infection. Reiter disease (and the closely related pustular psoriasis) is characterized by white circinate papules that can be difficult to distinguish from cutaneous candidosis (Fig. 11-34). Occasionally, white erosions of herpes simplex virus infection are nearly indistinguishable from candidosis.

CANDIDOSIS:	Diagnosis

- Red patches with white exudate, or papules of white, macerated epithelium on mucous membrane or modified mucous membranes of the vulva, glans penis, prepuce, or skin folds
- Fungal preparation or culture showing yeast
- Biopsy not required

Management

Topical therapy with azoles or nystatin vaginal suppositories and creams is often all that is required for uncomplicated cases of candidosis, but if there is a background dermatitis this must also be treated. One dose of oral fluconazole, 150 mg, is as effective for vulvovaginal candidosis as topical therapies and lacks the irritating effects of the preservatives that topical creams have on inflamed skin.

CANDIDOSIS:	Management

- Control of any underlying process (antibiotics, immunosuppression, incontinence)
- Oral fluconazole, or any topical azole, nystatin

Human Papillomavirus Infection

Genital warts and intraepithelial neoplasia generally present as skin-colored or hyperpigmented tumors, but many are often white (see Chapter 12 for primary discussion, as well as Chapter 13 for additional morphologies). The hyperkeratotic epithelia of warts, intraepithelial neoplasia, and squamous cell carcinomas can become white with the hydration that occurs due to the dampness in this occluded site. The application of 5% acetic acid (white vinegar) accentuates this whitening or produces whiteness in skin-colored lesions. Acetowhitening is not diagnostic of viral warts or neoplasia but is useful to accentuate subtle abnormalities to highlight the most suitable site for biopsy.

Genital Warts

Anogenital warts (condylomata acuminata) are benign epidermal tumors produced by any of several human papillomavirus (HPV) types. HPV types 6 and 11 are responsible for most anogenital warts and are recognized as *low-risk* viruses as malignant transformation is rare. HPV types 16, 18, 31, and 33 are *high risk* and are involved in the genesis of intraepithelial neoplasia and squamous cell

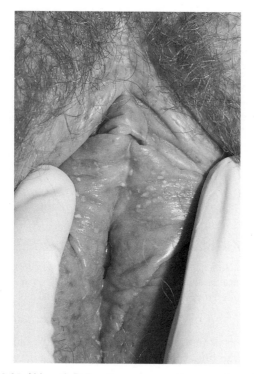

FIG. 11-34. Although Reiter disease normally occurs in male patients, these white solid and annular papules on the modified mucous membranes of a vulva with Reiter disease are similar to those seen on the glans penis.

carcinoma. Anogenital HPV infection is a sexually transmitted disease and usually presents as skin-colored or white papules and nodules (Fig. 11-35). Therapies include physical destruction by liquid nitrogen, electrocautery, and laser; chemical destruction by trichloroacetic acid and podofilox; promoting the local skin immunity with immune response–modulating creams such as imiquimod.

The new vaccines now available will hopefully provide immunity against these viruses in the future (23).

Intraepithelial Neoplasia

Intraepithelial neoplasia is still referred to as Bowen disease and Bowenoid papulosis when arising on the male genitalia and perianal skin, but these names have been changed for the female genitalia. The term vulval intraepithelial neoplasia (VIN) has been introduced to replace these clinical terms. Currently, there are two types of VIN. *Usual undifferentiated type* which is two thirds to full-thickness atypia and associated with HPV infection usually 16, 18, 31, and 33 and *differentiated type* which is atypia confined to the lower third of the epithelium with normal epithelial differentiation above. There is no strong link with HPV in this type. Both these types of VIN can be associated with white lesions. This entity is also discussed in Chapters 6, 12, and 13.

Usual, undifferentiated VIN may present as well-demarcated white, red, or skin-colored flat-topped papules and plaques. Any area of the anogenital skin can be affected by these HPV-induced lesions (Figs. 11-36 and 11-37). Undifferentiated VIN may also be seen in association with typical viral warts. Lesions of intraepithelial neoplasia may be enhanced with 5% acetic acid and can be a useful technique to locate or highlight subtle lesions. Female patients need to have cervical and vaginal screening for warts or intraepithelial neoplasia as up to two thirds of patients have cervical involvement at some stage. If there are perianal lesions, then the anal canal should also be screened.

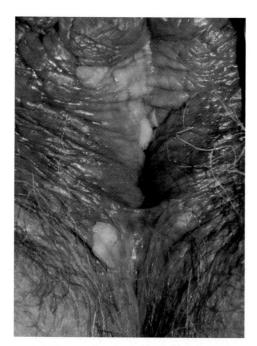

FIG. 11-35. Genital warts have overlying hyperkeratosis, so they appear white when hydrated because of their moist location.

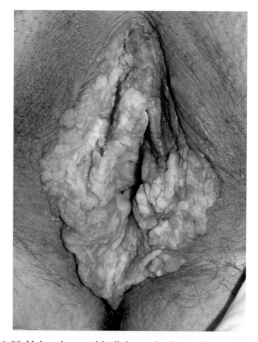

FIG. 11-36. Vulvar intraepithelial neoplasia can be erosive or hyperkeratotic. When hydrated, the hyperkeratotic form is manifested by hypopigmentation.

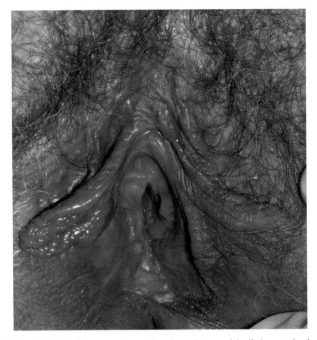

FIG. 11-37. Subtle papules of vulvar intraepithelial neoplasia over fourchette.

The diagnosis of intraepithelial neoplasia is made by the morphologic appearance with confirmation on biopsy, which shows full-thickness dysplasia. The differential diagnosis for lesions of white intraepithelial neoplasia includes lichen planus, lichen sclerosus, and basal cell carcinoma.

Management includes an evaluation of other sites prone to involvement including the cervix, vagina, and rectal canal. The treatment of intraepithelial neoplasia depends on the site and the extent of involvement. Unifocal disease undifferentiated and differentiated VIN is usually amenable to surgery and this is still the first-line treatment. Multifocal undifferentiated disease is more of a challenge but some surgical excision is still the first-line management, providing this will not be physically mutilating. If very widespread, then a combination of surgery and other medical treatment is employed. The main medical management is the use of the immune-modulating cream imiquimod (Aldara). In the past, 5-flurouracil was used more extensively but is now reserved for those cases where imiquimod is unsuccessful or not tolerated.

Cryotherapy, carbon dioxide laser, local interferon-α, and photodynamic therapy with levulinic acid have all been tried with limited success and a high rate of recurrence. The successful treatment of intraepithelial neoplasia is easier in men than in women. The affected skin of men is most often non–hair bearing, whereas in women the areas affected have deep adnexal structures and therefore superficial therapies may not be effective and recurrence is common.

White Sponge Nevus

The white sponge nevus is an uncommon but characteristic condition that occurs on mucous membranes/ modified mucous membranes.

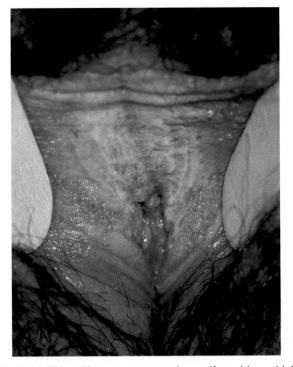

FIG. 11-38. This white sponge nevus is manifested by a thickened white plaque on the anterior modified mucous membranes of the vulva.

Clinical Manifestation

Vulvar involvement alone is extremely rare, and white sponge nevus of the vulva is usually seen in association with extragenital lesions sited in the oral cavity, esophagus, nasal mucosa, and perianal skin. The lesions are characteristically plaques of white hyperkeratotic epithelium (Fig. 11-38).

Diagnosis

The diagnosis is made from the clinical findings and pathologic examination. The biopsy shows an epidermis that is thickened, and there is a thick parakeratotic layer. Except for basal cells, many of the epithelial cells are large and clear, and many lack a nucleus or exhibit a very small nucleus.

All the white lesions described in this chapter can sometimes resemble a white sponge nevus. Warts, intraepithelial neoplasia, and hyperkeratotic lesions of lichen sclerosus or lichen planus are especially likely to be mistaken for a white sponge nevus, although the multimucosal nature of this disease eliminates warts and lichen sclerosus as serious possibilities.

WHITE SPONGE NEVUS:	**Diagnosis**

- White hyperkeratotic epithelium of vulva in association with similar lesions of oral cavity, esophagus, nasal mucosa, and/or perianal skin
- Confirmed on biopsy; epidermal thickening, with a thick parakeratotic layer, and epithelial cells that are large and clear, with no or a very small nucleus

Pathophysiology

White sponge nevus is an autosomal dominant condition with no evidence to date of HPV infection.

Management

There is no recognized treatment for the genital lesions, but tetracycline mouthwash results in improvement of oral lesions.

WHITE SPONGE NEVUS:	Management
• None	

WHITE PAPULES AND NODULES

Epidermal (Epidermoid, Epidermal Inclusion) Cysts and Milia

Epidermal cysts are common benign papules and nodules that occur when hair follicle structures become obstructed, and the deep portion of the follicle is gradually expanded by desquamated cells shed from the follicular epithelium (see also Chapters 7, 8, and 12). They can arise at any age, but they are seen most frequently in midlife and appear most often on the labia majora, labia minora, penile shaft, scrotum, and perianal area. They do not occur in the vestibule. The cysts appear as dome-shaped, white, yellow, or skin papules or nodules, often with a central plug (Fig. 11-39). They are usually asymptomatic but can become inflamed and tender. Very small 1- to 2-mm

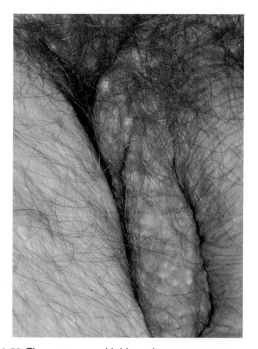

FIG. 11-39. The scrotum and labia majora are common areas for epidermoid cysts, formed by occluded follicles filled with white keratin debris of desquamated follicular epithelium.

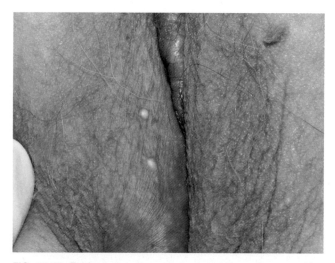

FIG. 11-40. Epidermal cysts appear as white, yellow, or skin-colored dermal nodules.

papules are referred to as milia (Fig. 11-40). Longstanding lesions can become calcified.

The diagnosis is made clinically, and it is easily confirmed if cheesy material is expressed. Histologic features are a cyst wall composed of stratified squamous epithelium surrounding a cavity that contains lamellar birefringent keratin and hair.

White nodules that can mimic epidermal cysts include enlarged sebaceous glands, steatocystomata, vellus hair cysts, and lesions of molluscum contagiosum. Vestibular cysts should be considered, but these are usually bluish, skin colored, or more yellow, and they are located in the vulvar vestibule.

Therapy generally is not needed for most cases but larger lesions that are troublesome can be excised and smaller cysts and milia can be extirpated, cauterized, or hyfrecated.

Molluscum Contagiosum

Mollusca contagiosa are skin lesions produced by a poxvirus and are usually sexually transmitted when they occur on the genitalia of adults. These can be skin-colored, pink, or white dome-shaped papules. Classically, at least some lesions have a central dell or depression. These are found on keratinized skin and, in immunocompetent people, are self-limited and self-resolving. These lesions involute spontaneously after any trauma, which includes extirpating with a sharpened orange stick, curettage, light cryotherapy, hyfrecation, and cantharidin. The topical immune-modulating cream imiquimod (Aldara) is also effective in the treatment of extensive lesions, particularly in children who will not tolerate the other methods.

Verrucous Carcinoma

Clinical Presentation

This unusual tumor occurs in older patients, often in their eighth or ninth decade, but there are anecdotal cases described in younger patients. The lesion appears as a slowly growing warty or papillomatous nodule, most commonly sited on the labia majora (Fig. 8-15), glans penis, and perianal skin. Verrucous carcinomas have also been described in the vagina, and on the cervix, penis, scrotum, rectum, and bladder, as well as in extragenital sites (i.e., the nasopharynx and esophagus).

Diagnosis

The diagnosis of verrucous carcinoma is often difficult in light of the rather banal histology, particularly in differentiating the lesion from a giant condyloma acuminatum. The histopathologic changes are undramatic and include marked hyperkeratosis and acanthosis with deeply penetrating, rounded, burgeoning rete ridges. The basal layer is intact and is clearly defined, and there is a striking lack of cellular atypia throughout the epithelium. A nonspecific inflammatory infiltrate is located around and beneath the tumor. A prominent granular layer with clear koilocytic cells is a frequent finding.

On occasion, a clear distinction is impossible, and a diagnosis rests on the natural history, age of the patient, and pattern of the clinical behavior; the verrucous carcinoma is generally more aggressive, with frequent recurrence after excision.

Other than a large wart, as discussed earlier, the main disease to be differentiated from verrucous carcinoma is typical squamous cell carcinoma. Histologic analysis should differentiate the two diseases.

VERRUCOUS CARCINOMA: **Diagnosis**

- Warty or papillomatous nodule
- Most often on the labia majora, glans penis, or perianal skin
- Biopsy required, but often banal and nonspecific, requiring a high index of suspicion and empiric diagnosis and therapy

---

Pathophysiology

Verrucous carcinoma is now considered to be a variant of well-differentiated squamous cell carcinoma. Despite its deceptively benign histologic appearance, the tumor growth is destructive and invasive locally. In some cases, there has been evidence of HPV infection, a history of genital warts, and sometimes a background of lichen sclerosus.

Management

Surgical excision is the treatment of choice and lymphadenectomy is rarely indicated because metastases to lymph nodes are very uncommon. Radiotherapy is not used because many tumors are not radiosensitive. An oral retinoid has been used successfully in one case (24).

VERRUCOUS CARCINOMA: **Management**

- Surgical excision

REFERENCES

1. Falabella R, Barona MI. Update on skin repigmentation therapies in vitiligo. *Pigment Cell Melanoma Res.* 2008;22:42–45.
2. James O, Mayes RW, Stevenson CJ. Occupational vitiligo induced by *p*-tert-butylphenol, a systemic disease? *Lancet.* 1977;310:1217–1219.
3. Serrao VV, Paris FR, Feio AB. Genital vitiligo-like depigmentation following use of imiquimod 5% cream. *Eur J Dermatol.* 2008;18:342–343.
4. Gawkrodger DJ. Guideline for the diagnosis and management of vitiligo. *Br J Dermatol.* 2008;159:1051–1076.
5. Ameen M, Exarchou V, Chu AC. Topical calcipotriol as monotherapy and in combination with psoralen plus ultraviolet A in the treatment of vitiligo. *Br J Dermatol.* 2001;14:476–479.
6. Chaudhry SI, Morgan PR, Neill SM. An unusual tongue. *Clin Exp Dermatol.* 2006;31:831–832.
7. Chan I, Oyama N, Neill SM, et al. Characterization of IgG autoantibodies to extracellular matrix protein 1 in lichen sclerosus. *Clin Exp Dermatol.* 2004;29:499–504.
8. Edmonds E, Mavin S, Francis N, et al. *Borrelia burgdorferi* is not associated with genital lichen sclerosus in men. *Br J Dermatol.* 2009;160:459–460.
9. Neill SM, Tatnall FM, Cox NH. Guidelines for the management of lichen sclerosus. *Br J Dermatol.* 2002;147:640–649.
10. Smith YR, Haefner HK. Vulvar lichen sclerosus: pathophysiology and treatment. *Am J Clin Dermatol.* 2004;5:105–125.
11. Dalziel KL, Wojnarowska F. Long-term control of vulval lichen sclerosus after treatment with a potent topical steroid cream. *J Reprod Med.* 1993;38:25–27.
12. Dahlman-Ghozlan K, Hedblad MA, von Krogh G. Penile lichen sclerosus et atrophicus treated with clobetasol dipropionate 0.05% cream: a retrospective clinical and histopathological study. *J Am Acad Dermatol.* 1999;40:451–457.
13. Oskay T, Sezer HK, Genc C, et al. Pimecrolimus 1% cream in the treatment of vulvar lichen sclerosus in postmenopausal women. *Int J Dermatol.* 2007;46:527–532.
14. Virgili A, Lauriola MM, Mantovani L, et al. Vulvar lichen sclerosus: 11 women treated with tacrolimus 0.1% ointment. *Acta Derm Venereol.* 2007;87:69–72.
15. Gupta S, Saraswat A, Kumar B. Treatment of genital lichen sclerosus with topical calcipotriol. *Int J STD AIDS.* 2005;16:772–774.
16. Fischer G, Bradford J. Topical immunosuppressants, genital lichen sclerosus and the risk of squamous cell carcinoma: a case report. *J Reprod Med.* 2007;52:329–331.
17. Beattie PE, Dawe RS, Ferguson J, et al. UVA1 phototherapy for genital lichen sclerosus. *Clin Exp Dermatol.* 2006;31:343–347.
18. Reichrath J, Reinhold U, Tilgen W. Treatment of genito-anal lesions in inflammatory skin diseases with PUVA cream photochemotherapy: an open pilot study in 12 patients. *Dermatology.* 2002;205:245–248.
19. Powell J, Wojnarowska F. Childhood vulvar lichen sclerosus: the course after puberty. *J Reprod Med.* 2002;47:706–709.

20. Setterfield JF, Neill SM, Shirlaw P, et al. The vulvo-vaginal ginigival syndrome: a severe subgroup of lichen planus with characteristic clinical features and a novel association with the class II HLADQB1*0201 allele. *J Am Acad Dermatol.* 2006;55: 98–113.

21. Scurry J, Dennerstein G, Brenan J, et al. Vulvitis circumscripta plasmacellularis. A clinicopathological entity? *J Reprod Med.* 1993;38:14–18.

22. Byrd JA, Davis M, Rogers RS. Recalcitrant symptomatic vulvar lichen planus. Response to topical tacrolimus. *Arch Dermatol.* 2004;140:715–772.

23. Garland SM, Hernandez-Avila M, Wheeler CM, et al. Quadrivalent vaccine against human papillomavirus to prevent anogenital diseases. *N Engl J Med.* 2007;356:1928–1943.

24. Mehta RK, Rytina E, Sterling JC. Treatment of verrucous carcinoma of vulva with acetretin. *Br J Dermatol.* 2000;142:1195–1198.

CHAPTER 12

Skin-Colored Lesions

PETER J. LYNCH

"Skin colored" refers to those lesions whose color is of the same hue as the patient's surrounding normal skin. Thus, in a darkly pigmented person, skin-colored lesions would be brown. Likewise, skin-colored lesions on a pink or red mucosal surface will also be pink or red. Although most skin-colored lesions match the adjacent normal skin color exactly, some may demonstrate a slight pink or tan hue. Skin-colored lesions may be benign or malignant.

GENITAL WARTS

Genital warts are caused by infection with human papillomavirus (HPV). They are common benign neoplasms that are significant because of their transmissibility, the association of some HPV types with the development of malignancy, and our current inability to eradicate latent HPV from infected tissue. In contrast with herpes simplex virus (HSV) where there are two viral types, HSV 1 and HSV 2, there are over 100 HPV types. These are usually divided on the basis of their oncogenic potential into low-risk and high-risk groups. Anogenital infection may occur with viruses from either of these groups.

Clinical Presentation

The data presented in a recent review regarding HPV prevalence and incidence indicate that anogenital infection due to HPV is extremely common. About 20% of women in their late teens and early twenties have polymerase chain reaction (PCR) evidence of HPV DNA infection (1). This rate decreases with age, declining to about 5% in older women. Not surprisingly, the rates are even higher in special groups such as prisoners and patients who attend an sexually transmitted disease (STD) clinic. The few studies carried out in men show great variability but the average prevalence appears similar to that in women.

HPV infection is quite transmissible and the major risk factor for acquisition of the virus relates to sexual activity. Specifically, the risk of infection correlates best with number of past sexual partners and the acquisition of a recent, new sexual partner. Most HPV transmission occurs by way of vaginal and anal intercourse but other forms of sexual activity also result in high transmission rates. In contrast, among children with anogenital warts, most transmission occurs through nonsexual contact (2). Incidence figures parallel prevalence data, and it is estimated that over a lifetime, 75% of all men and women will have contracted HPV infection. This observation suggests that HPV infection is the most common of all sexually transmitted infections. Condom use and male circumcision appear to decrease the risk of transmission (3).

Most anogenital HPV infections occur at a subclinical level and only a small percentage of those infected will develop the clinical lesions in the form of genital warts. The prevalence of genital warts in Western countries varies but the rate lies between 0.1% and 1% (4,5).

There are four major morphologic variants of genital warts. Those found in persistently moist areas tend to be skin colored, filliform (e.g., tall and narrow) with or without a brush-like tip (Fig. 12-1). This variant is appropriately termed "condylomata accuminata" and, strictly speaking, is the only variant for which this term should be used. The second variant occurring in the anogenital area is verruca vulgaris (common warts) (Fig. 12-2). These are skin colored and similar in appearance to hand warts. They are about as wide (5 to 10 mm) as they are tall and typically have palpable, if not visible, surface roughness due to the presence of scale. They are located on the drier aspects of the anogenital tissue. Smooth-surfaced, flat-topped papules (wider than they are tall) represent the third variant (Fig. 12-3). These are usually 3 to 15 mm in diameter and are wider than they are tall. They can occur on either moist or dry surfaces. While often skin colored, these flat-topped warts may also be pink, red, brown, or black. Large globular warts, 2 to 4 cm in diameter, correspond to the fourth variant (Fig. 12-4). They have a smooth, but often cauliflower-like surface and are skin colored, pink, or red in hue. This type of lesion is often termed a giant condyloma or Buschke–Lowenstein tumor.

Genital warts occur most often in individuals between the ages of 16 and 25 years. Although genital warts are usually asymptomatic, they occasionally produce itching and irritation. The number and size of lesions in an infected individual presumably depend on the immunologic resistance that the host can mount against the infecting virus. Thus, some individuals with very good immune response may have only a few small lesions that

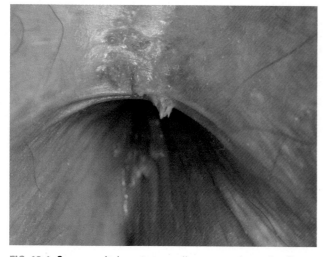

FIG. 12-1. Some genital warts are spiky, or acuminate, leading to the term condylomata accuminata. There are small lobular warts just above these pointed lesions.

respond readily to treatment, whereas other patients exhibit numerous small and large lesions that are very resistant to almost all attempts at therapy.

In men, most genital lesions involve the shaft of the penis and, less frequently, the glans, foreskin, scrotum, groin, and periurethral or intraurethral area. Perianal warts occur more commonly in homosexual men but also can develop in heterosexual men. In women, genital warts occur most commonly around the vaginal introitus, the

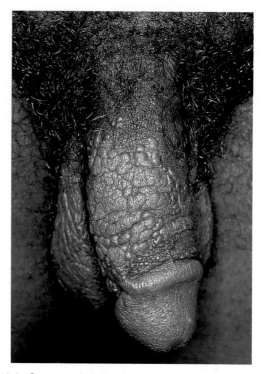

FIG. 12-3. Some genital warts are flat; this morphologic type should be examined by biopsy to rule out intraepithelial neoplasia.

vulvar vestibule, and surrounding anogenital skin. Fifty percent of women with vulvar warts have evidence of cervical HPV infection. Women may develop perianal warts and, not surprisingly, their presence at this site is especially likely in those who practice receptive anal intercourse.

Diagnosis

A diagnosis of anogenital warts is generally made on a clinical basis. However, biopsy is required for two types of warts, flat-topped, smooth-surface lesions and giant condylomata. This is so because in situ or invasive

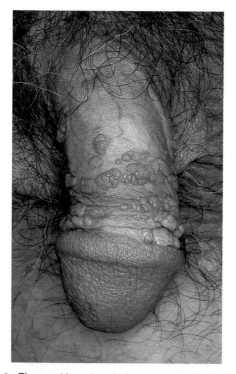

FIG. 12-2. These skin-colored, brown and slightly hypopigmented, lobular papules on the penis are a very common morphology of genital warts.

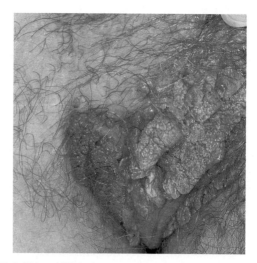

FIG. 12-4. This multilobular, verrucous genital wart is unusually large and raises the possibility of verrucous carcinoma.

squamous cell carcinoma may be present histologically in these types of otherwise normal-appearing warts. Some clinicians apply 5% acetic acid (common vinegar) to the anogenital area for several minutes prior to visual examination. Whitening occurs where warts are present but unfortunately neither the specificity nor sensitivity of this procedure is high enough for this technique to be recommended. Gynecologists sometimes examine the anogenital area with high magnification using a culposcope. I believe this has little usefulness and greatly increases the duration and cost of the examination. Cytologic preparations, similar to those used for cervical smears, are helpful in the diagnosis of suspected anal HPV infection and are highly recommended in the anal examination of immunosupressed patients. This is especially true for men who have sex with men (MSM) and are human immunodeficiency virus (HIV) positive.

Biopsy can confirm a clinical diagnosis of genital warts. The histologic hallmarks include variable acanthosis often with some elongation of the rete ridges. The presence of koilocytosis (vacuolated cells with dark pyknotic nuclei) is particularly helpful. True koilocytosis occurs throughout most of the epidermis. Pathologists who are not expert in cutaneous pathology often overcall this feature, failing to recognize that scattered vacuolated cells (usually without nuclear change) are normally present in anogenital tissue.

Tests for determining the HPV type are commercially available. However, this adds significant cost and rarely changes either the treatment or the follow-up of the patient. This testing is not currently recommended by the Centers for Disease Control (CDC). Viral cultures cannot be carried out as HPV does not grow in artificial media.

Many conditions must be considered in the list of differential diagnoses for genital warts. In women, vestibular papillomatosis can easily be confused. Patients with this condition have closely set, minute, hemispherical papules, arranged in a cobblestone-like pattern, within the vulvar vestibule (Fig. 12-5). This is a normal physiologic variant that needs no therapy. The equivalent variant in men consists of one or two rows of pearly penile papules encircling the corona of the glans penis (Figs. 12-6 to 12-8). Other conditions to be considered include molluscum contagiosum, common skin tags, lymphangiectasia, and enlarged sebaceous glands (Fordyce spots) (Figs. 12-9 and 12-10). As indicated above, both in situ and invasive squamous cell carcinoma may have an identical appearance as flat-topped or large globular warts (Fig. 12-11).

Pathophysiology

Genital warts are caused by the alpha group of HPV. This group contains about 60 HPV types and all of these can infect both mucous membranes and keratinizing epithelium. This group can be subdivided on the basis of

GENITAL WARTS:	Diagnosis

- Sexually active individuals 15 to 30 years of age
- Four clinical variants: filliform warts, verruca vulgaris, flat-topped papules/plaques, and large globular nodules
- Lesions may be pink, red, brown, black, or skin colored
- Biopsy to confirm diagnosis and to rule out malignancy
- Look for cervical involvement in women and anal involvement in MSM

their oncogenic potential into approximately 20 high-risk and 40 low-risk types. About 90% of genital warts are due to four HPV types. The vast majority of infections are caused by low-risk types HPV 6 and 11 and the remainder are mostly due to high-risk types 16 and 18. It is not possible clinically to determine which of these HPV types represents the cause of genital warts. Coinfection with multiple HPV types is quite common.

Information on the duration of HPV infection in untreated women is restricted almost entirely to data regarding cervical infection in immunocompetent women (6). These data indicate that for cervical infection, 50% to 90% of women will clear their infection spontaneously within 1 year. Clearance appears to take place more quickly with low-risk HPV infection than that it does with high-risk HPV infection. Men with asymptomatic HPV infection have similar or even more rapid clearance rates (1).

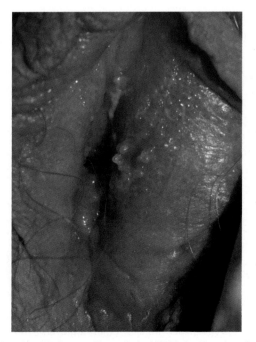

FIG. 12-5. Vestibular papillae mimic HPV infection, but the tips are rounded, and individual papillae are discrete to the base.

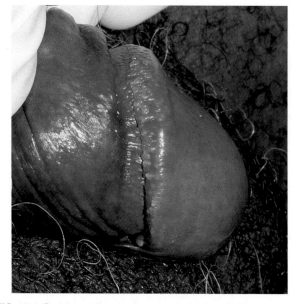

FIG. 12-6. Pearly penile papules are most common in uncircumcised patients and consist of monomorphous papules around the corona.

Data regarding the clearance of asymptomatic genital HPV infection are not available due to the lack of simple inexpensive tools for screening patients with latent disease. Likewise, the natural history of genital warts is not well established due to the almost universal treatment of clinically expressed infection. By analogy with warts in other sites, it is likely that most anogenital warts will resolve with the passage of time and there is some evidence to suggest that half of the anogenital warts occurring in children will resolve spontaneously (7).

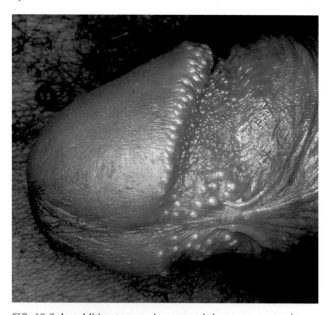

FIG. 12-7. In addition to papules around the corona, pearly penile papules sometimes are seen on the shaft, particularly near the frenulum.

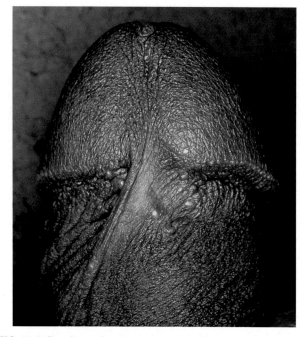

FIG. 12-8. Pearly penile papules can be differentiated from genital warts by their location and uniform size.

Spontaneous resolution occurs when an HPV-specific immune response develops. Antibodies to HPV gradually appear and can be measured. Cell-mediated immune (CMI) response, as judged by the presence of lymphocytes in biopsies of warts that subsequently resolve, also occurs. CMI response is more important than humoral response. This is based on two observations. First, the

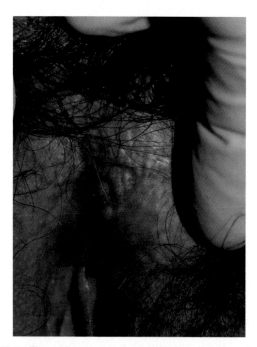

FIG. 12-9. The skin-colored but yellowish, lobular, discrete papules on the modified mucous membranes of the vulva are normal Fordyce spots (enlarged sebaceous glands).

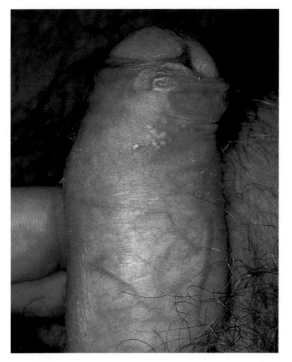

FIG. 12-10. Fordyce spots are also normal findings on the shaft of the penis.

titer and timing of antibody response do not correlate very well with resolution of warts, and second, many patients with visible lesions are not seropositive and many patients who are seropositive do not currently have clinically detectable infection (1).

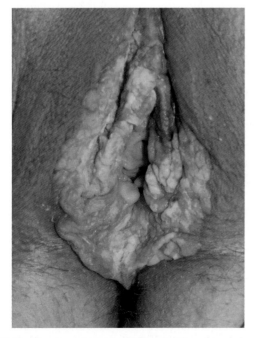

FIG. 12-11. These exuberant confluent skin-colored, hypopigmented, and brown warts showed VIN 3 (squamous cell carcinoma in situ) on biopsy.

Management

As noted above, genital warts may resolve spontaneously, especially in children and young adults. Contrarily, those occurring in immunosupressed patients are likely to remain in place indefinitely. In spite of the potential for resolution, nearly all anogenital warts should be treated to reduce contagion through sexual activity. This is particularly important because it is not possible to determine clinically which warts contain high-risk HPV types.

Before considering treatment options, clinicians should consider whether or not biopsy of one or more lesions should be undertaken. As indicated above, flat-topped warts (regardless of color) and large globular warts should be biopsied because of the possibility that in situ or invasive squamous cell carcinoma may be present. Shave biopsy is acceptable for flat-topped warts, whereas shave excision is preferred for large globular warts because of the greater risk of sampling error in these large lesions. Filliform lesions and those mimicking hand warts (see above) may be treated without biopsy due to the very low likelihood that dysplasia will be present.

Multiple approaches to treatment are available (8,9). Treatment needs to be individualized for each patient as no single therapy is universally preferable. One of the first priorities in the treatment process is the education of patients regarding the contagious aspects of the viral infection, the likelihood of recurrence after therapy, and, in some instances, the potential for malignant transformation. After this has been accomplished, input from the patient should be sought as to whether the treatment is to be undertaken by the patient (patient-based therapy) or by the clinician (clinician-based therapy).

There are three medications available for patient-based therapy: application of 0.5% podofilox, 5% imiquimod, or green tea polyphenon E. Podofilox (Condylox) solution or gel is applied to the warts twice daily for 3 days followed by 4 to 7 days without treatment. Imiquimod (Aldara) cream is applied once daily three times per week on alternate days. For both products, the cycle is repeated as necessary. A meta-analysis comparing these two products found that they were approximately equal in efficacy with clinical cure rates of 50% to 55% (10). However, the severity of adverse effects was slightly greater with podofilox (10). The Food and Drug Administration (FDA) has recently approved a green tea extract (Veregen), marketed as 15% ointment, to be applied to warts t.i.d. Data to support Veregen's use are limited. Three randomized, double-blind, placebo-controlled studies have been carried out with complete clearance rates of 50% to 60% (11). Adverse effects of redness, burning, pain, and erosion occur with all three of these products though possibly to a slightly lesser degree with the green tea extract.

Clinician-based therapy can be either medical or procedural. Two *medical* approaches are available. With the first, 25% podophyllin is applied to the warts once weekly or every other week. This approach is less used today than it was in the past due to nonstandardized podophyllin preparations, highly variable cure rates, and significant problems with irritation and pain. With the second, trichloroacetic acid can be applied (carefully!) in the office at 2- or 3-week intervals. Clearance rates of 70% to 80% have been reported after six applications (9). Burning on application is troublesome for patients but it is a reasonable approach when the warts are relatively nonkeratotic and the number and size of the lesions are small (12).

Clinician-based *procedural* therapy includes cryotherapy, electrosurgical destruction, laser destruction, and surgical excision. With cryotherapy, liquid nitrogen is sprayed (or applied with cotton-tipped applicators) at 2- to 3-week intervals. Clearance rates of about 80% are achieved with three to six treatments (9,13). Electrosurgical destruction (electrofulguration, electrodessication) is usually carried out using the ConMed Hyfrcator under local anesthesia. Other electrosurgical approaches using loop excision or a bipolar Bovie-type apparatus can also be used. Laser therapy, generally with a CO_2 laser, can also be considered but the cost of this equipment, and thus the treatments, is very high. Surgical excision is most often accomplished with a shave or scissors-snip technique; rarely elliptical excision might be considered. All three of these ablative approaches result in clearance rates of somewhat over 80% (9,14). Drawbacks, however, are the requirement for local anesthesia, the possibility of secondary infection, and potentially long healing times.

The choice of which medical or procedural approach is taken depends on patient preference and on the experience level of the clinician. For most patients, I prefer either electrosurgical destruction or shave removal with very light electrosurgery to the base. These two approaches are time honored, inexpensive, and do not depend on patient compliance. Moreover, only a single clinic visit is generally necessary and the patient leaves the clinic with the knowledge that he or she is free of all of the visible lesions. Of course, if the number and size of the warts are large, staged eradication at monthly intervals may be necessary.

The recurrence rate with all forms of therapy is very high, running generally in the 25% to 45% range. This presumably is the result of latent virus left in the perilesional skin after clinical visible lesions have been successfully treated.

Anogenital warts in children present a special problem because of the concern that sexual abuse may have taken place. However, for children under the age of two, it is very unlikely that the transmission occurred through sexual contact (7). Anogenital warts in these very young children may have arisen through normal parental contact or by way of contagion from an infected birth canal. A greater level of concern exists for those over the age of

four and, in any case, inquiry by an experienced clinician or by other skilled interviewers must be carried for all children with anogenital warts.

The best approach for genital warts is to prevent them for occurring in the first place. A quadrivalent vaccine (Guardasil) directed against HPV types 6, 11, 16, and 18 has been approved by the FDA for use in 9 to 26 year old children and adults of both sexes. The possibility of using this vaccine for women over the age of 26 is under consideration by the FDA currently. A bivalent (Cervarix) vaccine directed at HPV 16 and 18 has also been approved for girls and women 10 to 25 years of age. Clinical trials and almost 4 years of experience has documented that both of these vaccines are highly efficacious, safe, and durable. In addition both vaccines have some, but limited, crossover effect against HPV types other than those toward which the vaccines are primarily directed (15). The cost remains high and some parental objection exists. These two factors somewhat limit the use of these vaccines in many situations.

Both vaccines appear to be nearly 98% effective in preventing cervical and vulvar intraepithelial neoplasia (CIN 2 and 3) due to HPV types 16 and 18 for up to 3 years in those who were naïve to these types at the time of vaccination (15–17). Efficacy in older women aged 24 to 45 was slightly lower but still excellent at 90% (18).

GENITAL WARTS: **Management**

- Home therapy with imiquimod, podofilox, or green tea extract
- Office therapy with liquid nitrogen or trichloroacetic acid
- Office therapy with electrosurgery, excision, or laser ablation
- Follow-up for recurrences and development of new warts
- Check for sexual abuse in children with anogenital warts

MOLLUSCUM CONTAGIOSUM

Infection with molluscum contagiosum virus (MCV) is common and self-limited. It can be viewed as more of a nuisance than a threat to health or well-being.

Clinical Presentation

Molluscum contagiosum is a common infection that occurs primarily in children (19). Incidence rates can be as high as 20% of children in lesser developed countries but are lower elsewhere. In a large series reported from Greece, children with this condition accounted for 3.2% of outpatient pediatric visits over a 6-year period (20), and in a series from India, they accounted for 1.9% of new patients visits in a dermatology/STD clinic (21). It has been estimated that in the United States, office visits for molluscum contagiosum account for about 0.2% of total outpatient visits (22). Males appear to be affected somewhat more often than females. Adults account for less than 10% of all MCV infections. Transmission occurs primarily by casual skin-to-skin contact in children, whereas sexual transmission accounts for most of the cases in adults. Molluscum contagiosum occurs more commonly, and presents with more lesions, in patients with atopic dermatitis and in those who are significantly immunocompromised such as those with HIV/acquired immunodeficiency syndrome (AIDS) (23,24).

The lesions of molluscum contagiosum are skin colored, pink, white, or, occasionally, translucent hemispherical papules 3 to 10 mm in diameter (Fig. 12-12). Rarely, and mostly in immunocompromised patients, giant lesions are encountered. Immunocompetent patients generally have 15 to 50 lesions at any one time. Most of the lesions develop on keratinizing epithelial skin but they rarely also occur on mucous membranes. The skin surrounding lesions is usually normal in appearance but redness and eczematous changes may occur circumferentially. Sometimes in the resolution stage the lesions develop brisk, red inflammation (Fig. 12-13).

The papules of molluscum contagiosum characteristically have a central depression or umbilication. However, many lesions, especially early and small lesions, lack this feature (Fig. 12-14). Although this umbilication may not be seen in every lesion, a careful examination usually shows at least some umbilicated lesions. Sometimes, the papules of molluscum contagiosum mimic vesicles, thus accounting for the lay term "water warts" (Fig. 12-15). Molluscum contagiosum is typically asymptomatic but some patients may experience low-grade pruritus. Lesions in children may be found anywhere on the skin but most often the

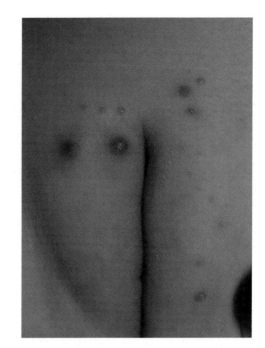

FIG. 12-13. As mollusca prompt an immune response, lesions sometimes become inflamed before resolving.

trunk is affected. Lesions in adults, because of sexual transmission, are most commonly located on the mons, the medial thighs, and the buttocks. They are less often found on the penis and on the labia.

Diagnosis

The diagnosis, especially when umbilicated lesions are present, is usually made on a clinical basis. Confirmation is possible through curettage of a lesion, which then reveals a small white "molluscum body." A shave biopsy may be appropriate if the clinical appearance is atypical. The

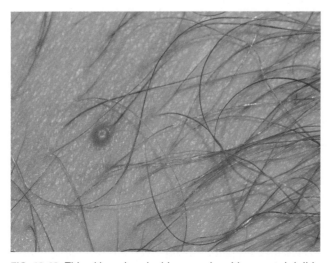

FIG. 12-12. This skin-colored, shiny papule with a cental dell is typical of molluscum contagiosum.

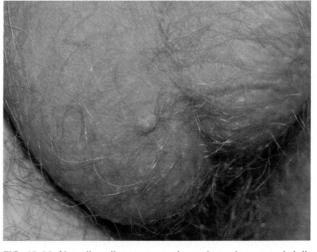

FIG. 12-14. Not all mollusca contagiosa show the central dell; this lesion is nonspecific and not diagnosable by morphology alone.

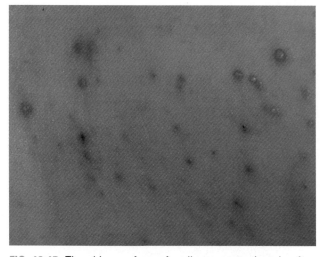

FIG. 12-15. The shiny surface of mollusca contagiosa is often reminiscent of vesicles, leading to the lay term "water wart."

histologic findings include pathognomonic features of intracytoplasmic inclusion bodies ("molluscum contagiosum bodies") made up of globular viral proteins.

The list of differential diagnoses includes HPV infection (genital warts), scabies, lichen nitidus, and lymphangiectasia. Genital warts are not usually hemispherical and often have a rough, rather than smooth, surface. The lesions of scabies occur in a characteristic distribution pattern (web spaces, axillary folds, areolae, and penis) and small linear burrows can usually be found. The lesions in lichen nitidus are more numerous, mostly flat-topped, and more morphologically homogenous. The small papules and vesicles of lymphangiectasia contain fluid when pierced with a needle.

MOLLUSCUM CONTAGIOSUM: **Diagnosis**

- Small, smooth, dome-shaped papules
- White, pink, translucent, or skin colored
- Umbilication at summit is characteristic in larger lesions
- Bright red color may occur when undergoing resolution
- Confirm by curettage for molluscum body

Pathophysiology

Molluscum contagiosum is caused by the MCV which is a very large DNA poxvirus. There are four virus types (c.f. two for HSV) of MCV (19). Most infections are caused by MCV 1. There are no significant differences in appearance or distribution for infections caused by the four types. As indicated above, transmission is primarily by skin-to-skin contact but a lesser role for fomites may also be likely. There is a long incubation period after inoculation of the virus. The time of this latency averages about 2 months but much longer intervals have been reported. MCV cannot be cultured using artificial media.

Resolution of the infection is associated with the development of both a humoral and a cell-mediated immune response. Antibodies to MCV are found in most, but not all, patients with molluscum contagiosum. However, the timing of their appearance and the titer levels do not closely parallel the severity or duration of the infection. The CMI response is much more important in allowing for resolution of the infection. The onset of the CMI is sometimes clinically apparent by the development of inflammation in and around individual lesions. Once such inflamed lesions are present, total resolution of the infection usually follows within a month or two.

Management

In immunocompetent patients, untreated individual lesions of molluscum contagiosum resolve spontaneously over a matter of 1 to 3 months. But, "seeding" of virus into surrounding skin or at distant sites occurs such that new lesions develop while old ones are resolving. The total duration of the infection, at least in children, averages 18 to 36 months. In immunocompromised persons, the number of lesions is larger and the variability in size is greater. Spontaneous resolution takes much longer and may not occur at all. On this basis, it seems prudent to check the HIV status in adults who develop lesions that are larger, more numerous, or last more than several months.

All of the treatments currently available are problematic in one way or another. For this reason, most clinicians advise "watchful waiting" rather than active therapy for pediatric patients. For adults and impatient patients, both medical and procedural approaches are possible. The most commonly used medical treatments include cantharidin, trichloroacetic acid, imiquimod, and potassium hydroxide. The first two are applied in the office by the clinician but the latter two can be used at home.

Cantharidin 0.7% solution is applied very carefully to prevent contact with the normal surrounding skin. Special care must be taken if cantharidin is used in intertriginous areas as the retained sweat can allow unwanted spread of the applied solution. For lesions in the anogenital area, it is useful to apply a loose bandage over the treated lesions to prevent spread of the cantharidin due to friction and retained sweat. Many clinicians advise that the cantharidin be washed off 6 to 8 hours after application but I have not found it necessary to do so. A blister develops at the cantharidin application site within 24 hours and the lesion is eventually sloughed off 4 or 5 days later when the blister roof peels away. Two to three office visits for repeat application are usually necessary. It is painlessness when initially applied, and for this reason, it is generally the treatment of choice for children. Mild pain and irritation may occur later. Clearance rates for individually treated lesions are about 90% and patient satisfaction is quite good (25,26).

Trichloroacetic acid 85% solution must be applied very carefully so that the solution does not run off of the papule onto normal skin. This approach is quite effective but it is somewhat painful at the time of application (27). Imiquimod may be used at home and the method in which it is used is identical to that described in the section above on genital warts. Home application reduces the number and expense of office visits but this approach is accompanied by considerable discomfort and the duration of treatment is long enough to hamper patient compliance. Potassium hydroxide (KOH) has only recently been described as a treatment modality. It can also be applied at home. In a recent study comparing 10% KOH solution with imiquimod, the two treatments were equally effective but KOH use was accompanied by more adverse effects (28).

The most commonly used procedural approaches are cryotherapy and curettage. Liquid nitrogen cryotherapy is used in the same manner as is used for actinic keratoses and warts. A total freeze time of about 10 seconds is recommended and this can be obtained either in a single freeze or in a freeze–thaw–freeze cycle. It is moderately painful. Curretage, in which the lesion is scraped away with the edge of a skin curet, is also moderately painful but the fact that treated lesions are completely removed leads to good patient satisfaction. Because of discomfort, both cryotherapy and curettage are best used when the number of lesions is small. In a randomized trial, comparing curettage with cantharidin and imiquimod, curettage was found to be the most efficacious and was associated with the fewest adverse effects (29).

MOLLUSCUM CONTAGIOSUM:	Management

- Consider observation without specific therapy in kids
- Office application of cantharidin is painless and effective
- Liquid nitrogen cryotherapy if lesion number is large
- Curretage for removal if lesion number is small
- Imiquimod or potassium hydroxide can be considered for home therapy

CONDYLOMA LATUM

Condyloma lata is the name used for the flat-topped papules and nodules that develop in the anogenital area during the secondary stage of syphilis. These lesions are uncommonly seen in conventional office practice but are, of course, encountered with some frequency in STD clinics. The primary coverage of syphilis is located in the section on chancre in Chapter 10 and only the clinical presentation and therapy of condyloma lata will be covered here.

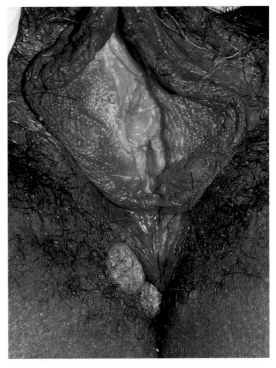

FIG. 12-16. Condylomata lata are often larger than genital warts and are flat topped.

Condylomata lata are sharply demarcated, large (1- to 2-cm), flat-topped, moist, skin-colored or pink papules (Fig. 12-16). When the lesions are located on a mucosal surface, they often exhibit a white surface because of retained moisture (Fig. 12-17). They are most commonly found on the vulva and the perianal area but can occur elsewhere on the genitalia and perigenital skin. As opposed to the other cutaneous lesions of secondary syphilis, the lesions of condyloma lata are teeming with spirochetes and pose a high risk for transmission to others. Condylomata lata are usually associated with other signs and symptoms of secondary syphilis such as fever, malaise, and generalized lymphadenopathy. Other skin findings such as slightly scaly red papules on the trunk, brown-red palmar and plantar papules, white patches on the oral mucous membranes, and patchy hair loss may also be present.

Patients with condylomata lata almost always exhibit a positive rapid plasma regain (RPR) or Venereal Disease Research Laboratory (VDRL) serologic test for syphilis. The only exceptions are those who are severely immunocompromised (e.g., HIV/AIDS) and those with such a high antibody titer that they exhibit the so-called prozone phenomenon. The lesions of condyloma lata can be confused with flat-topped HPV-induced warts and intraepithelial neoplasia of the vulva, penis, and scrotum. If there is any question about the correct identity, a serologic test for syphilis as well as a biopsy should be obtained. The treatment for secondary syphilis as recommended by the CDC is a single 2.4 million unit IM injection of benzathine penicillin G (Bicillin L-A) (30).

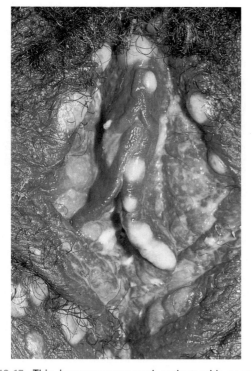

FIG. 12-17. This immunosuppressed patient with secondary syphilis shows large, skin-colored, flat-topped condyloma lata as well as some lesions that are white because of the hydrated, thickened epithelium.

LYMPHOGRANULOMA VENEREUM

Until recently, lymphogranuloma venereum (LGV) was rarely encountered in Western countries. However, during the last 5 years, there has been a significant rise in the number of cases reported from the United Kingdom and Europe and a smaller rise in the United States. Nearly all of this increase is accounted for by infections occurring in MSM. Currently, the prevalence of LGV serovars in the rectum in UK MSM is about 1% (31). LGV occurs very rarely in women.

Nearly all (90% to 95%) of the patients with LGV have presented with proctitis and most of the others have had inguinal adenitis (31). Transient genital ulcers together with appreciable lymphadenopathy occur in a minority of patients (32).

A discussion of proctitis, with or without perianal ulcers, falls outside the scope of this textbook and the rarely encountered ulcers are not well described in the literature. The most striking feature is likely to be impressive lymphadenopathy (buboes). The inguinal lymph nodes are most commonly affected though in some cases femoral nodes are also involved. When both sets of nodes are affected, Poupart ligament (ligamentum inguinale) creates a characteristic grove between the two groups of nodes. The enlarged nodes are usually bilateral and they are exquisitely tender. In untreated patients, nodes that have been present for some time undergo liquefaction with attendant fluctuance. Eventually, breakdown of the overlying

skin occurs, resulting in the presence of chronic purulent draining sinuses. Massive genital edema (elephantiasis) frequently develops. Patients with untreated proctitis develop rectal stenosis, strictures, and perianal abscess formation. The latter may be mistaken for Crohn disease.

LGV is caused by the L1, L2, or L3 serovars of the bacterium, *Chlamydia trachomatis*. Nearly all of the newly reported cases have been with the L2 serovar. The diagnosis is usually suspected on a clinical basis but similar adenopathy can occur in chancroid. Confirmation of the diagnosis requires identification of a LGV-type serovar from the site of infection. Previously, this had been accomplished primarily with bacterial cultures, but today molecular techniques are more widely used. In situations where these tests are not available, serologic techniques can be used but there are many problems with sensitivity and specificity.

The CDC guidelines recommend treatment with oral doxycycline 100 mg twice daily for 3 weeks (30). In an attempt to obtain better compliance, single dose or short course azithromycin has also been used but there is insufficient evidence of efficacy to support the use of this medication on a regular basis (30). Fluctuant lymph nodes should be aspirated.

EPIDERMAL CYSTS (EPIDERMOID CYSTS)

Epidermal cysts are commonly, but erroneously, termed sebaceous cysts. They are the most common type of cysts found in the anogenital area. They occur as firm, slope-shouldered, smooth-surfaced, white, yellow-white, slightly pink or skin-colored papules or nodules (Fig. 12-18). Very small cysts (1 to 2 mm) are called milia but these are not commonly seen in the anogenital area. The average diameter for genital lesions is 0.5 to 2.0 cm. Noninflamed

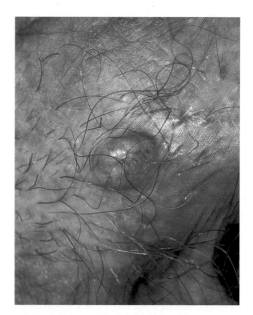

FIG. 12-18. This epidermal cyst on the base of the shaft of the penis is firm as a result of compact keratin within the distended follicle.

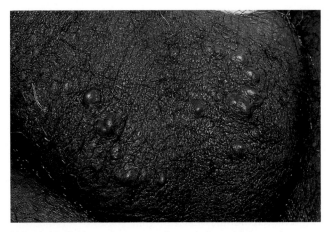

FIG. 12-19. Epidermal cysts are frequently multiple on the scrotum and the hair-bearing surface of the labia majora.

cysts are asymptomatic. Epidermal cysts are primarily found on the hair-bearing aspects of the genitalia. They are most commonly located on the scrotum in men and the labia majora in women. One or several may be present; rarely there are 10 to 20 clustered lesions (Figs. 12-19 and 12-20). The diagnosis is usually made on the basis of clinical appearance. Confirmation, if necessary, can be obtained when white cyst contents are visualized after incising and gently squeezing the lesion. Syringomas arising on the labia majora may be confused with epidermal cysts. The lesions of molluscum contagiosum may mimic epidermal cysts but the lesions of molluscum contagiosum are more superficial and appear to sit on the surface, rather than within the skin. Enlarged sebaceous glands (Fordyce spots) on mucosal aspects of the genitalia may resemble milia.

So-called "inclusion cysts" arise when bits of epithelium are implanted in the skin during the course of a surgical procedure or as a result of trauma sufficient to break the surface of the skin. The much more common, typical epidermoid cyst found on the genitalia, develops from the remnant of an anatomically malformed pilosebaceous unit that lacks a fully adequate outlet to the surface of the skin. These cysts may have a black dot, representing a comedone ("blackhead"), at the summit of the cyst. The white material located within an epidermal cyst is keratin that is produced by keratinocytes located in the lining of the cyst wall.

Epidermal cysts are medically unimportant and cause no problems unless the cyst wall leaks or ruptures. If this occurs, cyst contents come into contact with the connective tissue surrounding the cyst where they engender a brisk foreign body inflammatory reaction. This inflammation causes the cyst contents to liquefy into pus-like material. In spite of the appearance and smell, this mixture of liquefied keratin and inflammatory cells almost always lacks pathogenic bacteria. Nevertheless, such lesions may clinically resemble a furuncle or an inflammatory pseudocyst as seen in hidradenitis suppurativa. No treatment is needed for uninflamed cysts. Inflamed cysts may be incised and drained. Most clinicians prescribe antibiotics for inflamed cysts but any beneficial effect that occurs is likely due to the anti-inflammatory, rather than the antimicrobial, properties of these antibiotics. Rarely, symptoms or patient insistence will result in a need for excisional removal of the entire cyst.

MUCINOUS VESTIBULAR CYSTS

Mucinous vestibular cysts are commonly found within the vulvar vestibule. They develop from anatomic abnormalities or obstruction of the minor vestibular glands. A buildup of gland secretion forms these 0.5- to 2-cm cysts (Fig. 12-21). They can be skin colored, translucent, yellow, or blue. Although vestibular cysts can be

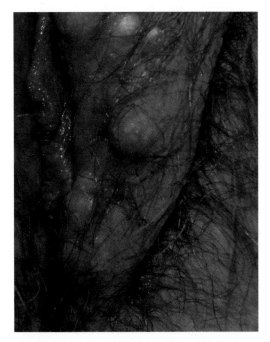

FIG. 12-20. These large epidermal cysts are both skin colored and yellowish, where the skin is thinned and stretched over follicles distended by yellow-white keratin.

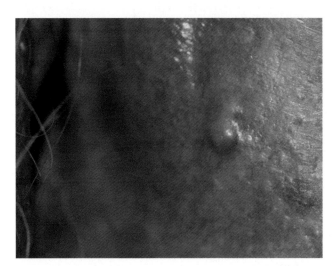

FIG. 12-21. Vestibular cysts can be skin colored, yellow, or bluish; however, translucent skin color is most common.

removed surgically, they are asymptomatic and therefore ordinarily require no treatment.

CYSTS OF THE MEDIAN RAPHE

A median raphe represents the midline embryonic joining point of two symmetrical tissues. In the anogenital area of men, a median raphe extends from the anus forward through the perineum, along the scrotum extending onto the underside of the penis and ending at the urethral meatus on the tip of the glans. The raphe is visible and palpable as a slight ridge that is skin colored or light brown. Cyst or canals can develop anywhere along this raphe but occur most commonly on the underside of the penis. Usually, only a solitary papule, representing a single cyst, is present but in some cases multiple cysts are found along the raphe. The lesions appear as dome-shaped skin-colored, yellow, or tan hemispherical papules that are 2 to 15 mm in diameter (Fig. 12-22). Presumably these are present from birth but slow growth and lack of symptoms generally mean they are not discovered until later in life. Rarely, they become inflamed as a result of trauma or infection. Histologically they may be lined with either columnar or stratified squamous epithelium. No treatment is necessary for asymptomatic lesions; inflamed or otherwise symptomatic lesions can be excised.

PILONIDAL SINUS (PILONIDAL CYST)

Though often termed pilonidal cyst, these lesions lack an epithelial cyst wall and therefore are more appropriately identified as a pilonidal sinus. They arise as an acquired lesion wherein hairs, trapped in folded areas of tissue, forcibly penetrate the skin and create a foreign body inflammatory reaction. Pilonidal sinus is most commonly located in the sacrococcygeal area in men but locations in other sites such as the axillae, webspaces of the hands, and genitalia have been reported (33). It appears that only about a dozen cases have reported to have involved the vulva and penis (33,34). Most of the vulvar cases have been located in a periclitoral site where they may develop into a clitoral or periclitoral abscess. In uncircumcised men, penile lesions have been located in the coronal sulcus.

Pilonidal sinus first develops as an asymptomatic, soft, skin-colored nodule that becomes red and very painful when as inflammation ensues. Hairs can sometimes be seen extruding from the surface of the lesion when the folds of skin around the lesion are separated. Accumulated pus within the lesion may drain from the sinus tract. Treatment is more difficult than might be expected. All of the inflamed tissue and the entire sinus tract must be completely excised. Even with careful, extensive surgery, the recurrence rate is fairly high.

BARTHOLIN CYSTS AND ABSCESSES

Bartholin glands (the major vestibular glands) open into the vulvar vestibule at about the 5 and 7-o'clock position, just distal to the hymeneal ring. They lie at the base of the labia minora and empty through ducts that are about 2 cm long. These glands provide a small amount of mucinous fluid during sexual activity. An extensive review of the cysts and abscesses that can develop in these structures has recently been published (35).

Bartholin duct cysts and abscesses are fairly common with a lifetime risk that is estimated at about 2%. They are most likely to occur during the third decade with the risk declining after that as the glands begin to involute. Dilation of the ducts to form a cyst-like structure occurs if the outlet of the duct becomes obstructed. This results in an asymptomatic skin-colored, smooth-surfaced, slope-shouldered nodule that ranges from about 1 to 5 cm in diameter. They arise at the lateral aspect of the vestibule under the labium minus (Fig. 12-23). The positioning of the labium minus directly over the approximate center of the cyst is a highly characteristic diagnostic feature. Bartholin cysts may become inflamed as a result of either infection or cyst rupture. The inflammation and swelling cause considerable pain and may be accompanied by fever. For infected cysts, the bacteria most often causing abscess formation include *Neisseria gonorrhoeae*, *Chlamydia trachomatis*, *Bacteroides* sp., and *Escherichia coli*.

The diagnosis is made on a clinical basis. Noninflamed cysts contain sterile, clear mucinous fluid. Pus is present within an abscessed cyst and sufficient purulent material for culture may be expressed from the ostium of the duct with gentle massage. If the lesion is too tender for such

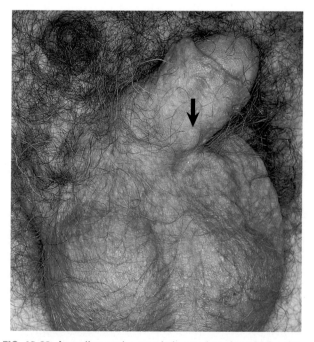

FIG. 12-22. A median raphe cyst is located on the middle of the ventral shaft of the penis, in this case near the base.

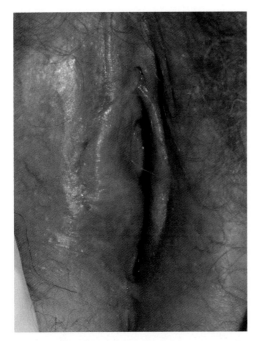

FIG. 12-23. This Bartholin gland duct cyst shows the typical deep, poorly demarcated swelling within the vestibule at about the 5-o'clock position.

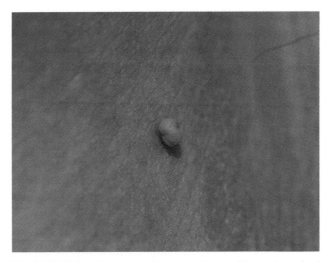

FIG. 12-24. This soft, pedunculated papule, or skin tag, is typical of a fibroepithelial polyp. Skin tags are most common in skin folds such as the crural crease and axillae.

manipulation, pus for culture can be obtained by needle aspiration or by incision and drainage. Noninflamed cysts do not require treatment unless they are large enough to cause discomfort. Inflamed cysts are generally treated with oral antibiotics and a fair number of these will then resolve spontaneously. Larger inflamed cysts can be incised and drained to relieve discomfort. Unfortunately, cysts treated in this manner frequently recur. Appreciable controversy exists regarding what represents the most definitive management of these lesions. Discussion of such therapy lies outside the scope of this textbook but has been recently reviewed (36). Carcinoma of Bartholin gland occurs occasionally in older women, so even for asymptomatic cysts, tissue taken from women over the age of 40 should be submitted for histologic examination.

SKIN TAG (ACROCHORDON, FIBROEPITHELIAL POLYP)

Skin tags are common benign skin growths that affect a large portion of the general population. Small lesions are referred to as skin tags, and large lesions are termed fibroepithelial polyps (Figs. 12-24 and 12-25). Skin tags occur most often in obese patients and in those with disturbances in insulin and glucose metabolism (37). Perianal skin tags are found more than would be expected in patients with inflammatory bowel disease.

Skin tags are soft, asymptomatic tan or skin-colored papules. They may be very small (2 to 3 mm long) or somewhat larger (1 cm long). The longer skin tags are pedunculated with a thin base and larger body. Most often

skin tags are numerous and somewhat clustered. They preferentially develop in the axillae, around the neck, and in the inguinal folds. They are rarely encountered on the penis, and they generally do not occur on the modified mucous membranes of the vulva. Larger, often solitary, fibroepithelial polyps have a predilection for the upper inner thighs, inguinal creases, and the buttocks. Polypoid edema of the labia minora may mimic the appearance of fibroepithelial polyps. The diagnosis of skin tags is made on a clinical basis. Rarely, they may be confused with genital warts, intradermal nevi, and isolated neurofibromas.

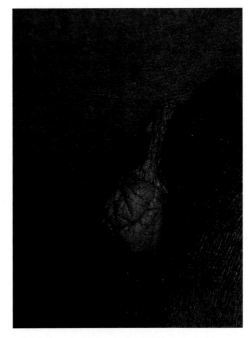

FIG. 12-25. This pedunculated fibroepithelial polyp is quite large, and sometimes becomes tender when caught in underwear.

Skin tags are always benign and no treatment is necessary unless they become inflamed and painful. In this situation, the lesions can be snipped with fine scissors. The slight bleeding that occurs can be stopped by the application of Monsel (ferric subsulfate) solution, aluminum chloride, or light electrocautery. Very small skin tags can be obliterated by liquid nitrogen cryotherapy or electrodessication. There is an effective home remedy in which a thread is tied tightly around the base of a lesion. A week or so later the skin tag undergoes necrosis and falls off.

INTRADERMAL NEVI (DERMAL NEVI)

Intradermal nevi are benign neoplasms demonstrating clusters of nevus cells (melanocytes) within the dermal connective tissue. They present as soft hemispherical papules 5 to 15 mm in diameter (Fig. 12-26). Color is variable and can be pink, tan, or skin colored. Intradermal nevi rarely occur on the penis, scrotum, or within the vulva but are encountered fairly commonly on the thighs, buttocks, and in the pubic area. These lesions need to be differentiated from basal cell carcinomas, genital warts, and isolated neurofibromas. In some instances, they are pedunculated enough to be confused with skin tags. They are always benign and are not precursors of melanoma. No treatment is necessary unless they are inflamed as a result of trauma. If removal is necessary, they can be shaved from the surface or excised.

NEUROFIBROMA

Neurofibromas are asymptomatic, remarkably soft, skin-colored or light tan nodules. Small neurofibromas may mimic fibroepithelial polyps and intradermal nevi. They are very occasionally found on the genitalia either as

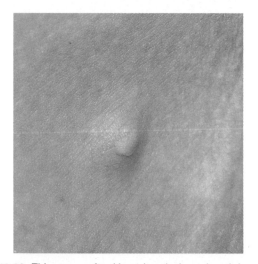

FIG. 12-26. This very soft, skin-colored, dermal nodule represents an intradermal nevus but is indistinguishable from a small neurofibroma.

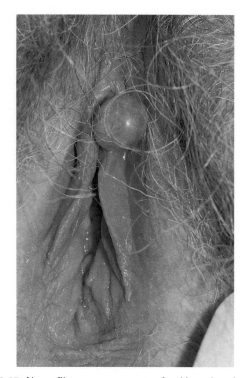

FIG. 12-27. Neurofibromas are very soft, skin-colored, superficial nodules that are most often sporadic rather than a sign of neurofibromatosis.

sporadic, solitary lesions (Fig. 12-27) or within the context of generalized (von Recklinghausen disease) (38). On the vulva, neurofibromas are most likely to be located in the periclitoral area or, less likely, on the labia majora. Penile lesions are rare. These cutaneous neurofibromas (as opposed to subcutaneous, plexiform neuromas) are benign lesions that do not evolve into sarcomas. Small lesions may be left untreated. Large lesions may be mechanically troublesome to the patient in which case they can be excised.

LIPOMA

Lipomas are a common hamartoma of fat. They can develop anywhere on the body as asymptomatic, lobular, soft, skin-colored, smooth, mobile nodules. Their size is variable but generally ranges from 2 to 5 cm (Fig. 12-28). In the vulva, lipomas are most often located in the periclitoral area and within the labia majora. The histology shows mature fat cells. Therapy is unnecessary, but surgical excision or liposuction may be appropriate if the lipoma is unduly troublesome.

PEARLY PENILE PAPULES

Pearly penile papules (PPP) are so common as to be considered a normal variant rather than as a disease (see also Chapter 1). They are estimated to be present in about 20% of men. Their prevalence is higher in uncircumcised

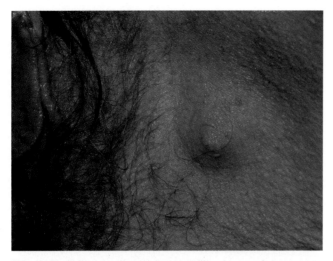

FIG. 12-28. Although a lipoma is normally a deep, subcutaneous, fatty tumor, in areas where there is little subcutaneous tissue, these can become large and pedunculated.

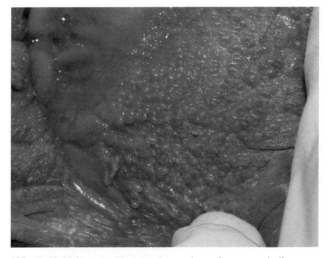

FIG. 12-29. Vulvar papillomatosis can be soft, grouped, discrete, usually closely set, elongated, fleshy papules with rounded tips, or they can be nearly confluent.

and African American men. These papules first appear during adolescence at which point they may cause some anxiety as the young men in whom they develop may fear that they represent a sexually transmitted disease. PPP are asymptomatic, small, skin-colored, whitish, or pink papules that can be either elongated (filliform) or globular (Fig. 12-6). The smallest lesions are only about 1 mm in diameter and height, while larger filliform lesions can be 2 mm wide and up to 4 to 5 mm in length. They are most commonly located on the corona of the penis where they often entirely encircle the glans. A single row of lesions may be present but it is not uncommon to encounter double rows. Less often they occur in the coronal sulcus or even on the distal shaft of the penis (Figs. 12-7 and 12-8).

The diagnosis is made on the basis of the characteristic morphology and location. They should be differentiated from enlarged sebaceous glands on the inner prepuce (Tyson glands) and on the distal shaft of the penis (Fordyce spots). Occasionally biopsy is needed to differentiate PPP from filliform genital warts. Treatment is unnecessary but if the patient is troubled by their presence they can be destroyed with electrosurgery or laser ablation.

VULVAR VESTIBULAR PAPILLOMATOSIS

Vulvar vestibular papillomatosis (VVP) is a normal anatomic variant. Early publications described a prevalence of only 1% but later reports, and our own clinical experience, indicate that they occur in about one third of premenopausal women (see also Chapter 1). The papillae in VVP are tissue colored which means that they are pink or red but similar in hue to the color of the vestibular tissue from which they arise. They are asymptomatic, soft, hemispherical or slightly elongated papules with a diameter of about 1 to 2 mm and a height that is usually about the same. However, some filliform lesions may be as tall as 5 mm.

Sometimes only a few papules are present but it is not uncommon to see hundreds such that the entire vestibule is carpeted with them (Figs. 12-5 and 12-29). The papules may be arranged in a cobblestone pattern but often, on close inspection, they can be seen as arranged in linear rows. VVP can be considered as the analog of pearly penile papules.

The papules in vestibular papillomatosis must not be confused with vestibular genital warts, as indeed they were until fairly recently. This differentiation is possible clinically based on the following characteristics of VVP: (1) the overall appearance is very homogenous with each papule being very similar in morphology to its neighbors; (2) the papules remain separate and remain discrete down to their base; (3) the papules are soft to touch; and (4) a linear pattern of arrangement can usually be discerned. Early on, the confusion with genital warts was engendered by reports that HPV DNA was frequently present within them. Today, however, there is consensus that HPV DNA is present no more often than it is found in vestibules of women with no VVP. If need be, biopsy can be carried out but the clinician should beware that pseudokoilocytic changes present in normal mucosal epithelium sometimes result in an incorrect diagnosis of HPV infection. The papules of VVP should also be differentiated from ectopic sebaceous glands (Fordyce spots) which are fewer in number, less elevated, and more yellow in color. Because the lesions are asymptomatic, no treatment needs to be undertaken.

FORDYCE SPOTS AND SEBACEOUS GLAND HYPERPLASIA

Fordyce spots (Fordyce granules) represent the appearance of ectopic sebaceous glands on mucosal surfaces. On the other hand, sebaceous gland hyperplasia occurs as appreciable enlargement of pilosebaceous units in nonectopic locations. They differ in clinical and histologic appearance

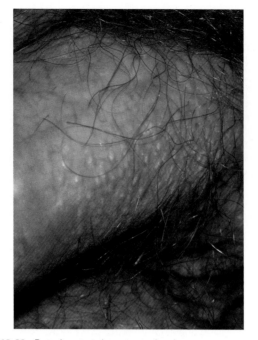

FIG. 12-30. Prominant sebaceous glands are common, skin-colored to yellow, grouped papules most often found on the proximal penile shaft.

such that with sebaceous gland hyperplasia, the lesions are larger, may be dimpled due to the follicular orifice at the summit, and, microscopically, there is an attached hair follicle (39).

Small numbers of sebaceous glands are commonly found anywhere on the shaft of the penis but their concentration is noticeably increased in the proximal quarter of the penile shaft (Fig. 12-30). These glands are very small, 1–2-mm papules that are skin colored or slightly yellow. A small dimple representing the follicle outlet may be visible in the center of the larger lesions. These glands (especially if they are small) are often mistermed Fordyce spots even though they are occurring on stratified squamous epithelium where pilosebaceous units would normally be found.

Ectopic sebaceous glands (Fordyce spots) similar to those that occur on the mucosal surface of the lips are very commonly encountered on the labia minora inside Hart line and on the non-hair bearing distal shaft of the penis (Fig. 12-10). They appear as small, barely raised, smooth, yellow, dome-shaped papules about 1 mm in diameter (Figs. 12-9 and 12-31). They become more obvious when the mucosa is stretched. None of these sebaceous glands has any clinical significance, except in those rare cases when an overanxious patient suddenly discovers them and becomes frightened that they may be warts. Reassurance is all that is needed.

TYSON GLANDS

These are small, modified sebaceous glands occasionally found on the underside of the penile foreskin where they are located at, or very near, the preputial sulcus. They

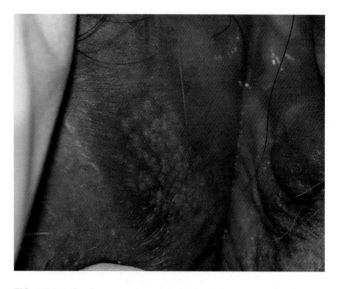

FIG. 12-31. Fordyce spots, or ectopic sebaceous glands, are normal findings most often found on the medial labia minora of premenopausal women.

are similar to, but different from, ordinary ectopic sebaceous glands (Fordyce spots) (40). As is true for Fordyce spots, these may be mistaken for small genital warts. At times, large Tyson glands may be confused with molluscum contagiosum. In the presence of clinical uncertainty, biopsy may be necessary. Since they are benign and asymptomatic, no treatment is necessary.

FOX–FORDYCE DISEASE

Fox–Fordyce disease (FFD) is an uncommon, highly pruritic, chronic inflammatory condition of apocrine glands. The condition is much more common in women than in men and African American individuals appear to be affected disproportionally often. Clinically, FFD appears as monomorphous, skin-colored, tan or brown dome-shaped, follicular papules. They are usually arrayed in a cobblestone pattern and located in sites such as the axillae, mammary areolae, and the anogenital region that contain apocrine gland-related follicles. The axillae are most often affected. In the anogenital region, lesions occur mainly on the labia majora in women and the pubic area in both sexes (Fig. 12-32). The onset is at puberty. The diagnosis is made by the distribution pattern and by the clinical morphology of the lesions. A suspected diagnosis can be confirmed by biopsy.

The pathogenesis of this condition is unknown. One hypothesis suggests that outlet obstruction of apocrine gland-related follicles leads to retention and dilatation of the apocrine duct and/or gland. Subsequent extravasation of apocrine sweat into the surrounding dermis could then lead to inflammation and itching. However, a recent microscopic study showed that most of the changes believed to be characteristic of FFD were also present in axillary skin from control patients (41). Interestingly, this same report,

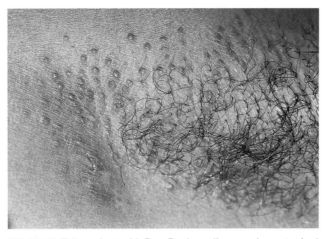

FIG. 12-32. This patient with Fox–Fordyce disease shows typical monomorphous, skin-colored, dome-shaped follicular papules within the pubic hair and surrounding skin.

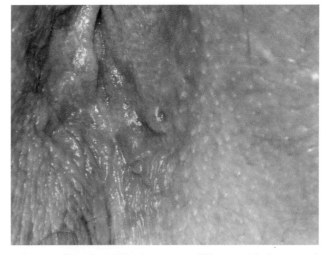

FIG. 12-33. A typical hidradenoma papilliferum with the central outlet.

together with observations from another study, identified a highly characteristic presence of both perifollicular foam cells and perifollicular mucin (41,42). The authors of the second study hypothesized that the foamy appearance of these cells developed as a result of phagocytosed mucin from extravasated apocrine sweat (42). While the cause of the initiating follicular obstruction is unknown, I believe that in at least some instances it is secondary to chronic rubbing of pruritic skin with subsequent hyperkeratinization and plugging of the follicular outlet.

There is no fully established therapy for FFD. The severity of the itching improves with pregnancy and while taking oral contraceptives. Topical steroids, topical tretinoin cream (which is often too irritating to use effectively), and oral isotretinoin may improve symptoms in some patients. At menopause, the condition appears to remit.

HIDRADENOMA PAPILLIFERUM (MAMMARY-LIKE GLAND ADENOMA)

Hidradenoma papilliferum is an uncommon tumor that exhibits a strong predilection for the anogenital area of postpubertal women. Clinically, it occurs as a 0.5- to 2-cm, smooth-surfaced, medium soft to firm asymptomatic nodule that is skin colored or red (Figs. 12-33 and 12-34). This lesion may have a somewhat translucent, cystic-type appearance. Some have an ulcerated surface. Most are asymptomatic but pruritus, bleeding, and mild pain occur in a minority of instances. In a recent review of 46 cases, these tumors were noted to occur entirely in women 30 to 90 years of age (43). All were located on the vulva; half occurred on the labia minora and most of the rest were on the labia majora (43).

These neoplasms were originally thought to be apocrine gland–derived tumors but they are now thought to be derived from the related, but separately identified,

mammary-like glands that are known to be located in the anogenital area of women (43). This new category of mammary-like gland adenomas may subsume other rare anogenital tumors such as syringocystadenoma papilliferum. Almost all of the tumors are benign and can be cured with local excision.

LICHEN NITIDUS

Lichen nitidus is an uncommon disease of children and adolescents. It is usually an asymptomatic eruption characterized by multiple, tiny (1 to 2 mm), shiny, flat-topped papules that are usually skin-colored or less often pink or white (Figs. 12-35 and 12-36). The lesions are most often asymptomatic though some patients report mild pruritus. This eruption usually involves the trunk and upper extremities. In males, the shaft of the penis is characteristically

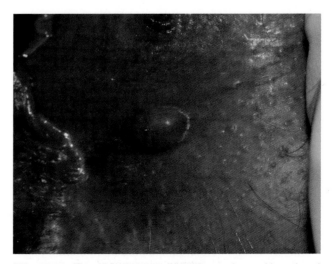

FIG. 12-34. The hidradenoma papilliferum is a skin-colored papule with a central pit; a drop of mucoid material can be seen at the opening.

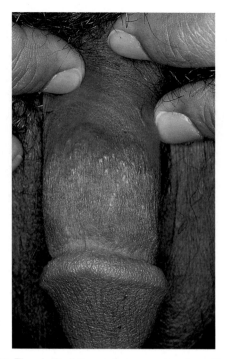

FIG. 12-35. The shaft of the penis is an area of predilection for lichen nitidus, consisting of tiny, closely set, dome-shaped papules.

involved. No cases involving the vulva appear to have been reported. The condition remits spontaneously after several years.

A clinical diagnosis is commonly confirmed by biopsy. Histologically, there is a unique picture of a lichenoid reaction with the presence of small, focal granulomas located in the papular dermis. These granulomas are partially or completely surrounded by tongues of downward proliferating epidermis ("ball in a claw" formation). The etiology of lichen nitidus is unknown. Originally some thought that it was a variant of lichen planus, and indeed

lichen planus and lichen nitidus can rarely develop concomitantly. Today, however, it is considered to be a separate, unique disease. No treatment is completely satisfactory though the application of high or superpotent topical steroids may hasten its resolution. But, since it is asymptomatic and tends to remit with time, it seems reasonable in most instances to leave it untreated.

SCLEROSING LYMPHANGITIS OF THE PENIS

Nonvenereal sclerosing lymphangitis usually presents as a very firm, linear, smooth-surfaced, rope-like nodule that is located at, or just proximal to, the coronal sulcus (Fig. 12-37). At this site, it partially or completely encircles the penis. Occasionally, the nodule branches such that there is a small perpendicular extension a short way along the shaft of the penis. The overlying skin is freely moveable over it.

The condition develops quite quickly, almost always shortly after a prolonged period of vigorous sexual intercourse or masturbation. It may occur in association with one or another sexually transmitted infection, but there is no evidence that infection plays a role in its etiology (44). Controversy exists as to whether this represents a thrombosis of lymphatic or venous vessels. Recent authors favor a venous origin that, if true, would then make sclerosing lymhangitis analogous, or even synonymous, with the similar appearing Mondor disease of the penis. Treatment of this benign condition is reduction of sexual activity. If this occurs, spontaneous resolution of the disease can be expected within several weeks.

SQUAMOUS CARCINOMA IN MEN

In both men and women, there are two distinct pathways through which squamous cell carcinoma (SCC) can develop: an HPV-related pathway and a non-HPV-related

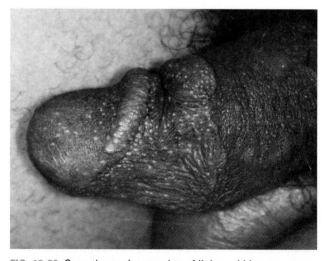

FIG. 12-36. Sometimes, the papules of lichen nitidus can occur in lines or groups, arising in scratches or other areas of injury or inflammation.

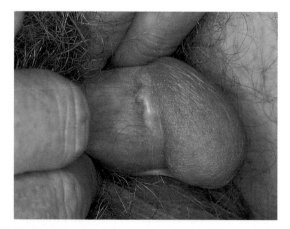

FIG. 12-37. This patient shows the classic skin-colored, cord-like nodule of sclerosing lymphangitis, located on the distal shaft parallel to the corona.

pathway. The lesions that develop through each of these routes have a different appearance and course. Those lesions that are HPV-related have a more variegated appearance (pink, red, brown, black, or skin-colored papules and plaques) and a more prolonged duration between the in situ and the invasive stage. On the other hand, those lesions that are non-HPV-related are less variegated (red, white, and skin-colored nodules) with a more rapid progression between the in situ and invasive stages. Obviously, with all of this variability, these malignancies could have been placed in any one of several chapters and our placement of the major discussion in this chapter is entirely arbitrary.

Clinical Presentation

The category of penile SCC includes both in situ, penile intraepithelial neoplasia (PIN) and invasive SCC. These are uncommon conditions in the United States. Overall, penile SCC accounts for only about 1% of all malignancies in men. The annual incidence of invasive SCC increases with age and is approximately 1/100,000 at age 50 and 5/100,000 at age 80 (45). Patients with in situ disease account for about one third of these reported figures (46). The annual incidence of PIN appears to be increasing, while that of invasive SCC appears to be decreasing (46). Rates are higher in lesser developed countries and are higher among Hispanics in the United States.

PIN can occur either on the prepuce or glans (where it was previously known as erythroplasia of Queyrat) or on the shaft (where it was previously known as Bowen disease and Bowenoid papulosis). An uncommon variant of PIN is pseudoepitheliomatous micaceous and keratotic balanitis in which the lesion appears as thick, heaped-up scale and crust (Fig. 12-38) (47). One or several lesions of PIN may be present. PIN occurs as flat-topped papules or plaques (Fig. 12-39). The latter may be as large as 2 or 3 cm in diameter. The papules and plaques on the shaft may be

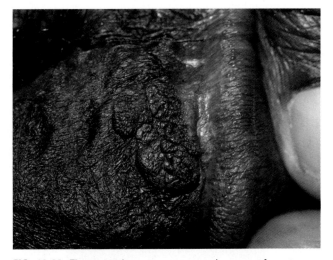

FIG. 12-39. Flat-topped warts represent the type of wart morphology most likely to show PIN as was true for this lesion.

pink, red, brown, or skin colored. Those on the glans and prepuce are usually white, pink, or red. The surface of PIN lesions is not ulcerated and may be smooth or slightly scaly.

Almost all invasive SCC of the penis occurs on the glans, prepuce, and coronal sulcus. Invasive SCC usually presents as a 1- to 3-cm solitary nodule that is usually red or white in color (Fig. 12-40). The surface may be ulcerated in which case friable tissue with bleeding may be present at the base of the ulcer. Verrucous carcinoma, which accounts for only a small percentage of cases, presents as a nonscaling, cauliflower-like, globular mass that is clinically indistinguishable from giant condyloma (Buschke–Lowenstein tumor) (Fig. 12-41). Regional lymphadenopathy, which is sometimes due to inflammation

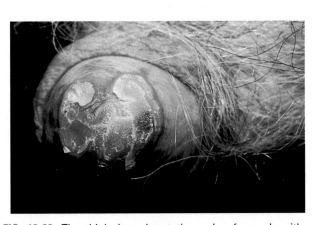

FIG. 12-38. The thick, hyperkeratotic scale of pseudoepitheliomatous, micaceous, and keratotic balanitis is characteristic of this probable premalignant condition.

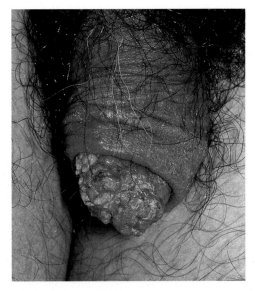

FIG. 12-40. This squamous cell carcinoma is skin colored and verrucous and was precipitated by human papillomavirus infection.

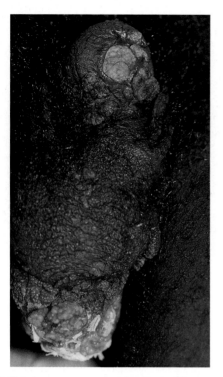

FIG. 12-41. This immunosuppressed patient with a carcinogenic human papillomavirus type has developed multiple verrucous, skin-colored nodules of squamous cell carcinoma.

SQUAMOUS CELL CARCINOMA IN MEN:	Diagnosis

HPV-related: flat-topped red, brown, or skin-colored papules and plaques; younger men; multiple lesions are present

- Location on penile shaft, pubis, and perianal tissue
- Biopsy shows in situ dysplasia (PIN); rarely invasive cancer

Non-HPV-related: pink, red, white or skin-colored papule, plaque ulcer or nodule; older men; only a solitary lesion is present

- Location on glans, coronal sulcus, inner aspect of prepuce
- Association with lichen sclerosus
- Biopsy shows either in situ dysplasia or invasive cancer

rather than metastases, is present in a majority of patients with invasive carcinoma.

Diagnosis

Though a diagnosis of penile SCC is frequently apparent on clinical findings, biopsy is always required for confirmation of the diagnosis. Histologically penile SCC is divided into in situ (PIN) cancer and invasive cancer. In a recent series, 20% of the specimens were in situ and 80% were invasive (48). Of the in situ lesions, 90% were positive for HPV DNA, and in the invasive lesions, 52% were positive for HPV DNA (48). Depending on various authors and their institutions, there are multiple histologic subtypes of penile SCC. Suffice it to say that those within the basaloid and warty category are highly likely to contain HPV DNA, whereas those in the keratinizing (differentiated) and verrucous carcinoma subtypes were much less likely to contain HPV DNA (48,49).

PIN on the shaft cannot clinically be differentiated from HPV-related warts. Likewise, verrucous carcinoma at any site cannot be clinically differentiated from HPV-related giant condyloma (Buschke–Lowenstein tumor). Seborrheic keratoses, psoriasis and lichen planus can appear very similar to PIN both on the shaft and on the glans and prepuce. Extramammary Paget disease also appears similar to PIN though the diameter of the plaques in the former is usually much greater.

Pathophysiology

There are multiple risk factors associated with the development of invasive penile SCC. The two most important in most studies have been smoking and phimosis (50). Other risk factors primarily relate to the acquisition of HPV and include early and numerous sex partners, penile–oral sex, and a history of anogenital warts (51).

As noted above, there appear to be two major pathways through which penile SCC develops: HPV-related and non-HPV-related. In the former, the same high-risk HPV types that are responsible for cervical carcinoma (notably HPV 16 and 18) appear to be responsible for nearly all of the PIN and about half of the invasive penile SCC. The situation for giant condylomata and verrucous carcinoma is more ambiguous. These two lesions are indistinguishable clinically and have many overlapping features histologically but low-risk HPV types (HPV 6 or 11) are almost always found in the giant condylomata, whereas the vast majority of verrucous carcinomas entirely lack HPV DNA (48).

The non-HPV pathway is less well understood but probably involves the presence of carcinogens (e.g., tobacco smoke, retained smegma) or underlying chronic inflammatory disease such as is found in lichen planus (52) and lichen sclerosus (balanitis xerotica obliterans) (53). The frequency with which lichen sclerosus transforms into penile cancer is hard to determine. Most series of patients with lichen sclerosus suggest that only a small proportion of patients go on to develop cancer (53), but in several studies of penile SCC, histologic evidence of lichen sclerosus was very frequently found in peritumoral tissue (54). This same conundrum occurs in vulvar SCC.

Management

Staging is appropriate for patients with penile SCC. This is carried out using the TNM staging system that has been in use since 1987 (55). Discussion in this chapter is restricted to in situ and minimally invasive carcinoma since the deeper forms require the involvement of oncologists and urologists. "Tis" is the TNM term used for the usual in situ carcinoma and "Ta" is used for in situ verrucous carcinoma. "T1" applies to carcinomas that invade only into subepithelial tissue without involving the corpus spongiosum or corpus cavernosum.

Local, wide excision represents the treatment of choice for Tis and Ta malignancies. Second-line therapy includes destructive methods (such as with laser ablation and electrosurgery) or possibly even topical therapy (such as fluorouracil and imiquimod) once biopsy has ruled out invasive disease. The problem of course with this approach is that one is depending on limited biopsy sampling to assume that invasion is not occurring elsewhere in the lesion.

Recurrence after excision is common, especially with verrucous carcinoma. Nevertheless, both Tis and Ta are expected to have essentially a 100% 5-year survival. Node dissections are not carried out for Tis and Ta malignancy. Excision represents the only acceptable treatment for T1 tumors. It is controversial as to whether sentinel node biopsy and/or node dissection should be offered to these patients. In any event, the 5-year disease-free survival rate remains very high with the exact rate depending on microscopic factors such as histologic grade and vascular and perineural invasion.

HPV infection tends to be multifocal, occurs in younger women, progresses from in situ disease more slowly, and has a better prognosis. On the other hand, invasive SCC not associated with HPV tends to be unifocal, occurs in older women, progresses more quickly from the in situ stage, and has a poorer prognosis.

Clinical Presentation

The category of vulvar SCC includes both in situ vulvar intraepithelial neoplasia (VIN) and invasive SCC. VIN and invasive SCC of the vulva account for slightly less than 1% of all cancers in women. The overall annual incidence of vulvar SCC in the United States is about 1.7/100,000 and this rate increases with age (56). The incidence of VIN cannot be determined accurately because controversy regarding terminology has led to data that is difficult to interpret. However, the rate is at least 1.2/100,000 and more likely double or triple this figure. VIN appears to increasing at a rate of about 3.5% per year, whereas the incidence of invasive SCC is nearly stable, rising only about 1% per year (57). Nearly all of the VIN increase is due to HPV-related VIN (58). VIN increases with age until about age 50 after which the incidence decreases (56,58). Unlike the situation for penile SCC, VIN and invasive SCC are more common in white women than in Blacks or Hispanics.

The clinical manifestations of VIN vary depending on whether they are HPV related or not. VIN associated with HPV infection occurs almost entirely in young women, 15 to 50 years of age. It is a multifocal process such that multiple lesions are present concomitantly (Fig. 12-42). The

SQUAMOUS CELL CARCINOMA IN MEN:	Management

In situ carcinoma (PIN)

- HPV-related: excision or destruction with electrosurgery, laser, or topical imiquimod
- Non-HPV-related: excision required

Invasive carcinoma

- Use TNM staging
- Excision for all
- If deep invasion, sentinel node biopsy; node dissection if positive

SQUAMOUS CELL CARCINOMA IN WOMEN

There are many similarities between squamous cell cancer of the genitalia in men and women. Specifically, both develop through two pathways: an HPV-related one and a non-HPV-related one. Invasive SCC associated with

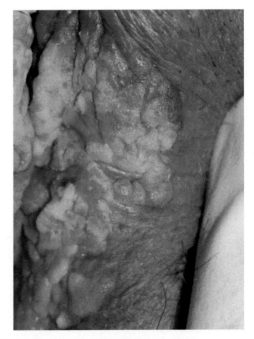

FIG. 12-42. Often, vulvar intraepithelial neoplasia shows several different morphologies; this patient has a confluent plaque of red, brown, whitened, and skin-colored papules.

lesions are flat-topped papules and plaques that vary in diameter from 0.5 to 3 cm. At times, these grow into confluence resulting in the presence of even larger plaques that may occupy a very large portion vulvar surface. The color is remarkably variable and may be pink, red, white, brown, black, or skin colored. The surface is usually smooth or slightly scaly but rarely can be slightly eroded. HPV-related VIN occurs both within the vestibule and on the keratinizing skin over the rest of the anogenital area. The lesions are usually asymptomatic.

Non-HPV-related VIN presents much differently. These lesions are most often solitary and occur more often in older women. They occur as plaques or nodules that are usually 2 to 5 cm in diameter. Palpable scale, erosion, and/or crusting are frequently present especially when VIN occurs on lesions of lichen sclerosus or lichen planus. The lesions are red, white, or brown in color and they occur mostly within the vestibule when VIN is associated with lichen sclerosus or lichen planus. In other settings, VIN can be found on keratinizing skin anywhere in the anogenital area. Lesions overlying concomitant lichen sclerosus and erosive lichen planus are usually associated with itching, burning, or pain. Lesions arising on normal appearing skin are usually asymptomatic.

Invasive SCC develops in association with untreated HPV-related VIN in at least 10% of patients (59). This progression is appreciably more common in women than it is in men with untreated HPV-related PIN. Early in its evolution minimally invasive SCC cannot be distinguished clinically from VIN. Non-HPV-related invasive SCC mostly occurs against a background of lichen sclerosus (Fig. 12-43) or lichen planus but rarely it can arise de novo

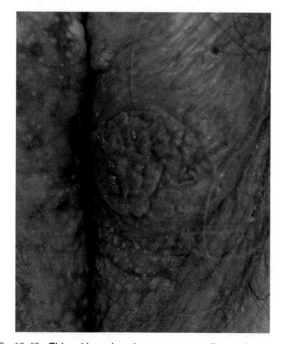

FIG. 12-43. This skin-colored squamous cell carcinoma occurred in a setting of lichen sclerosus in an elderly woman.

from normal-appearing mucous membrane or skin. Advanced lesions occur as white, red, or skin-colored plaques or nodules. The surface is often ulcerated with the ulcer cavity containing friable tissue that bleeds easily. Itching and/or pain may occur in some patients.

Verrucous carcinoma is identical in clinical appearance to giant condylomata (Buschke–Lowenstein tumors). At one time it was thought that verrucous carcinoma represented malignant transformation of HPV-related giant condylomata but this hypothesis has fallen into disfavor for two reasons: (1) giant condylomata are associated only with low-risk HPV types (mostly HPV 6 and 11) and thus should not progress to cancer and (2) polymerase chain reaction (PCR) studies of verrucous carcinoma rarely reveal the presence of any HPV DNA.

Diagnosis

Clinically it is not possible to differentiate nonulcerated forms of HPV-related VIN from anogenital warts and thus these lesions must be biopsied. If the lesions are nodular or ulcerated, a diagnosis of invasive SCC is likely, but here too, biopsy is necessary. Because of potential sampling error, it is advisable to take several biopsies from different parts of the lesion or from different lesions if multiple lesions are present. It is especially important to biopsy any persistently elevated or eroded area in lichen sclerosus and lichen planus that has not responded to appropriate therapy within a month or so.

Microscopically, and by analogy with cervical in situ carcinoma, VIN was originally subdivided into VIN 1, VIN 2, and VIN 3. However, in 2004 the International Society for the Study of Vulvovaginal Disease (ISSVD) adopted a new classification (60). This new classification instituted a number of changes. First, it deleted the category of VIN 1 based on three considerations: VIN 1 was not a reproducible histologic finding, it was almost always related to infection with low-risk HPV, and it uncommonly progressed to in situ or invasive cancer. Second, VIN 2 and VIN 3 were combined into a single category of ungraded VIN based on the recognition that the separate identification of VIN 2 and VIN 3 was not very reproducible when sections were viewed by multiple pathologists. Third, VIN itself was divided into two categories: "usual" VIN and "differentiated" VIN. The committee indicated that usual VIN was mostly HPV-related, multifocal, and slowly progressive, whereas differentiated VIN was usually non-HPV-related, progressed more rapidly, and commonly occurred superimposed on a background of lichen sclerosus. This new classification has become accepted by some, but certainly not by all, clinicians. Some experts favor the concepts contained in it but others favor the use of a modified Bethesda classification (low-grade VIN for VIN 1 lesions and high-grade VIN for VIN 2 and 3), while still others would like to continue on with the current WHO classification of VIN 1, 2, and 3 (61).

In terms of differential diagnosis, VIN arising from normal skin must be differentiated from anogenital warts, psoriasis, lichen planus, and seborrheic keratoses. It is difficult to separately identify VIN overlying lichen sclerosus and lichen planus from those diseases themselves. In all of these situations, biopsy is required. The well-developed nodular and ulcerated lesions of VSCC are usually clinically distinctive but here, too, biopsy is necessary.

SQUAMOUS CELL CARCINOMA IN WOMEN:	Diagnosis

HPV-related: flat-topped red, brown, or skin-colored papules and plaques; younger women; multiple lesions are present

- Location on vestibule, labia majora, perivulvar, and perianal sites
- Biopsy shows in situ carcinoma (VIN); invasion occasionally present

Non-HPV-related: pink, red, or white papule, nodule, or ulcer; older women; only a solitary lesion is present

- Location within vestibule and labia minora; occasionally elsewhere
- Frequent association with lichen sclerosus or lichen planus
- Biopsy often shows invasion

Pathophysiology

As indicated above, there are two pathways relating to the development of vulvar SCC: an HPV-related pathway and a non-HPV-related pathway (62). These two pathways correlate well, but not perfectly, with separate histologic patterns: a warty/basaloid pattern in HPV-related disease and a differentiated (keratinizing) pattern for non-HPV-related disease (61).

The HPV-related pathway involves infection with the same high-risk HPV types (especially that of HPV 16) responsible for cervical carcinoma (63,64). This type of infection leads first to the development of warty and/or basaloid VIN followed in some cases by the development of invasive carcinoma with those same histologic features. PCR studies reveal HPV DNA to be resent in the vast majority of warty and basaloid VIN and in a somewhat smaller percentage of invasive carcinomas with warty or basaloid histology.

The non-HPV-related pathway is less clear. Some, but not all, differentiated VIN arises in the setting of lichen sclerosus or erosive lichen planus (61,62,65). It is possible that there is an association with other chronic inflammatory disease as well. In this regard, there is a very high frequency of squamous cell hyperplasia (the acanthotic changes found in lichen simplex chronicus, LSC) in the peritumoral tissue in some malignancies, thus raising the possibility that long-term inflammation from chronic scratching might be involved (62). However, an alternative explanation is possible. It is quite difficult to reliably separate the histologic appearance of early differentiated VIN from that of the squamous cell hyperplasia present in LSC, and for this reason it is possible that what has been termed "squamous hyperplasia" is in reality early differentiated VIN. It also should be noted that DNA for high-risk HPV types is found in a small percentage of cases of differentiated VIN and associated invasive SCC but it is not known what role, if any, they might play in causation.

There are multiple clinical risk factors associated with the development of VIN and invasive SCC. Smoking is the most important of these for both HPV-related and non-HPV-related malignancy. Factors specifically important for HPV-related VIN revolve around behavior likely to lead to HPV infection such as early age at sexual debut, multiple sex partners, history of abnormal Pap smears, and history of previous anogenital warts. Factors specifically important for non-HPV-related VIN include the presence of lichen sclerosus and erosive lichen planus.

Management

Spontaneous regression of HPV-related VIN has been reported in both some women under age 35 and in some patients following parturition (59). This, along with a very low likelihood of malignant progression in this relatively young population, suggests that it would be reasonable to follow very young patients without treatment for up to 1 year. For those over 30 or 35 years of age, and for differentiated type VIN, local excision shortly after diagnosis is the treatment of choice. There is controversy regarding the appropriate width of margins for these excisions. Wider margins may be theoretically preferable but this must be balanced by considerations regarding greater architectural distortion and its effect on patient quality of life (66). Generally, it is recommended that differentiated VIN be treated with more aggressive surgery, including wider margins, than would be used for HPV-related VIN (67). Regardless of margin width, recurrence rates are high and re-excision will fairly frequently be required (68).

Laser ablation may be considered for HPV-related VIN, but generally the results are inferior to those obtained by excision (67). There are scattered reports of successful treatment with photodynamic therapy and medical therapy using topical imiquimod. These approaches offer potential benefits in terms of tissue sparing and the prevention of architectural distortion but it currently appears that the results are less good than with excision (69).

The prognosis for VIN depends on patient age, immunocompetency, and whether the VIN is HPV-related or is of the differentiated type. As noted above, spontaneous resolution occurs with some frequency in the youngest patients and following some pregnancies but is unlikely after the age of 35 (59). Patients who are immunocompromised and those with differentiated VIN appear to have an appreciably poorer prognosis. There are two large series and one meta-analysis describing the prognosis of VIN after excisional surgery (59,67,68). The data in these studies indicate that for those patients with clear margins, there was a 15% to 20% chance of recurrence. About 5% of patients thought to have VIN, and who were treated with excision, were found to have invasive cancer once the entire surgical specimen had been microscopically sectioned. Approximately 4% to 7% of patients followed prospectively after treatment of VIN developed invasive carcinoma.

When invasive SCC is discovered on biopsy, staging should be carried out using the newly revised International Federation of Gynecology and Obstetrics (FIGO) guidelines (70). Stage Ia patients (those with lesions confined to the vulva, less than 2 cm in diameter and with 1 mm or less of invasion) have minimal risk of nodal metastases and have an excellent prognosis (71). Thus, local excision as is carried out for VIN is sufficient. Patients with Stage Ib carcinoma (those with lesions still confined to vulvar tissue but with larger than 2 cm or more than 1 mm of invasion) should be offered sentinel node biopsy, as this procedure offers a sensitive and specific means of determining the presence or absence of node metastases. Patients with negative nodes have a very good prognosis and these patients probably do not require lymphadenectomy (72). Treatment of patients with positive nodes and those with Stages II, III, or IV disease falls outside of the scope of this chapter.

As indicated in two recent studies, the prognosis for patients with invasive SCC depends on several factors (73,74). Older patients do less well with a sharp fall in survival after age 70. And, not surprisingly, those with positive lymph nodes had a much worse survival than those with negative nodes. Other important adverse factors included tumor size, ulceration of the initial lesion, and TNM classification grade. Cancers arising on a background of usual VIN (HPV-related VIN) had a lower recurrence rate than those arising from differentiated VIN (75). This difference was even more notable when an associated vulvar disease such as lichen sclerosus was concurrently present in the perilesional tissue of differentiated VIN (75).

An even better approach to the problem of HPV-related SCC would be to prevent it from occurring in the first place. Some optimism in this regard is warranted. A bivalent and a quadrivalent vaccine designed to prevent infection from HPV16 and HPV18, the two most common and most important high-risk HPV types, are now available. These are expected to both prevent infection and also to prevent the development of in situ and invasive SCC associated with those infections. In a recent large, placebo-controlled trial, the quadrivalent vaccine was 100% effective in preventing VIN 1, 2, and 3 (16). These are somewhat preliminary results but the future appears very promising. Additional material regarding HPV vaccines can be found in the section on genital warts.

SQUAMOUS CELL CARCINOMA IN WOMEN:	Management

In situ carcinoma (VIN)

- HPV-related (usual VIN): excision; consider electrosurgery, laser ablation, or topical imiquimod after biopsy; 1-year observation OK under age 30
- Non-HPV-related (differentiated VIN): excision only

Invasive carcinoma

- Use FIGO staging
- Excision for all
- If greater than 1 mm invasion, sentinel node biopsy, node dissection if positive

BASAL CELL CARCINOMA

Basal cell carcinoma (BCC), the most frequently diagnosed of all skin tumors on sun exposed skin, is uncommonly encountered on the genitalia.

Clinical Presentation

BCC occurring on the anogenital skin is encountered infrequently though the incidence, possibly due to better surveillance, seems to be increasing (76). These tumors account for about 2% to 3% of all vulvar cancers and 0.3% to 2% of BCC located at all sites. Women appear to be affected somewhat more frequently than men. BCC is more often found in the older population. The average age at diagnosis is about 70 and lesions tend to have been present for a long period of time prior to diagnosis. The age at diagnosis seems to be decreasing presumably due to better awareness and surveillance (77). Almost all lesions are solitary and they usually appear as skin-colored or pink 1.0- to 3.0-cm plaques or nodules. Occasionally tan or even brown hues are noted due to increased melanin pigmentation (Fig. 12-44) (78). Intact lesions are smooth surfaced but about 30% of the tumors are ulcerated with rolled margins. Most are asymptomatic though occasionally mild pruritus or bleeding is noted. BCC occur only on nonmucosal surfaces of the genitalia. In women, they are mostly located on the labia majora, usually on the lateral side (Fig. 12-45). In men, scrotal lesions are more common than penile shaft lesions (Fig. 12-46). In both sexes, BCC may occur in the perianal area.

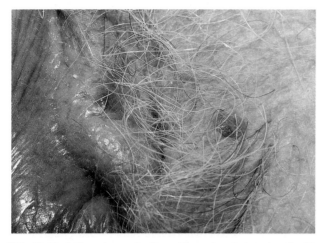

FIG. 12-44. Although most often skin colored, basal cell skin cancers may have flecks of pigment or even grayish color.

Diagnosis

Occasionally the correct diagnosis is suspected clinically but most lesions require biopsy for identification. The histologic appearance is usually quite characteristic, but occasionally the pathologist has trouble distinguishing BCC from other hair follicle-derived tumors. Disorders commonly considered in differential diagnosis include SCC and intradermal nevi. Less often other skin-colored lesions described in this chapter will need to be considered.

BASAL CELL CARCINOMA:	Diagnosis

- Older men and women
- Solitary pink or skin-colored plaque, papule, or nodule
- Lesion may be ulcerated
- Occurs only on keratinizing (nonmucosal) skin
- Location: labia majora in women; penis and scrotum in men; perianal area for both sexes
- Biopsy for confirmation

Pathophysiology

Chronic ultraviolet light exposure plays a very important role for those BCC that occur on sun-exposed skin. Obviously this is not the situation for genital lesions. All patients with Gorlin syndrome (nevoid basal cell carcinoma syndrome) and many with sporadic BCC have mutations in genes (especially the patched and smoothened genes) that are part of the sonic hedgehog signaling pathway and it is likely that patients with anogenital BCC also do. In this regard, it is interesting that at least one patient with a genital BCC developed it in the setting of Gorlin syndrome (79). It is likely that such mutations act in

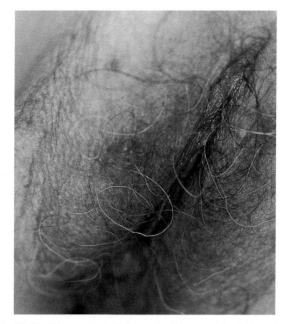

FIG. 12-45. This pearly nodule on the labium majus is basal cell carcinoma despite the lack of chronic sun exposure.

concert with other environmental factors such as chronic irritation and inflammation to induce the development of malignancy.

Management

Excision represents the treatment of choice. The recurrence rate is fairly high but most recurrences develop in cases where the histologic margins were not clear (77).

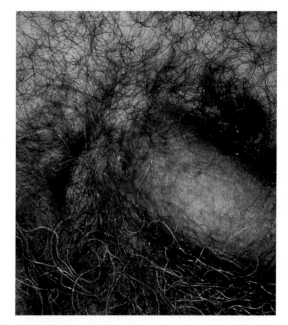

FIG. 12-46. Skin-colored basal cell carcinomas can be secondarily inflamed when ulceration occurs, as has occurred here at the base of the shaft of the penis.

For this reason, Mohs micrographic surgery should be considered as it combines maximum tissue sparing with the ability to obtain microscopically documented tumor-free margins at the time of the initial procedure. Topical application of imiquimod cream is theoretically attractive on the basis of excellent cosmetic outcome but it is not approved for nodular BCC and experience with its use for genital BCC is limited.

The overall prognosis for BCC occurring at nongenital sites is excellent as it rarely results in metastasis. However, metastases have been reported in about a dozen patients with genital BCC. This number seems to be excessively high given the relative infrequency with which genital BCCs occur. However, this apparent excess may be explained by the observation that patients with genital BCCs seem to have had their tumors longer, present with larger lesions, and are appreciably older than patients with lesions on other parts of the body.

BASAL CELL CARCINOMA:	**Management**

- Excision for all
- Consider Mohs micrographic surgery for excision as recurrence rates are fairly high
- Risk of metastasis is small
- No sentinel node biopsy
- No node dissection

GENITAL EDEMA

Genital edema occurs as a result of fluid build-up in the subcutaneous tissue of the genitalia. The fluid may be related to plasma or lymph. The former is termed angioedema and is generally transient (acute genital edema), whereas the latter is termed lymphedema and is persistent (chronic genital edema). The term elephantiasis is often used for lymphedema that is chronic and massive. In some instances, especially when vessel-damaging inflammation is present, angioedema may transition into lymphedema blurring the line of identification between these two forms of edema.

For the most part, the clinical presentation in both forms of edema is quite similar in that the tissue of the genitalia is distended to greater or lesser degree. However, in acute genital edema, the tissue on palpation is softer, "pits" more easily, and is more variable in duration and extent. Chronic lymphedema, on the other hand, is more firm on palpation, pits less easily, lasts longer, and is more likely to be stable in severity and extent.

Both forms of edema are usually asymptomatic though with sudden distention, stretching of the tissue may lead to some pain. Acute genital edema due to allergic reactions may be associated with varying degrees of itching.

Acute Genital Edema (Angioedema)

Most instances of acute genital edema are due to allergic reactions as a result of topical applications or systemic ingestion of products to which the patient, because of prior exposure, has developed immune reactivity. This form of edema develops over minutes to hours and evolves over hours to days. The tissue returns to its former normal size and appearance after each episode of edema.

The most important and dangerous forms of acute genital edema are those that occur as a result of immunoglobulin E (IgE) reactions. Individuals with such reactions are potentially liable to develop anaphylaxis. The two most common allergens causing genital IgE-mediated reactions are latex and semen. Latex allergy occurs in about 4% of health care workers and about 1% of the general public (80). Awareness of the problem caused by latex allergy has led to a decrease in the use of latex products, notably latex-containing examination gloves, and the prevalence of latex reactions seem to be decreasing. However, latex still is present in most condoms and some contraceptive diaphragms and therefore genital edema due to these sources is still a potential problem. Confirmation of suspected latex allergy as a cause for genital edema can be obtained through radioallergosorbent (RAST) testing and skin prick tests.

There are somewhat fewer than 100 reports of genital edema in women who were allergic to their male partner's semen (seminal plasma) but it is probably much more prevalent than this figure suggests (81). Semen allergy should be suspected when vulvovaginal symptoms, especially that of vulvar swelling, occur shortly after unprotected coitus. A suspected diagnosis can usually be confirmed through the observation that no reaction occurs after an intercourse in which a condom is used. Irritant and allergic reaction to *Candida* sp. should be considered in the differential diagnosis of suspected semen allergy. Treatment can be carried out by means of subcutaneous immunotherapy or intravaginal graded challenge (81).

Genital edema as part of a more widespread reaction can also occur with IgE allergy to ingested foods such as peanuts and shell fish. Prophylactic and/or therapeutic use of oral antihistamines may be of some help in these IgE-mediated reactions but they are seldom sufficient by themselves. Consultation with an allergist is usually desirable.

Genital edema also occurs in patients with presumed non-IgE allergic reactions to topically applied products. This type of reaction generally develops a type 4, cell-mediated immune response. Most often, this presents as a form of contact dermatitis with attendant eczematous morphology but a few cases of anaphylaxis have occurred due to the application of the common topical antibiotics, neomycin and bacitracin. Such reactions can result in genital edema but they differ from the IgE reactions in that they occur many hours after exposure, are accompanied by more redness, and may have an eczematous appearance in addition to the genital swelling. These types of contact dermatitis and the products that most frequently cause them are covered in Chapter 4.

Patients with hereditary angioedema due to a deficiency in C1 inhibitor may develop acute genital edema as part of a more widespread systemic reaction. Genital edema can also occur in the setting of infection most notably cellulitis in both sexes and in women with vulvovaginal candidiasis and males with epididymitis. Genital edema accompanied by malaise, chills, fever, and WBC elevation may indicate the initial symptoms and signs of necrotizing fasciitis (Fournier gangrene). This represents an impending medical emergency that should result in hospitalization and consultation with experts.

Rarely, acute genital edema occurs in settings of trauma, notably that due to long stints of bicycle riding. Traumatic edema is usually apparent from history but can also occur as a result of unrecognized hair coiling and "strangulation." This most often involves the clitoris in women and the glans penis in men. Other infrequently encountered instances of acute genital edema occur through increased hydrostatic fluid pressure such as may be present in peritoneal dialysis and pregnancy, especially pregnancy with preeclampsia. Vulvar edema frequently is seen in the immediate postpartum period and occasionally this persists for quite long time. A few cases of nonallergic genital edema occurring after the oral ingestion of an angiotensin-converting enzyme inhibitor have been reported.

Acute idiopathic scrotal edema (AISE) is an uncommon condition that has mostly been reported in the urology literature (82). It occurs in mid to late childhood and presents with an acute onset of asymptomatic redness and edema of the scrotal sac. The involvement is unilateral in 90% of the cases and the entire process generally resolves spontaneously in a matter of a few days. The cause is unknown and there is no specific recommended therapy. It must be differentiated from testicular torsion, another common cause of scrotal swelling in young boys.

Chronic Genital Edema (Elephantiasis)

Chronic genital edema occurs as a result of lymphatic flow disruption secondary to infection, noninfectious inflammation, surgery, radiation therapy, congenital abnormalities, and as a seemingly idiopathic process. In all of these situations, the process is disfiguring and extraordinarily troublesome to patients both physically and psychologically. Unfortunately, treatment is never curative and is only rarely of significant help.

Congenital Abnormalities

Milroy disease is a rare congenital abnormality in which the lymph vessels of the lower portion of the body fail to develop correctly. The legs are primarily involved and the problem becomes clinically apparent shortly after birth or in adolescence (lymphedema praecox). Interestingly, edema only rarely occurs in the genitalia.

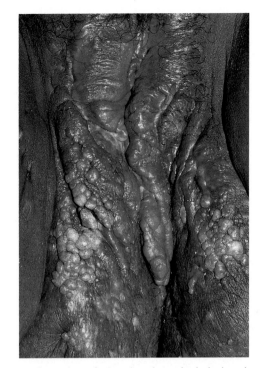

FIG. 12-47. Sequelae of chronic edema include lymphangiectasias, dilated lymphatic vessels that protrude through the surface and appear as vesicles. In this extreme case, these dilated lymphatic channels look like multilobular genital warts.

Lymphangioma circumscriptum is a congenital abnormality in which embryonic lymphatic sacs do not connect appropriately to the lymph vessels. It occurs anywhere in the body but sometimes arises in the inguinal region where it can involve the genitalia. Clinically it appears as a localized cluster of small superficial vesicles containing clear, or sometimes bloody, fluid. This condition may be associated with deep underlying lymphatic abnormalities (cavernous lymphangioma) in which case superficial destruction of lymphatic vessels will be regularly followed by recurrence of the cutaneous vesicles. Patients with this process are very prone to the development of bacterial infection. When this occurs, lymph vessels are further compromised and genital edema is quite likely to develop. An acquired form of lymphangioma circumscriptum (more appropriately termed lymphangiectasia) can arise in any setting of underlying chronic edema (Fig. 12-47). It seems to occur with particular frequency in patients with anogenital cutaneous Crohn disease.

Surgery and Radiation

Surgery involving the lower abdomen, pelvis, inguinal, or anogenital areas can result in lymphatic vessel disruption. This is particularly true when the surgery is extensive such as might be undertaken for malignancy occurring in these areas. Radiation alone, but more commonly when used in conjunction with surgery, can cause similar problems. The resultant chronic lymphedema can then become a focus for recurring bacterial infection that compounds the problem.

Infection

When lymphedema is present, there is a local reduction in immune response to bacterial infection (83). As such, lymphedema can be viewed as a *locus minoris resistentiae*. When cellulitis develops, as it frequently does, there is further destruction of lymphatics and a vicious cycle ensues. Surprisingly, the cutaneous infection appears to arise spontaneously without requiring a break in the overlying skin or the presence of appreciable trauma. These recurring episodes of cellulitis are primarily due to streptococcal infection. The involved area becomes pink and slightly tender. Usually there are no systemic symptoms and signs; if they do occur, they are very mild. As a result, patients are often unaware that the area of lymphedema is recurrently infected. Unfortunately, documenting the presence of infection is difficult as there is no reliable way of obtaining cultures. The cellulitis responds very well to antibiotics such as dicloxacillin or cephalexin, but by the time the treatment is started, another round of damage to lymphatic vessels has occurred. I agree with others that the best approach is to place these patients on constant antibacterial treatment with either oral or intramuscular penicillin (84). It is my belief that this infectious problem is both one of the most frequent and one of the most unrecognized causes of "idiopathic" chronic genital edema.

In lesser developed countries, infection with the nematode *Wuchereria bancrofti* causes filariasis with resultant elephantiasis of the male genitalia. Chronic, untreated infection with *Chlamydia trachomatis* (lymphogranuloma venereum) and *Klebsiella granulomatis* (granuloma inguinale) regularly lead to genital edema.

Noninfectious Inflammation

Two disorders, *hidradenitis suppurativa* and *Crohn disease*, when they occur in the anogenital area are notoriously likely to cause chronic genital inflammation and significant genital edema (Figs. 12-48 and 12-49). These diseases are covered elsewhere in this book and review of those sections will provide information on their clinical manifestations, prognosis, and therapy.

Sarcoidosis is rarely encountered in the anogenital area but when it does occur in this location, it may be confused histologically with Crohn disease and thus be inaccurately described as a cause of genital edema. The granulomas in some of the patients with *Melkersson–Rosenthal syndrome* (see below) can be very similar microscopically with those occurring in sarcoidosis and Crohn disease. It is not clear what, if any relationship Melkersson–Rosenthal syndrome has with these two conditions.

Idiopathic Chronic Genital Edema

Melkersson–Rosenthal syndrome (orofacial granulomatosis) was originally described as a syndrome involving

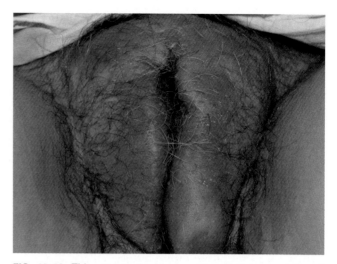

FIG. 12-48. This woman had only a few draining nodules of hidradenitis suppurativa, but she has impressive firm edema.

granulomatous swelling (usually unilateral) of the upper lip, lingua plicata, and facial nerve palsy. Asymptomatic granulomatous edema of the lip, without the other two components, is believed to be a monosymptomatic form of the disease and is encountered fairly frequently. Identical granulomatous edema involving the genitalia has been reported in about 30 patients. Many of these patients also had orofacial involvement, suggesting that that these two processes are all part of the same syndrome (85).

The majority of the patients described in the medical literature have been women with vulvar involvement; there have been only a few cases involving the male

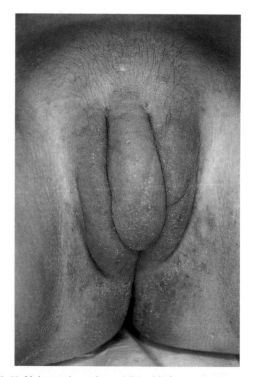

FIG. 12-49. Vulvar edema in a child with Crohn disease.

genitalia (85). In the often-overlooked report of Murphy et al., most of the patients had, or subsequently developed, Crohn disease (85). This association is further supported by a recent report in which 30% of patients with orofacial involvement also had Crohn disease (86). These data suggest the possibility that both "idiopathic" orofacial and genital granulomatous disease represent a forme fruste of Crohn disease. For this reason, patients without symptomatic Crohn disease at the time that genital granulomatous edema is first recognized must be followed with the realization that in some instances Crohn disease will eventually develop.

The best treatment for the Melkersson–Rosenthal form of genital granulomatous edema is repeated intralesional injections of triamcinalone acetonide (Kenalog) with or without accompanying oral administration of nonsteroidal anti-inflammatory agents such as dapsone, clofazamine, dapsone, hydroxychloroquine, metronidazole, or methotrexate (86,87). If this approach fails, oral prednisone or IV infliximab might be considered.

REFERENCES

1. Trottier H, Burchell AN. Epidemiology of mucosal human papillomavirus infection and associated diseases. *Public Health Genomics*. 2009;12:291–307.

2. Doerfler D, Bernhause A, Kottmel A, et al. Human papilloma virus infection prior to coitarche. *Am J Obstet Gynecol*. 2009;200:487.e1–487.e5.

3. Tobian AA, Serwadda D, Quinn TC, et al. Male circumcision for the prevention of HSV-2 and HPV infections and syphilis. *N Engl J Med*. 2009;360:1298–1309.

4. Castellsagué X, Cohet C, Puig-Tintoré LM, et al. Epidemiology and cost of treatment of genital warts in Spain. *Eur J Public Health*. 2009;19:106–110.

5. Garland SM, Steben M, Sings HL, et al. Natural history of genital warts: analysis of the placebo arm of 2 randomized phase III trials of a quadravalent human papillomavirus (types 6, 11, 16, and 18) vaccine. *J Infect Dis*. 2009;199:805–814.

6. Insinga RP, Dasbach EJ, Elbasha EH. Epidemiologic natural history and clinical management of human papillomavirus (HPV) disease: a critical and systematic review of the literature in the development of an HPV dynamic transmission model. *BMC Infect Dis*. 2009;9:119.

7. Mammas IN, Sourvinos G, Spandidos D. Human papilloma virus (HPV) infection in children and adolescents. *Eur J Pediatr*. 2009;168:267–273.

8. Cook K, Brownell I. Treatments for genital warts. *J Drugs Dermatol*. 2008;7:801–807.

9. Scheinfeld N, Lehman DS. An evidence-based review of medical and surgical treatments of genital warts. *Dermatol Online J*. 2006;12:5.

10. Yen J, Chen SL, Wang HN, et al. Meta-analysis of 5% imiquimod and 0.5% podophyllotoxin in the treatment of condylomata accuminata. *Dermatology*. 2006;213:218–223.

11. Meltzer SH, Monk BJ, Tewari KS. Green tea catechins for treatment of external genital warts. *Am J Obstet Gynecol*. 2009;200:233.e1–233.e7.

12. Taner ZM, Taskiran C, Onan AM, et al. Therapeutic value of trichloroacetic acid in the treatment of genital warts on the external female genitalia. *J Reprod Med*. 2007;52:521–525.

13. Strefanski C, Katzouranis I, Lagogianni E, et al. Comparison of cryotherapy to imiquimod 5% in the treatment of anogenital warts. *Int J STD AIDS*. 2008;19:441–444.

14. Aynaud O, Buffet M, Roman P, et al. Study of persistence and recurrence rates in 106 patients with condyloma and intraepithelial neoplasia after CO_2 laser treatment. *Eur J Dermatol*. 2008;18:153–158.

15. Paavonen J, Naud P, Salmeron J, et al. Efficacy of human papillomavirus (HPV)-16/18 ASO4-adjuvanted vaccine against cervical infection and precancer caused by oncogenic HPV types (PATRICIA): final analysis of a double-blind, rondomised study in young women. *Lancet*. 2009;375:301–314.

16. Majewski S, Bosch FX, Dillner J, et al. The impact of a quadrivalent human papillomavirus (types 6, 11, 16, 18) virus-like particle vaccine in European women aged 16–24. *J Eur Acad Dermatol Venereol*. 2009;23:1147–1155.

17. Future II Study Group. Quadrivalent vaccine against human papillomavirus to prevent high-grade cervical lesions. *N Engl J Med*. 2007;356:1915–1927.

18. Muñoz N, Manalastas R Jr, Pitisuttithum P, et al. Safety, immunogenicity, and efficacy of quadrivalent human papillomavirus (types 6, 11, 16, 18) recombinant vaccine in women aged 24–45 years: a randomized, double-blind trial. *Lancet*. 2009;373:1949–1957.

19. Brown J, Janniger CK, Schwartz RA, et al. Childhood molluscum contagiosum. *Int J Dermatol*. 2006;45:93–99.

20. Kyriakis KP, Palamaras I, Terzoudi S, et al. Case detection rates of molluscum contagiosum. *Pediatr Dermatol*. 2007;24:198–199.

21. Laxmisha C, Thappa DM, Jaisankar T. Clinical profile of molluscum contagiosum in children versus adults. *Dermatol Online J*. 2003;9:1.

22. Reynolds MG, Holman RC, Christensen KLY, et al. The incidence of molluscum contagiosum among American Indians and Alaska Natives. *PLoS ONE*. 2009;4:e5255.

23. Dohil MA, Lin P, Lee J, et al. The epidemiology of molluscum contagiosum in children. *J Am Acad Dermatol*. 2006;54:47–54.

24. Gur I. The epidemiology of molluscum contagiosum in HIV-seropositive patients: a unique entity of insignificant finding. *Int J STD AIDS*. 2008;19:503–506.

25. Cathcart S, Colos J, Morrell DS. Parental satisfaction, efficacy, and adverse events in 54 patients treated with cantharidin for molluscum contagiosum infection. *Clin Pediatr (Phila)*. 2009;48:161–165.

26. Coloe J, Morrell DS. Cantharidin use among pediatric dermatologists in the treatment of molluscum contagiosum. *Pediatr Dermatol*. 2009;26:405–408.

27. Bard S, Shiman MI, Bellman B, et al. Treatment of facial molluscum contagiosum with trichloroacetic acid. *Pediatr Dermatol*. 2009;26:425–426.

28. Metkar A, Pande S, Khopkar U. An open, nonrandomized, comparative study of imiquimod 5% cream versus 10% potassium hydroxide solution in the treatment of molluscum contagiosum. *Indian J Dermatol Venereol Leprol*. 2008;74:614–618.

29. Hanna D, Hatami A, Powell J, et al. A prospective randomized trial comparing the efficacy and adverse effects of four recognized treatments of molluscum contagiosum in children. *Pediatr Dermatol*. 2006;23:574–579.

30. Workowski KA, Beerman SM. Sexually transmitted diseases treatment guidelines, 2006. *MMWR*. 2006;55:1–94.

31. White JA. Manifestations and management of lymphogranuloma venereum. *Curr Opin Infect Dis.* 2009;22:57–66.

32. Sethi G, Allason-Jones E, Richens J, et al. Lymphogranuloma venereum presenting as a genital ulceration and inguinal syndrome in men who have sex with men in London, UK. *Sex Transm Infect.* 2009;85:165–170.

33. Sion-Vardy N, Osyntsov L, Cagnano E, et al. Unexpected location of pilonidal sinuses. *Clin Exp Dermatol.* 2009;34:e599–e601. [Epub ahead of print].

34. Baker T, Barclay D, Ballard C. Pilonidal cyst involving the clitoris: a case report. *J Low Genit Tract Dis.* 2008;12:127–129.

35. Patil S, Sultan AH, Thakar R. Bartholi's cysts and abscesses. *J Obstet Gynaecol.* 2007;27:241–245.

36. Wechter NE, Wu JM, Marzano D, et al. Management of Bartholin duct cysts and abscesses: a systematic review. *Obstet Gynecol Surv.* 2009;64:395–404.

37. Jowkar F, Fallahi A, Namazi MR. Is there any relation between serum insulin and insulin-like growth factor-1 in non-diabetic patients with skin tag? *J Eur Acad Dermatol Venereol.* 2010;24:73–74.

38. Pascual-Castroviejo I, Lopez-Pereira P, Savasta S, et al. Neurofibromatosis type 1 with external genitalia involvement presentation of 4 patients. *Pediatr Surg.* 2008;43:1998–2003.

39. Al-Daraji WI, Wagner B, Ali RBM, et al. Sebaceous hyperplasia of the vulva: a clinicopathological case report with a review of the literature. *J Clin Pathol.* 2007;60:835–837.

40. Ena P, Origa D, Massarelli G. Sebaceous gland hyperplasia of the foreskin. *Clin Exp Dermatol.* 2009;34:372–374.

41. Bormate AB Jr, LeBoit PE, McCalmont TH. Perifollicular xanthomatosis as the hallmark of axillary Fox–Fordyce disease: an evaluation of histopathologic features of 7 cases. *Arch Dermatol.* 2008;144:1020–1024.

42. Macarenco RS, Garces JC. Dilation of apocrine glands. A forgotten but helpful histopathological clue to the diagnosis of axillary Fox–Fordyce disease. *Am J Dermatopathol.* 2009;31:393–397.

43. Scurry J, van der Putte SC, Pyman J, et al. Mammary-like gland adenoma of the vulva: review of 46 cases. *Pathology.* 2009;41:372–378.

44. Rosen T, Hwong H. Sclerosing lymphangitis of the penis. *J Am Acad Dermatol.* 2003;49:916–918.

45. Hernandez BY, Barnholtz-Sloan J, German RR, et al. Burden of invasive squamous cell carcinoma of the penis in the United States, 1998–2003. *Cancer.* 2008;113:2883–2891.

46. Rippenstrop JM, Joslyn SA, Konety BR. Squamous cell carcinoma of the penis: evaluation of the data from the surveillance, epidemiology, and end results program. *Cancer.* 2004;101:1357–1363.

47. Perry D, Lynch PJ, Fazel N. Pseudoepitheliomatous, keratotic, and micaceous balanitis: a case report and review of the literature. *Dermatol Nurs.* 2008;20:117–120.

48. Krustrup D, Jensen HL, van den Brule AJC, et al. Histological characteristics of human papilloma-virus-positive and negative invasive and *in situ* squamous cell tumors of the penis. *Int J Exp Pathol.* 2009;90:182–189.

49. Backes DM, Kurman RJ, Pimenta JM, et al. Systematic review of human papillomavirus prevalence in invasive penile cancer. *Cancer Causes Control.* 2009;20:449–457.

50. Daling JR, Madeleine MM, Johnson LG, et al. Penile cancer: importance of circumcision, human papillomavirus and smoking in in situ and invasive disease. *Int J Cancer.* 2005;116:606–616.

51. Madsen BS, van den Brule AJ, Jensen HL, et al. Risk factors for squamous cell carcinoma of the penis—population-based case–control study in Denmark. *Cancer Epidemiol Biomarkers Prev.* 2008;17:2683–2691.

52. Hoshi A, Usui Y, Terachi T. Penile carcinoma originating from lichen planus on glans penis. *Urology.* 2008;71:816–817.

53. Ranjan N, Singh SK. Malignant transformation of penile lichen sclerosus: exactly how common is it? *Int J Dermatol.* 2008;47:1308–1309.

54. Pietrzak P, Hadway P, Corbishley CM, et al. Is the association between balanitis xerotica obliterans and penile carcinoma underestimated? *BJU Int.* 2006;98:74–76.

55. Leijte JAP, Gallee M, Antonini N, et al. Evaluation of current TNM classification of penile carcinoma. *J Urol.* 2008;180:933–938.

56. Saraiya M, Watson M, Wu X, et al. Incidence of in situ and invasive vulvar cancer in the US, 1998–2003. *Cancer.* 2008;113:2865–2872.

57. Bodelon C, Madeleine MM, Voigt LF, et al. Is the incidence of invasive vulvar cancer increasing in the United States? *Cancer Causes Control.* 2009;20:1779–1782.

58. Van de Nieuwenhof HP, Massuger LF, van der Avoort JA, et al. Vulvar squamous cell carcinoma development after the diagnosis of VIN increases with age. *Eur J Cancer.* 2009;45:851–856.

59. Van Seters M, van Beurden M, de Craen AJ. Is the assumed natural history of vulvar intraepithelial neoplasia III based on enough evidence? A systematic review of 3322 published patients. *Gynecol Oncol.* 2005;97:645–651.

60. Sideri M, Jones RW, Wilkinson EJ, et al. Squamous vulvar intraepithelial neoplasia. 2004 modified terminology, ISSVD Vulvar Oncology Subcommittee. *J Reprod Med.* 2005;50:8807–8810.

61. McCluggage WG. Recent developments in vulvovaginal pathology. *Histopathology.* 2009;54:156–173.

62. Van de Nieuwenhof HP, van der Avoort IA, de Hullu JA. Review of squamous premalignant vulvar lesions. *Crit Rev Oncol Hematol.* 2008;68:131–156.

63. De Vuyst H, Clifford GM, Nascimento MC, et al. Prevalence and type distribution of human papillomavirus in carcinoma and intraepithelial neoplasia of the vulva, vagina, and anus: a meta-analysis. *Int J Cancer.* 2009;124:1626–1636.

64. Smith JS, Backes DM, Hoots BE, et al. Human papillomavirus type-distribution in vulvar and vaginal cancers and their associated precursors. *Obstet Gynecol.* 2009;113:917–924.

65. Kennedy CM, Peterson LB, Galsk RP. Erosive vulvar lichen planus: a cohort at risk for cancer? *J Reprod Med.* 2008;53:781–784.

66. Likes WM, Stegbauer C, Tillmanns T, et al. Correlates of sexual function following vulvar excision. *Gynecol Oncol.* 2007;105:600–603.

67. Preti M, van Seters M, Sideri M, et al. Squamous vulvar intraepithelial neoplasia. *Clin Obstet Gynecol.* 2005;48:845–861.

68. Jones RW, Rowan DM, Stewart AW. Vulvar intraepithelial neoplasia: aspects of the natural history and outcome in 405 women. *Obstet Gynecol.* 2005;106:1319–1326.

69. Bruchim I, Gotlieb WH, Mahmud S, et al. HPV-related vulvar intraepithelial neoplasia: outcome of different management modalities. *Int J Gynaecol Obstet.* 2007;99:23–27.

70. Pecorelli S. Revised FIGO staging for carcinoma of the vulva, cervix, and endometrium. *Int J Gynecol Obstet.* 2009;105:103–104.

71. Yoder BJ, Rufforny I, Massoll NA, et al. Stage IA vulvar squamous cell carcinoma: an analysis of tumor invasive characteristics and risk. *Am J Surg Pathol.* 2008;32:765–772.

72. Van der Zee AG, Oonk MH, De Hullu JAQ, et al. Sentinel node dissection is safe in the treatment of early-stage vulvar cancer. *J Clin Oncol.* 2008;26:884–889.

73. Ayhan A, Velipasaoglu M, Salman MC, et al. Prognostic factors for recurrence and survival in primary vulvar squamous cell cancer. *Acta Obstet Gynecol Scand.* 2008;87:1143–1149.

74. Blecharz P, Karolewski K, Bieda T, et al. Prognostic factors in patients with carcinoma of the vulva—our own experience and literature review. *Eur J Gynaecol Oncol.* 2008;29:260–263.

75. Eva LJ, Ganesan R, Chan KK, et al. Vulval squamous cell carcinoma occurring on a background of differentiated vulval intraepithelial neoplasia is more likely to recur: a review of 154 cases. *J Reprod Med.* 2008;53:397–401.

76. Wright JL, Morgan TM, Lin DW. Primary scrotal cancer: disease characteristics and increasing incidence. *Urology.* 2008;72:1138–1143.

77. DeAmbrosis K, Nicklin J, Yong-Gee S. Basal cell carcinoma of the vulva: a report of four cases. *Aust J Dermatol.* 2008;49:213–215.

78. Lui PC, Fan YS, Lau PP, et al. Vulvar basal cell carcinoma in china: a 13 year review. *Am J Obstet Gynecol.* 2009;200:514.e1. [Epub February 6, 2009].

79. Giuliani M, Di Stefano L, Zoccali G, et al. Gorlin syndrome associated with basal cell carcinoma of the vulva: a case report. *Eur J Gynaecol Oncol.* 2006;27:519–522.

80. Bousquet J, Flahault A, Vandenplas O, et al. Natural rubber latex allergy among health care workers: a systematic review of the literature. *J Allergy Clin Immunol.* 2006;118:447–454.

81. Lee-Wong M, Collins JS, Nozad C, et al. Diagnosis and treatment of human seminal plasma hypersensitivity. *Obstet Gynecol.* 2008;111:538–539.

82. Weinberger LN, Zirwas MJ, English JC III. A diagnostic algorithm for male genital edema. *J Eur Acad Dermatol Venereol.* 2007;21:156–162.

83. Keeley VL. Lymphedema and cellulitis: chicken or egg? *Br J Dermatol.* 2008;158:1175–1176.

84. Vignes S, Dupuy A. Recurrence of lymphedema-associated cellulitis (erysipelas) under prophylactic antibiotherapy: a retrospective cohort study. *J Eur Acad Dermatol Venereol.* 2006;20:818–822.

85. Murphy MJ, Kogan B, Carlson JA. Granulomatous lymphangitis of the scrotum and penis. Report of a case and review of the literature of genital swelling with sarcoidal granulomatous inflammation. *J Cutan Pathol.* 2001;28:419–424.

86. Ratzinger G, Sepp N, Vogetseder W, et al. Cheilitis granulomatosa and Melkersson–Rosenthal syndrome: evaluation of gastrointestinal involvement and therapeutic regimens in a series of 14 patients. *J Eur Acad Dermatol Venereol.* 2007;21:1065–1070.

87. Sobjanek M, Wlodarkiewicz A, Zelazny I, et al. Successful treatment of Melkersson–Rosenthal syndrome with dapsone and triamcinalone injections. *J Eur Acad Dermatol Venereol.* 2008;22:1028–1029.

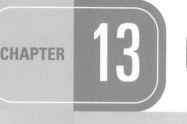

Pigmented Disorders

PETER J. LYNCH

Pigmented lesions are present on the skin of the genitalia in approximately 10% to 12% of women and a slightly smaller proportion of men. The etiologic basis for these pigmented lesions includes physiologic hyperpigmentation, postinflammatory hyperpigmentation, some infections, and benign and malignant neoplasms. The brown and black colors usually arise as a result of melanin pigmentation. Melanin pigment is made within cytoplasmic organelles (melanosomes) in melanocytes that lie along the basement membrane of the epithelium. The amount of color in both normal skin and various lesions is determined by several factors: the density of melanocytes, the amount of melanin produced per melanocyte, and the transfer rate of the melaninized melanosomes to the 30 or so keratinocytes that surround each melanocyte. The density of melanocytes does not vary appreciably in people of different racial backgrounds but it does vary by site. Genital tissue, for instance, has about 50% more melanocytes per unit of area than does trunkal skin. The development of increased pigmentation is partially dependent on genetic factors (variability in racial groups) and partly on acquired factors such as ultraviolet light, the presence of inflammation (especially that involving basal layer damage), and some kinds of infection (notably human papillomavirus [HPV] infection in the genital and perigenital areas). Increased pigmentation also occurs when there is proliferation in the number of normally melanized keratinocytes (epithelial hyperplasia) and/or when there is an increased retention of normally melanized keratinocytes in the stratum corneum. For a few disorders in this chapter, heme pigment rather than melanin explains the presence of a dark color.

PHYSIOLOGIC HYPERPIGMENTATION

Physiologic hyperpigmentation occurs as symmetrical, flat, smooth-surfaced, asymptomatic darkening of the skin. The most commonly affected sites include the scrotum in male patients and the labia majora and outer edges of the labia minora in female patients (Fig. 13-1). The perianal skin in both genders usually displays some degree of physiologic hyperpigmentation. Appreciable variation in hue occurs across racial groups and also from person to person even within a given racial group. The

degree of hyperpigmentation can be so light that it is hardly noticeable or may be so dark as to be almost black in color.

The diagnosis of physiologic hyperpigmentation is made on a clinical basis. The differential diagnosis includes postinflammatory hyperpigmentation but the latter tends to be patchier and is often less symmetrically distributed. If biopsy is carried out because of either patient or clinician concern, increased melanin will be found in both the melanocytes and keratinocytes which line the basal layer of the epithelium. Hyperpigmentation occurs preferentially in genital skin because of the greater density of melanocytes in this tissue compared to the surrounding skin. These areas of hyperpigmentation will darken further under the influence of both endogenous and exogenous sex hormones. This is particularly notable during pregnancy. Darkening will also occur due to the presence of increased melanocyte-stimulating hormone (MSH) in neonates and in patients with disorders such as Addison disease due to the marked disturbance in pituitary–adrenal axis function.

Treatment is not necessary or even desirable. However, it is worth noting that obsession with anogenital hyperpigmentation has led to the provision of bleaching services by both licensed and unlicensed practioners.

ACANTHOSIS NIGRICANS

Acanthosis nigricans was an uncommon disorder 50 year ago, but it has become very prevalent in recent years due to the epidemic of obesity, especially in children. In a recent survey of pediatric practices, obesity (body mass index > 95th percentile) was found in about 32% of the children and teenagers. Of these overweight patients, more than 62% were noted to have acanthosis nigricans and it was particularly prominent in the Hispanic and African American children (1). While acanthosis nigricans is most often found in those who are obese, it can also occur with various endocrinopathies, malignancies, and with the use of medications such as niacin, topical fusidic acid, and prednisone.

Acanthosis nigricans appears as poorly demarcated light-brown to dark-brown lesions around the neck, in the axillae, and in the crural folds (Figs. 13-2 and 13-3).

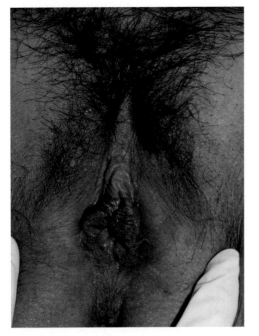

FIG. 13-1. Physiologic hyperpigmentation of the vulva may be most marked on the labia minora and, sometimes, on the posterior fourchette.

Rarely, it develops in other folded areas of the body. The background of hyperpigmentation may be flat but characteristically there are elevated linear ridges running parallel to one another. The surface of the lesions is slightly "bumpy" and, on palpation, is often velvety or very slightly rough. Acanthosis nigricans is asymptomatic but is very troubling to the patient because it suggests the

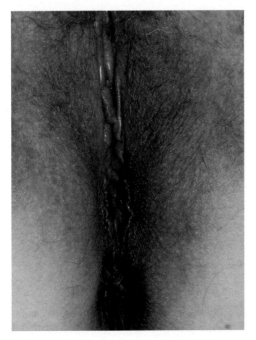

FIG. 13-2. Acanthosis nigricans is manifested by hyperpigmentation in skin folds, often with a velvety appearance.

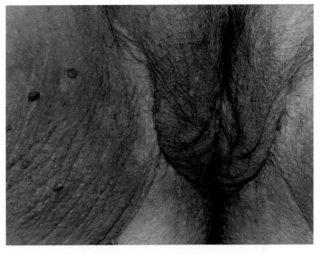

FIG. 13-3. Acanthosis nigricans is most common in overweight individuals, and more severe acanthosis nigricans shows not only more thickened appearing skin but may also be associated with skin tags.

appearance of dirty skin. The diagnosis is established clinically. The major disorder to be considered in the list of differential diagnoses is those instances of lichen simplex chronicus in which postinflammatory hyperpigmentation has occurred.

There is no dermatologic therapy for acanthosis nigricans but the appearance can be improved through weight loss or treatment for any associated endocrinopathy. Medical evaluation of patients with acanthosis nigricans is usually desirable because of the frequently associated presence of insulin resistance, abnormal glucose homeostasis, hypertension, and elevated cholesterol (2). Very rarely acanthosis nigricans is associated with the development of systemic malignancy, especially that involving the gastrointestinal tract. This association should be considered in those individuals who are nonobese, lack endocrinopathy, and/or have a recent history of unintentional weight loss.

POSTINFLAMMATORY HYPERPIGMENTATION

Inflammation affects melanocytes in two ways. Severely damaged melanocytes discontinue the production of melanin with resulting hypopigmentation. Conversely, mildly damaged ("irritated") melanocytes react with increased melanin production and hyperpigmentation. Postinflammatory hyperpigmentation develops at the site of previous inflammation. This inflammation may be either an inherent component of a skin disease or the inflammation may develop at the site of trauma such as might occur following the use of liquid nitrogen or trichloroacetic acid. Postinflammatory hyperpigmentation is clinically recognized as light- to dark-brown, nonpalpable macules and patches occasionally displaying hues of gray, blue, or black (Fig. 13-4). The

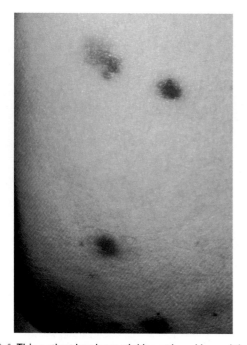

FIG. 13-4. This patient has been picking at her skin, and the open excoriation is accompanied by healed lesions that show poorly demarcated brown-pink macules of postinflamamtory hyperpigmentation.

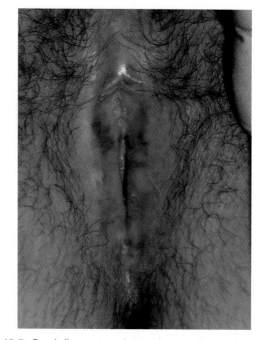

FIG. 13-5. Postinflammatory hyperpigmentation occurs occasionally on modified mucous membranes following lichen planus or lichen sclerosus. This woman has partially treated lichen sclerosus.

distribution, location, and intensity of hyperpigmentation are dependent on the underlying cause.

Diseases such as lichen sclerosus and lichen planus, in which inflammation preferentially damages the epithelial basal layer, are likely to develop darker pigmentation than occurs with other inflammatory disorders (Figs. 13-5 and 13-6). Not surprisingly, patients with racially or nationally darker skin are more likely to develop exaggerated postinflammatory hyperpigmentation. Similarly, because normal genital color is often darker than surrounding skin, inflammation in genital tissue is particularly likely to cause postinflammatory hyperpigmentation.

Although a history of prior trauma or inflammation is an important diagnostic clue, often such a history cannot be evoked. This is particularly true in lichen planus and lichen sclerosus where the extraordinarily long-lasting hyperpigmentation may first be noted a very long time after the inflammation has resolved. In this situation, the coexistence of architectural damage and pigmentation may identify the nature of the process. In some instances, a biopsy will be necessary to confirm a clinical diagnosis of postinflammatory hyperpigmentation. This is particularly true for pigmented macules or patches where the pigment is variable in density or where gray or black hues are present (see the sections on melanosis and nevi).

Because postinflammatory hyperpigmentation usually resolves over several months, no treatment is necessary. However, the hyperpigmentation sometimes obscures continuing low-grade inflammation and when there is

any suspicion of this possibility, anti-inflammatory treatment, such as with topical steroids, should be administered. Topical fading agents, such as hydroquinone, may improve pigmentation where the excess melanin is confined to the epidermis but are of no use

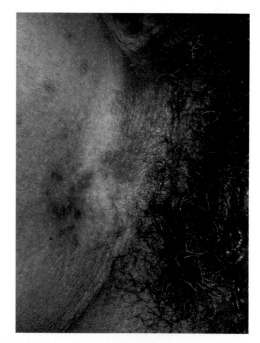

FIG. 13-6. Lichen planus is associated with prominent postinflammatory hyperpigmentation, the underlying etiology in this patient.

for pigment lying below the epithelium in dermal melanophages.

SEBORRHEIC KERATOSES

Seborrheic keratoses are extremely common benign growths. Most individuals over the age of 40 have at least one lesion and often 50 to 100 are present. Most are located on the trunk but occasionally they are noted on the proximal limbs and genitalia. Seborrheic keratoses present as sharply marginated, square-shouldered, tan, brown, or black papules 10 to 15 mm wide and 2 to 10 mm tall (Figs. 13-7 and 13-8). These attributes contribute to a characteristic "stuck on" appearance. The surface often contains visible scale and is usually rough on palpation. However, in some instances, the surface has a smooth and "waxy" feeling. In these smooth lesions, the presence of scale can be identified when the surface is gently scraped with a blade held perpendicular to the top of the lesion. The presence of scale is a very helpful point in distinguishing seborrheic keratoses from nevi, lentigines, and melanomas. Small characteristic surface pits may be found when magnification is used in the course of examination.

Genital seborrheic keratoses may be quite difficult to differentiate from both pigmented genital warts and HPV-related intraepithelial neoplasia. The number of lesions present is a helpful clue. Genital seborrheic keratoses are generally solitary, whereas HPV-related lesions are almost always more numerous. Seborrheic keratoses may also resemble pigmented basal cell carcinomas, nor-

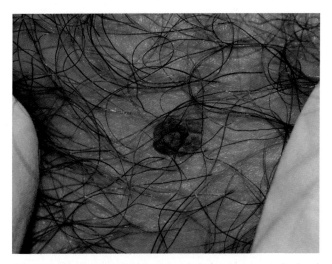

FIG. 13-8. On dry genital skin, seborrheic keratoses can be hard and keratotic.

mal nevi, dysplastic nevi, and melanomas. Scale is, of course, not present in these latter lesions, but when scale is absent or sparse, differentiation is not easy. For all of these reasons, unless they are completely typical in appearance, there ought to be a low threshold for biopsy. Support for this statement is offered by the observation that in a large study of biopsied lesions thought to be seborrheic keratoses, 0.5% turned out to be melanomas (3).

The cause of seborrheic keratoses is unknown but frequent presence of familial patterns regarding both age at onset and number of lesions suggests that both genetic and aging factors play a role. Growth factors may also be important even as they are in many other cutaneous neoplasms. Specifically, a small proportion of seborrheic keratoses contain mutations in the fibroblast growth factor receptor 3 (*FGFR3*) gene and a larger proportion demonstrates activation of the same normal (nonmutated) gene (4). Beta-type (epidermodysplasia verruciformis–associated) HPV is found more commonly in seborrheic keratoses than in normal skin but the meaning of this is not clear (5). In many previous reports, seborrheic keratoses occurring in and around the genitalia were found to contain alpha-type HPV (mucocutaneous wart type) and thus presumably were in reality pigmented genital warts (6).

No therapy is necessary for clinically typical seborrheic keratoses. Lesions that are irritated by clothing and those that are particularly bothersome to the patient may be treated with liquid nitrogen.

PIGMENTED WARTS

Genital warts of the flat-topped type are frequently tan, brown, or black in color (Figs. 13-9 and 13-10). These lesions are covered along with other morphologic types of warts in Chapter 12.

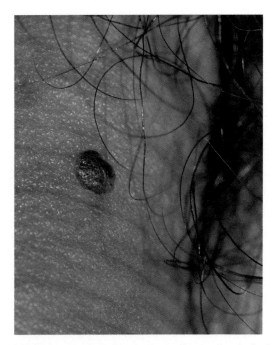

FIG. 13-7. The seborrheic keratosis on the penile shaft shows typical well-demarcated borders, and the surface is slightly stippled with pinpoint dark keratin plugs.

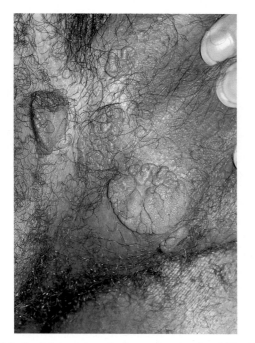

FIG. 13-9. Genital warts can be hyperpigmented and identical to seborrheic keratoses, but the multifocal nature is more suggestive of wart infection. Black patients regularly exhibit pigmented warts.

GENITAL INTRAEPITHELIAL NEOPLASIA

HPV-related vulvar, penile, and scrotal intraepithelial neoplasia is frequently tan, brown, or black in color (Figs. 13-11 and 13-12). These conditions are discussed in Chapter 12.

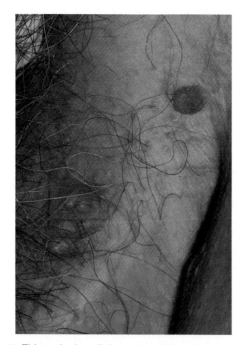

FIG. 13-10. This typical, well-demarcated, flat-topped pigmented wart is accompanied by grouped blisters of recurrent herpes simplex virus infection. Brown, flat warts are morphologically identical to intraepithelial neoplasia and should be biopsied in light-complexioned patients.

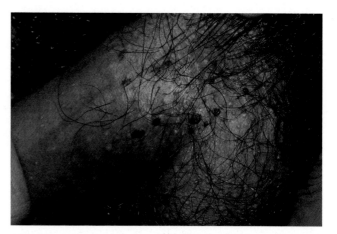

FIG. 13-11. These brown, flat-topped papules on the shaft showed penile intraepithelial neoplasia on biopsy; any pigmented genital lesion without an obvious morphologic diagnosis should undergo biopsy. (Courtesy of Errol Craig, MD.)

PIGMENTED BASAL CELL CARCINOMA

Basal cell carcinomas are normally skin colored but a small proportion contain sufficient melanin to be at least partially brown, blue, or black in color (Fig. 13-13). These lesions are covered in Chapter 12.

ANGIOKERATOMAS

Genital angiokeratomas are usually light to dusky red in color but those occurring on the vulva are sometimes blue, purple, or black (Figs. 13-14 and 13-15). These lesions are covered in Chapter 7.

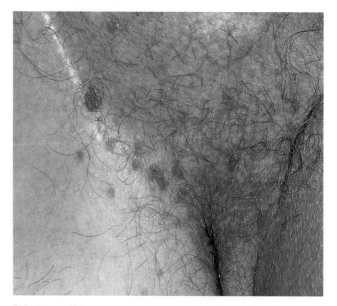

FIG. 13-12. When a person of light complexion has hyperpigmented, flat-topped genital warts, intraepithelial neoplasia is extremely likely, as is true in this patient.

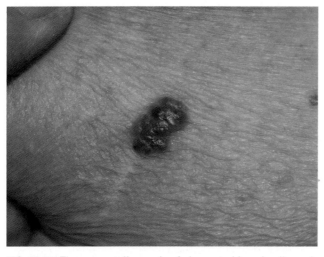

FIG. 13-13. The correct diagnosis of pigmented basal cell carcinoma can be suspected by the nearly translucent nature that sometimes mimics a fluid-filled lesion.

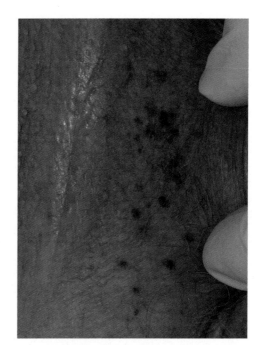

FIG. 13-15. When multiple lesions are present, angiokeratomas are more easily diagnosed, as at least some lesions usually reveal the underlying vascular nature by red or purple color.

KAPOSI SARCOMA

The nodules of Kaposi sarcoma occurring on the trunk and genitalia are usually medium to dusky red in color. Less often they are darker in color and may have blue, purple, or even black hues (Fig. 13-16). This neoplasm is discussed in Chapter 7.

GENITAL VARICOSITIES

Varicose veins occur on the vulva with some frequency in pregnant women and they often resolve following parturition (7). Varicosities are less common on the penis and scrotum. The varicosities may be small or large. Larger lesions are usually blue in color (Figs. 13-17 and 13-18). Very

small diameter vessels ("spider veins") are more likely to be medium to dark red. On the scrotum, tiny angiokeratomas may overlie these fine, red telangiectatic vessels. Varicosities are identified by their disappearance following compression with a glass slide (diascopy). No treatment is ordinarily necessary but bleeding following trauma may require electrosurgery or even excision.

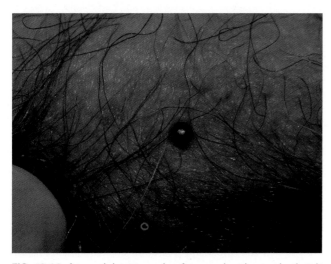

FIG. 13-14. An angiokeratoma is often so deeply purple that it appears black. This lesion must be differentiated from a nodular melanoma.

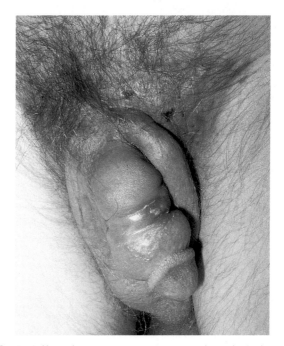

FIG. 13-16. Kaposi sarcoma presents as purple or dusky brown-red nodules.

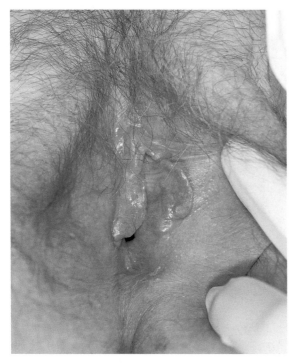

FIG. 13-17. This purple, tortuous vessel on the vulva is a varicose vein.

GENITAL MELANOSIS (LENTIGINOSIS)

Clinical Presentation

The terms genital melanosis and genital lentiginosis are often used interchangeably by clinicians but, strictly

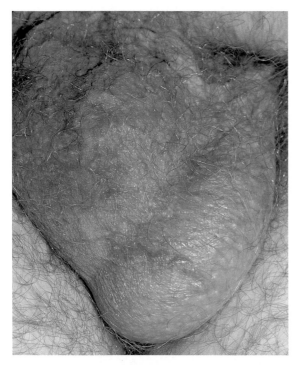

FIG. 13-18. Varicosities also occur on the scrotum and appear identical to those on the vulva.

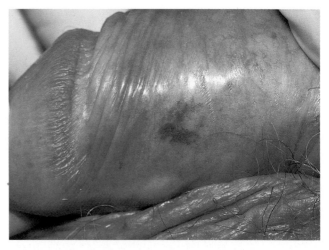

FIG. 13-19. Genital lentiginosis is characterized by poorly demarcated or irregular, macular hyperpigmentation.

speaking, the latter term is only applicable to those lesions that demonstrate a lentigo-like histologic pattern on biopsy. Since this is not present in all cases, we prefer the term genital melanosis. Pigmented lesions of melanocytic type are common on the genitalia, with a prevalence estimated to be about 10% to 15% in women and in a slightly lower percentage in men (8). In women, histologic examination of flat pigmented patches reveals that about one third of the lesions are nevi with the remainder representing vulvar melanosis (9,10).

Genital melanosis consists of nonpalpable, nonelevated macules and patches of dark, usually black, pigmentation (Figs. 13-19 through 13-21). This pigmentation occurs on both keratinizing skin and mucous membranes but is more common at the latter site. Genital melanosis is particularly likely to arise from a background of lichen sclerosus (Fig. 13-22). Lesions may be either solitary or

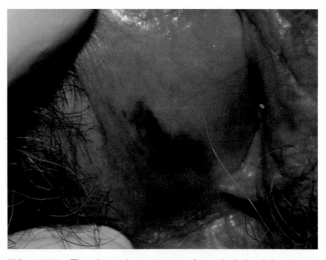

FIG. 13-20. The irregular nature of genital lentiginosis or melanosis is often suggestive of melanoma, so any lesion with this appearance should undergo biopsy.

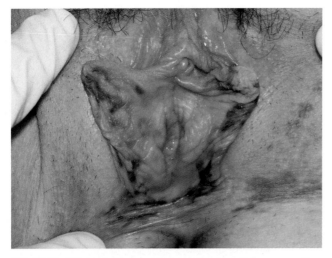

FIG. 13-21. Although brown, black, and gray patches are rather wild in appearance, large number of discrete lesions suggests a benign nature.

multifocal with the latter occurring more frequently. Lesions may be as small as 5 mm but most are considerably larger with diameters up to 2 cm. Asymmetry in distribution is common and the configuration is at times quite angular. The color may be tan, brown, blue, or, most commonly, black. Often there is considerable variation in pigment density within the lesions. The borders may be either diffusely or sharply marginated. In men, given the ready visibility of the penis, there may be a history of long duration with little or no change in appearance but for

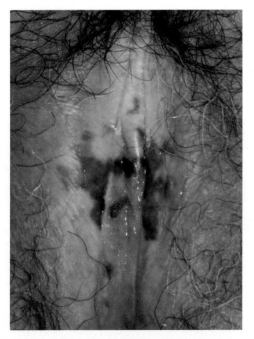

FIG. 13-22. Genital lentiginosis sometimes occurs in association with lichen sclerosus, as demonstrated by these brown and black patches within the white epithelium and resorption of the labia minora in a patient with lichen sclerosus.

women the duration is often unknown. In women, the pigmented patches are most often found on the labia minora. The labia majora are less frequently involved and vaginal and perineal lesions are only rarely encountered. In men, most lesions occur on the glans and inner aspects of the prepuce but penile shaft involvement is possible.

Most cases of genital melanosis develop in adult life with an average reported age of about 40 (8). When young patients present with genital melanosis, the oral mucous membranes should be inspected for the presence of similar pigmentation. When this is found, consideration should be given to the possibility of any one of a number of rarely encountered conditions such as Peutz–Jehgers syndrome, Laugier–Hunziger syndrome, Bannayan–Riley–Ruvalcaba syndrome, LEOPARD syndrome, and the several syndromes in which lentigines and cardiocutaneus myxomas are found.

Diagnosis

The diagnosis can be made on a clinical basis in many cases but, unless a long history of stable appearance is available, biopsy should be undertaken to rule out postinflammatory hyperpigmentation, pigmented intraepithelial neoplasia, dysplastic nevus, lentigo maligna, lentigo maligna melanoma, and superficial spreading melanoma.

Histologically most, but not all, specimens of genital mucinosis demonstrate lentiginous elongation of the rete ridges with slight hyperproliferation of benign-appearing melanocytes within the basal layer. Pigmented melanophages are commonly found in the dermis.

MELANOSIS:	Diagnosis

- Dark (usually black) flat, smooth, 5- to 25-mm patch
- Asymmetric or angular configuration
- Located primarily on nonkeratinizing (mucosal) tissue
- History of an unchanged appearance if the patient has previously been aware of the lesion
- Incisional biopsy to rule out dysplasia and malignancy

Pathophysiology

In most instances, the cause of genital melanosis is not known. Usually, there is no history of any preceding disorder, but in a minority of instances genital lentigines have arisen in a setting of previously existing lichen sclerosus (11,12). Historically and before coverage of the genitalia was offered for men receiving psoralen and ultraviolet light (PUVA) therapy penile lentigines were noted fairly often. As indicated above, genital lentigines may occur in a number of heritable disorders.

Management

Genital melanosis is believed to be a benign condition. Once a diagnosis of genital melanosis is histologically confirmed, further therapy is not required. Essentially all of the reported patients remained free of malignancy at least up until the time of publication but, because of the small number of patients and relatively short duration of reported follow-up, there is no absolute certainty regarding the natural history of these lesions. As a case in point, there is one instance of melanoma developing in the bladder in a patient with vulvar melanosis. Long-term follow-up of these patients seems advisable but periodic rebiopsy is not necessary unless either the patient reports a changed appearance or the clinician notes a change at the time of examination.

MELANOSIS:	Management

- Depends on biopsy results:
  - If dysplasia or malignancy, excision of entire lesion
  - If no dysplasia or malignancy, observation is appropriate
- Benign course with little or no change is expected
- But since data on the natural history is meager, periodic observation is desirable

MELANOCYTIC NEVUS (MOLE, PIGMENTED NEVUS)

Pigmented lesions are noted on the vulva in approximately 15% of women (8). Of these, 35% to 50% are melanocytic nevi. An older study indicated that the overall prevalence of vulvar nevi was about 2%. Corresponding data for men seem not to be available. Genital nevi fall into four categories: common nevi, dysplastic nevi, atypical nevi genital type, and nevi arising in lichen sclerosus.

Clinical Presentation

Common Nevus

Common nevi account for about 90% of genital nevi. They are found more frequently in women than in men. A classic benign melanocytic nevus appears as a symmetric macule (junctional nevi) or papule (compound and intradermal nevi), smaller than 10 mm in diameter with well-demarcated borders and a homogenous tan or brown color (Figs. 13-23 through 13-27). Less often, papular nevi of the intradermal type may be skin colored. Papular nevi are fairly soft on palpation, a feature that helps to distinguish them from more ominous neoplasms. Occasionally, a single atypical feature such as a notched border or slight pigment variegation may be present (Fig. 13-28). Common nevi may be located on either mucosal or hair-bearing skin and they may be present at birth or acquired later in life (Figs. 13-29 and 13-30).

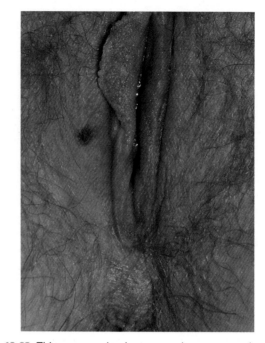

FIG. 13-23. This common benign nevus shows reassuring signs of sharply demarcated borders and even pigmentation.

Dysplastic Nevus

Dysplastic nevi occur in both men and women and account for about 5% of genital nevi. Most often these occur as part of the dysplastic nevus syndrome in which multiple family members have large numbers (>60) of nevi with clinically atypical features. These nevi are flat or only slightly elevated and characteristically have some degree of asymmetry, indistinct margination, and variegation of pigment density. They may be brown or black and, fairly often, red, white, and blue hues may be present (Figs. 13-31 through 13-33). Most dysplastic lesions are large with an average diameter of 7 to 15 mm. It is important to recognize that melanomas develop in a small percentage of dysplastic nevi.

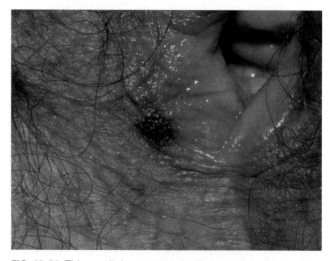

FIG. 13-24. This small, brown, evenly pigmented papule is characteristic of a common nevus, but it mimics pigmented intraepithelial neoplasia as well.

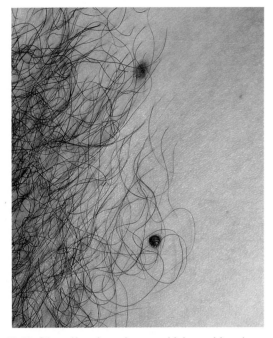

FIG. 13-25. Often, if patients have multiple nevi in other areas, they have multiple nevi in the genital area.

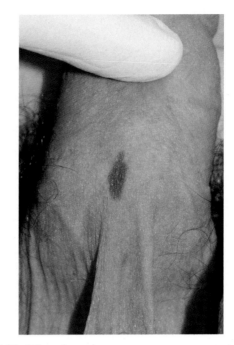

FIG. 13-27. Although nevi are more common on extragenital skin, they can occur on the penis.

Atypical Melanocytic Nevus of Genital Type

Atypical genital nevus (AGN) was identified as a specific subtype of nevus about 30 years ago. Previously these lesions, when biopsied, were often mistakenly thought to be melanomas. AGN are not restricted specifically to the genitalia and may also occur along the anatomic milk line, especially in the axillae and on the breasts of women. A series of 56 cases has recently been reported and the information in this publication has clarified many of the clinical and histologic aspects of these unusual lesions (13). AGN occur almost only in women where they make up about 5% of the nevi found in the anogenital area. They are identified mostly in older children, adolescents, and young women. The lesions tend to be larger (6 mm mean

diameter) than common nevi and may have a polypoid surface. Mildly atypical clinical features, as noted above for dysplastic nevi, are occasionally present. Most AGN are located on the labia minora and labia majora but lesions may occur on the mons pubis, clitoris, and perineum.

Nevi Arising in Lichen Sclerosus

Nevi have been reported to occur in association with the lesions of genital lichen sclerosus. Most of these have been described with vulvar lichen sclerosus but a few have also occurred in men (11,14). Most of the lesions have been described as small (3- to 6-mm) black macules but a few larger ones have also been reported. The dark-black color of

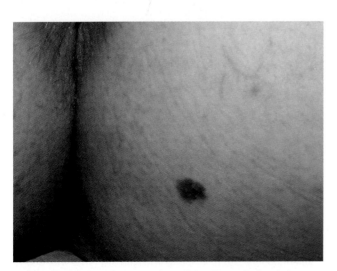

FIG. 13-26. This common nevus has minimal irregularity of pigment.

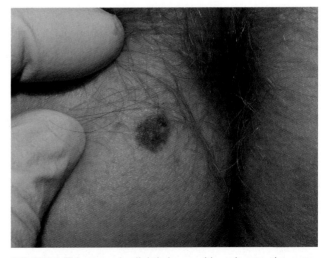

FIG. 13-28. This nevus is slightly large with variegate pigmentation; a biopsy shows a benign nevus, demonstrating the continuum from classically benign to abnormal.

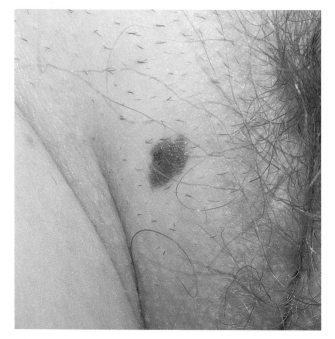

FIG. 13-29. A congenital nevus, as seen here, often is larger and more irregular without necessarily signifying malignancy.

these lesions often suggests the possibility of melanoma and for this reason excisional biopsy is almost always necessary.

Diagnosis

The situation regarding the necessity of biopsy for pigmented genital lesions is controversial. Experienced dermatologists may be satisfied with a clinical diagnosis for those lesions showing no clinical atypicality, whereas less experienced clinicians will generally prefer to biopsy all pigmented lesions. For both types of clinicians, biopsy is probably mandatory for any lesion presenting with atypical

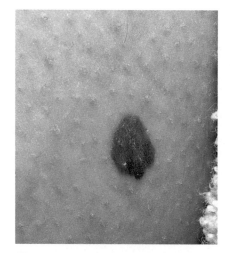

FIG. 13-31. The large size and irregular border and variegate color are typical of a dysplastic nevus.

features and for all patients presenting with pigmented lesions arising within areas of lichen sclerosus.

The histologic features of common nevi and dysplastic nevi are well understood by most pathologists and therefore biopsied lesions will be correctly diagnosed. However, the situation for AGN and those nevi arising in lichen sclerosus is different. The histology of AGN reveals many changes that are regularly present in melanoma such as appreciable junctional melanocytic proliferation (either in a lentiginous pattern or in the form of large oval nests), pagetoid spread into the mid epidermis, and appreciable cytologic atypia. In one series of pigmented vulvar lesions reviewed in a tertiary center, one third of the AGN had erroneously been previously diagnosed as melanoma (15).

A similar situation occurs with nevi arising in patients with genital lichen sclerosus. In this situation, the presence of lentiginous melanocytic proliferation, confluence of junctional nests, pagetoid upward spread of melanocytes,

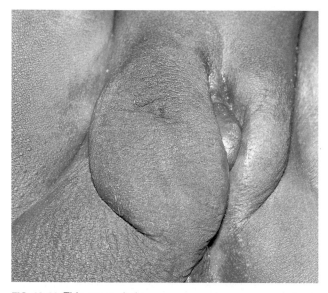

FIG. 13-30. This congenital nevus covers a large area and also is deep; she was originally evaluated for amgibuous genitalia.

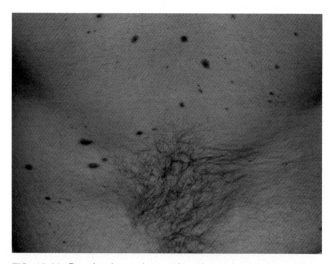

FIG. 13-32. Dysplastic nevi are often found in a setting of increased numbers of nevi, many of which are large with poorly demarcated or irregular borders, and irregular color.

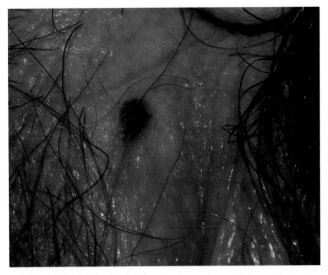

FIG. 13-33. Although this lesion is a normal size, the remarkable irregular black color suggests a melanoma. However, a biopsy showed a dysplastic nevus.

nests of melanocytes trapped within encircling dermal fibrosis, and peritumoral lymphocytic inflammation can easily be confused with both so-called "persistent" nevi and with melanomas (14). With this in mind, and since both childhood melanomas and vulvar melanomas in general are rare, it seems likely that some, maybe even most, cases of childhood vulvar melanoma arising in lichen sclerosus are in reality only atypical nevi (14).

The differential diagnosis of nevi includes dysplastic nevi, melanoma, pigmented basal cell carcinoma, pigmented intraepithelial neoplasia, mucosal melanosis, and postinflammatory hyperpigmentation.

MELANOCYTIC NEVUS: **Diagnosis**

- Common nevus
  - Tan to brown, smooth-surfaced, 3- to 10-mm macule or papule
  - Borders are sharp, color is even, shape is symmetrical
- Dysplastic nevus
  - Brown, smooth-surfaced, 6- to 20-mm macule or papule
  - One or more atypical features: diffuse margination, speckling of color, additional red, white, or blue hues, asymmetry
- Atypical nevus, genital type
  - Similar to the common nevus but often larger (6 to 15 mm)
  - Surface may be polypoid (mammillated, "bumpy")
- Nevus arising from a background of lichen sclerosus
  - Black, smooth-surfaced, 5- to 20-mm macule, patch, or papule

---

Pathophysiology

Nevi are thought to be either developmental hamartomas or benign proliferations of melanocytes that have acquired some growth advantage over normal melanocytes. However, the exact reason why they arise is not known. Genetic factors appear to play a role for the development of nevi as there is often a familial pattern regarding their clinical appearance and number. Ultraviolet light exposure plays an important role in nevi arising on sun-exposed surfaces, but this is clearly not the case for genital nevi. Hormonal factors are likely important especially for the development of AGN since these lesions arise almost entirely in women and occur only within the milk line. Mutations in *BRAF*, which are commonly present in nevi on sun exposed skin are present, but not so often found, in nevi from sun protected sites such as both typical and atypical genital nevi (16). Increased activity in the tumor suppressor gene, *IGFBP7*, may explain why these lesions remain benign in outcome (16).

Management

Nevi with a benign histology can appropriately be left in place as there is little or no likelihood of progression to melanoma. Dysplastic nevi with histologic confirmation of atypicality should be excised because adequate follow-up for such genital lesions is difficult and there is a small possibility of progression to melanoma. AGN, in spite of their suspicious histologic appearance, have a low recurrence rate and do not appear to progress to melanoma (13). However, given the sparsity of follow-up information about them, excision is recommended. Nevi arising in lichen sclerosus in the elderly, once demonstrated to be benign by biopsy, can be left untreated. On the other hand, histologic uncertainty regarding a diagnosis of melanoma in those that arise in younger patients suggests that these lesions should be excised with histologically clear margins (14).

MELANOCYTIC NEVUS: **Management**

- Common nevus
  - If no clinical atypicality, no biopsy is needed
- Dysplastic nevus
  - Excisional biopsy if size is small, incisional biopsy if large
- Atypical nevus, genital type
  - If diagnosis is suspected, excisional biopsy is desirable
  - If diagnosis not suspected (looks like a common nevus), observation is okay since course is benign
- Nevus arising from a background of lichen sclerosus
  - Excisional biopsy is necessary in children and young women
  - Excisional biopsy is desirable in older adults

MELANOMA

Melanoma of the anogenital region accounts for less than 1% of all melanomas and for this reason they will very rarely be encountered in most clinical practices. Remarkably, while the incidence of melanoma at other cutaneous sites is increasing, the incidence of genital melanomas is stable or decreasing. Most of the reported anogenital melanomas have occurred in women with approximately 2000 cases of vulvar melanoma having been published (17). Genital melanomas occur extremely rarely in men. Penile melanoma has been reported in about 70 patients and scrotal melanoma in about 20 patients. Anal melanoma is more common than genital melanoma but it is still rarely seen. As opposed to genital melanoma, there is evidence that the incidence of anorectal melanoma is increasing (18). This increase seems predominantly due to an increased incidence in young men living in places where there is a large gay population (18).

Anogenital melanomas differ from cutaneous melanomas in multiple ways. First, with the exception of anal melanoma, there is a decreasing rather than increasing incidence. Second, it occurs in an appreciably older age group. Third, it is obviously not related to ultraviolet light–related DNA damage. Fourth, there is less often an association with a contiguous nevus. Fifth, the proportion of melanomas that are amelanotic is higher. Sixth, in a large proportion of cases, it occurs on glaborous (mucosal) surfaces and thus the histologic pattern is much more often that of mucosal lentiginous melanoma, rather than superficial spreading melanoma. Seventh, the outcome, probably related to delayed diagnosis, is appreciably worse. Eighth, there is somewhat less racial disparity in incidence compared to the marked predominance of whites diagnosed with nongenital cutaneous melanoma.

Unfortunately, because of the infrequency with which anogenital melanoma is seen, all of the published reports consider both those tumors arising on mucous membrane (mucosal lentiginous melanoma) and those arising on keratinizing skin within a single group. It seems likely that there are major differences between these two groups of melanoma but data to support this supposition are lacking at this time.

Clinical Presentation

Vulvar Melanoma

Melanoma is the second most common malignancy arising in the vulva but nevertheless it only accounts for about 5% of all malignant vulvar neoplasms and 2% to 3% of all of the melanomas occurring in women. The incidence of vulvar melanoma is stable or is slightly decreasing in frequency. It is disproportionally more common in the white population and it occurs predominantly in older women with a mean age at diagnosis of 68 (19). Importantly, those few reported vulvar melanomas arising in children and very

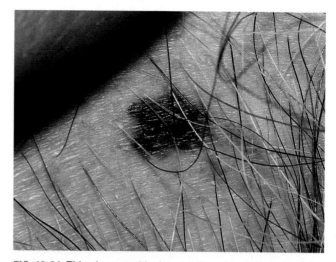

FIG. 13-34. This pigmented lesion shows more striking irregularity of color and border, with an unusually dark central area. On biopsy, this showed a fairly superficial melanoma.

young women have occurred almost entirely in a setting of lichen sclerosus. However, as noted above, some, or maybe even most, of these may have been markedly atypical nevi rather than true melanomas (12,14,20).

Most vulvar melanomas have an appearance similar to atypical nevi and melanomas occurring at other cutaneous sites. Suspicious features includes large size, dark-black pigmentation, dark speckling of pigment against a lighter background, color variegation with red, white and blue hues, nonsharp borders, and a configuration that is asymmetric (Figs. 13-34 through 13-38). In contrast to cutaneous melanomas, approximately 20% of vulvar melanomas are multifocal, 25% are amelanotic (Fig. 13-39), and 75% occur on a mucosal surface or glabrous skin (17,21,22). Most vulvar melanomas are asymptomatic but when symptoms and signs are present, they most commonly include pruritus, presence of a palpable lesion, bleedings, and visual change in a preceding lesion (21).

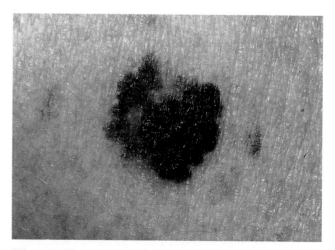

FIG. 13-35. The very large size and wildly irregular pigmentation with regression are typical of cutaneous melanoma.

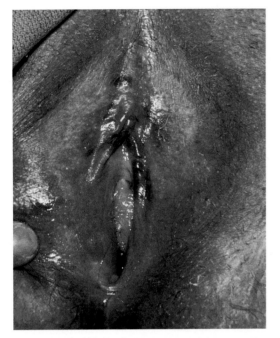

FIG. 13-36. The deep gray-black, irregular pigment on the vulva is a classic sign of either melanoma or genital lentiginosis—in this case, melanoma.

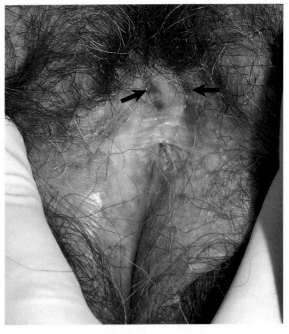

FIG. 13-38. This patient with lichen sclerosus showed a recalcitrant thickened area with minor flecks of pigmentation *(arrows)* that represented a spindle cell melanoma on biopsy. In patients with lichen sclerosus probably even bland pigmented lesions should be biopsied.

Tumors are most often found on the labium majus and labium minus but location on the clitoris and periclitoral area is also fairly common. Reflecting their large size and presumed long duration before discovery, ulceration of the surface occurs with considerable frequency (21). At the time of diagnosis, about 50% of the women have

localized disease without evidence of regional or distant spread (19). Nodular and mucosal lentiginous types of melanoma are overrepresented compared to the very high frequency of superficial spreading melanomas found at other cutaneous sites.

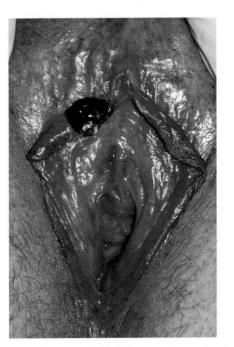

FIG. 13-37. This nodular melanoma has not shown the classic irregularity of color and outline, but rather a black, large nodule that is already quite advanced. (Courtesy of Ron Jones, MD.)

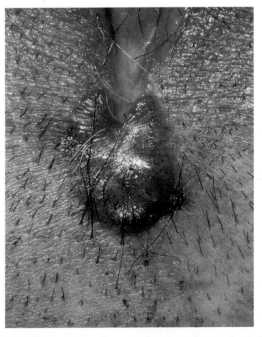

FIG. 13-39. There are a disproportionate number of relatively amelanotic melanomas on the vulva. The overriding color here is pink, but flecks of pigment are discernible to the careful observer. (Courtesy of Ron Jones, MD.)

Penile and Scrotal Melanoma

As noted above, penile melanomas are very rarely encountered. The average age at diagnosis is about 60 (23). Most lesions occur on the glans and inner prepuce but involvement of the penile shaft or the urethra is also possible (24). Lesions may be flat or raised and many are polypoid. About 40% are ulcerated (23). As is true for vulvar melanoma, it appears that a larger than expected number of penile melanomas are amelanotic. The majority of patients have localized disease at the time of diagnosis (23).

Scrotal melanoma occurs even more rarely with fewer than 20 reported cases in the literature. Some male genital melanomas present with a pigmented macule or papule, while others are exophytic, often with overlying ulceration (25).

Anal Melanoma

Anal melanoma occurs infrequently but the number of tumors pertinent to dermatologists is uncertain because most series group patients with anal melanoma and those with rectal melanoma into the single category of anorectal melanomas. Probably about one third of these occur in the anus and thus might initially be brought to the attention of a dermatologist (18). More anorectal melanomas occur in women than in men reversing the situation for cutaneous melanomas (18). The ratio of white patients to black patients was more nearly even than the marked dominance of cutaneous melanoma in white patients (18). As is true for genital melanoma, anorectal melanoma occurs predominantly in an older population with a reported median age of 66 at the time of diagnosis (26).

The most frequent presenting symptoms and signs were rectal bleeding, anal pain, and the presence of a mass (26,27). Less frequently patients noted pruritus or a change in bowel habits (26,27). The majority of patients have metastatic disease at the time of diagnosis (27). As is true for genital melanomas, a sizeable proportion (about 20%) of these melanomas is amelanotic (27). Other information such as the clinical appearance, size of the tumors, percentage that is ulcerated, etc. is not readily available in the recently published reviews.

Diagnosis

Anogenital melanomas may be flat, plaque-like, nodular, or polypoid. A clinical diagnosis is usually possible on the basis of dark, often variegated, pigmentation which may be intermingled with other blue, gray, red, or white hues (Figs. 13-34 through 13-37); however, amelanotic tumors which account for about 20% to 25% of anogenital melanomas, are more easily missed (Fig. 13-39). Diseases to be considered in the differential diagnosis include atypical nevi, vascular lesions, lentiginosis, seborrheic keratoses, pigmented basal cell carcinomas, and both pigmented and nonpigmented forms of squamous cell carcinoma.

A suspected clinical diagnosis must, of course, be confirmed with biopsy. Excisional biopsy is preferred, but for large lesions incisional biopsy is appropriate. The diagnosis is usually apparent with routine hematoxylin and eosin (H&E) stain. However, in some cases, especially for amelanotic melanoma, special stains such as S-100, HMB-45, and Mart-1 may be required (22). Presumably due to delayed recognition, the usual Breslow depth of anogenital melanomas is around 2 to 3 mm (21). Interestingly, and in contrast to cutaneous melanomas, a contiguous nevus is essentially never found in the microscopic examination of melanomas arising on mucous membranes.

MELANOMA: **Diagnosis**

- Older patient (50 to 80) with black exophytic mass
- Atypical color features: color variegation (red, white, or blue hues); consider amelanotic melanoma if color is pink or red
- Surface may be friable or ulcerated
- Symptoms (pruritus, pain) and signs (palpable mass); history of rapid growth may or may not be present
- Biopsy any lesion for which there is the slightest suspicion

---

Pathophysiology

Genetic factors are important in etiology. A positive family history for melanoma is present in 15% to 30% of vulvar melanomas and clinically atypical nevi, located at other sites, occur in 20% to 60% of patients with vulvar melanoma (17,21). These generalized atypical nevi are recognized as part of the inherited dysplastic nevus syndrome. Patients with familial forms of nongenital cutaneous melanoma have a fairly high frequency of mutations in the *CDKN2A* and *CDK4* genes and, while this has not specifically been looked at in anogenital melanomas, it seems likely that this might be true for melanomas at these sites as well.

Mutations in other genes such as *BRAF*, *MC1R*, *ASIP*, *TYR*, *TYR1*, *NRAS*, and *KIT* occur in varying proportions of sporadic cutaneous melanomas (28). However, it is apparent that the molecular profile is quite different in mucosal and non-mucosal anogenital melanomas. These melanomas have a much lower frequency of BRAF and NRAS mutations and a somewhat higher frequency of KIT mutations compared to nongenital cutaneous melanomas (29).

Considerable controversy exists regarding what, if any, role HPV viral infection plays in melanoma formation. This controversy revolves around the fact that both normal human skin and melanomas frequently demonstrate the presence of HPV, especially the beta types of HPV that were originally identified in patients with epidermodysplasia verruciformis (30). Overall, it seems likely that there is no specific etiologic role for HPV infection but it remains possible that some types of HPV infection might be important in certain subtypes of melanoma (30).

The presence of chronic inflammation is well known to play a role in the development of squamous cell carcinoma. This has been amply demonstrated in the situation of genital lichen planus and lichen sclerosus. Melanoma probably occurs with a somewhat greater than expected frequency in patients (especially children) with vulvar lichen sclerosus, but it is unclear what proportion of these putative melanomas are in fact only severely atypical benign nevi (12,14,20) (Fig. 13-38).

Management

Once a diagnosis has been documented, staging of the tumor should be undertaken. Most often the 2002 American Joint Committee on Cancer (AJCC) melanoma staging system is used and currently seems to be the best of the several staging systems available (18,31). However, this system was not specifically designed for the staging of anogenital melanoma. A revision is expected sometime in 2010 and hopefully it will address melanomas at these sites. Breslow depth of invasion, measured in millimeters, represents the single most important prognostic factor and, importantly, this measurement is contained within the AJCC staging protocol (31).

A study using multivariate analysis indicated that older age, advanced stage, and positive lymph nodes were significant factors adversely influencing prognosis for vulvar melanoma (19). Other factors such as tumor ulceration, tumor size, and the number of positive nodes also probably play a role in prognosis (19,23). Sufficient specific information regarding prognostic factors for anorectal and male genital melanomas is not readably available but presumably they would be similar to those for vulvar carcinoma. Currently, sentinel node biopsy is not required for AJCC staging but there is increasing interest in its use even if, as for cutaneous melanoma, it appears to offer mostly prognostic, rather than therapeutic, information (31).

Multiple studies have shown that wide local excision for all types of anogenital melanoma offers results at least as good as were obtained with the more radical procedures carried out in the past (19,24,27,32). There is general agreement that neither prophylactic nor therapeutic lymphadenectomy is warranted as this procedure does not appear to improve 5-year survival (17,22,23,27). However, as experience is gained with sentinel node biopsies, this position may require reinvestigation (31). There may be a minor role for radiotherapy in certain patients (31).

Despite therapy, the outcome for anogenital melanoma is dismal. For women with vulvar melanoma, the overall 5-year survival is less than 55% though for patients with localized disease it may be as high as 70% to 75% (17,19).

The prognosis for penile and anorectal carcinoma is even worse. Overall, 5-year survival for penile melanoma appears to be about 30% and is only slightly higher at 39% for those with localized disease (23). For anorectal melanoma, the overall 5-year survival is approximately 20% (32). These figures are appreciably worse than for cutaneous melanoma probably because there is a longer duration before recognition and this leads to consequently larger size and significantly deeper levels of invasion at the time the diagnosis is finally established.

MELANOMA: **Management**

- Carry out staging (see the text)
- Consider sentinel node biopsy for lesions that are more than 1 mm in depth
- Wide local excision is the surgical procedure of choice
- Radical surgery seldom is indicated
- Consider radiation therapy or chemotherapy in selected cases

---

REFERENCES

1. Brickman WJ, Binns HJ, Jovanovic BD, et al. Acanthosis nigricans: a common finding in overweight youth. *Pediatr Dermatol.* 2007;24:601–606.
2. Brickman WJ, Huang J, Silverman BL, et al. Acanthosis nigricans identifies youth at high risk for metabolic abnormalities. *J Pediatr.* 2010;156:87–92.
3. Izikson L, Sober AJ, Mihm MC Jr, et al. Prevalence of melanoma clinically resembling seborrheic keratosis: analysis of 9204 cases. *Arch Dermatol.* 2002;138:1562–1556.
4. Hida Y, Kubo Y, Arase S. Activation of fibroblast growth factor receptor 3 and oncogene-induced senescence in skin tumors. *Br J Dermatol.* 2009;160:1258–1263.
5. Li YH, Chen G, Dong XP, et al. Detection of epidermodysplasia verruciformis-associated human papillomavirus DNA in non-genital seborrheic keratosis. *Br J Dermatol.* 2004;151:1060–1065.
6. Bai H, Cviko A, Granter S, et al. Immunophenotypic and viral (human papillomavirus) correlates of vulvar seborrheic keratosis. *Hum Pathol.* 2003;34:559–564.
7. Bell D, Kane PB, Liang S, et al. Vulvar varices: an uncommon entity in surgical pathology. *Int J Gynecol Pathol.* 2007;26:99–101.
8. Barnhill RL, Albert LS, Shama SK, et al. Genital lentiginosis: a clinical and histologic study. *J Am Acad Dermatol.* 1990;22:453–460.
9. Mannon F, De Giorgo V, Cattaneo A, et al. Dermoscopic features of mucosal melanosis. *Dermatol Surg.* 2004;30:1118–1123.
10. Ferrari A, Buccini P, Covello R, et al. The ringlike pattern in vulvar melanosis. A new demoscopic clue for diagnosis. *Arch Dermatol.* 2008;144:1030–1034.
11. El Shabrawi-Caelen L, Soyer HP, Schaeppi H, et al. Genital lentigines and melanocytic nevi with superimposed lichen

sclerosus: a diagnostic challenge. *J Am Acad Dermatol.* 2004;50: 690–694.

12. Schaffer JV, Orlow SJ. Melanocytic proliferations in the setting of vulvar lichen sclerosus: diagnostic considerations. *Pediatr Dermatol.* 2005;22:276–278.

13. Gleason BC, Hirsch MS, Nucci MR, et al. Atypical genital nevi. A clinicopathologic analysis of 56 cases. *Am J Surg Pathol.* 2008;32:51–57.

14. Carlson JA, Mu XC, Slominski A, et al. Melanocytic proliferations associated with lichen sclerosus. *Arch Dermatol.* 2002; 138:77–87.

15. Clark WH Jr, Hood AF, Tucker MA, et al. Atypical melanocytic nevi of the genital type with a discussion of reciprocal parenchymal–stromal interactions in the biology of neoplasia. *Hum Pathol.* 1998;29(1 suppl 1):S1–S24.

16. Nguyen LP, Emley A, Wajapeyee N, et al. BRAF V600E mutation and the tumor suppressor IGFBP7 in atypical genital nevi. *Br J Dermatol.* 2010;162:677–680.

17. De Simone P, Silipo V, Buccini P, et al. Vulvar melanoma: a report of 10 cases and review of the literature. *Melanoma Res.* 2008;18:127–133.

18. Coté TR, Sobin LH. Primary melanomas of the esophagus and anorectum: epidemiologic comparison with melanoma of the skin. *Melanoma Res.* 2009;19:58–60.

19. Sugiyama VE, Chan JK, Shin JY, et al. Vulvar melanoma. A multivariable analysis of 644 patients. *Obstet Gynecol.* 2007;110:296–201.

20. Rosamilia LL, Schwartz JL, Lowe L, et al. Vulvar melanoma in a 10 year-old girl in association with lichen sclerosus. *J Am Acad Dermatol.* 2006;54(2 suppl):S52–S53.

21. Wechter ME, Gruber SB, Haefner HK, et al. Vulvar melanoma: a report of 20 cases and review of the literature. *J Am Acad Dermatol.* 2004;50:554–562.

22. An J, Li B, Wu L, et al. Primary malignant amelanotic melanoma of the female genital tract: report of two cases and review of literature. *Melanoma Res.* 2009;19:267–270.

23. van Geel AN, den Bakker MA, Kikels W, et al. Prognosis of primary mucosal penile melanoma: a series of 19 Dutch patients and 47 patients from the literature. *Urology.* 2007;70:143–147.

24. Sanchez-Ortiz R, Huang SF, Tamboli P, et al. Melanoma of the penis, scrotum and male urethra: a 40-year single institution experience. *J Urol.* 2005;173:1958–1965.

25. Lillis JV, North J, Vetto JT, et al. Primary scrotal melanoma presenting as a large, amelanotic, exophytic mass. *Arch Dermatol.* 2009;145:1071–1072.

26. Droesch JT, Flum DR, Mann GN. Wide local excision or abdominoperineal resection as the initial treatment for anorectal melanoma? *Am J Surg.* 2005;189:446–449.

27. Heyn J, Placzek M, Ozimek A, et al. Malignant melanoma of the anal region. *Clin Exp Dermatol.* 2007;32:603–607.

28. Meyle KD, Guldberg P. Genetic risk factors for melanoma. *Hum Genet.* 2009;126:499–510.

29. Sekine S, Nakanishi Y, Ogawa R, et al. Esophageal melanomas harbor frequent NRAS mutations unlike melanomas of other mucosal sites. *Virchows Arch.* 2009;454:513–517.

30. Ruer JB, Pépin L, Gheit T, et al. Detection of alpha- and beta-human papillomavirus (HPV) in cutaneous melanoma: a matched and controlled study using specific multiplex PCR combined with DNA microarray primer extension. *Exp Dermatol.* 2009;18:857–862.

31. Piura B. Management of primary melanoma of the female urogenital tract. *Lancet Oncol.* 2008;9:973–981.

32. Iddings DM, Fleisig AJ, Chen SL, et al. Practice patterns and outcomes for anorectal melanoma in the USA, reviewing three decades of treatment: is more extensive surgical resection beneficial in all patients? *Ann Surg Oncol.* 2010;17:40–44.

CHAPTER 14

Pediatric Genital Disease

LIBBY EDWARDS

Genital complaints produce anxiety in patients generally, with fears of malignancy, sexual functioning, fertility, and sexually transmitted diseases. Genital symptoms and abnormalities in children are fraught with even more anxiety in parents, who feel responsibility for their child's disease, while being unable to alleviate it. Often, providers have investigated the possibility of sexually transmitted disease, or have broached the subject of sexual abuse, producing even more anxiety, defensiveness, and anger. Or, a parent's overattention to the child's symptoms can lead to either anxiety on the part of the child or enjoyment of the attention with subsequent manipulation.

The primary therapy for parents of children with genital complaints is reassurance, and words of caution regarding information they will find on the Internet. Printed handouts are supportive, as the written word is perceived as authoritative, and assures the parent that the problem is one recognized and shared by others. Their child is not alone, and both information and treatment of the condition are available. Specific reassurance that their condition is not the parent's fault, and that it will not affect fertility, sexual functioning, or the development of malignancy is crucial to many families.

NORMAL GENITALIA

The appearance of the prepuberal external genitalia varies with the age of the child and with the normal differences among individuals. Generally, clinicians do not examine the genitalia carefully after the newborn examination unless there are questions of abuse or disease. Therefore, the range of normal is often not appreciated, and, except for the hymen, there is little information on the normal variants and changes in the external genitalia.

Females

Newborn female genitalia reflect the effects of maternal hormones (Fig. 14-1). The presence of estrogen produces generous labia minora, which extend beyond puffy labia majora. The mucosa is pink, resilient, and moist, with thick hymenal folds covering the small vaginal and urethral openings. Milky, physiologic secretions are often present.

By 8 weeks of life, the effect of maternal hormones has diminished. The labia majora lose the full, puffy appearance, and the underlying labia minora and hymen are thin and flat. The labia minora are vestigial, and generally represent only anterior remnants of the clitoral frenulum. The vaginal opening is easily viewed, without a need for separation of the labia minora. The thin hymenal ring is present within the vaginal opening. There are several normal variations of the appearance and shape of the hymen. The mucosa is now thin and atrophic, often with a red and irritated appearance that worries parents. Friction, urine, stool, over-washing, soaps, etc. produce irritation in this atrophic, fragile skin. Tissues lack elasticity in early childhood, and this contributes to tearing with trauma. I believe that many children also experience adhesions of the clitoral hood to the clitoris simply as a result of this mild vulvar irritation, just as midline labial adhesions occur. Both processes generally reverse in later childhood. However, a recent study has reported that a third of college women exhibit synechiae of variable severity of the clitoris to the clitoral hood (1).

With the onset of puberty, there is thickening of all vulvar and vaginal tissues, and midline hair growth is noted. The labia majora become puffy with fat deposition, and the labia minora develop a rounded, thickened appearance. The clitoris enlarges, and the hymen thickens with enlargement of the central opening. As in infancy, the mucosa becomes pink, soft, elastic, and moist. White discharge is common as endogenous estrogens stimulate vaginal secretions, and puritus occurs in some girls as a result of the constant and unaccustomed wetness.

Males

The influence of maternal hormones on male genitalia is less pronounced. Newborn boys often exhibit swelling of the scrotum resulting from fluid collection in the tunica vaginalis during the birthing process or a hydrocele (see section "Hydrocele"). Hyperpigmentation of the scrotum and penile shaft may be more prominent at birth, especially in darkly pigmented races. A study of 10,421 newborns showed that all exhibited at least partial phimosis, with an inability to retract the foreskin (2). By adolescence, only 6.8% of boys could not retract the foreskin.

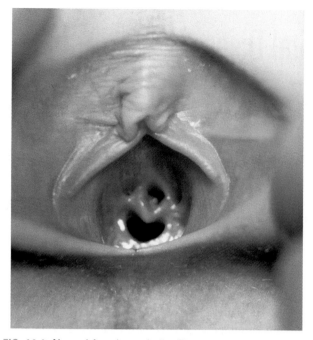

FIG. 14-1. Normal female genitalia. The labia majora are being retracted. The clitoris is visible superiorly. The labia minora do not fully cover the vaginal opening, thus allowing a clear view of the hymenal ring.

Before puberty, the penis is short and thin (Fig. 14-2). Pigmentation is similar to the general body pigment. The scrotum is less pendulous, and the skin is soft, thin, and pink, with few rugae. Both testes are palpable as soft masses within the scrotal sac. Small milia may be present on the scrotum.

At puberty, there is enlargement of the phallus both in length and circumference, with thickening and development of the glans. The scrotal sac and testes also enlarge and become more pendulous. The skin of the scrotum darkens and thickens, developing a coarse texture and folding into rugae. Pubic hair is noted first along the base of the shaft and then extending into the inguinal creases and onto the medial thighs as it becomes darker, coarser, and curlier.

CONGENITAL ABNORMALITIES

Hypospadias and Chordee

Hypospadias is a developmental anomaly in which the opening of the urethra is abnormally positioned on the undersurface of the penis. It can also occur in girls, with the urethral canal opening into the vagina. About 1 in 500 newborns are affected with hypospadias.

Hypospadias can be mild, with the urethral meatus opening on the ventral aspect of the glans, or more severe, with a larger opening more proximally on the shaft (Fig. 14-3). When the opening occurs at the penoscrotal junction, the penis is curved ventrally (chordee), and the penile urethra is very short. In the most extreme cases of hypospadias, the urethra opens into the perineum, the scrotum is bifid, and the chordee is extreme.

Testes are undescended in 10% of boys with hypospadias, and there may be an associated inguinal hernia, but other anomalies of the genitourinary tract are rare.

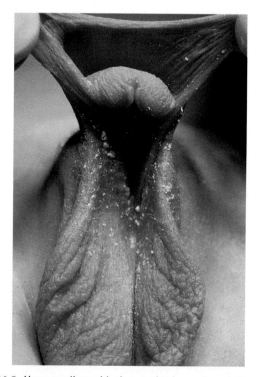

FIG. 14-3. Hypospadias with the urethral opening at the penoscrotal junction. The penis is curved ventrally (chordee).

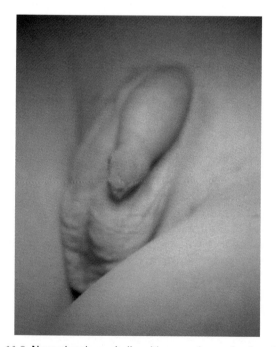

FIG. 14-2. Normal male genitalia with an uncircumcised penis.

However, severe cases of hypospadias can be confused with ambiguous genitalia, especially masculinization of female infants as a result of congenital adrenal hyperplasia.

Treatment for hypospadias and chordee is surgical and usually takes place in the first year of life. Mild cases are repaired for cosmetic reasons and to allow the child to void in a standing position. However, repair of severe hypospadias and chordee is essential to allow for normal sexual function. Newborns with hypospadias should not be circumcised because the foreskin will be used for the reconstructive procedure.

Hydrocele

A congenital hydrocele is a collection of fluid in the scrotum surrounding the testes (Fig. 14-4). It occurs when the processus vaginalis remains patent, connecting the abdominal cavity to the tunica vaginalis in the scrotum. If the connection is narrow, only peritoneal fluid collects in the tunica vaginalis, causing scrotal swelling and making the testis difficult to palpate. If it is large, a loop of intestine or the omentum can enter the processus vaginalis, forming an inguinal hernia. When the herniated viscera extend into the scrotum, a complete indirect inguinal hernia is present. Scrotal swelling resulting from a hydrocele can be distinguished from an inguinal hernia by transillumination of the scrotum; the former transilluminates brightly but the latter does not.

Small hydroceles often disappear in the first year of life. If the amount of fluid in the scrotum varies with time, a patent processus vaginalis with connection to the peritoneal cavity is present. This requires surgical correction, which is usually accomplished in the first year of life.

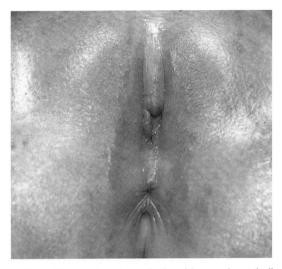

FIG. 14-5. Ambiguous female genitalia with an enlarged clitoris and interlabial fusion.

Larger hydroceles that do not vary in size often require surgical correction as well.

Ambiguous Genitalia

Either virilization of the female fetus or incomplete virilization of the male fetus *in utero* produce ambiguous genitalia (Fig. 14-5). There are several different abnormalities that can lead to these developmental anomalies.

Clinical Presentation

Female infants are born as pseudohermaphrodites with varying degrees of masculinization. Enlargement of the clitoris and labial fusion are usual. Sometimes, the clitoris can be so enlarged that it resembles a penis. The urethral opening below is attributed to hypospadias, with cryptorchidism resulting in incorrect gender assignment. In boys, newborns are either phenotypically female or have varying degrees of virilization from labioscrotal fusion to perineal hypospadias and cryptorchidism.

Diagnosis

The identification of ambiguous genitalia is made on the clinical examination, but the diagnosis of the underlying cause requires laboratory testing, and is discussed in section "Management."

Pathophysiology

The most common cause of female virilization is congenital adrenal hyperplasia. In this condition, there is an inherited enzymatic defect in the production of cortisol, usually resulting from a 21-hydroxylase deficiency. Deficiency of cortisol results in an increased secretion of corticotropin and stimulation of adrenocortical hyperplasia with overproduction of intermediate metabolites in the cortisol pathway. In the classic form of the disease,

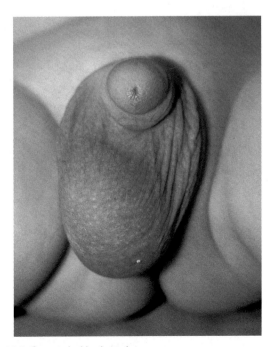

FIG. 14-4. Congenital hydrocele.

patients are also salt losers, a potentially life-threatening condition when not recognized. Four other enzymatic defects of cortisone production as well as virilizing adrenocortical tumors in the mother can also result in ambiguous genitalia in the newborn female.

In the male fetus, the situation is even more complex. Male pseudohermaphroditism can result from chromosomal deletion of the male-determining genes that are present on both arms of the Y chromosome, from aplasia or hypoplasia of Leydigs cells, from genetic defects in the synthesis of testosterone or in the production of other androgens such as dihydrotestosterone, or from peripheral cellular resistance to the action of these hormones.

Management

Ambiguous genitalia in a newborn should be addressed immediately. Chromosomal analysis should be undertaken at once. For female patients, studies of adrenal hormones should be done to rule out salt-losing adrenogenital syndrome. Ultrasound of internal organs to determine the presence of uterus and ovaries is indicated, as well as endoscopic examination of the vagina if possible.

For male patients, it is necessary to determine whether testicular androgen production is normal and whether there is normal conversion of testosterone to dihydrotestosterone. If a microphallus is present, it may be possible to stimulate growth with testosterone injection. If this is unsuccessful, boys are usually raised as girls. Gender assignment should take place early to avoid psychologic problems. Reconstruction of the external genitalia to create a functional female is more easily accomplished than creating a functional male phallus. Male testes are removed during surgery because of the increased incidence of gonadal malignancy in pseudohermaphrodites.

Labial Adhesions

Clinical Presentation

Labial adhesions appear as midline fusion of the introitus. This is the most common form of vaginal obstruction seen in prepubertal girls. Adhesions are posterior in 79% to 93% of affected girls (Fig. 14-6), sometimes with mid- or anterior adhesions forming (3). Uncommonly, the vulvar vestibule fuses entirely, covering the urethra (Fig. 14-7). Patients with labial agglutination are asymptomatic unless urinary retention or infection occurs behind the adhesions. Occasionally, even incomplete adhesions are bothersome as urine can become partially trapped above the synechiae, with dribbling when the child stands.

Diagnosis

The diagnosis is made by the clinical appearance. The smooth, flat surface that overlies the introitus can suggest absence of the vagina, but it is distinguished by the presence of a central thin translucent line of fibrous tissue at the site of fusion.

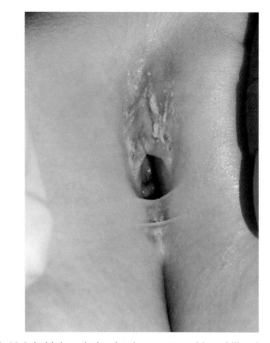

FIG. 14-6. Labial agglutination has occurred by midline fusion of the posterior vestibule.

Pathophysiology

Synechiae caused by chronic inflammation of the vulvar skin, resulting from mechanical trauma, infection, or skin disease, including lichen sclerosus or irritant dermatitis. Some have suggested that, because topical estrogen generally lyses labial adhesions, low estrogen levels

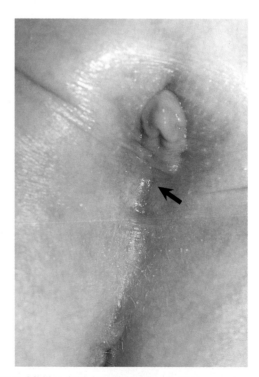

FIG. 14-7. Midline labial agglutination in this case has nearly completely fused the labia, leaving only a pinpoint opening that nonetheless produces no significant urinary obstruction (arrow).

may play a role in the formation of these adhesions. However, serum levels of estrogen in girls with labial adhesions are the same as those in girls without adhesions (4). Still, the normal infantile estrogen-deficient (compared to postpubertal girls) vulvar epithelium is thin, easily irritated, and more likely to scar compared to well-estrogenized vulvar skin. Vulvar epithelium scars easily in general, and even more so in atrophic prepubertal skin.

Management

Generally, no treatment beyond robust reassurance is required, as adhesions regularly resolve by puberty. Complete or symptomatic adhesions are treated with local application of estrogen cream combined with gentle massage and good hygiene, or a topical corticosteroid, especially if there is clinical underlying skin disease. Although the classic treatment is a topical estrogen, a recent retrospective chart review showed that a potent topical corticosteroid produced lysis of adhesions in an average of 1.3 months, with a lower recurrence rate, as compared to 2.2 months with the use of estrogen. Side effects with the estrogen were vaginal bleeding and breast budding, as compared to local irritation with the corticosteroid (5). Another chart review reported successful lysis of adhesions in 15 of 43 children treated with topical estrogen, with 19 lost to followup (6), and a third chart review of children treated with topical estrogen showed success in 79% of children, but 41% experienced recurrence of labial adhesions (7). A retrospective survey of girls treated with a potent topical corticosteroid showed success in 68% of children (8). A topical potent corticosteroid ointment (such as clobetasol or betamethasone dipropionate) is applied very sparingly once or twice a day, with monthly followup.

Occasionally, surgical separation is required because of pain, infection, or urinary retention. In a cooperative child, this can be done using topical anesthesia with lidocaine/prilocaine; the frightened child is best treated under general anesthesia/conscious sedation. A well-lubricated cotton swab sometimes can be used to separate the labia. More difficult scarring can be separated by peeling the synechiae apart following a nick of the edge of the line of fusion with a #15 blade. Estrogen cream or a corticosteroid ointment should be applied afterward to prevent reformation of the adhesions that is otherwise likely to occur immediately. The area should be re-evaluated every few days initially by the clinician to detect early recurrence during healing.

RED PLAQUES AND PAPULES

Diaper Dermatitis (napkin dermatitis)

Diaper dermatitis is best viewed as a combination of dermatoses that result from the unique environment of the diaper area. Diaper dermatitis must be differentiated

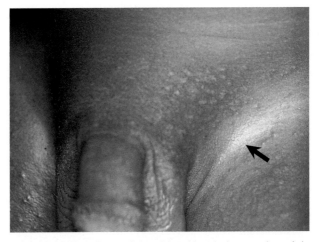

FIG. 14-8. Irritant diaper dermatitis with relative sparing of the inguinal creases *(arrow)*, and papules on the convex surfaces of the mons and thighs.

from other skin diseases that preferentially occur in this area.

Clinical Presentation

Diaper dermatitis is characterized by scaling, erythematous plaques that sometimes exhibit maceration and erosion when severe. Often, there are several factors that produce this occluded dermatitis, and the features depend on the causes playing a role in that child.

Irritant diaper dermatitis is characterized by dermatitis occurring on the more convex surfaces that directly contact urine and stool, and sparing of the skin creases (Figs. 14-8 and 14-9). The perineum, buttocks, lower abdomen, and upper thighs are most commonly involved. Sharp margination where the diaper ends is typical. The skin is pink to bright red, often with edema and superficial erosions that produce a shiny, glazed appearance.

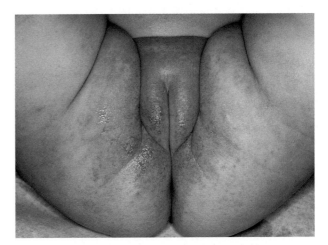

FIG. 14-9. Irritant diaper dermatitis with shiny, glazed buttocks, fissures, and erosions that are covered with superficial erosions.

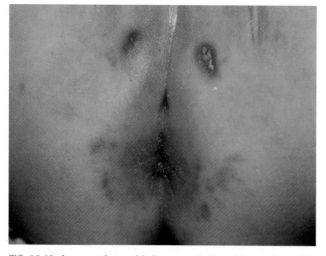

FIG. 14-10. Jacquet dermatitis is severe irritant diaper dermatitis with characteristic eroded nodules; early changes of this condition are evident here.

Eroded skin is tender and painful, especially when it is in contact with irritating substances such as alcohol or propylene glycol that are contained in diaper wipes.

A severe form of irritant dermatitis is termed diaper dermatitis of Jacquet, granuloma gluteale infantum, or pseudowarts (see section "Granuloma Gluteale Infantum"). This is characterized by sharply marginated, red nodules, often with overlying erosion that confers an umbilicated appearance. These typically affect the labia majora, perianal skin, and the glans penis (Figs. 14-10 and 14-11). Crusting of the urinary meatus can make voiding difficult and painful.

Frictional dermatitis is most pronounced on the inner thighs, under the fastening tabs and waistband of the diaper, and on other surfaces that rub against the diaper. It consists of mild erythema and papules that wax and wane and respond quickly to diapering more often so that moisture is minimized.

Intertrigo from moisture and friction occurs within the skin folds of the diaper area, but also can occur in the neck creases, under the axilla, and between the fat rolls on the thighs. A sharp cutoff where the dry skin begins is noted. Affected areas are oozing, macerated, and red. Superficial sloughing of white hydrated skin is common.

When *Candida albicans* complicates diaper dermatitis, the infection preferentially affects the skin folds, with deep, bright erythema showing surrounding peripheral scale (Fig. 14-12). Satellite collarettes or round erosions are characteristic.

Diagnosis

The diagnosis of diaper dermatitis is made by the presence of erythema and scale, with or without erosions and maceration in the diaper area. Specific dermatoses other than irritant dermatitis and candidiasis should be excluded. A biopsy is not indicated, but a fungal preparation of affected skin can help to elucidate the role of *C. albicans*.

Response to therapy helps to confirm the diagnosis. Any diaper rash that is properly managed with barriers, frequent diaper changes, low-potency corticosteroids, and antifungal agents should resolve over 1 to 2 weeks.

An inflammatory disease that occurs in the diaper area and resembles diaper dermatitis is psoriasis. Silvery scale in drier areas and sharply demarcated borders suggest this diagnosis. Often, typical plaques on other skin surfaces and nail changes support a diagnosis of psoriasis. Seborrhea

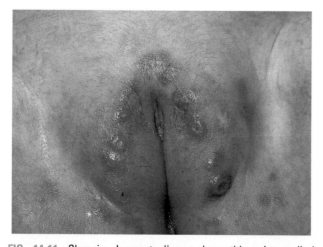

FIG. 14-11. Chronic Jacquet diaper dermatitis, also called pseudowarts, granuloma gluteale infantum, and papulonodular irritant dermatitis, exhibits more well-formed, firm nodules with the classic umbilicated center, again most marked on convex surfaces.

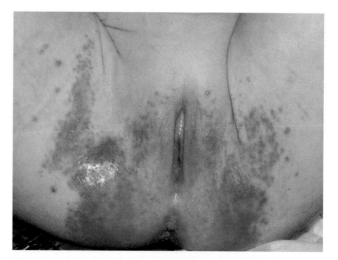

FIG. 14-12. The shiny, glazed appearance of buttocks, and the coalescing satellite papules and pustules are characteristic of *Candida* diaper dermatitis. This is confirmed by microscopic examination or culture.

mimics diaper dermatitis, but these babies have scalp disease as well. The presence of lichenification suggests atopic dermatitis. Atopic dermatitis of the diaper area is generally accompanied by pruritic eczematous plaques on the cheeks, dorsal arms, and legs. The presence of vesicles suggests allergic contact dermatitis, and a history of application of a potential allergen supports this diagnosis.

Acrodermatitis enteropathica is a rare disease that is a manifestation of zinc deficiency. This is characterized by diarrhea, alopecia, and well-demarcated red, crusted plaques of the anogenital skin and perioral area.

Langerhans cell histiocytosis and granuloma gluteale infantum occur in the diaper area as well (see section "Granuloma Gluteale Infantum").

Pathophysiology

Diaper dermatitis is multifactorial but primarily irritant contact, sometimes with candidiasis (Table 14-1). The irritants include wetness and friction of a diaper over skin exposed to urine and stool. Occasionally, atopic dermatitis plays a role (Fig. 14-13).

Irritant contact diaper dermatitis occurs when there is prolonged contact of the skin in the diaper area with irritating substances such as urine and feces. Infrequent diaper changes combined with heat and maceration of the skin under the diaper contribute to the severity of this dermatitis. It is often precipitated by the loose, frequent stools that accompany viral illnesses in infancy. Concentrated urine, proteolytic enzymes, and the high pH of stool that occurs with malabsorption are particularly problematic for sensitive skin. In addition, heightened efforts to cleanse the diaper area using harsh soaps and detergents expose already inflamed skin to further

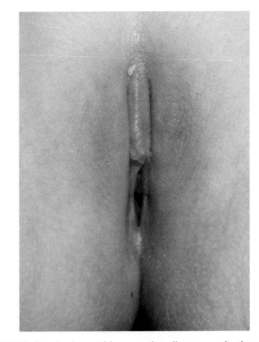

FIG. 14-13. Atopic dermatitis occasionally occurs in the diaper area, as manifested here by lichenification. However, the diaper area is often spared of atopic dermatitis because the environment is not dry, and diapers protect from rubbing and scratching. This condition is generally associated with typical eczematous lesions on the extremities.

irritation and can set up a vicious cycle that is difficult to break.

Intertrigo, irritant dermatitis from chronic moisture and friction between skin folds, occurs more commonly in hot weather and is often accompanied by miliaria, or prickly heat. It is localized to the skin folds, where sweat and moisture are trapped, causing maceration and oozing.

Management

Treatment of diaper dermatitis is primarily aimed at changing the environment to eliminate common causes and re-evaluating the dermatitis that remains. Regardless of cause, all diaper dermatitis improves with elimination of irritating substances and a decrease in friction and maceration. This can best be accomplished with frequent diaper changes, the use of gel-containing disposable diapers that diminish direct contact of body substances with the skin, and the application of barrier cream to the involved areas. Pastes containing high concentrations of impervious zinc oxide or petroleum jelly are most effective (9). Copious quantities must be applied to the skin with each diaper change, and avoidance of further irritation from cleansing soaps and older, irritating wipes is critical (Fig. 14-14A, B). Newer emollient wipes may be better tolerated than water and a soft cloth (10). However, adherent stool is best removed by gently rinsing the perianal area with warm water and patting the skin dry. The application of a

TABLE 14.1	Diaper dermatitis: a multifactorial eruption

Factors include some or all:
Irritant contact dermatitis
  Urine
  Feces
  Soap
  Water
  Wipes
  Fragrances
  Creams
Frictional dermatitis (rubbing of diapers and skin folds)
Intertrigo (skin-fold irritation from heat, moisture of sweat and excrement, and sometimes *Candida albicans*)
Candida albicans infection

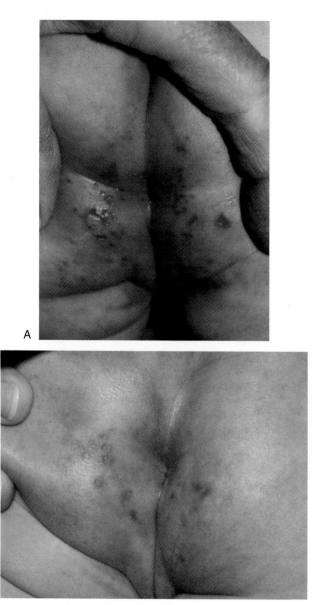

FIG. 14-14. A: This severely erosive diaper dermatitis occurs each time this child develops diarrhea, an extraordinarily corrosive, alkaline substance. **B:** After 10 days of the use of a heavy barrier with zinc oxide and petrolatum and hydrocortisone ointment, the dermatitis is improved, and the infant is more comfortable.

barrier cream to anogenital skin is more effective than the aggressive removal of feces by rubbing or the use of harsh cleansers. Mild corticosteroid preparations such as 1% or 2.5% hydrocortisone ointment (not cream) hastens resolution of inflammation when applied twice daily and covered with barrier cream or ointment. Potent corticosteroids should not be applied under diaper occlusion, which enhances the effect of the medication. Adrenal suppression and deaths due to immunosuppresion have been reported in several infants treated with ultrapotent corticosteroids under diaper occlusion (11,12). Anticandidal agents should be added if there is a question of yeast.

Nystatin is available in an ointment base and is less irritating than the azole creams. When disease is severe and erosions are present, antifungal medication should be administered orally until healing begins.

Persistence of dermatitis when these measures are taken usually indicates an ongoing irritant process or an alternative diagnosis. Chronic diarrhea is a common cause for persistence of dermatitis, and this predisposes to yeast. An evaluation of the child's diet and growth parameters and a search for underlying disease such as infection or malabsorption are indicated. In the absence of diarrhea, a skin biopsy may be helpful to identify other primary cutaneous disease.

Seborrheic Dermatitis

Seborrheic dermatitis is a common form of dermatitis in infants and adolescents.

Clinical Presentation

Seborrheic dermatitis first occurs at about 4 to 6 weeks of life, but rarely after a year of age. Scalp seborrhea is common after puberty, but genital involvement does not occur. In infants, the areas most commonly involved are the scalp, the face, the postauricular area, and the intertriginous folds including the neck, axillae, inguinal area, and between fat rolls. The scalp is usually involved first, with greasy, yellow scales with minimal inflammation. The diaper area is the second most common area to develop a rash. Seborrheic diaper dermatitis consists of erythematous, sharply marginated scaling plaques with greasy, macerated scales (Figs. 14-15 and 4-22). *Candida* frequently superinfects the area. The inguinal creases are more severely affected, but in many cases the groin and perineum are confluently involved. Spread to other flexural areas and even onto the trunk as isolated scaly plaques can occur (Fig. 14-15). Unlike atopic dermatitis, seborrheic dermatitis is nonpruritic.

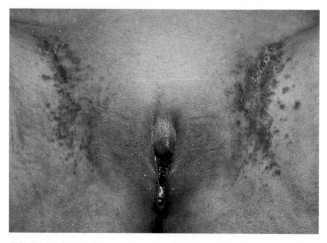

FIG. 14-15. Seborrheic diaper dermatitis exhibits greasy, yellow, crusted scales in the inguinal creases.

Diagnosis

The diagnosis of seborrheic dermatitis is usually made on a clinical basis, in an infant with scalp and intertriginous erythema and yellowish scale. The age of onset and distribution are the most helpful clinical features. A biopsy is rarely required for the diagnosis, and the histologic features of seborrheic dermatitis are nondiagnostic. Spongiosis with parakeratosis, moderate acanthosis, and exocytosis of neutrophils are seen. There is a superficial perivascular lymphohistiocytic infiltrate.

The differential diagnosis of seborrheic dermatitis includes atopic dermatitis, intertrigo, and Langerhans cell histiocytosis. Psoriasis can mimic seborrhea, by exhibiting well-demarcated scaly plaques in the groin. Involvement of the periumbilical area and well-demarcated plaques on the posterior scalp, rather than diffuse scalp involvement, can help to distinguish these two entities. Biopsy of seborrheic dermatitis can be similar to that of psoriasis and is not helpful.

Pathophysiology

Seborrheic dermatitis affects the areas of the skin where there is an abundance of sebaceous glands, including the scalp, face, and postauricular and intertriginous areas. The cause of seborrheic dermatitis is unknown. An abnormal reaction in the skin to a commensural yeast, *Pityrosporum ovale*, has been implicated in the pathogenesis of this dermatitis, because treatment with topical and oral antifungal agents causes improvement, although topical corticosteroids are even more effective. It is not known whether the observed effects of these agents result from their anti-inflammatory properties or their antifungal properties, however. Impaired function of the enzyme γ-6-desaturase was implicated in the pathogenesis of infantile seborrheic dermatitis by causing an alteration of essential fatty acids.

Management

The treatment of seborrhea of the diaper area consists of low-potency hydrocortisone ointment and barrier creams or ointments. Antifungal therapy can be helpful in the event of candidiasis. The scalp should be treated for maximal improvement; this can be achieved by removing scale with mineral or baby oil. Antiseborrheic shampoos or mild baby shampoos, and mild topical steroid scalp solutions, such as hydrocortisone 1% or 2.5% to reduce recurrent inflammation, are also helpful. Scrubbing and shampoos with acids should be discouraged.

Atopic Dermatitis

Atopic dermatitis is an extremely pruritic eruption that occurs when irritation precipitates rubbing and scratching, which, in turn, cause erythema, lichenification, and excoriation (Fig. 14-16A, B) (see Chapter 4). The diaper area is relatively spared in infants because the skin is covered and remains moist, and the diaper helps to protect the skin

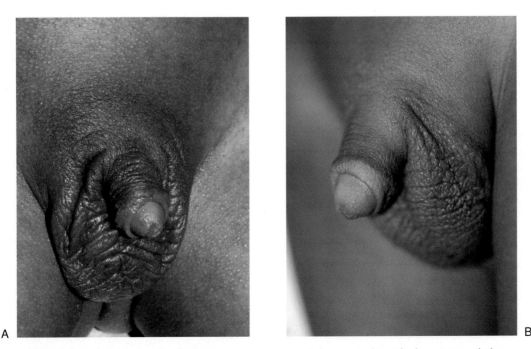

FIG. 14-16. A: Lichenified atopic dermatitis of the scrotum and penis in a young boy who has extragenital eczema as well. Shiny, monomorphous papules of papular atopic dermatitis can be seen on the proximal thighs. **B:** After several weeks of a potent topical corticosteroid (but not under diaper occlusion), the penis is normal and scrotal lichenfication is much improved.

from rubbing and scratching. Treatment consists of a topical corticosteroid and avoidance of irritants.

Psoriasis

Psoriasis is a skin condition that is relatively uncommon in children in the genital area (see Chapter 6). This is a skin disease characterized by increased turnover of epidermal cells, so the skin becomes thickened and covered by dense scale. It preferentially affects irritated or injured skin, so the genitalia and diaper area are often affected.

Plaques are red, well demarcated, and thickened (Figs. 14-17 and 14-18). Often, psoriasis also affects the umbilicus, scalp, and gluteal cleft, and the fingernails may exhibit small pits. Often, however, there are no pathognomonic signs of psoriasis. Psoriasis of the skin folds and diaper area can mimic seborrheic dermatitis as well as cutaneous candidiasis, which is often a secondary factor. Even a biopsy is characteristic but often not diagnostic. In unclear cases, the course of the disease eventually provides a diagnosis, because psoriasis is chronic and other areas of the skin nearly always become involved, showing typical psoriatic lesions.

Treatment consists of careful local care and topical corticosteroids. For the occasional unfortunate child with severe or widespread disease, systemic therapy may be required.

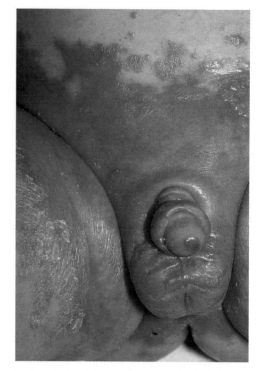

FIG. 14-18. Psoriasis also sometimes exhibits a glazed appearance in the diaper area and generally differs from atopic dermatitis in its very sharp borders and frequent extragenital involvement of other skin surfaces.

Perianal Streptococcal Dermatitis (perianal streptococcal cellulitis)

Perianal streptococcal dermatitis is a red, tender rash that classically occurs in the perianal area, sometimes encompassing the vulva and penis. Although primarily a childhood disease, this occurs also in adults on occasion. See also Chapter 6.

Clinical Presentation

Perianal streptococcal dermatitis typically occurs in 3- to 5-year-old children, and it is more common in boys than in girls. Most commonly, 2- to 3-cm of erythema extends outward around the anus with minimal induration (Fig. 14-19). In other individuals, this erythema is accompanied by painful anal fissuring and a mucoid discharge that makes defecation painful. Constipation and withholding of stool are common, and it is often unclear whether the fissure was produced by the primary disease or by passage of hard stool. Finally, well-demarcated, scaly, beefy red, crusted dermatitis with maceration of the anal verge can occur. In addition, induration of the perianal skin and satellite crusted plaques can be seen. Bleeding from the area is common. Girls can exhibit vulvar and vaginal involvement, and boys can experience penile involvement, so a change in name to perineal streptococcal disease has been suggested (Fig. 14-20).

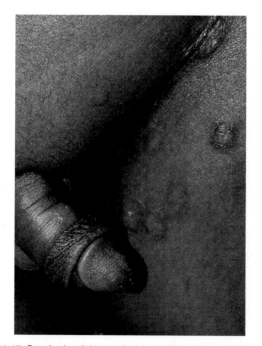

FIG. 14-17. Psoriasis of the genital area, like extragenital psoriasis, is classically manifested by inflamed (appearing hyperpigmented in darker skin) well-demarcated plaques. Scale is often subtle due to the moist environment of the genital skin.

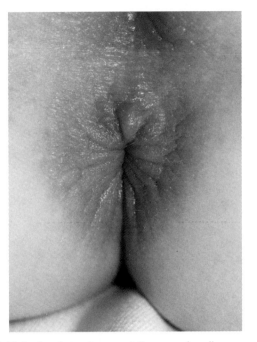

FIG. 14-19. Perianal streptococcal disease primarily causes erythema, edema, subtle scaling, and fissuring perianal skin. Note the protrusion of perianal skin at 12 o'clock, representing a mild infantile perianal pyramidal protrusion, which can be seen with any inflammation, or even as a normal finding.

In all forms of anogenital streptococcal dermatitis, pruritus, excoriations, and lichenification from scratching and rubbing are common. These superimposed eczematous changes can delay the diagnosis.

Diagnosis

The diagnosis of perianal streptococcal dermatitis is made on clinical grounds and is confirmed by a routine culture of the surrounding skin that yields group A β-hemolytic *Streptococcus* on blood agar. It is important to ask the

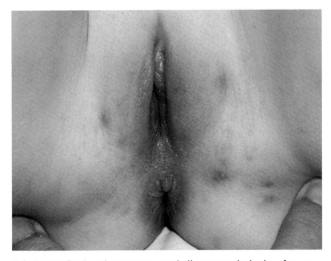

FIG. 14-20. Perianal streptococcal disease relatively often extends to affect the vulva and produces vaginitis (or balanitis in male patients).

laboratory to culture for *Streptococcus* because most laboratories select for enteric pathogens from perianal swabs. Culture of the throat often yields the same organism.

The differential diagnosis of perianal *Streptococcus* includes pinworm infestation, irritant or *Candida* dermatitis, atopic dermatitis, psoriasis, inflammatory bowel disease, perianal staphylococcal dermatitis, and sexual abuse. Scratching and rubbing of the skin resulting from pruritus are common and can confuse the diagnosis. All perianal dermatitis should be cultured to rule out perianal *Streptococcus* as a possible pathogen.

Pathophysiology

Bacterial skin infection of the perianal skin, most often with group A β-hemolytic *Streptococcus*, produces distinctive this dermatitis in children. Many patients diagnosed with perianal streptococcus have throat cultures positive for the organism without symptoms of pharyngitis. Presumably, digital contamination of the anus from the infected pharynx or other body site is the source of the infection.

Managment

The treatment of choice for group A β-hemolytic *Streptococcus* has been penicillin V 5 mg/kg/day orally in four divided doses for 10 days. More recently, a trial comparing penicillin to cefuroxime showed such superiority of the cefuroxime that the study was discontinued; cultures of those treated with penicillin were positive for persistent streptococci in 7 of 15 patients as compared to positive culture in only 1 of 14 patients treated with cefuroxime (13). Because recurrences are common, some clinicians support antibiotic therapy for as long as 21 days to allow for the skin to heal before discontinuation of medication (14). Mupirocin ointment applied two to four times a day may minimize recurrences as well. Stool softeners can be useful in children with painful defecation due to perianal inflammation and fissures, and hydrocortisone 1% or 2.5% ointment can minimize pain while awaiting improvement with the antibiotic.

Pinworm

Pinworms infection is a common cause of perianal pruritus in small children.

Clinical Presentation

Pinworms produce no symptoms during infestation except transient dermatitis and pruritus of the perianal skin or vulva. Excoriations are often more prominent than obvious redness and scaling. Complaints of nighttime pruritus are the greatest complaint, and may be severe enough to wake the child. Occasionally, a child describes pain rather than itching. Rarely, the worms migrate to the vagina in girls and cause vulvar dermatitis and a vaginal discharge, or produce balanitis in boys.

Diagnosis

The diagnosis of pinworms is made in the setting of an unexplained perianal or vulvar pruritus, with or without a mild dermatitis, and is confirmed by response to therapy. Pinworms are usually difficult to find for diagnostic evaluation. At night, adult worms are occasionally seen on the perineum or in the anal canal when it is gently everted. Eggs can usually be collected using clear tape placed over the anus first thing in the morning before the eggs are disturbed. The eggs can be viewed adherent to the tape as thick-walled, ovoid structures most easily seen by light microscopy under low power.

The differential diagnosis of pinworm infection includes perianal streptococcal dermatitis, atopic dermatitis, irritant dermatitis, and candidiasis. The presence of severe nighttime symptoms of perianal pruritus with minimal inflammation can help to distinguish this disorder from other forms of dermatitis.

Pathophysiology

Pinworm infestation is the most common form of helminth infestation seen in humans, and is produced by infestation with *Enterobius vermicularis*. Pinworms are much common in children than in adults, with more than 20% of school-aged children acquiring this ubiquitous infestation.

Pinworm infestation begins by ingestion of eggs, usually on fingers that have contacted perianal skin or dirt with eggs. Eggs hatch in the duodenum and mature during passage through the intestines. Migration to the perianal skin occurs, and gravid females deposit their eggs on the anal verge, causing pruritus. Four to six hours after the eggs are deposited, they become infectious, and when the eggs are swallowed, the cycle begins again.

Management

Treatment of pinworms is with mebendazole 100 mg in a single dose, and application of a mild topical steroid ointment for any dermatitis that is present. Pyrantel pamoate, in a single dose of 11 mg/kg, can also be used. Multiple family members are often affected at the same time, necessitating widespread simultaneous treatment to cure the infestation. Reinfection is common in school-aged children.

Retreatment in 2 to 3 weeks is recommended because neither drug is effective against ova that may have been ingested at the time of the first treatment.

Acrodermatitis Enteropathica and Acrodermatitis-like Eruptions

Acrodermatitis enteropathica is a rare skin disease produced by zinc deficiency, showing characteristic findings. These findings are also associated with nutritional deficiencies and several other uncommon metabolic disorders.

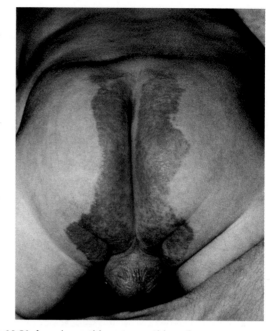

FIG. 14-21. Acrodermatitis enteropathica often causes severe involvement of the diaper area.

Clinical Presentation

The classic presentation of acrodermatitis enteropathica is a triad of periorificial dermatitis, diarrhea, and alopecia. Infants are irritable and have severe failure to thrive.

The dermatitis consists of periorificial erythematous, well-demarcated, and scaling plaques. At times, the skin may exhibit vesicopustular plaques and crusting (Figs. 14-21 and 14-22). It is most pronounced around the mouth, eyes, and genital area. Neck folds are often involved in infants, and the acral extremities may have similar scaly, erythematous, well-marginated plaques, especially in older children and adults. The diaper der-

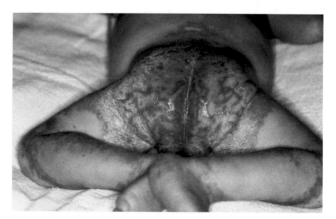

FIG. 14-22. This child with acrodermatitis enteropathica exhibits psoriasiform lesions present on the extremities as well as the buttocks.

matitis is usually severe and refractory to standard therapy. Secondary infections with *Staphylococcus* and *Candida* are common. Nail dystrophy and paronychia are also common, as is stomatitis.

Diagnosis

The diagnosis of acrodermatitis enteropathica is suspected based on the classical triad of dermatitis in a peri-orificial and acral distribution, alopecia, and diarrhea, and it is confirmed by low serum levels of zinc, alkaline phosphatase, and lipids. A skin biopsy is characteristic but not diagnostic. In early lesions, the upper part of the epidermis appears pale because of the presence of clear cells with balloon-like cytoplasm and loss of normal basophilia. Subcorneal vesicles may be present in the upper epidermis, and there is diffuse parakeratosis. Hyperplasia of the epidermis and parakeratosis are seen in older lesions in a nonspecific pattern.

Similar acral dermatitis is seen in other nutritional-deficiency states including biotin, protein, and essential fatty acid deficiency. These occur with cystic fibrosis, anorexia nervosa, chronic illness, and Crohn disease (15). Organic acidemias also produce these skin findings, including maple syrup urine disease, methylmalonic acidemia, and phenylketonuria (16). When screening for zinc deficiency is normal, serum metabolic screening can differentiate among these diseases.

Severe cases of seborrheic dermatitis or psoriasis, especially those complicated by superinfection with *Candida*, can have a similar appearance, but accompanying extragenital skin is often pathognomonic. The presence of scalp dermatitis suggests seborrhea, and normal laboratory findings rule out acrodermatitis enteropathica.

Pathophysiology

Acrodermatitis enteropathica is the classic manifestation of zinc deficiency. It occurs as a rare autosomal recessive disease or in nutritional deficiency states. Iatrogenic zinc deficiency can also result from parenteral nutrition. It is endemic in the adolescent population in some Middle Eastern countries.

All patients with acrodermatitis enteropathica have low levels of plasma zinc and other zinc-dependent metalloproteins such as alkaline phosphatase. In the inherited disease, there is a defect in zinc transport across the intestinal wall, and the responsible gene, SLC39A4, has been identified (17).

Symptoms of acrodermatitis enteropathica usually do not appear in breast-fed infants until weaning. A zinc-binding ligand that may be absent from the newborn's intestine appears to be present in breast milk, thus accounting for this observation. In Middle Eastern adolescents, the defect develops as a result of ingestion of high quantities of phytate, which binds zinc and prevents intestinal absorption.

Management

Treatment for acrodermatitis enteropathica consists of supplementation of zinc. Oral supplementation using zinc gluconate, acetate, or sulfate in doses of 5 mg/kg/day is recommended. Symptoms improve within 1 to 2 days of supplementation, and a response is noted in the dermatitis by 3 to 4 days. Hair growth begins in 2 to 4 weeks. After resolution of the disease symptoms, supplementation should be continued, in the inherited form of the disease, with measurement of serum zinc levels one or twice yearly. The acrodermatitis-like eruptions produced by other nutritional deficiencies are managed by identification of the cause of the deficiencies, and correction of these, just as the therapy of each metabolic disorders requires its unique management.

Letterer–Siwe Disease

Letterer–Siwe disease is the infantile form of Langerhans cell histiocytosis, formerly called histiocytosis X. Other forms of Langerhans cell histiocytosis are not characterized by genital skin disease.

Clinical Presentation

Letterer–Siwe disease usually manifests in children aged 3 years or younger. Skin features are the presenting signs in most children, and systemic manifestations typically occur in weeks to months after the onset of the cutaneous disease.

Affected infants develop an erythematous, scaly rash in the intertriginous areas, mimicking seborrheic dermatitis, but generally with induration not found in other scaling eruptions of the genitals in children (Fig. 14-23). The scalp, posterior auricular area, axilla, and inguinal creases are prominently involved. In infants, the diaper area is always severely affected. Moist scale and crust

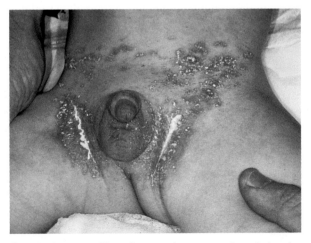

FIG. 14-23. Letterer–Siwe disease always prominently involves the diaper area. These skin findings can be differentiated from candidiasis and seborrheic dermatitis by their more infiltrated morphology and unresponsiveness to treatment for these conditions.

often cover the papules, but the reddish brown or purpuric nature of the lesions can usually be appreciated. Ulcerations are common and may be present on the oral mucous membranes. Purpuric nodules on the palms and soles are a poor prognostic sign.

Letterer–Siwe disease is a systemic process, with dissemination of abnormal histiocytes into the skin and extracutaneous locations including the liver, bone marrow, lymph nodes, and central nervous system. This fulminant process can be fatal, even with early treatment. Infiltration into the pituitary gland can lead to diabetes insipidus, and orbital infiltrates produce exophthalmos. Fever, anemia, thrombocytopenia, hepatosplenomegaly, and adenopathy are typical. Bony tumors may be hard to appreciate clinically. Some infants have a typical histologic appearance and never develop extracutaneous manifestations. These patients retrospectively have what is called self-healing reticulohistiocytosis.

The prognosis depends on the age of onset, the duration of symptoms, and the degree of systemic involvement. Onset after 6 months of age, the absence of thrombocytopenia and lung involvement, the lack of extensive systemic involvement, and the lack of purpuric skin lesions are all good prognostic signs.

A skin biopsy reveals infiltration with foamy histiocytes with a kidney-shaped nucleus. The infiltrate can be bandlike or nodular in plaque lesions or epidermotropic, producing the clinical petechiae and erosions. Immunohistochemistry is needed to identify the type of histiocytes present in the infiltrate. In Langerhans cell histiocytosis, cells are S100 and CD1 positive. Lymphomas can also contain histiocytes with these markers; so if the clinical diagnosis is unclear, ultrastructural analysis using electron microscopy can be used to demonstrate the presence of Birbeck granules, a finding that confirms the disease.

Diagnosis

The diagnosis of Letterer–Siwe disease is made with skin biopsy. Immunohistochemistry and occasionally electron microscopy can be used to confirm the diagnosis.

The rash of Letterer–Siwe disease most closely resembles severe seborrheic dermatitis. Any infant with a seborrheic-like rash that is purpuric, ulcerated, indurated, or poorly responsive to topical therapy should be examined by biopsy to rule out this disease. Intertrigo can also be seen in this distribution, but lack of involvement of the scalp, trunk, or extremities allows distinction from Langerhans cell histiocytosis. The presence of nodular and ulcerated lesions in the groin also suggests scabies. The absence of a history of scabies or other lesions suggestive of this diagnosis should warrant a skin biopsy.

Pathophysiology

Letterer–Siwe disease is produced by infiltration of the skin and other organs with histiocytes displaying Langerhans cell markers. The pathogenesis and origin of

this disease remain obscure, although studies have demonstrated that lesions in Letterer–Siwe disease comprise cells that are clonal. The reasons for localization of the disease process in the other forms of Langerhans cell histiocytosis are also unknown.

Management

All patients with a diagnosis of cutaneous Langerhans cell histiocytosis should undergo a complete survey for systemic disease by an oncologist. The skin disease can be treated with topical steroids, emollients, antibiotic ointments, and good local care. Topical nitrogen mustard has also been used in patients with severe skin involvement with good success. Spontaneous resolution of skin lesions occurs over time in many of these patients. Patients with systemic involvement are treated by an oncologist.

Scabies

Scabies is a fairly common mite infection that is extraordinarily itchy, and preferentially affects skin folds.

Clinical Presentation

Scabies manifests as an extremely pruritic dermatitis that is widespread in infants and young children. The pathognomonic skin burrow is difficult to find because of the presence of excoriations and crusted dermatitis in most patients. Other primary lesions include vesicles and papules that are similarly obliterated by most patients. The greatest clue to diagnosis in young infants and children is the presence of skin lesions on the fingers, hands, wrists, penis, buttocks, and in skin folds of the axillae and groin (Fig. 14-24).

Many infants and young children develop nodular lesions that are reddish brown and infiltrated, particularly on the glans penis, and in the genital area, the inguinal area, and the axilla (Fig. 14-25). These lesions represent hy-

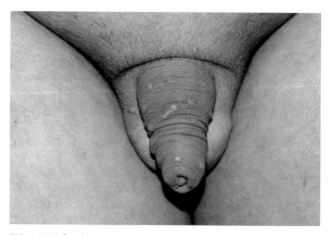

FIG. 14-24. Scabies prominently affects the genitalia, expecially the penis, as evidenced by these burrows. (Courtesy of Errol Craig, MD.)

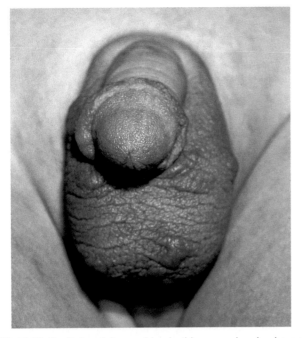

FIG. 14-25. Genital nodular scabies in this young boy is characterized by infiltrated, red, extremely pruritic lesions on the scrotum and penile shaft.

persensitivity reactions to the mite and have a very atypical appearance on biopsy that can be mistaken for histiocytosis or lymphoma. These nodules can persist for months after treatment.

In older children and adolescents, the typical distribution of lesions involves the web spaces, wrists, intergluteal cleft, elbows, belt line, under watch bands and rings, and around the nipple and genitals. The scalp and face are never involved in patients older than 2 years of age unless the child is immunosuppressed or bedridden.

Scabies is often complicated by a prolonged course as a result of misdiagnosis. Administration of topical corticosteroids can mask the infestation and can contribute to the spread of the mites by suppressing the immune hypersensitivity reaction that produces symptoms. Superinfection of the excoriated, eczematized lesions with *Staphylococcus aureus* produces crusting and pustules. Urticaria can also be seen.

Diagnosis

The diagnosis of scabies is made with the combination of clinical features in the typical distribution and microscopic evidence of infestation on mineral oil examination. Hand lesions, burrows, and nodular lesions are quite pathognomonic when present in infants and young children.

Scrapings of skin lesions and nail debris viewed microscopically in mineral oil are used for diagnosis. Mites and mite parts, eggs, and scybala (feces) are identified under 10× to 40× magnification. Ova are egg-shaped and translucent centrally. Scybala are much smaller and

are round or oval, often golden brown, and present in groups. On biopsy, histology reveals a nondiagnostic spongiotic dermatitis. Occasionally, a burrow or mite may be identified, but this is rare. Nodular lesions demonstrate intense inflammation with atypical histiocytes and lymphocytes. These can be mistaken for Langerhans cell histiocytosis or lymphoma in young children. It is important to consider scabies as a cause of nodular lesions in infants, even when there is little else clinically to suggest the diagnosis.

The differential diagnosis of scabies includes other eczematous dermatoses such as seborrheic dermatitis, atopic dermatitis, and even histiocytosis X. Multiple skin scrapings, a strong clinical suspicion, and, on occasion, a skin biopsy may be required to establish a diagnosis. Questioning and examining other family members for symptoms and signs of the infestation can often be helpful. Although the symptoms of scabies may lessen with topical corticosteroid application, resurgence with withdrawal of this treatment is usual.

Pathophysiology

Scabies is caused by infestation of the skin by *Sarcoptes scabiei*. This minute mite is unique to humans and endemic in the population. Intimate contact is necessary for spread of the mite, but it is usual for most family members to acquire the infestation once it is present and undiagnosed in the household.

The infestation begins with a newly fertilized female mite that burrows into the skin and lays eggs. There is a preference for skin that has a thin stratum corneum and few pilosebaceous glands. In children, the scalp can be involved, whereas infestation is confined to the area below the neck in adults, probably as a result of this skin preference.

The adult mite is approximately 0.5 mm in length with eight legs and an oval, translucent, gray body when viewed with the naked eye. Children are infested with large numbers of mites compared with adults, a finding perhaps relating to the immune reaction to the parasite. Symptoms of scabies infestation typically occur in 4 weeks to 4 months after acquiring the mite because sensitization of the host to the mite, feces, and eggs must occur before clinical symptoms develop.

Management

Treatment of scabies is accomplished with widespread application of a topical permethrin 5% cream. Care must be taken to cover all body areas, including the scalp in infants younger than 2 years old. The cream must be left in place overnight. Bathing before application is discouraged because this may increase percutaneous absorption. Fingernails should be cut and cleaned. Clothing and bedding that have been in contact with the patient or family members in the previous 24 hours should be washed, including outergarments. Treatment of all family members at once is essential to avoid reinfestation. An 89% cure rate is noted 1 month following a single treatment with permethrin. Retreatment of symptomatic patients and family members after 1 month may occasionally be necessary. Persistence of symptoms relates more commonly to inadequate treatment or reinfestation than to treatment failure.

Oral ivermectin in a single dose has been shown to be highly effective against scabies. This includes the hyperinfestation states seen with Norwegian scabies, and larger series have shown this agent to be safe in children. Use of this oral treatment may replace topical treatment in the future.

Granuloma Gluteale Infantum (pseudowarts, Jacquet diaper dermatitis)

Granuloma gluteale infantum is an uncommon reaction to a strong and chronic irritant in the anogenital area. More common in infants, this has been recognized in adults, with the tentative name of granuloma gluteale adultorum.

Clinical Presentation

Granuloma gluteale infantum is a nodular, skin-colored to red-brown eruption that develops in the diaper area (Figs. 14-10, 14-11, and 14-26). The individual lesions are indurated, flattopped papules that may exhibit central erosion, and are often monomorphous in appearance. They are usually multiple and occur primarily on the anterior surface of the genital area, mons, and perineum. The buttocks are usually spared, although perianal skin can be involved. Typically, granuloma gluteale infantum is preceded by irritant diaper dermatitis that was treated with a potent topical corticosteroid. Often, there is a concomitant *Candida* infection.

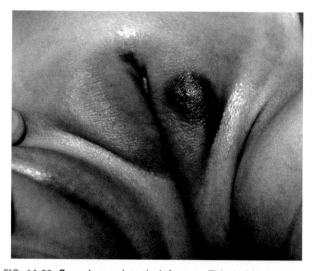

FIG. 14-26. Granuloma gluteale infantum. This red-brown nodules on the labia majora of this patient resemble cutaneous lymphoma or Kaposi sarcoma, and is atypical in that it is solitary.

Diagnosis

A history of a preceding diaper rash, especially one treated with potent topical steroids, can be helpful in the diagnosis. In cases of clinical uncertainty, the diagnosis can be confirmed with a skin biopsy. Histology of granuloma gluteale infantum reveals intensely infiltrated nodules with a hyperplastic epidermis with parakeratosis. There is exocytosis of neutrophils. The dermis is composed of a dense infiltrate of neutrophils, lymphocytes, histiocytes, plasma cells, eosinophils, giant cells, and hemorrhage. Fibrous spindle cells and mitoses are rare.

The differential diagnosis of granuloma gluteale infantum includes granulomatous processes such as infectious granulomas, talc or zirconium granulomas, or foreign body reactions. Scabetic nodules can have a similar appearance. Kaposi sarcoma, lymphomas, and histiocytic infiltrates such as those seen in Langerhans cell histiocytosis can present in a similar manner in the diaper area.

The clinical picture of a healthy infant with a diaper rash that progresses to nodules is usually adequate for diagnosis. If any uncertainty exists, a skin biopsy can be performed. Lack of spindle cell proliferation and mitoses can help to differentiate this disorder from sarcomatous and lymphomatous processes.

Pathophysiology

Granuloma gluteale infantum is believed to be an irritant dermatitis unique to the moisture and maceration of the local environment. This is especially likely to occur in the setting of chronic diarrhea in infants, but can occur as a response to other irritants and allergens (18). The use of potent topical steroids in the setting of an infection may play a role in the pathogenesis; I believe that topical corticosteroids are not important in the pathogenesis, but rather most recalcitrant diaper rashes have been treated with corticosteroids.

Management

Lesions of granuloma gluteale infantum usually resolve spontaneously over several months once the local environment of maceration and inflammation is treated.

Infantile Perianal Pyramidal Protrusion

Infantile perianal pyramidal protrusions are puffy protrusions, usually in young girls, located in the midline anterior to the anus. They appear on the median raphe as a pyramidal soft tissue swelling, covered by smooth, slightly erythematous skin (Figs. 14-19 and 14-27–14-30). Most are noted in the first 2 years of life and are asymptomatic (19).

This configuration can be seen with any irritation, and, sometimes, in normal anogenital skin. Mechanical irritation from wiping after defecation is presumed to be a cause of an increase in the size or swelling of the protrusion, and this has been seen in children with lichen sclerosus (20).

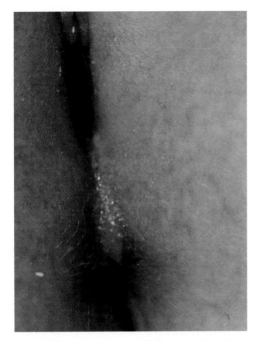

FIG. 14-27. Infantile perianal pyramidal protrusion of the midline anterior to the anus is a fairly common condition, as seen in this girl with no signs of genital inflammation.

Biopsy of these lesions demonstrates an acanthotic epidermis with marked edema of the upper dermis and an inflammatory infiltrate in the lower dermis.

Spontaneous resolution of these protrusions can occur without any treatment over several years. There is no need for treatment, as these are asymptomatic beyond any underlying irritation. It is important to recognize this entity, to avoid concern that this represents a sign of sexual abuse.

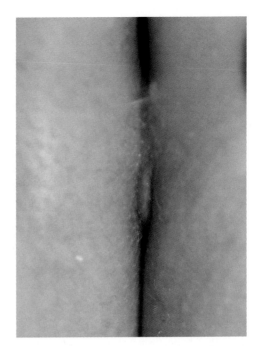

FIG. 14-29. Another young girl, although not an infant, with lichen sclerosus and infantile perianal pyramidal protrusion.

Urethral Prolapse

Urethral prolapse occurs most commonly in black prepubertal girls. The distal urethra is structurally dependent on the surrounding tissue for support. Before puberty, these estrogen-dependent tissues are diminutive and atrophic. Prolapse can occur with any activity that increases abdominal pressure, such as straining to defecate, crying,

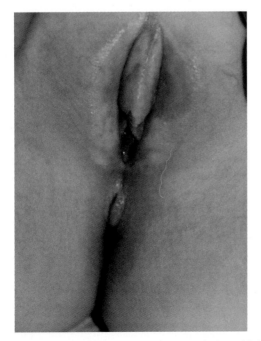

FIG. 14-28. Lichen sclerosus is a common association with infantile perianal pyramidal protrusions.

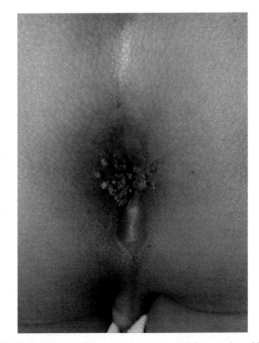

FIG. 14-30. This boy with perianal warts exhibits unrelated infantile perianal pyramidal protrusion.

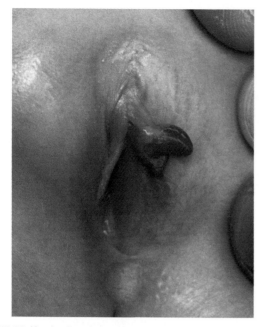

FIG. 14-31. Urethral prolapse is characterized by eversion of the urethral mucosa.

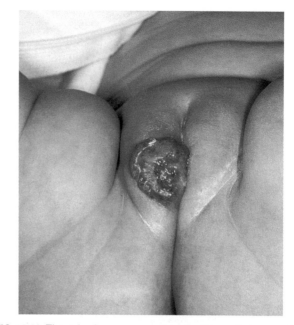

FIG. 14-32. The vulva is a common place for this well-demarcated, bright red hemangioma, which, in this case, has begun to ulcerate.

or coughing. Spontaneous occurrence is also possible. The exposed mucosa is very friable and easily irritated and eroded (Fig. 14-31). It can be mistaken for vaginal bleeding or trauma. Pain is usually absent, but urination may be difficult, especially in the presence of edema.

Diagnosis can be established by inserting a catheter into the bladder. There are no associated urogenital anomalies.

Most cases of prolapse resolve spontaneously with puberty and the onset of endogenous hormone production. Sitz baths can help to reduce swelling so the prolapse can be manually corrected, and topical estrogen may help to strengthen the tissue to minimize the risk of recurrence. Complications are rare. If vulvar bleeding is recurrent, surgical excision with reapproximation of the mucosal edges is curative.

Capillary Hemangiomas

Hemangiomas are benign, proliferative vascular tumors that occur in infancy. They are more common in girls and in premature infants. The cause of these lesions is unknown. Most are absent at birth or are noted as a faint pink flush on the skin until 2 to 3 weeks of life. Rapid growth then commences that lasts approximately 4 months. Slower growth can continue up until 1 year of age, when gradual involution begins. Half of hemangiomas resolve by 5 years of age. Most of the remainder continues to involute up until 9 years of age. Congenital hemangiomas involute more rapidly than lesions acquired after birth, and they usually resolve by 2 years of age.

Although the most common sites for hemangiomas are on the face and scalp, these are fairly common on the genitalia, especially the vulva (Fig. 14-32). Established hemangiomas are bright red, well-demarcated nodules or plaques. Hemangiomas can be both superficial and deep in the skin.

Complications of hemangiomas often relate to their location on the body and their size. Ulcerations are a common complication of genital hemangiomas, producing pain. These are often very painful, and they are easily infected, resulting in residual scarring with involution. Withholding of stool and urine can occur as a response to severe pain.

If a genital hemangioma does not obstruct an orifice, ulceration is absent, and lesions are reasonably sized, observation rather than active therapy is the usual therapy. Oral prednisone, antibiotics both topically and orally, intralesional steroids, and pulsed dye laser are all used to help heal ulcerated or otherwise complicated hemangiomas and to diminish pain. Interferon-α has been used for hemangiomas in children, but longlasting neurologic sequelae have been reported in some patients. More recently, a reaction to the vesicle rather than to the interferon itself has been suggested.

When larger hemangiomas involute, permanent skin changes often remain. Especially in the case of deep hemangiomas, the overlying skin can be atrophic, telangiectatic, and baggy, with abnormal texture. Fibrofatty tissue may be deposited during the resolution phase of the hemangioma, so the deep component appears to resolve incompletely. Intervention with surgery or laser may be indicated when involution is complete, to improve the cosmetic appearance, especially on the face.

SKIN-COLORED LESIONS

Anogenital Warts (genital warts, Condylomata acuminata, venereal warts, human papilloma virus infection)

Genital warts are relatively common infections in young children. The primary issues are concerns regarding childhood sexual abuse, and the least painful and stressful means of management. For the primary discussion of anogenital wart infection, see Chapter 12.

Genital warts are an increasingly common and difficult problem in infants and young children, probably reflecting the increased incidence of infection with this virus in the adult population. Genital warts in infants and children usually present in a perianal location (Fig. 14-30). Less frequently, the vulva and vaginal area and the penis are affected. Warts uncommonly develop on other mucous membranes such as the oral cavity, the nasopharynx, and the conjunctiva.

There are several methods of acquiring genital warts in childhood. For teenagers and adults, acquisition is almost always by sexual contact. Young infants often, acquire the virus passively and innocently during passage through the birth canal or even by upstream contamination of amniotic fluid in infants born by cesarean section to infected mothers. In addition, innocent transmission from mother or caregiver to child of both genital wart types and common hand wart viruses can occur during routine diaper changing and bathing. Studies have demonstrated HPV 2, the cause of human hand warts, to be commonly associated with anogenital warts, a finding suggesting that autoinoculation and heteroinoculation from cutaneous warts are a common means of acquiring anogenital warts (21). Despite all this, the presence of condylomata acuminata in a child should alert the caregiver to the possibility of sexual abuse.

For infants who develop lesions by the age of 3, perinatal acquisition is highly likely. The incubation period of the virus acquired perinatally is not known, but it can be up to several years. Laryngeal papillomatosis, infection of the airway by HPV acquired at birth, typically does not manifest until the age of 2 to 4 years with stridor, hoarseness, and a weak cry. A possibility of sexual abuse should be considered in a child older than 3 years with new onset of anogenital warts. HPV typing does not determine the mode of transmission of the virus, and cannot be used to determine sexual abuse. Any virus type can be transmitted by abuse, innocent contact, or vertical transmission.

The differential diagnosis of condyloma acuminatum includes condylomata lata, mollusca contagiosa, and acrochorda. With condylomata lata, other manifestations of syphilis are usually present, especially in infants. Pseudowarts, or granuloma gluteale infantum, can also resemble warts. If any doubt, a biopsy can confirm the diagnosis.

Spontaneous resolution of genital warts occurs in more than half of affected children within 5 years of age (22). Treatment of warts by the various destructive modalities often is followed by recurrence for many years. Morbidity, from pain with defecation and with repeated treatment, is considerable. More gentle, conservative treatment of the warts in childhood is recommended. The most important aspect of therapy is education of the parent. The difficulties of therapy, the frequency of recurrences, modes of transmission, and the phenomenon of latency should be discussed.

I prefer treating genital warts in children with the least painful method available. I use imiquimod applied topically overnight three times a week, titrating the frequency to the degree of inflammation. Otherwise, podofilox is another minimally invasive therapy whose frequency of application can be adjusted to the severity of inflammation. I do not use painful genital therapies without the use of topical anesthetics. Otherwise, the same treatments can be used for children as are used for adults.

Molluscum Contagiosum

Molluscum contagiosum is a very common childhood infectious dermatosis caused by a DNA pox virus, and discussed primarily in Chapter 12. Preschool and elementary school children are most frequently infected. This condition is not suggestive of sexual transmission in prepubertal children. Mollusca contagiosa are common and more severe in immunocompromised children and adults. Single lesions are usually gone within a year, and the entire infection rarely lasts longer than 2 years in healthy children (Fig. 14-33). Therefore, avoidance of scarring or very painful procedures, as well as parent education are the most important aspects of therapy. Many parents insist on therapy even after learning of the predictable spontaneous resolution. Sometimes, childcare providers require therapy of exposed lesions because of the infectious nature of molluscum contagiosum.

Removal of the core, or molluscum body, is followed by spontaneous resolution of the lesion, and this can be achieved in several ways. Cantharidin is a minimally painful treatment that can be applied to the surface to create a superficial blister. This medication is not commercially available in the United States. However, its extreme usefulness for some skin lesions makes compounding the medication by a pharmacist for office use very reasonable for any clinician who cares for children or treats molluscum contagiosum. A single test lesion on genital skin should be performed before larger numbers are treated, because of the possibility of a large and painful blister. Care must be taken to remove the cantharidin if any symptoms develop or within 4 hours of application, to avoid large blisters and unnecessary complications. Imiquimod applied overnight two or three times weekly and titrated to irritation can be useful. An

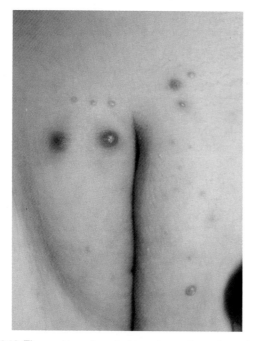

FIG. 14-33. These skin-colored, shiny, dome-shaped papules are characteristic of molluscum contagiosum; spontaneous resolution is often preceded by the appearance of red or pustular lesions, signifying an immunologic response to the virus.

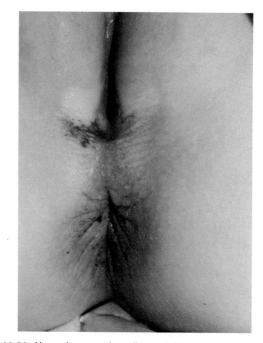

FIG. 14-34. Hypopigmentation, fine crinkling, and purpura are pathognomonic of lichen sclerosus.

open-label trial evaluating a 2-month course of oral cimetidine has suggested that this agent may be effective and is especially helpful in children with hundreds of lesions. Other treatments are painful.

WHITE LESIONS

Lichen Sclerosus

Lichen sclerosus is discussed primarily in Chapter 11. This genital skin disease characterized by white, crinkled, fragile, pruritic skin is found most often in post-menopausal women, but occurs with regularity also in prepubertal girls, and in boys.

Lichen sclerosus of childhood most often begins before the age of 7 years. Misdiagnosis as sexual abuse is common in childhood lichen sclerosus. Although many children with lichen sclerosus have no symptoms, others experience itching or irritation. Severe constipation has been reported in 67% of girls with lichen sclerosus, who regularly experience perianal involvement that produces splitting and pain with defecation that can result in retention of feces (23). This does not occur in boys.

Lichen sclerosus classically presents in the anogenital area in young girls as sharply demarcated, white plaques of crinkled skin. Underlying erythema is common as well. The outline of the plaque, which encompasses the vulva and perianal skin connected by a narrower area of involvement on the perineal body, is often described as an hourglass-like or figure-of-eight configuration around

the vulva and perianal skin. Atrophy of the skin, manifested by a shiny texture or crinkling, is typical. Hemorrhage, erosions, and fissuring occur as a result of fragility that allows for tearing and bruising with scratching (Figs. 14-28, 14-34, and 14-35). As the disease progresses,

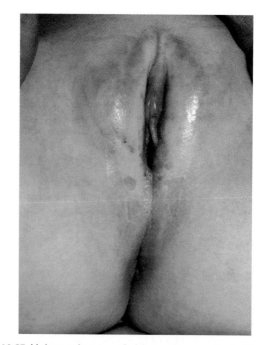

FIG. 14-35. Lichen sclerosus of girls is often manifested by waxy or smooth, shiny hypopigmentation rather than the more classic crinkling.

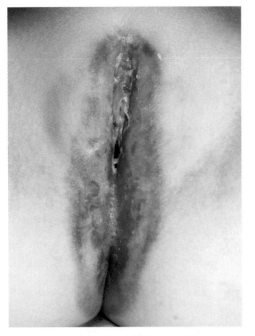

FIG. 14-36. Secondary infection of lichen sclerosus is common, as has occurred in this child pictured in Figure 14-35.

scarring occurs, including agglutination (resorption) of the labia minora and covering of the clitoris by the clitoral hood. Bacterial superinfection is especially common in girls, and is responsible for some of the associated irritation (Fig. 14-36). Vaginal discharge from secondary bacterial vaginitis may be present.

Genital lichen sclerosus generally affects only the glans penis and prepuce of boys, and it never affects the perianal skin. This disease is a prominent cause of phimosis in boys, accounting for about 40% of phimosis requiring circumcision (24).

Usually, lichen sclerosus affects only the genitalia, but extragenital lesions sometimes develop in both genders. Lichen sclerosus can be difficult to diagnose in pale children who already exhibit thin, smooth skin compared to adults. Also, prepubertal girls have only vestigial labia minora, and at least minor midline agglutination of the clitoral hood is common, so that resorption due to disease is more difficult to detect. Excoriations, maceration, irritation, and concurrent infection can further complicate the clinical picture. When clinical features are nondiagnostic, a skin biopsy is sometimes helpful. Unfortunately, when the clinical features are incomplete, the histologic features may be nondiagnostic. Sometimes, the diagnosis cannot be made, and the child must be treated empirically with close followup.

The differential diagnosis in the genital area includes irritant dermatitis with postinflammatory pigment loss, pinworm infestation, and sexual abuse. Lichenification from lichen simplex chronicus can appear white at times. Vitiligo can produce similar whitening but lacks the atrophy and hemorrhage seen in lichen sclerosus.

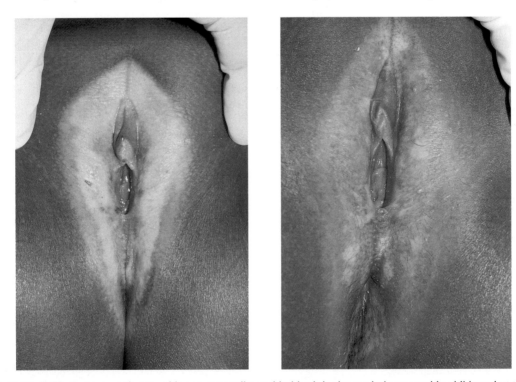

FIG. 14-37. **A:** Ultrapotent corticosteroids are generally avoided both in the genital area and in children, but this is the treatment of choice for lichen sclerosus in children. Before treatment, this patient shows a white plaque with purpura and midline fusion of the clitoral hood. **B:** Following 2 months of treatment with clobetasol, the symptoms of the patient in Figure 14-37A have disappeared, the texture has reverted to normal, and normal pigment is beginning to return.

Extragenital lesions may be mistaken for vitiligo, morphea, or lichen planus.

Treatment of childhood lichen sclerosus is the same as for adults with lichen sclerosus. Circumcision is curative in the overwhelming majority of boys with phimosis due to lichen sclerosus (24). Otherwise, the treatment of choice is the application of daily ultrapotent topical steroids. This usually results in dramatic improvement in symptoms in a few days, and the clearing of lesions over several months (Fig. 14-37A, B). Maintenance with an ultrapotent steroid applied one to three times a week or the regular use of a less potent topical steroid is required for persistent improvement. There is no benefit to topical testosterone, progesterone, or estrogen therapy in this disease beyond their lubricating effects.

Vulvar lichen sclerosus is often superinfected, and this superinfection is sometimes the immediate cause of itching and pain associated with lichen sclerosus (Fig. 14-36). A 1-week course of an antistaphylococcal/antistreptococcal antibiotic is warranted in girls with very inflamed or exudative skin.

Although lichen sclerosus was once believed to resolve at puberty in girls, more recent data show that persistence is common, although symptoms may improve significantly. Of 21 postpubertal girls with lichen sclerosus, 16 had signs of persistent lichen sclerosus, whereas 5 had cleared (25). The appearance of estrogen and resulting thickening of genital skin may account for this symptomatic improvement. However, these patients remain at risk of scarring and obliteration of vulvar architecture, with strictures of the introitus and dyspareunia. Although malignancy as a sequela of lichen sclerosus is extremely rare in childhood, those children who reach adulthood and have persistent lichen sclerosus are at risk of squamous cell carcinoma.

REFERENCES

1. Wiesmeier E, Masongsong EV, Wiley DJ. The prevalence of examiner-diagnosed clitoral hood adhesions in a population of college-aged women. *J Low Genit Tract Dis.* 2008; 12:307–310.

2. Yang C, Liu X, Wei GH. Foreskin development in 10 421 Chinese boys aged 0–18 years. *World J Pediatr.* 2009;5:312–315.

3. Jaresová V, Hrochová V, Sottner O, et al. [Synechia vulvae infantum—incidence on Department of Obstetric/Gynaecology, Teaching Hospital Na Bulovce, the First Medical Faculty of Charles University in Prague, Czech Republic from 2001 through 2005]. *Ceska Gynekol.* 2007;72:131–135.

4. Cağlar MK. Serum estradiol levels in infants with and without labial adhesions: the role of estrogen in the etiology and treatment. *Pediatr Dermatol.* 2007;24:373–375.

5. Mayoglou L, Dulabon L, Martin-Alguacil N, et al. Success of treatment modalities for labial fusion: a retrospective evaluation of topical and surgical treatments. *J Pediatr Adolesc Gynecol.* 2009;22:247–250.

6. Kumetz LM, Quint EH, Fisseha S, et al. Estrogen treatment success in recurrent and persistent labial agglutination. *J Pediatr Adolesc Gynecol.* 2006;19:381–384.

7. Schober J, Dulabon L, Martin-Alguacil N, et al. Significance of topical estrogens to labial fusion and vaginal introital integrity. *J Pediatr Adolesc Gynecol.* 2006;19:337–339.

8. Myers JB, Sorensen CM, Wisner BP, et al. Betamethasone cream for the treatment of pre-pubertal labial adhesions. *J Pediatr Adolesc Gynecol.* 2006;19:407–411.

9. Xhauflaire-Uhoda E, Henry F, Piérard-Franchimont C, et al. Electrometric assessment of the effect of a zinc oxide paste in diaper dermatitis. *Int J Cosmet Sci.* 2009;31:369–374.

10. Visscher M, Odio M, Taylor T, et al. Skin care in the NICU patient: effects of wipes versus cloth and water on stratum corneum integrity. *Neonatology.* 2009;96:226–234.

11. Semiz S, Balci YI, Ergin S, et al. Two cases of Cushing's syndrome due to overuse of topical steroid in the diaper area. *Pediatr Dermatol.* 2008;25:544–547.

12. Güven A, Gülümser O, Ozgen T. Cushing's syndrome and adrenocortical insufficiency caused by topical steroids: misuse or abuse? *J Pediatr Endocrinol Metab.* 2007;20:1173–1182.

13. Meury SN, Erb T, Schaad UB, et al. Randomized, comparative efficacy trial of oral penicillin versus cefuroxime for perianal streptococcal dermatitis in children. *J Pediatr.* 2008; 153:799–802.

14. Herbst R. Perineal streptococcal dermatitis/disease: recognition and management. *Am J Clin Dermatol.* 2003;4:555–560.

15. Gehrig KA, Dinulos JG. Acrodermatitis due to nutritional deficiency. *Curr Opin Pediatr.* 2010;22:107–112.

16. Tabanlıoğlu D, Ersoy-Evans S, Karaduman A. Acrodermatitis enteropathica-like eruption in metabolic disorders: acrodermatitis dysmetabolica is proposed as a better term. *Pediatr Dermatol.* 2009;26:150–154.

17. Schmitt S, Küry S, Giraud M, et al. An update on mutations of the SLC39A4 gene in acrodermatitis enteropathica. *Hum Mutat.* 2009;30:926–933.

18. Robson KJ, Maughan JA, Purcell SD, et al. Erosive papulonodular dermatosis associated with topical benzocaine: a report of two cases and evidence that granuloma gluteale, pseudoverrucous papules, and Jacquet's erosive dermatitis are a disease spectrum. *J Am Acad Dermatol.* 2006;55(5 suppl):S74–S80.

19. Kayashima K, Kitoh M, Tomomichi O. Infantile perianal pyramidal protrusion. *Arch Dermatol.* 1996;132:1481–1484.

20. Cruces MJ, de la Torre C, Losada A. Infantile pyramidal protrusion as a manifestation of lichen sclerosus et atrophicus. *Arch Dermatol.* 1998;134:1118–1120.

21. Handley J, Hants E, Armstrong K, et al. Common association of HPV2 with anogenital warts in prepubertal children. *Pediatr Dermatol.* 1997;14:339–343.

22. Allen AL, Siegfried EC. The natural history of condyloma in children. *J Am Acad Dermatol.* 1998;39:951–955.

23. Maronn ML, Esterly NB. Constipation as a feature of anogenital lichen sclerosus in children. *Pediatrics.* 2005; 115:e230–e232.

24. Kiss A, Király L, Kutasy B, et al. High incidence of balanitis xerotica obliterans in boys with phimosis: prospective 10-year study. *Pediatr Dermatol.* 2005;22:305–308.

25. Powell J, Wojnarowska F. Childhood vulvar lichen sclerosus. The course after puberty. *J Reprod Med.* 2002;47:706–709.

SUGGESTED READINGS

Ferreira LM, Emerich PS, Diniz LM, et al. [Langerhans cell histiocytosis: Letterer–Siwe disease—the importance of dermatological diagnosis in two cases]. *An Bras Dermatol*. 2009; 84:405–409.

Fleet SL, Davis LS. Infantile perianal pyramidal protrusion: report of a case and review of the literature. *Pediatr Dermatol*. 2005;22:151–152.

Humphrey S, Bergman JN, Au S. Practical management strategies for diaper dermatitis. *Skin Therapy Lett*. 2006;11:1–6.

Mammas IN, Sourvinos G, Spandidos DA. Human papilloma virus (HPV) infection in children and adolescents. *Eur J Pediatr*. 2009;168:267–273. [Department of Virology, School of Medicine, University of Crete, Heraklion, 71100, Crete, Greece.]

Scheinfeld N. Diaper dermatitis: a review and brief survey of eruptions of the diaper area. *Am J Clin Dermatol*. 2005; 6(5):273–281.

Sinal SH, Woods CR. Human papilloma virus infections of the genital and respiratory tracts in young children. *Semin Pediatr Infect Dis*. 2005;16:306–316.

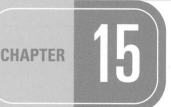

CHAPTER 15

Vaginitis and Balanitis

LIBBY EDWARDS

Vaginitis and balanitis are nonspecific terms that refer to inflammation of the vagina or the glans penis. Because these epithelial surfaces are variably moist (in men, depending on the presence or absence of the prepuce), the clinical manifestations of common diseases are often altered, and diseases unique to warm, wet areas may occur.

VAGINITIS

Although cutaneous innervation within the vagina has a limited capacity to transmit pain, vaginal inflammation is often very symptomatic. Irritating or infected vaginal secretions drain onto the vulva, which is exquisitely sensitive to sensations of burning, irritation, stinging, and itching. Copious or irritating vaginal secretions produce irritant contact dermatitis of the vestibule and sometimes a larger area of the modified mucous membrane (Fig. 15-1).

Nonneoplastic vaginal abnormalities can be classified into one of the two overlapping categories: vaginitis or vaginosis. Vaginitis is characterized by signs of inflammation, such as redness and vaginal secretions containing an increase in leukocytes. Vaginosis is characterized by abnormalities unaccompanied by erythema or a purulent vaginal discharge. An example is bacterial vaginosis, in which signs and symptoms of inflammation are notably absent. However, not all instances of *Candida* vaginitis are accompanied by visible erythema or an increase in white blood cells. In addition, patients with cytolytic vaginosis and *Lactobacillus* vaginosis characteristically report symptoms of inflammation, particularly itching.

Before the vagina and vaginal secretions can be evaluated, the examiner must be aware of the appearance of normal vaginal epithelium and normal vaginal secretions (see Chapter 3). The normal premenopausal but postmenarchal vagina is pink and wet, with prominent folds, or rugae. Prepubertal girls and postmenopausal women exhibit pale, smooth vaginal epithelium with a loss of these rugae.

The normal vaginal secretions of a well-estrogenized woman are notable for three obvious characteristics (Fig. 15-2). First, desquamated epithelial cells are mature, shed from a resilient, normally thickened epithelium. These cells are large and flat with a small nucleus and crisp borders that are often folded to reveal the flattened nature of the cell. Second, abundant lactobacilli are present, providing an acid pH lower than 5. Finally, the presence of white blood cells is expected, but white blood cells should not greatly outnumber epithelial cells.

Infectious Vaginal Disease

Most clinicians presume the term *vaginitis* to be synonymous with infection. In fact, many clinicians oversimplify further and expect all vulvovaginal symptoms, especially when accompanied by abnormal secretions, to be caused by yeast, *Trichomonas*, or bacterial vaginosis. Certainly, these are the most common, striking, or easily diagnosable forms of vaginitis, but other less well-described processes also occur.

Candida Vaginitis

Candida vaginitis, particularly that produced by *Candida albicans*, is extremely common. It also generally takes the initial blame for any vulvovaginal itching or burning, whether or not yeast actually is identified on microscopic smears or cultures. At least half of patients referred to specialty clinics for chronic or recurrent candidiasis actually experience symptoms on the basis of another process.

Clinical Presentation Itching is the usual presentation of vaginitis caused by *C. albicans* and *C. tropicalis*. Chronic infection or colonization with *C. albicans* produces irritation or burning in a much smaller subset of women. Although *C. albicans* vaginitis classically is accompanied by a white, clumped, cottage cheese-like discharge that is often not particularly copious, vaginal secretions often appear normal clinically. Vestibular erythema is usual, and some patients develop more extensive erythema, skin-fold fissures, and scale, as well as peripheral satellite pustules, erosions, or collarettes (Fig. 15-3).

Vaginitis produced by non-albicans yeast, including *C. glabrata*, *C. parapsilosis*, *C. krusei*, and *Saccharomyces cerevisiae*, are most often asymptomatic. When vaginal cultures were performed in 223 symptomatic and asymptomatic women, 17% of cultures positive for yeast in asymptomatic women showed *C. glabrata*, whereas 4% of cultures in symptomatic women showed *C. glabrata* (1). When symptoms occur, women generally report irritation and burning more than itching. Vaginal secretions are clinically unremarkable,

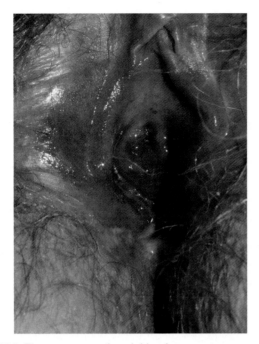

FIG. 15-1. The symptoms of vaginitis often occur as a result of contact dermatitis from irritating vaginal secretions that inflame the introitus and modified mucous membranes of the vulva. This is manifested by nonspecific redness and edema, so that the cause of the vaginitis often cannot be ascertained from the appearance of the vulva.

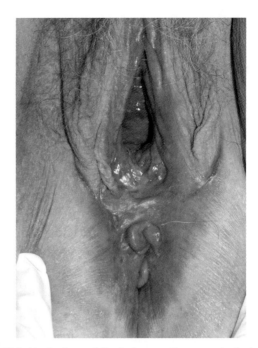

FIG. 15-3. Vaginal candidiasis frequently secondarily infects the vulva, and this redness, fissuring, and shininess are characteristic.

and microscopically show subtle budding yeasts without hyphae or pseudohyphae. Vulvar manifestations are limited to vestibular erythema or no objective abnormalities; scaling, fissuring, and satellite pustules do not occur.

Diagnosis The diagnosis of a *C. albicans* infection requires identification of the organism on a microscopic examination of vaginal secretions. This can be achieved by an experienced examiner on a microscopic smear. However, the

ease of this examination is generally underestimated by the nondermatologist; when the index of suspicion is high but a smear is negative, or a smear is positive but the patient does not improve as expected, a vaginal culture should be performed.

The identification of non-*albicans Candida* on microscopic smear is much more difficult. Only *C. albicans* and *C. tropicalis* exhibit hyphae, pseudohyphae, and budding yeasts that are normally seen with the 10× objective (Fig. 15-4). Non-*albicans Candida* infections reveal only tiny, budding yeasts that can be seen best with the 40× objective (Figs. 15-5 and 15-6). However, a non-*albicans Candida*

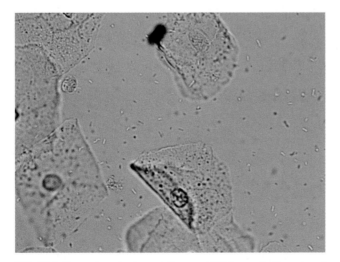

FIG. 15-2. Normal vaginal secretions exhibit large, flattened and folded mature squamous epithelial cells, one or fewer white blood cells for each epithelial cell, and abundant lactobacilli.

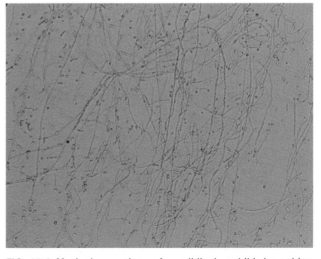

FIG. 15-4. Vaginal secretions of candidiasis exhibit branching pseudohyphae and tiny, budding yeasts on a microscopic examination of vaginal secretions.

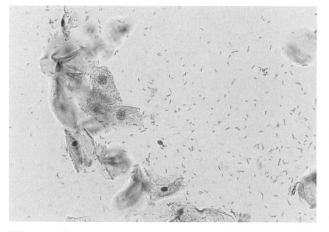

FIG. 15-5. Wet mounts of vaginal secretions of patients with non-albicans Candida vaginal infection show tiny, budding yeasts seen best with a higher power objective such as 40×. This shows the classic "bowling pin" appearance of C. glabrata.

infection usually exhibits multiple budding yeasts, so nearly every field shows at least one yeast form. The presence of non-*albicans Candida* is best evaluated on a saline preparation rather than a smear treated with potassium hydroxide. Debris from the lysis of cells by potassium hydroxide can obscure the small budding yeasts.

Biopsies of yeast vaginitis are performed only if the diagnosis is not suspected by the clinician, because less expensive and painful methods of diagnosis are usual. However, a typical tissue sample of acute vaginal candidiasis reveals inflammation consisting primarily of lymphocytes with some plasma cells and neutrophils, with stromal edema and spongiosis. Fungal elements are often seen within the most superficial portions of the vaginal epithelium. Less inflammation is seen in chronic candidiasis.

C. albicans vaginitis often coexists with, precipitates, and drives eczema. Therefore, *C. albicans* vaginitis should be considered in the differential diagnosis of eczema or

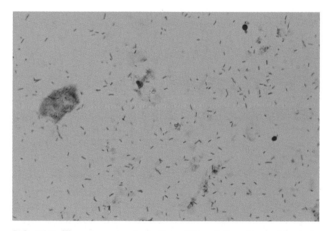

FIG. 15-6. The very round configuration of these yeast buds is characteristic of S. cerevisiae. Although non-albicans Candida yeast forms are harder to identify because there are no mycelia, they generally are distributed throughout the wet mount so the trained eye can identify them fairly quickly.

any other itchy vulvovaginal disease. Vulvar psoriasis and lichen sclerosus are other itchy dermatoses that are often misdiagnosed as *Candida* vaginitis.

C. ALBICANS VAGINITIS: **Diagnosis**

- Pruritus, often of the vestibule, occasionally extending to the entire vulva, perianal skin, and crural creases
- Changes that range from a normal vulva or vestibular erythema and vaginal redness with vaginitis alone, to generalized redness, peripheral peeling, satellite papules, pustules or collarettes, and fissures when the vulva is affected
- Vaginal secretions that range from normal clinically to clumped, "dry" secretions
- pH below 5
- Wet mount showing hyphae/pseudohyphae/budding yeast
- Culture (when recurrent or recalcitrant) revealing *C. albicans*

FREQUENTLY RECURRENT, OR RECALCITRANT, C. ALBICANS VAGINITIS: **Diagnosis**

- Culture that shows yeast; wet mount and symptoms should be confirmed by culture if patient does not respond

---

Non-*albicans Candida* infection tends to produce burning, so the usual diseases considered in the differential diagnosis of vulvodynia should be considered in patients suspected with non-*albicans Candida* infection. Vulvodynia is a primary condition in the differential diagnosis of this condition, as are erosive dermatoses such as lichen planus, and other vaginal infectious and inflammatory processes should be considered such as desquamative inflammatory vaginitis (DIV).

NON-*ALBICANS* CANDIDA VAGINITIS: **Diagnosis**

- Usually, no symptoms. Occasionally, irritation, burning, rawness
- Normal vulva and vagina
- Vaginal secretions that are normal clinically
- pH below 5
- Wet mount showing budding yeast without hyphae or pseudohyphae
- Culture C. glabrata, C. parapsilosis, C. lusitaniae, C. krusei, Saccharomyces cerevisiae, etc.

Pathophysiology The most common cause of vulvovaginal yeast infections is *C. albicans*, but the proportion of non-*albicans Candida* is increasing. A study of 223 Australian women showed that of the 21% of women colonized with yeast, 73% were found to have *C. albicans* (2). In another study, 44.2% exhibited *C. albicans*, 28% had *C. glabrata*, and 16.2% had *S. cerevisiae* (1). Although most physicians in the United States do not find that non-*albicans Candida* infections represent this large a proportion of all infections, the fact that non-*albicans Candida* is usually asymptomatic and these organisms are relatively resistant to therapy leads to underdiagnosis. Older women may be more likely to experience non-*albicans Candida* than younger women (3).

The simple presence of *C. albicans* does not provide a diagnosis of *Candida* vaginitis. A recent study showed 21% of normal, asymptomatic women show evidence of vaginal *Candida* by culture (2). A yeast infection is produced by higher numbers of organisms and an inflammatory response to these organisms. Cutaneous vulvar candidiasis is associated with superficial invasion of the epithelium by yeast.

Several known factors contribute to the development of a yeast infection. Patients who are immunosuppressed by virtue of medication or disease are more likely to develop a symptomatic yeast infection. A common local immunosuppressing medication is a topical corticosteroid. Systemic antibiotic medications also predispose women to *Candida* vaginitis, and the combination of corticosteroids and antibiotics is especially likely to provoke a yeast infection. Patients with diabetes mellitus are at increased risk of the development of *Candida* infections, as are pregnant women (4).

Management There are multiple effective and safe options for treating *C. albicans* vaginitis. Oral or topical azoles are the most frequently prescribed medications (Table 15-1). A one-time dose of fluconazole 150 mg orally produces the same rate of success as a course of a topical azole. In addition to the convenience and high compliance rate with one-dose therapy, this medication has the advantage of avoiding irritation from the alcohols, preservatives, and stabilizers in topical creams, and it also has the advantage of treating both the vulva and vagina simultaneously. The most common side effects are headache, occurring in about 13% of patients (as compared with 7% of those receiving placebo), and nausea, occurring in 7% of patients. Oral ketoconazole is rarely used for this condition now, because of the risk of hepatotoxicity and the availability of fluconazole. Itraconazole is another oral azole that is known to be effective but does not have indication approval for vulvovaginal candidiasis. This medication has the additional disadvantage of several important medication interactions. In addition, both ketoconazole and itraconazole require multiple doses to eradicate vulvovaginal yeast.

Topical azoles are equally beneficial as compared with oral fluconazole and effect symptom control slightly faster. There are multiple similar products available, with dosing ranging from one vaginal suppository (clotrimazole vaginal troche 500 mg) to suppositories or creams inserted daily for 7 days. Advantages include the availability of clotrimazole and miconazole without a prescription and the avoidance of exposure to an oral medication. Generic, over-the-counter preparations are effective and very inexpensive, whereas some prescription topical azoles are the most expensive of all available anticandidal therapies. When significant vulvar candidiasis is present,

---

TABLE 15.1 Oral medications for vulvovaginal yeast infections

Medication	Dosing	Comments[a]
Fluconazole	150 mg once for uncomplicated infection; recommended by the Centers for Disease Control and Prevention in weekly dosing for frequently recurrent candidiasis	Headache 13%, uncommon medication interaction
Itraconazole[b]	200 mg b.i.d. once; 200 mg daily × 2; 200 mg daily × 3	Medication interactions, theoretically significant effect against non-*albicans Candida*
Ketoconazole[b]	200 mg b.i.d. × 5 days	Medication interactions, idiosyncratic hepatotoxicity

[a]All have potential hepatotoxicity, ranging from life-threatening idiosyncratic disease with ketoconazole to only theoretic disease produced by weekly fluconazole. All have potential medication interactions; ketoconazole and itraconazole have the largest number of potential interactions.

[b]Not approved by the United States Food and Drug Administration for the treatment of vulvovaginal candidaisis, although shown to be very effective. There are several different regimens shown to be effective.

an anticandidal cream should be applied to the vulva two to four times a day, in addition to the topical vaginal medication, until the skin is clear.

Nystatin is a time-honored therapy for *C. albicans* infection, but generally it is not used. This medication is less effective than the newer azoles, although its availability in a soothing, ointment base is a distinct advantage for patients with significant inflammation, and I use this regularly in combination with fluconazole for women with prominent vulvar involvement. Nystatin ointment or vaginal tablets are inserted into the vagina daily for 2 weeks. When significant vulvar disease is present, nystatin cream or ointment should be applied to the vulva four times a day until the skin is clear.

C. ALBICANS VAGINITIS: **Management (see Table 15-1)**

- Fluconazole 150 mg once (80% cure), may repeat in 1 week if symptoms persist
- Any topical azole suppository or cream, per package insert
- Topical azole or nystatin twice daily to vulva when needed

FREQUENTLY RECURRENT C. ALBICANS: **Management**

- Fluconazole 150 mg weekly for 3 to 6 months; rarely needed q 3 days (confirm persistent yeast with a culture) or
- Vagina azole or boric acid 600 mg per vagina 2 to 3 times a week for 3 to 6 months if fluconazole is contraindicated
- May continue longer than 6 months if needed
- Probiotic and diet have not been shown beneficial, except diet control for diabetes

---

Unfortunately, many non-*albicans* Candida infections, especially those caused by *C. glabrata* and *S. cerevisiae*, are unresponsive to azole therapy, including fluconazole, terconazole, and butoconazole, despite in vitro sensitivities that would indicate sensitivity to these medications (4). These yeast forms sometimes are extraordinarily difficult to eradicate (Table 15-2). Although an azole can be tried first for these non-*albicans* Candida infections, patients should be advised that their infection likely will not clear. The occurrence of resistant non-*albicans* Candida organisms is related to characteristics of the organism rather than the presence of immunosuppression in the host. However, resistant *C. albicans* is uncommon except in immunosuppressed patients. Resistance to therapy increases during treatment, so low-dose or intermittent therapy should be avoided.

Before aggressive anticandidal therapy is instituted under the assumption that poor response to therapy is the result of resistance, a fungal vaginal culture should be performed to confirm the diagnosis. Some clinicians also advocate sensitivities, whereas others state that sensitivities are unreliable because they are based on expected concentrations of medication achievable in blood rather than that occurring in the vagina.

An alternative therapy shown to be effective for non-*albicans* Candida infections resistant to azole is boric acid capsules, which are prescribed by instructing a pharmacist to place 600 mg of boric acid in a gelatin capsule (5). This capsule is inserted in the vagina daily for 2 weeks. Boric acid capsules are irritating in some patients, particularly those who are already irritated by their infection. Most women experience significant improvement but not necessarily cure, with symptoms recurring off therapy, requiring maintenance therapy with boric acid. Nystatin vaginal tablets or ointment are sometimes more beneficial than azoles.

Arguably most effective is intravaginal flucytosine. Fourteen 500-mg capsules of flucytosine are dissolved in 45 g of a hydrophilic cream base, and a 6.4-g vaginal applicator filled with cream is inserted in the vagina daily for a week. This is extremely expensive and many compounding pharmacies will not provide this due to the cost of the medication, which must be bought in large quantities. Pharmalogics, Inc; phone number (248) 552-0070 currently will fill and mail this medication. Resistance occurs quickly.

Amphotericin cream is available commercially and can be inserted daily, but it is sometimes irritating. A compounded 80-mg amphotericin vaginal suppository is less irritating to some patients, but there are no data on the effectiveness of intravaginal amphotericin. There are several recipes for these suppositories, and these are generally available from any compounding pharmacy. I have treated five patients and cleared one of a non-*albicans* Candida infection. One report described a compounded suppository of amphotericin and flucytosine. Although butoconazole has demonstrated in vitro activity against non-*albicans* Candida, I have not had success with this medication in the treatment of recalcitrant vulvovaginal non-*albicans* Candida infections.

Gentian violet is another potent fungicidal substance. Unfortunately, this is also an extreme irritant in some patients, occasionally producing even blisters and erosions. It is also extremely messy. The usual regimen consists of a weekly application of a 1% solution painted on the vaginal walls with a saturated gauze swab. However, to avoid the occasional blistering reaction to a higher concentration of gentian violet, I use a 0.25% solution for the first treatment, followed by 0.5% a few days later, and then 0.75% solution before graduating to a full 1.0% solution. Medication is applied weekly in the office for 4 to 6 weeks, while the patient is maintained on daily topical therapy with nystatin or boric acid.

TABLE 15.2 Therapies for resistant non-*albicans Candida* vaginal infections

Medication	Dosing	Advantages	Disadvantages[a]
Boric acid vaginal capsules	600 mg inserted b.i.d. × 2–4 weeks	Inexpensive, fairly effective	Sometimes irritating, poisonous if ingested orally
Nystatin vaginal tablets or ointment	Insert b.i.d. × 1 month	Inexpensive, nonirritating	
Gentian violet	Painting in the office weekly	One of the more effective medications	Can produce erosive contact dermatitis, stains skin and clothing
Flucytosine fourteen 500-mg capsules dissolved in 45 g of hydrophilic cream base	6.4 g inserted hs × 1–2 weeks	Well tolerated, fairly effective	Expensive
Amphotericin suppositories	Insert hs for 2–4 weeks	—	Expensive, can be irritating
Amphotericin/flucytosine vaginal suppositories	Insert hs	—	Expensive, can be irritating

hs, at bedtime.

[a]All are often ineffective, and often several in sequence or together must be used for the best chance of success.

[b]All except nystatin are unavailable commercially and must be compounded. Terconazole and butoconazole have been shown in a laboratory setting to exhibit increased activity against non-*albicans Candida*; this has not been confirmed in patients in published clinical trials, and this author has not found them to be useful.

The average patient with *C. albicans* vaginitis experiences resolution of symptoms within 2 or 3 days. Immediate recurrence is not usual but it is relatively common. Patients who have had severe vulvovaginal candidiasis can require longer time for their symptoms to resolve, and an occasional patient experiences frequently recurrent yeast infections. When recurrence of *C. albicans* is documented, further recurrences can be prevented with once weekly dosing of fluconazole 150 mg (6). This medication, in my experience, can be discontinued after several months without recurrence once the skin has completely healed and barrier function has returned. There is evidence, however, that long-term therapy with fluconazole sometimes leads to decreased sensitivity of *C. albicans* to this medication (7).

The use of probiotics has been a popular means of preventing vulvovaginal yeast for years. Although common wisdom dictates that the presence of lactobacilli protects from vulvovaginal candidiasis, vaginal yeast is rarely seen in those patients who have no lactobacilli; atrophic vagina, bacterial vaginosis. A recent study suggests that numerous lactobacilli on wet mount increase rather than decrease the risk of vulvovaginal candidiasis (8). This has

not been confirmed, and there are studies that suggest benefit of lactobacillus therapy, and others that show no benefit (9).

NON-*ALBICANS CANDIDA* VAGINITIS: **Management**

- Trial of fluconazole 150 mg once; may repeat in 3 days; or, any topical azole suppository or cream, per package insert
- For failures (frequent), see Table 15-2
  - Boric acid capsules 600 mg b.i.d. PER VAGINA for 2 to 4 weeks
  - Nystatin ointment per vagina b.i.d. for 2 to 4 weeks
  - Flucytosine ointment per vagina 7 to 14 days
  - Amphotericin suppositories, amphotericin/flucytosine suppositories
  - Gentian violet
  - Combinations of the above

Trichomonas Vaginitis

Clinical Presentation *Trichomonas* vaginitis produces extreme itching and irritation. Dysuria and lower abdominal pain are common, and most patients experience a copious yellow or green vaginal discharge.

Bright red erythema of the vestibule is usual on physical examination. The vagina is inflamed also, and the cervix often is red and covered with discrete, punctate, bright red, and hemorrhagic macules and papules, producing the classic but nonspecific "strawberry cervix." A copious, purulent, frothy vaginal discharge is typical. The vaginal pH is high, as occurs with most extremely inflammatory vaginal diseases and conditions characterized by an absence of lactobacilli.

Trichomonas can occur in men, but it is generally asymptomatic. A purulent urethral discharge occurs in some patients.

Diagnosis This diagnosis is often made easily on a wet mount if it is examined immediately under high power. The presence of trichomonads is often obvious when they are active, but the diagnosis sometimes is more difficult. Trichomonads are approximately the size of a white cell, but these flagellate organisms are teardrop shaped rather than round and they are extremely active, so their motion is not missed easily. However, as trichomonads cool, they lose their characteristic teardrop shape, becoming round and still, making differentiation from white blood cells very difficult. Neutrophils are abundant. However, a recent study showed, compared to cultures, a false negative rate of 36.93% in a group of 200 women, with no false positives (10). A similar study shows 81% to 85% sensitivity of the diagnosis on wet mount as compared to diagnosis with a DNA probe (11). Therefore, when there is a high index of suspicion, cultures or DNA probes are indicated in the absence of a positive wet mount. There are no specific histologic findings on biopsy.

Trichomonads are sometimes reported on Papanicolaou smears. Although the accuracy of this is dependent on the individual examiner, some series show good correlation of this report with the presence of trichomoniasis (12,13).

The differential diagnosis of *Trichomonas* vaginitis includes all causes of a purulent vaginitis, including DIV and inflammation associated with an atrophic vaginal epithelium, an intravaginal foreign body, or any erosive vaginal skin disease.

Pathophysiology Trichomoniasis is caused by the protozoan *Trichomonas vaginalis*. This disease is always sexually transmitted. The vagina is the primary area of involvement, but the organism is sequestered in other areas in both men and women, including the paraurethral ducts, the urethra, and Skene glands. Circumcision reduces infection rate with trichomonads in men (14).

***TRICHOMONAS* VAGINITIS:** **Diagnosis**

- Discharge, irritation, itching, burning
- Red mucous membranes and modified mucous membranes; sometimes a classic "strawberry cervix"
- White or yellow copious vaginal secretions
- pH higher than 5
- Wet mount showing motile trichomonads; if negative and high index of suspicion, DNA probe/polymerase chain reaction for trichomonads

---

Management Trichomoniasis must be treated orally because topical therapies do not eliminate organisms sequestered within the urethra and paraurethral ducts. In addition, sexual partners must be treated to prevent immediate reinfection. Oral metronidazole, at a dose of 500 mg twice a day for 1 week or a single 2-g dose, is usually effective, as is tinidazole as a one-time dose of 2 g. Women should be warned about the disulfiram-like effect of metronidazole with alcohol consumption in some patients, but tinidazole is better tolerated. In addition, some level of resistance to metronidazole was encountered in 1.16% of women in a genitourinary clinic in the United Kingdom (15); either tinidazole or a prolonged course of metronidazole generally effects cure in these patients (15,16).

An occasional patient is allergic to metronidazole, or does not clear with one of these medications. Acetarsol pessaries, furazolidone, fenticonazole, and naturopathic treatments with plant extracts have been used (15,17–19). Other topical azoles can provide some measure of comfort as well. Most patients improve rapidly without recurrence.

***TRICHOMONAS* VAGINITIS:** **Management**

- Metronidazole 500 mg b.i.d. for 1 week, or metronidazole or tinidazole 2 g once
- Topical azoles can provide some comfort but not cure

Bacterial Vaginosis

Bacterial vaginosis is a common, unpleasant, but generally benign, disruption in the population of the normal premenopausal vaginal flora.

Clinical Presentation Women with bacterial vaginosis report an increased volume of vaginal secretions and an unpleasant fishy odor, especially after contact with alkaline semen during intercourse. In spite of the increased volume of theoretically irritating alkaline secretions, itching and burning are generally absent or mild, and there is no vaginal or introital redness. The notable clinical complication of symptomatic bacterial vaginosis is an increased risk of preterm labor.

Diagnosis The diagnosis of bacterial vaginosis is made by the presence of three or more of the following: a profuse, milky vaginal discharge; a vaginal pH greater than 5; the presence of a fishy odor when secretions are exposed to 10% or 20% potassium hydroxide (positive whiff test); and the presence of clue cells on microscopic examination of vaginal smears (Fig. 15-7). Clue cells are squamous epithelial cells covered by coccobacilli that give the cytoplasm a ground-glass appearance and obscure the crisp margins of the cell, leaving ragged borders. Bacterial vaginosis is also characterized by the absence of lactobacilli and no increase in white blood cells. For practical purposes, a high vaginal pH and the milky nature of the vaginal discharge are nonspecific, and the diagnosis should not be made without the presence of clue cells and the absence of lactobacilli. DNA probes are also available for diagnosis. Vaginal biopsies are not performed for this disease but they are presumably normal.

Poor hygiene producing odor and a heavy but normal physiologic discharge can mimic bacterial vaginosis, but the high pH and characteristic microscopic findings are diagnostic. *Trichomonas* can produce a heavy discharge and pH greater than 5, as can DIV, but these conditions exhibit an increase in white blood cells on wet mount, no clue cells, and a negative whiff test.

Pathophysiology This common disease associated with an unpleasant vaginal discharge is characterized by an

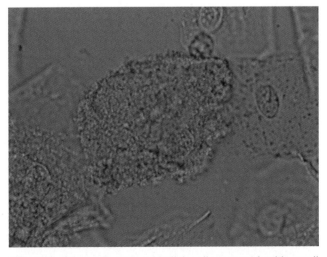

FIG. 15-7. Clue cells are epithelial cells covered with small bacteria that obscure the sharp, crisp borders of the cells, thus producing a granular, ragged edge as seen here. A lack of lactobacilli is another important finding on wet mount.

BACTERIAL VAGINOSIS:	Diagnosis

- Discharge and odor, especially following sexual intercourse; occasional itching, irritation
- pH of 5 or higher
- Wet mount showing clue cells, lack of lactobacilli, lack of increased white blood cells
- Positive whiff test

overgrowth of organisms often present as part of the normal vaginal flora. Although bacterial vaginosis occurs in women who are sexually active, and some clinicians believe that this is a sexually transmitted disease, the epidemiology of the disease and the unimportance of treating sexual partners in preventing recurrence suggest otherwise. The characteristic odor of bacterial vaginosis is produced by the release of bacterial amines following exposure to an alkaline substance such as potassium hydroxide or semen.

Management Metronidazole 500 mg twice daily for 7 days or 2 g in one dose usually clears these symptoms, although the single-dose therapy is slightly less effective (Table 15-3). Topical metronidazole, inserted twice daily for 5 days, and clindamycin 2% vaginal cream, inserted at bedtime for 3 to 7 days, are equally beneficial, with fewer side effects compared to oral metronidazole (20). Oral clindamycin has not been studied widely, but also is effective and, with oral metronidazole, was recently shown to produce better outcomes in high-risk pregnant women as compared to topical therapy (21). More recently, tinidazole has been used, and some believe this may be marginally more effective than metronidazole (22). Probiotics are sometimes used for bacterial vaginosis; these have been studied as a means to enhance the repopulation of normal lactobacilli to prevent recurrence (23,24), but evidence also exists for using lactobacilli for initial treatment (25,26). Other trials show no benefit. Recurrence is common until lactobacilli repopulate the vagina. When these measures fail, prolonged therapy is reasonable. Although there are no data, I have prescribed prolonged clindamycin, 150 mg twice daily for several months, with careful education regarding the slight risk of *Clostridium difficile* with success.

Although treatment of asymptomatic bacterial vaginosis is not needed in women who are not pregnant, there is a known increased risk of preterm labor when this condition occurs in pregnant women. However, a recent large trial suggests that the treatment of asymptomatic bacterial vaginosis in low- or normal-risk pregnancies is not beneficial (27). There is also a suggestion that the preterm labor is more related to the absence of lactobacilli than the bacterial vaginosis, as preterm labor occurs in other

TABLE **15.3** Therapy of bacterial vaginosis[a]		
Medication	Dosing	Approximate efficacy at 1 month (%)
Metronidazole gel	1 applicator per vagina hs × 1 week	70–80
Metronidazole tablets	500 mg b.i.d. × 1 week; or	70–80
	2 g once orally	65–70
Clindamycin tablets	300 mg b.i.d. × 5–7 days	65–70
Clindamycin vaginal ovules	100 mg hs × 3 days	65–70

b.i.d., twice daily; hs, at bedtime.

[a]Bacterial vaginosis clears in most patients with any of these therapies, but recurrence is common. Long-term suppressive therapy or probiotics are sometimes useful for those patients who experience prompt recurrence.

conditons that are characterized by absent lactobacilli, including an atrophic vagina (28).

BACTERIAL VAGINOSIS: Management

- Metronidazole or tinidazole 2 g once, or 500 mg b.i.d. for 7 days
- Metronidazole, 1 g inserted per vagina b.i.d. for 5 days
- Clindamycin, one applicatorful per vagina hs for 3 to 7 days
- Clindamycin 300 mg b.i.d. for 1 week (not FDA approved for this indication)
- For recurrent disease, longer courses, add probiotics; treating partners not shown to be beneficial

---

Bacterial Vaginitis

Bacterial vaginitis is an uncommon condition whose name is sometimes confused with bacterial vaginosis. However, inflammation is associated with bacterial vaginitis, and a specific bacterial organism is identified.

Clinical Presentation Vulvovaginal redness, irritation, rawness, and soreness, associated with a yellow or yellow-green vaginal secretions, are typical complaints of women with bacterial vaginitis. Dyspareunia is common.

On physical examination, vulvar erythema is common, often associated with a slightly glazed texture to the vulvar skin. Although subtle scale and fissures within skin folds are common, the vulva sometimes appears entirely normal. The vaginal epithelium is generally red, and vaginal secretions are grossly and microscopically purulent, with a remarkable increase in neutrophils on wet mount (Fig. 15-8). Often, many epithelial cells are immature parabasal cells, signifying erosions or the increased turnover of epithelial cells that would be manifested as scale on dry, keratinized epithelium. Also common but not uniformly present are a

decrease in lactobacilli and a resulting pH of greater than 5. Sometimes, especially when the organism is group B *Streptococcus* (GBS), chains of cocci are seen (Fig. 15-9).

Diagnosis The diagnosis is made by clinical suspicion and is confirmed by bacterial culture showing a pure growth of a pathogen, and by a good response to therapy. Frequently, especially when *Streptococcus agalactiae* (GBS) is the identified organism, appropriate antibiotic therapy does not resolve signs or symptoms, and the organism can be considered a coincidental colonizer (29). Histology has not been described, but a biopsy would presumably exhibit an acute inflammatory infiltrate with stromal and epidermal edema.

The signs and symptoms of symptomatic bacterial vaginitis can be identical to those associated with an inflamed vagina atrophic from estrogen deficiency due to age, pregnancy, or breast-feeding, from DIV, and from an inflammatory erosive dermatosis such as lichen planus. These diseases are distinguished by their setting, negative cultures, and response to appropriate therapy such as

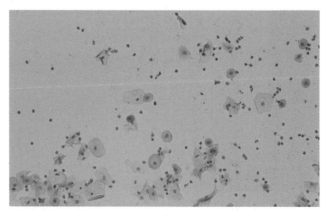

FIG. 15-8. Bacterial vaginitis, not to be confused with bacterial vaginosis, is characterized microscopically by an increase in neutrophils and parabasal cells (immature epithelial cells), both frequent signs of inflammation.

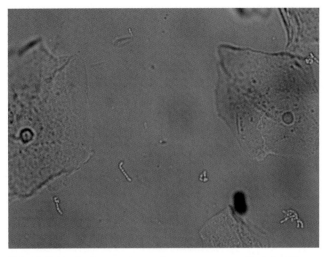

FIG. 15-9. Vaginal secretions of some women with infection or colonization with GBS (Streptococcus agalactiae) show chains of cocci.

local estrogen therapy. As noted earlier, these diseases not only resemble bacterial vaginitis, but also can be complicated by a secondary bacterial infection.

Pathophysiology Bacterial vaginitis is an infection with a specific bacterial organism. Group A β-hemolytic streptococcus (GAS) infection is relatively common in children (see Chapter 14), but sometimes found in adult women as well (30). Asymptomatic carriage from male partners has been implicated as a cause of recurrent GAS vaginitis (31). Although the existence of vaginitis produced by GBS is controversial, many clinicians are confident that this entity exists, although it is uncommon (32). Clinicians who care for vaginitis report the occasional patient who exhibits purulent vaginal secretions, symptoms of irritation, a culture yielding GBS, and immediate remarkable improvement with antibiotics. However, the overwhelming majority cultures that yield GBS represent colonization only. *Staphylococcus aureus* usually occur in a predisposing setting (such as a retained tampon), and often is associated with bacterial vulvitis or surrounding staphylococcal folliculitis. *Escherichia coli* sometimes produces vaginitis, but this and other enterics are more often contaminants, and treatment does not effect improvement.

Management The treatment of bacterial vaginitis includes amelioration of predisposing conditions including atrophic vaginitis or erosive vaginal disease and identification and removal of a foreign body. The patient should be treated with an antibiotic known to be active against the organism identified on culture. Often, prolonged therapy may be required while any underlying condition is adequately treated. GBS is recognized as extremely difficult to eradicate, and treatment with penicillin V potassium or oral clindamycin is often followed by immediate recur-

rence. Theoretically, the use of newer probiotics may help to minimize this recurrence.

A topical corticosteroid such as triamcinolone ointment applied twice a day to modified mucous membranes of an irritated vulva can improve comfort more quickly because this is a nonspecific anti-inflammatory medication.

Because some women tend to develop candidiasis with antibiotic use, particularly in combination with topical steroids, I treat with fluconazole once weekly to prevent intercurrent yeast while they are taking an antibiotic and topical corticosteroid. This oral medication avoids the irritation of a topical antifungal in an already irritated vulva and vagina.

Vaginal Diseases Associated with Increased Levels of Lactobacilli

Lactobacilli are normal inhabitants of the vagina of women with normal levels of estrogen. These bacteria help to create the normal acid environment of this area. A few clinicians believe that unusually large numbers of lactobacilli can, however, produce symptoms, but this remains very controversial. In addition, although the diseases discussed here are both termed vaginosis, indicating a lack of inflammation, they are characterized by inflammatory symptoms of itching or irritation.

Cytolytic Vaginosis (Döderlein Cytolysis)

Although the existence of this vaginal condition remains in debate, a recent review of 2947 wet mounts in patients with symptoms of candidiasis described 54 as having cytololytic vaginosis based on cytologic criteria (33).

Clinical Presentation Patients present with symptoms similar to those of a yeast infection. Women describe itching, irritation, and a thick, clumped, white vaginal discharge. On physical examination, the skin appears normal without redness. There is a normally acid vaginal pH.

Diagnosis The diagnosis of cytolytic vaginosis is made by the constellation of symptoms in a setting of an acid vaginal pH and by characteristic findings on a cytologic examination of vaginal secretions (34). Microscopically, there are large numbers of epithelial cells, many with nuclei that have been stripped of surrounding cytoplasm. These nuclei can be difficult to distinguish from white blood cells, but they can be identified by phase microscopy. In addition, lactobacilli are extremely abundant, yeast forms are absent, and white blood cells are not increased in number. There are no specific histologic findings, and a biopsy is not indicated.

Candida vaginitis is the major disease to be differentiated from cytolytic vaginosis, and *Lactobacillus* vaginosis also produces the same symptoms and characteristic discharge. However, these entities can be differentiated by the respective presence of yeast forms or elongated lactobacilli and by the absence of cytolysis.

CYTOLYTIC VAGINOSIS (EXISTENCE CONTROVERSIAL):   **Diagnosis**

- Vulvovaginal itching, irritation
- Dry, clumped discharge
- pH less than 5
- Wet mount showing abundant lactobacilli, no yeast forms, no clue cells, but many nuclei of epithelial cells with loss of cytoplasm
- Negative culture for yeast

Pathophysiology The cause of cytolytic vaginosis is postulated by some physicians to be an abnormal increase in lactobacilli and resulting lactic acid, whereas a recent report suggests that an increased production of hydrogen peroxide is causative (35), and other clinicians believe this to result from hyperproliferation of vaginal epithelium of unknown cause (Eduard Friedrich, Jr, MD, personal communication, 1987).

Management The treatment for cytolytic vaginosis consists of alkaline douches with a dilute solution of sodium bicarbonate. Thirty to 60 g of baking soda is mixed with 1 L of warm water. Patients douche two or three times a week, until they are comfortable. This therapy does not eliminate cytolytic vaginosis, and douching once or twice a week may be needed to control symptoms.

CYTOLYTIC VAGINOSIS: **Management**

- Sodium bicarbonate douche two to three times a week to manage symptoms; 30 to 60 g of baking soda in 1 L of warm water

---

Vaginal Lactobacilliosis (Lactobacilliosis)

There has been little acknowledgement of this condition associated with high levels of lactobacilli since its introduction by Horowitz et al. (36).

Clinical Presentation Women with *Lactobacillus* vaginosis report itching and irritation, which they generally assume to be caused by yeast. In addition, these patients often describe a yeast-like, white, thick, cheesy discharge. Physical examination reveals a normal vulva and vagina. A curd-like white discharge is often present, and the pH of these vaginal secretions is normally acid.

Diagnosis The diagnosis of this condition is based on the symptoms of itching and irritation in combination with characteristic microscopic findings of vaginal secretions

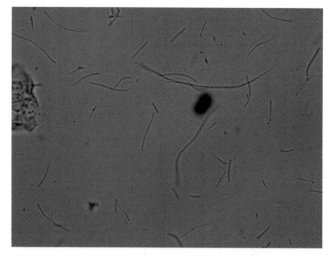

FIG. 15-10. Lactobacilli sometimes line up from end to end, to form long filaments formerly and erroneously called leptothrix. These can be confused with the long pseudohyphae of candidiasis, but the caliber of the filaments is much smaller than that of yeasts.

(36). These reveal very elongated lactobacilli, formerly called leptothrix. There is no increase in white blood cells microscopically, and there are no yeast forms (Fig. 15-10). The histopathology of the vagina has not been described and is not important in the diagnosis. A normal biopsy would be expected.

The diseases most often confused with *Lactobacillus vaginosis* are vaginal candidiasis and cytolytic vaginosis. However, the microscopic appearance of the elongated lactobacilli is distinctive, and yeast forms are absent, as is cytolysis.

VAGINAL LACTOBACILLIOSIS (EXISTENCE CONTROVERSIAL):   **Diagnosis**

- Vulvovaginal itching, irritation
- Dry, clumped discharge
- pH less than 5
- Wet mount showing abundant elongated lactobacilli, no yeast forms, no clue cells
- Negative culture for yeast

Pathophysiology An increase in numbers of lactobacilli is believed to produce this controversial condition. *Lactobacillus* vaginosis tends to occur in a setting of recent anticandidal therapy. Whether the therapy for yeast is causative or whether empiric anticandidal therapy is inevitable as first-line treatment for women with these symptoms is not known.

Management Both eradication of symptoms and elimination of elongated lactobacilli can be achieved with either doxycycline (100 mg twice daily for 2 weeks), amoxicillin/clavulanic acid (500 mg twice daily), or ciprofloxacin 250 mg twice daily for a week.

Oral doxycycline 100 b.i.d., amoxicillin/clavulanic acid b.i.d., ciprofloxacin 250 b.i.d. for 1 week

Noninfectious Inflammatory Vaginal Diseases

Although the most common cause of vaginitis is an infection, chronic symptoms of vaginitis usually are not infectious in nature (37).

Atrophic Vagina and Vaginitis

An atrophic vagina exhibits pallor, dryness, and a pH greater than 5. When the vagina becomes irritated or eroded as a result of the thin, dry vaginal walls, redness appears, and white blood cells are seen on wet mount; this is referred to as atrophic vaginitis.

Clinical Presentation The atrophic vagina has become extremely common since systemic estrogen was withdrawn from many women in the early 2000s. Atrophic vaginitis is characterized by a sensation of dryness, irritation, and sometimes itching. Sexual intercourse is painful and exacerbates symptoms. On physical examination, the modified mucous membranes of the vulva are often pale and smooth. The normal coarse, wet, pink vaginal rugae are replaced by pale, flat, dry mucosa. Occasionally, a grossly purulent, although generally scant, vaginal discharge is present. More severe disease is accompanied by patchy erythema that represents vaginal erosions, in which fragile epithelium has been abraded by friction from intercourse or pressure from a vaginal wall that has been distended by a cystocele or a rectocele. Symptomatic atrophic vaginitis occurs when symptoms or signs of inflammation, such as vaginal erythema and white blood cells in vaginal secretions, develop as a result of erosions or secondary infection.

Diagnosis The diagnosis of an atrophic vagina is made by the setting of estrogen deficiency in association with characteristic smooth, pale vaginal epithelium and a typical microscopic appearance of vaginal secretions. These secretions exhibit small, round, immature parabasal cells that have been shed from thinned, atrophic epithelium rather than the mature, large, flat epithelial cells that are normally shed from the surface of well-estrogenized vaginal skin (Fig. 15-11). Lactobacilli are absent, and the vaginal pH measures greater than 5. These signs all suggest estrogen deficiency. Atrophic vaginitis occurs when significant inflammation from erosions or superinfection occurs, and white cells are abundant on wet mount. The diagnosis is confirmed by normalization of symptoms and signs after a few weeks of estrogen therapy. A vaginal biopsy is not a routine test for the diagnosis of atrophic vaginitis, nor is it indicated. Histologically, however, the tissue shows epithelial thinning. In addition, the absence

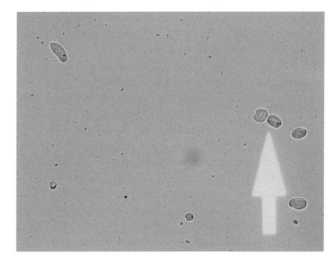

FIG. 15-11. An estrogen-deficient vagina is manifested on wet mount by small, round, immature squamous epithelial cells (parabasal cells) shed from the surface of a thin vaginal epithelium. Often, in high estrogen-deficient women, the vaginal fluid is almost acellular.

of normal maturation with progressive flattening of epithelial cells closer to the surface is characteristic.

DIV presents similarly to atrophic vaginitis, with parabasal cells, purulent vaginal secretions, and a negative culture. However, the history of a woman with atrophic vaginitis should reveal estrogen deficiency, and estrogen should quickly correct the abnormalities. Bacterial (aerobic) vaginitis is also identical on presentation, but a culture should reveal an organism, and the appropriate antibiotic should clear the abnormality.

ATROPHIC VAGINA/VAGINITIS: **Diagnosis**

- Sometimes asymptomatic, sometimes burning, dryness, dyspareunia
- Pale, smooth, dry vagina (atrophic vagina); red, smooth vagina (atrophic vaginitis)
- No discharge (atrophic vagina), or yellow discharge (atrophic vaginitis)
- pH higher than 5
- Wet mount showing parabasal cells, decreased lactobacilli, no clue cells, no yeast (atrophic vagina); increased white blood cells also (atrophic vaginitis)

Pathophysiology The vaginal epithelium requires estrogen for normal maturation of squamous cells. In the absence of estrogen, there are fewer cell layers in the epithelium, and the epithelium becomes fragile. The atrophic vagina is at higher risk of erosions and secondary bacterial infection, with resulting inflammation producing pain and irritation. Interestingly, those women who engage in regular coitus after menopause are relatively well protected from vaginal atrophy.

Management Atrophic vaginitis can be treated equally effectively with either systemic or local estrogen replacement. Local replacement can be accomplished by cream, vaginal tablet, or ring. Either a gram of estradiol (Estrace) or conjugated equine estrogen (Premarin) is inserted in the vagina 3 nights a week, with improvement beginning within a week. Some clinicians find conjugated equine estrogen to be more irritating than estradiol. A healthy vaginal epithelium can then be maintained with one to three intravaginal applications of estrogen each week.

Less messy and less irritating are the estradiol vaginal tablets (Vagifem), also inserted with an applicator thrice weekly, or via estradiol released slowly from an inert, nonirritating ring inserted into the upper vagina every 3 months (ESTring). A review of 37 trials comparing these methods of local estrogen replacement showed them to be equally effective; uterine thickening, bleeding, and breast tenderness were found in some trials to be greater with conjugated equine estrogen as compared with estradiol tablets and ring (38). The ring was most acceptable to women because of comfort and ease of use (38). Obviously, patients who use topical estrogen derive only local benefit, and, generally, only local side effects. Systemic estrogen replacement also normalizes vaginal mucosa.

Patients with atrophic vaginitis do very well with long-term or intermittent estrogen replacement therapy. However, some patients do not require ongoing therapy to remain comfortable, particularly those who may have had a specific, correctable event such as an infection or local erosion that precipitated symptoms, and those who are not sexually active.

Desquamative Inflammatory Vaginitis

DIV is an arguably common syndrome of vaginal erythema, profuse purulent vaginal secretions, and a vaginal culture that yields no relevant infection.

Clinical Presentation The symptoms of DIV consist of irritation, burning, dyspareunia, and, sometimes, itching. Patients often describe a yellow or green vaginal discharge. Symptoms of inflammation of other mucosae, such as the oral mucosa and gingivae, are absent.

DIV occurs at any age, both pre- and postmenopausal. On physical examination, these women exhibit a variably red vestibule, as a result of irritation from purulent vaginal secretions (Fig. 15-12). The vagina is red; sometimes this is striking, sometimes mild, but erosions are not present (Figs. 15-13 and 15-14). The vaginal epithelium sometimes exhibits small, red papules similar to the classic "strawberry cervix" of trichomoniasis. At other times, the vagina is uniformly red. There is no scarring of the vulva or vagina.

More severe cases exhibit poorly demarcated, mild erythema of the entire modified mucous membranes of the vulva and edema of the labia minora. However, these vulvar abnormalities are nonspecific and are sometimes fairly mild.

ATROPHIC VAGINA/VAGINITIS:	Management

- Topical estrogen replacement
  - Estradiol vaginal cream or conjugated equine estrogen 1 g per vagina three times a week
  - Estradiol vaginal tablets per vagina three times a week
  - Estradiol ring changed every 3 months
- Systemic estrogen replacement
  - Oral
  - Patch
- Consider oral fluconazole weekly or vaginal azole cream two to three times a week the first month to prevent secondary candidiasis

Vaginal secretions of DIV are characteristic but not specific, being identical to those of atrophic vaginitis, bacterial vaginitis, and erosive vaginitis such as that caused by lichen planus, and cicatricial pemphigoid (Fig. 15-15). Some of the epithelial cells seen with DIV are parabasal cells; these are round, small, and immature, having been shed from an epithelium that is too rapidly proliferating for maturation of the upper layer into the usual large, flattened cells to occur. Inflammation usually recruits multiple white blood cells as well, and lactobacilli are generally absent, with a vaginal pH greater than 5.

Diagnosis DIV is diagnosed by the findings of vaginal erythema and characteristic secretions in the setting of adequate estrogen, absence of other skin and mucous

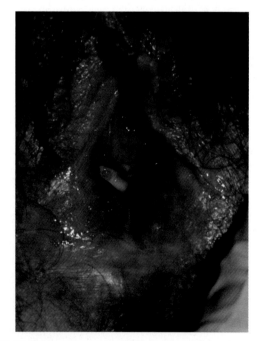

FIG. 15-12. DIV is characterized by red modified mucous membranes from irritation produced by purulent vaginal secretions. This is a characteristic but nonspecific picture.

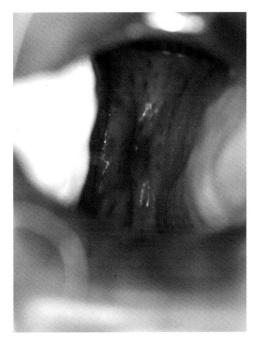

FIG. 15-13. The vaginal mucosa of DIV sometimes shows small red macules, similar to the "strawberry cervix" that is classic for trichomonads.

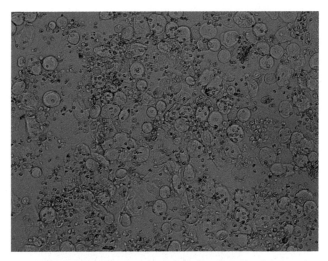

FIG. 15-15. Both DIV and any erosive skin disease of the vagina show vaginal secretions with a marked increase in white blood cells, parabasal cells, and a concomitant decrease in lactobacilli.

membrane disease, and negative cultures. The histologic findings of DIV fall into one of two groups, either a lichenoid infiltrate without basement membrane changes or a nonspecific mixed inflammatory infiltrate with lymphocytes, eosinophils, and plasma cells (39). A few of these patients revealed direct immunofluorescent biopsies showing nonspecific but distinct fine, granular C3 along the basement membrane. Whether these nonspecific findings are variants of the same process or represent two processes is not known. The lichenoid findings probably are indicative of the lichenoid vaginitis described by Dr Edward Wilkinson, or perhaps this lichenoid pattern is

only a common nonspecific reaction pattern characteristic of any inflammation on genital mucous membrane and modified mucous membrane skin.

The differential diagnosis includes atrophic vaginitis, when secondarily inflamed or infected because of erosions and fragility of the epithelium, erosive vaginitis of lichen planus or ciciatricial pemphigoid, bacterial vaginitis, and inflammation or infection associated with a retained foreign body.

DESQUAMATIVE INFLAMMATORY VAGINITIS:	Diagnosis

- Introital irritation, burning, dyspareunia
- Variably red vagina, often red, puffy vestibule, sometimes labia minora
- Yellow/green discharge
- pH usually higher than 5
- Wet mount showing parabasal cells, increased white blood cells, decreased lactobacilli
- Negative culture, negative trichomonads, adequate estrogen, no erosive skin disease of vagina, vulva or mouth

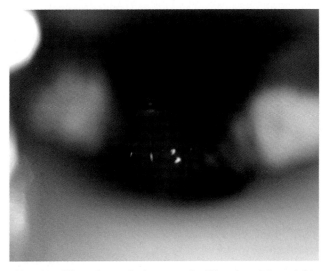

FIG. 15-14. Often, the vaginal mucosa is diffusely red, in variable degrees; there are never erosions.

Pathophysiology There are several different concepts of the term desquamative inflammatory vaginitis. Publications are few, and these have been limited to opinion or clinical observation. In the past, some experienced clinicians believed that DIV, like desquamative inflammatory gingivitis, was a clinical picture resulting from any noninfectious erosive mucosal skin disease, especially lichen planus, occurring within the vagina (Fig. 15-16). However, most physicians now feel that DIV is distinct from these erosive diseases because erosive lichen planus and ciciatrical

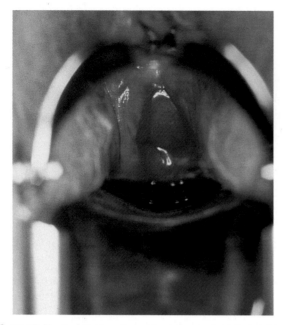

FIG. 15-16. Vaginal lichen planus is characterized by bright red vaginal erosions that sometimes progress to synechiae of the vaginal walls and shortening of the vagina. (Courtesy of Gordon Davis, SW Vulvar Clinic, Phoenix, AZ.)

pemphigoid occur primarily in postmenopausal women, erosions and scarring are not found, and DIV is unaccompanied by oral mucosal and vulvar disease. More providers now believe that DIV is a specific disease, presenting as noninfectious erythema without erosions and occurring in a different population from lichen planus, likely autoimmune or hypersensitivity in origin, because of its response to corticosteroids and clindamycin cream, an antibiotic known for its anti-inflammatory effects.

Management First, any estrogen deficiency should be corrected, including premenopausal women with estrogen levels suppressed by oral contraceptives. In addition, any accompanying infection should be treated.

First-line specific therapies for DIV are topical clindamycin cream (40) or hydrocortisone acetate 25-mg rectal suppositories inserted per vagina. I instruct patients to insert an applicatorful of clindamycin cream nightly and I re-evaluate in 1 month. Theoretically, oral clindamycin would be a better choice, lacking the potentially irritating properties of a topical medication. Actually, however, topical clindamycin is not irritating and the oral preparation does not produce a significant clinical benefit. The frequency of application can be tapered in those patients whose condition clears or who improve remarkably, and medication can be discontinued altogether in many patients. In those women who do not respond to topical clindamycin, a hydrocortisone acetate suppository is used nightly, tapering the frequency of use when improvement occurs. The risk of candidiasis is fairly high with vaginal corticosteroid use, and I prescribe oral fluconazole, 150 mg/week, to prevent this infection. For women who

do not respond to these regimes, a compounded 500-mg vaginal suppository can be compounded, or the ultrapotent corticosteroid clobetasol propionate 0.05% ointment can be inserted. Also, a combination of clindamycin cream and a corticosteroid can be used.

Often, a vaginal culture yields GBS. I treat these women with inflammatory vaginitis and a culture showing GBS with oral penicillin or clindamycin, in case of the very uncommon occurrence of GBS vaginitis.

DESQUAMATIVE INFLAMMATORY VAGINITIS: **Management**

- Topical clindamycin cream, ½ to 1 applicatorful in vagina hs for 2 weeks; or
- Hydrocortisone acetate 25-mg rectal suppository per vagina hs for 2 weeks. If uncontrolled with either, then
- Both hydrocortisone suppositories and clindamycin cream hs for 2 weeks. If uncontrolled,
- Consider compounded hydrocortisone 500-mg suppositories, or clobetasol ointment 1 g hs (long-term use may cause adrenal suppression). Anytime controlled,
  - Taper frequency to lowest frequency that controls the condition
  - Discontinue and wait for recurrence systemic estrogen replacement
- Consider weekly fluconazole to prevent secondary candidiasis

---

Erosive Vaginitis due to Specific Skin Disease

Several erosive skin diseases show a predilection for mucous membranes, to include the vagina and, often, the mucous membranes and modified mucous membranes of the vulva. These are primarily discussed in Chapter 9.

Lichen planus is far and away the most common of these diseases. Other mucosal erosive diseases include cicatricial pemphigoid, pemphigoid vulgaris, and erythema multiforme. These diseases exhibit frank erosions. Other mucous membranes are also regularly affected, expecially the oral mucosa. In addition, most of these diseases exhibit lesions of extragenital dry, keratinized skin surfaces as well.

The diagnosis is made by the constellation of findings, and by both routine histology from the edge, or an erosion, and direct immunofluorescent biopsies from nearby but unaffected epithelium.

Vestibulodynia (Vulvar Vestibulitis Syndrome, Localized Provoked Vulvodynia)

Vulvar vestibulitis is not a vaginal disease, but it is often mistaken for vaginitis because of introital redness

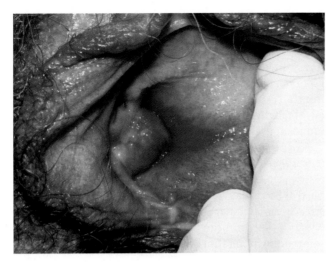

FIG. 15-17. Although not vaginitis, the vulvar vestibulitis syndrome presents similarly, with introital irritation and pain to touch, accompanied by erythema in the vestibule, especially around the ostia of the vestibular glands. However, wet mounts and cultures are normal.

and symptoms of irritation and burning (see Chapter 3 for primary discussion) (Fig. 15-17).

Physiologic Discharge

A common complaint of premenopausal women is that of excess discharge, sometimes associated with odor. These patients occasionally report irritation manifested by itching or rawness, but more often the presence of the unpleasant discharge is the primary feature. Generally, the patient is convinced that infection is the cause of the secretions, and she often has been diagnosed with infections by previous physicians.

A physical examination is normal, except, at times, vaginal secretions are copious, but normal in color and consistency. The pH is normal, and a wet mount shows no evidence of yeast, clue cells, trichomonads, or increased white blood cells. There are abundant lactobacilli. A whiff test is negative, and vaginal secretions produce normal odor.

The "diagnosis" of physiologic discharge is made by the complaint of increased secretions, a normal wet mount, and a negative culture. The differential diagnosis includes all other vaginitis, especially bacterial vaginosis. In addition, an occasional patient experiences "discharge" and odor on the basis of excessive sweating from the groin area. This can be diagnosed by response to antiperspirant with a deodorant.

The management of physiologic secretions rests in patient education (see patient handout). Either patients accept the results of the evaluation, sometimes with relief, or, more often, with annoyance that there is no answer, or they refuse to believe that their secretions are normal.

Some women are remarkably distressed by their secretions and perceived odor, and continue to request re-evaluation and empiric treatment. Occasionally, pa-

PHYSIOLOGIC DISCHARGE:	**Diagnosis**

- Complaints of heavy discharge, uncomfortable wetness, sometimes odor
- Normal vulva and vagina, possibly mild erythema of modified mucous membranes
- Variably heavy discharge, white or clear, normal odor
- Wet mount showing mature epithelial cells, no clue cells, no yeast forms, no increase in white blood cells
- Negative culture
- No response or brief, partial response to antimicrobials

tients are crippled by their symptoms, believing that others can smell them; they avoid work and social activities. These women experience a body dysmorphic disorder, and are best treated with counseling and psychotrophic medications, but they generally are resistant to this route (see Chapter 16).

PHYSIOLOGIC DISCHARGE:	**Management**

- Patient education (see handout)
- Reassurance
- Re-evaluate for flares once or twice for reassurance

BALANITIS

Balanitis refers to inflammation of the glans penis. The term *balanoposthitis* is used when inflammation includes the prepuce. Because an intact prepuce provides a damp, occluded, warm space that is a favorable environment for some organisms, balanitis of all kinds is far more common in men who are uncircumcised.

Infectious Balanitis/Balanoposthitis

Balanoposthitis is often an infectious condition. Although yeast is the organism most often diagnosed, cultures reveal that other microbes are common causes as well. One hundred men with balanoposthitis showed 18% with *Candida*, 19% with *Staphylococcus aureus*, 9% with *Streptococcus agalactiae*, and 23% with *Malassezia*, as compared to controls who also showed 23% with *Malassezia*, and 7.7% with *Candida* (41).

Candida Balanitis

Clinical Presentation *Candida* balanitis presents as red papules, superficial erosions, or white papules (Fig. 15-18). Erosions are discrete and round, but these can become more confluent and less well demarcated as a result of the

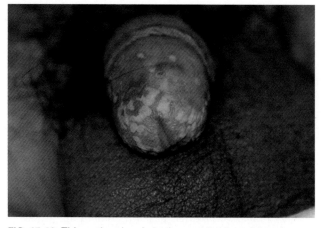

FIG. 15-18. This patient has irritation and itching of the glans as a result of Candida balanitis. (Courtesy of Errol Craig, MD.)

very fragile, occluded nature of this skin and resulting maceration. White papules representative of a yeast infection, like those of oral thrush, can be removed by gentle scraping. Unless the patient is incontinent, the dry external prepuce and shaft of the penis are spared, but the moist crural creases and gluteal cleft may be affected. Gluteal cleft involvement often is characterized by fissuring.

Diagnosis The diagnosis is confirmed by the identification of fungal elements from white material scraped from the skin or from the edge of an erosion. This can be accomplished either by culture or by examination of a microscopic smear. Biopsies are not indicated but are occasionally performed when the diagnosis is not suspected. A subcorneal pustule with infiltration of the stratum corneum by hyphae and pseudohyphae is usual. A circumcised man sometimes experiences irritation from yeast following sexual intercourse with an infected partener. Most often, this is manifested by subtle transient erythema and symptoms of irritation. This is self-limited, resolving quickly without treatment.

Candida balanitis should be included in the differential diagnosis of any inflammation of the uncircumcised glans penis. Not only is it a very common cause, it also complicates inflammation of other causes, such as psoriasis or herpes simplex virus infection. Lichen planus and penile intraepithelial neoplasia (erythroplasia of Queyrat, Bowen disease) can mimic *Candida* balanitis.

CANDIDA BALANITIS: **Diagnosis**

- Irritation and itching
- Redness, erosion, white papules and plaques removed with a cotton-tipped applicator, in uncircumcised man
- Fungal preparation of white material shows yeast forms
- Otherwise, culture showing Candida

Pathophysiology Penile candidiasis is almost limited entirely to uncircumcised men. Colonization is fairly high, occurring in 26.2% of 478 men attending a sexually transmitted disease clinic, and over 18% exhibited *Candida* balanitis (42). *C. albicans* from the bowel or from a sexual partner provides the organisms, and risk factors include an age greater than 60 years, diabetes, immunosuppression, and incontinence.

Management Topical therapy with an azole cream such as clotrimazole, miconazole, econazole, or ketoconazole applied twice a day is usually curative. Men with extreme erosive disease may experience burning with a cream. Nystatin ointment can be used for those patients, but it is sometimes macerating. An alternative treatment is oral therapy, using fluconazole.

Bacterial Balanitis/Balanoposthitis

Again occurring primarily in uncircumcised men, bacterial infection can cause inflammation of the glans and prepuce. Bacterial balanitis can be accompanied by perianal infection as well. Erythema, purulence, and pain of the glans and foreskin are common clinical findings, particularly in a setting of *Streptococcus pyogenes* (42). Most patients with *S. pyogenes* in one study were found to have contracted their infection via fellatio with a commercial sex worker (42). Other bacteria found on culture include *Streptococcus agalactiae* and *Staphylococcus aureus*.

CANDIDA BALANITIS: **Management**

- Topical azole cream once or twice a day if not eroded
- Nystatin ointment one to four times a day if eroded or painful, or
- Fluconazole 100 to 200 mg daily until clear
- Treat any yeast in partner; manage, when possible, diabetes, incontinence, obesity, etc.
- Use medication of choice with the first onset of recurrrence

The diagnosis is made by culture and response to therapy. Management includes oral antibiotics according to sensitivities reported on culture, and the avoidance of known contactants.

BACTERIAL BALANITIS AND BALANOPOSTHITIS: **Diagnosis**

- Irritation and pain
- Redness, erosion, exudation, in uncircumcised man
- Culture showing *Streptococcus pyogenes, Staphylococcus aureus, Streptococcus agalactiae*

BACTERIAL BALANITIS AND BALANOPOSTHITIS: **Management**

• Oral antibiotics per culture

Noninfectious Balanitis/Balanoposthitis

Circinate Balanitis (Reiter Syndrome)

Lesions of Reiter syndrome on the glans penis are called circinate balanitis (see Chapter 8). These lesions are indistinguishable clinically and histologically from those of the closely related disease, pustular psoriasis. Uncircumcised men exhibit white, annular papules that sometimes coalesce into arcuate plaques (Fig. 15-19). Circumcised men generally experience relatively well-demarcated scaling, crusted papules, and plaques (Fig. 15-20). Patients with Reiter syndrome and those with pustular psoriasis often have associated circumscribed crusted plaques on the palms and feet, and sometimes these generalize to cover larger areas. Treatment consists of topical corticosteroids, oral etretinate, and oral methotrexate.

Pseudoepitheliomatous, Micaceous, and Keratotic Balanitis

Clinical Presentation Pseudoepitheliomatous, micaceous, and keratotic balanitis presents as indolent, relatively asymptomatic, hyperkeratotic, and sometimes crusted plaques on the glans (Figs. 15-21 and 15-22). This condition

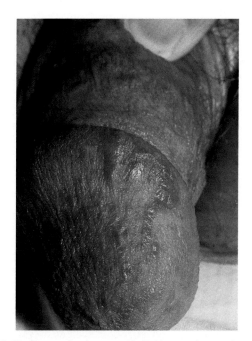

FIG. 15-20. Circumcised men with Reiter syndrome show morphology more consistent with psoriasis, with well-demarcated, inflamed, scaling papules.

is found most often in older men, often who have been circumcised late in life (43).

Diagnosis The diagnosis is made by the clinical appearance and is confirmed by biopsy. A skin biopsy shows a moderately well-differentiated epithelium, with pseudoepitheliomatous hyperplasia, and a normal dermis with a mild chronic inflammatory infiltrate.

The main and most dangerous disease in the differential diagnosis is squamous cell carcinoma, which usually is distinguishable on biopsy.

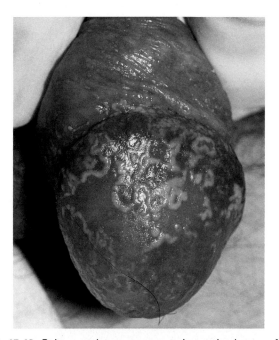

FIG. 15-19. Reiter syndrome on an uncircumcised man often shows annular, sometimes coalescing or red papules, resulting in the term circinate balanitis. (From Lynch P, Edwards L. Genital Dermatology. New York: Churchill Livingstone; 1994, with permission.)

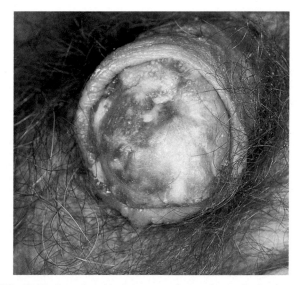

FIG. 15-21. Pseudoepitheliomatous, keratotic, and micaceous balanitis is characterized by thickened hyperkeratotic plaques.

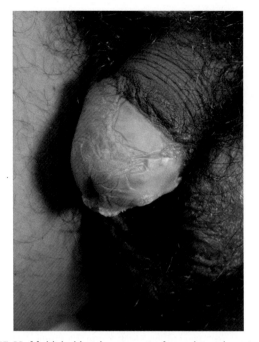

FIG. 15-22. Multiple biopsies were performed to rule out squamous cell carcinoma before a diagnosis of pseudoepitheliomatous, keratotic, and micaceous balanitis was made. He is still followed very carefully.

Pathophysiology The origin of this disease is not known, but it is postulated to be a premalignant condition with a high likelihood to progress into invasive squamous cell carcinoma (44).

Management Although the lesion can be followed carefully, removal by excision is preferred, both to prevent possible malignant transformation and to ensure adequate tissue for histology. Topical fluorouracil has also been used successfully.

Plasma Cell Balanitis (Zoon Balanitis)

Plasma cell balanitis is an uncommon, distinctive dermatosis of unknown etiology. This condition is discussed primarily in Chapters 6 and 9. Plasma cell balanitis presents as a well-demarcated, red, glistening plaque (Fig. 15-23). Although it is largely asymptomatic, mild pruritus or tenderness may occur.

The diagnosis is made by correlating the clinical and histologic presentations and by ruling out diseases similar in appearance, including lichen planus, candidiasis, Bowen disease, and psoriasis. The histology of plasma cell balanitis is characteristic, showing a dense plasma cell infiltrate in the upper dermis. Plasma cell balanitis can mimic many inflammatory processes, especially in uncircumcised men. Lichen planus, candidiasis, Bowen disease, and psoriasis are the most common processes to exclude.

Although the cause of this inflammatory disease is unknown, plasma cell balanitis does not appear to be infectious or neoplastic. Topical corticosteroids, topical retinoids, and laser therapy have all been reported useful.

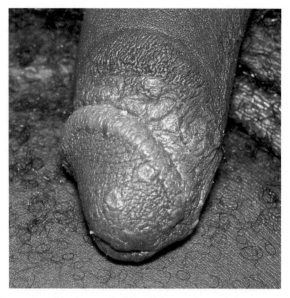

FIG. 15-23. Plasma cell (the Zoon balanitis) shows well-demarcated, red, moist-appearing plaques most common on the glans.

However, this is a chronic process that tends to recur if ablated, and only improve with topical therapy.

Other Noninfectious Causes of Balanitis: lichen planus, psoriasis, penile intraepithelial neoplasia (Bowen disease, erythroplasia of Queyrat)

Other diseases can preferentially affect the glans penis. Common benign skin diseases are psoriasis and lichen planus (Fig. 15-24). These diseases are red, usually

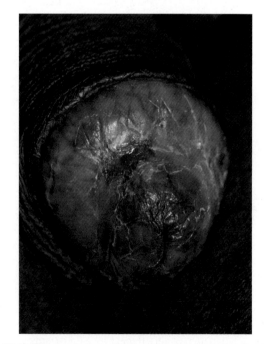

FIG. 15-24. The penis is a relatively common location for lichen planus, which can mimic candidiasis, psoriasis, and intraepithelial neoplasia.

well-demarcated papules and plaques that show a predilection for the glans on uncircumcised men (discussed primarily in Chapter 6). These often appear nonspecific and can be confused with red papules of intraepithelial neoplasia (Bowen disease, erythroplasia of Queyrat) and candidiasis. An examination of other skin surfaces often shows more specific morphology of psoriasis or lichen planus, but a biopsy is often required.

Penile intraepithelial neoplasia (also called squamous cell carcinoma in situ, Bowen disease, or erythroplasia of Queyrat) can produce red papules on the glans as well. Chronic, unresponsive red papules or plaques on the glans should be examined by biopsy to ensure that neoplastic processes do not go undetected and untreated.

REFERENCES

1. Corrêa Pdos R, David PR, Peres NP, et al. Phenotypic characterization of yeasts isolated from the vaginal mucosa of adult women. *Rev Bras Ginecol Obstet.* 2009;31:177–181.

2. Pirotta MV, Garland SM. Genital Candida species detected in samples from women in Melbourne, Australia, before and after treatment with antibiotics. *J Clin Microbiol.* 2006;44: 3213–3217.

3. Vermitsky JP, Self MJ, Chadwick SG, et al. Survey of vaginal-flora Candida species isolates from women of different age groups by use of species-specific PCR detection. *J Clin Microbiol.* 2008;46:1501–1503.

4. García Heredia M, García SD, Copolillo EF, et al. Prevalence of vaginal candidiasis in pregnant women. Identification of yeasts and susceptibility to antifungal agents. *Rev Argent Microbiol.* 2006;38:9–12.

5. Ray D, Goswami R, Dadhwal V, et al. Prolonged (3-month) mycological cure rate after boric acid suppositories in diabetic women with vulvovaginal candidiasis. *J Infect.* 2007;55:374–377.

6. Sobel JD, Wiesenfeld HC, Martens M, et al. Maintenance fluconazole therapy for recurrent vulvovaginal candidiasis. *N Engl J Med.* 2004;26(351):876–883.

7. Shahid Z, Sobel JD. Reduced fluconazole susceptibility of Candida albicans isolates in women with recurrent vulvovaginal candidiasis: effects of long-term fluconazole therapy. *Diagn Microbiol Infect Dis.* 2009;64:354–356.

8. Abad CL, Safdar N. The role of lactobacillus probiotics in the treatment or prevention of urogenital infections—a systematic review. *J Chemother.* 2009;21:243–252.

9. Falagas ME, Betsi GI, Athanasiou S. Probiotics for prevention of recurrent vulvovaginal candidiasis: a review. *J Antimicrob Chemother.* 2006;58:266–272.

10. Hegazi MM, Makhlouf LM, Elbahey MA, et al. Polymerase chain reaction versus conventional methods in the diagnosis of vaginal trichomoniasis. *J Egypt Soc Parasitol.* 2009;39:11–21.

11. Lowe NK, Neal JL, Ryan-Wenger NA. Accuracy of the clinical diagnosis of vaginitis compared with a DNA probe laboratory standard. *Obstet Gynecol.* 2009;113:89–95.

12. Heller DS, Pitsos M, Skurnick J. Does the presence of vaginitis on a Pap smear correlate with clinical symptoms in the patient? *J Reprod Med.* 2008;53:429–434.

13. Aslan DL, McKeon DM, Stelow EB, et al. The diagnosis of trichomonas vaginalis in liquid-based Pap tests: morphological characteristics. *Diagn Cytopathol.* 2005;32:253–259.

14. Sobngwi-Tambekou J, Taljaard D, Nieuwoudt M, et al. Male circumcision and Neisseria gonorrhoeae, Chlamydia trachomatis and Trichomonas vaginalis: observations after a randomised controlled trial for HIV prevention. *Sex Transm Infect.* 2009;85:116–120.

15. Waters LJ, Dave SS, Deayton JR, et al. Recalcitrant Trichomonas vaginalis infection—a case series. *Int J STD AIDS.* 2005;16: 505–509.

16. Kissinger P, Secor WE, Leichliter JS, et al. Early repeated infections with Trichomonas vaginalis among HIV-positive and HIV-negative women. *Clin Infect Dis.* 2008;46:994–999.

17. Goldman LM, Upcroft JA, Workowski K, et al. Treatment of metronidazole-resistant Trichomonas vaginalis. *Sex Health.* 2009;6:345–347.

18. Veraldi S, Milani R. Topical fenticonazole in dermatology and gynaecology: current role in therapy. *Drugs.* 2008;68:2183–2194.

19. El-Sherbini GT, El Gozamy BR, Abdel-Hady NM, et al. Efficacy of two plant extracts against vaginal trichomoniasis. *J Egypt Soc Parasitol.* 2009;39:47–58.

20. Chen JY, Tian H, Beigi RH. Treatment considerations for bacterial vaginosis and the risk of recurrence. *J Womens Health (Larchmt).* 2009;18:1997–2004.

21. Darwish A, Elnshar EM, Hamadeh SM, et al. Treatment options for bacterial vaginosis in patients at high risk of preterm labor and premature rupture of membranes. *J Obstet Gynaecol Res.* 2007;33:781–787.

22. Dickey LJ, Nailor MD, Sobel JD. Guidelines for the treatment of bacterial vaginosis: focus on tinidazole. *Ther Clin Risk Manag.* 2009;5:485–489.

23. Larsson PG, Stray-Pedersen B, Ryttig KR, et al. Human lactobacilli as supplementation of clindamycin to patients with bacterial vaginosis reduce the recurrence rate; a 6-month, double-blind, randomized, placebo-controlled study. *BMC Womens Health.* 2008;8:3.

24. Petricevic L, Witt A. The role of Lactobacillus casei rhamnosus Lcr35 in restoring the normal vaginal flora after antibiotic treatment of bacterial vaginosis. *BJOG.* 2008;115:1369–1374.

25. Martinez RC, Franceschini SA, Patta MC, et al. Improved cure of bacterial vaginosis with single dose of tinidazole (2 g), Lactobacillus rhamnosus GR-1, and Lactobacillus reuteri RC-14: a randomized, double-blind, placebo-controlled trial. *Can J Microbiol.* 2009;55:133–138.

26. Mastromarino P, Macchia S, Meggiorini L, et al. Effectiveness of Lactobacillus-containing vaginal tablets in the treatment of symptomatic bacterial vaginosis. *Clin Microbiol Infect.* 2009; 15:67–74.

27. Nygren P, Fu R, Freeman M, et al.; U.S. Preventive Services Task Force. Evidence on the benefits and harms of screening and treating pregnant women who are asymptomatic for bacterial vaginosis: an update review for the U.S. Preventive Services Task Force. *Ann Intern Med.* 2008;148:220–233.

28. Donders GG, Van Calsteren K, Bellen G, et al. Predictive value for preterm birth of abnormal vaginal flora, bacterial vaginosis and aerobic vaginitis during the first trimester of pregnancy. *BJOG.* 2009;116:1315–1324.

29. Shaw C, Mason M, Scoular A. Group B streptococcus carriage and vulvovaginal symptoms: causal or casual? A case-control study in a GUM clinic population. *Sex Transm Infect.* 2003;79: 246–248.

30. Bray S, Morgan J. Two cases of group A streptococcal vulvovaginitis in premenopausal adults in a sexual health setting. *Sex Health.* 2006;3:187–188.

31. Sobel JD, Funaro D, Kaplan EL. Recurrent group A streptococcal vulvovaginitis in adult women: family epidemiology. *Clin Infect Dis.* 2007;44:e43–e45.

32. Donders GG, Vereecken A, Bosmans E, et al. Definition of a type of abnormal vaginal flora that is distinct from bacterial vaginosis: aerobic vaginitis. *BJOG.* 2002;109:34–43.

33. Demirezen S. Cytolytic vaginosis: examination of 2947 vaginal smears. *Cent Eur J Public Health.* 2003;11:23–24.

34. Cerikcioglu N, Beksac MS. Cytolytic vaginosis: misdiagnosed as candidal vaginitis. *Infect Dis Obstet Gynecol.* 2004;12: 13–16.

35. Shopova E, Tiufekchieva E, Karag'ozov I, et al. Cytolytic vaginosis—clinical and microbiological study. *Akush Ginekol (Sofiia).* 2006;45(suppl 2):12–13.

36. Horowitz BJ, Mårdh PA, Nagy E, et al. Vaginal lactobacillosis. *Am J Obstet Gynecol.* 1994;170:857–861.

37. Nyirjesy P, Peyton C, Weitz MV, et al. Causes of chronic vaginitis: analysis of a prospective database of affected women. *Obstet Gynecol.* 2006;108:1185–1191.

38. Suckling J, Lethaby A, Kennedy R. Local oestrogen for vaginal atrophy in postmenopausal women. *Cochrane Database Syst Rev.* 2006;(4):CD001500.

39. Murphy R, Edwards L. Desquamative inflammatory vaginitis: what is it? *J Reprod Med.* 2008;53:124–128.

40. Sobel JD. Desquamative inflammatory vaginitis: a new subgroup of purulent vaginitis responsive to topical 2% clindamycin therapy. *Am J Obstet Gynecol.* 1994;171:1215–1220.

41. Alsterholm M, Flytström I, Leifsdottir R, et al. Frequency of bacteria, Candida and malassezia species in balanoposthitis. *Acta Derm Venereol.* 2008;88:331–336.

42. Lisboa C, Santos A, Dias C, et al. Candida balanitis: risk factors. *J Eur Acad Dermatol Venereol.* 2009. [Epub ahead of print.]

43. Perry D, Lynch PJ, Fazel N. Pseudoepitheliomatous, keratotic, and micaceous balanitis: case report and review of the literature. *Dermatol Nurs.* 2008;20:117–120.

44. Child FJ, Kim BK, Ganesan R, et al. Verrucous carcinoma arising in pseudoepitheliomatous keratotic and micaceous balanitis, without evidence of human papillomavirus. *Br J Dermatol.* 2000;143:183–187.

SUGGESTED READINGS

Abad CL, Safdar N. The role of lactobacillus probiotics in the treatment or prevention of urogenital infections—a systematic review. *J Chemother.* 2009;21:243–252.

Alsterholm M, Flytström I, Leifsdottir R, et al. Frequency of bacteria, Candida and malassezia species in balanoposthitis. *Acta Derm Venereol.* 2008;88:331–336.

De Seta F, Schmidt M, Vu B, et al. Antifungal mechanisms supporting boric acid therapy of Candida vaginitis. *J Antimicrob Chemother.* 2009;63:325–336.

Demirezen S. Cytolytic vaginosis: examination of 2947 vaginal smears. *Cent Eur J Public Health.* 2003;11:23–24.

Horowitz BJ, Mårdh PA, Nagy E, et al. Vaginal lactobacillosis. *Am J Obstet Gynecol.* 1994;170:857–861.

Lisboa C, Santos A, Dias C, et al. Candida balanitis: risk factors. *J Eur Acad Dermatol Venereol.* 2009. [Epub ahead of print.]

Newbern EC, Foxman B, Leaman D, et al. Desquamative inflammatory vaginitis: an exploratory case-control study. *Ann Epidemiol.* 2002;12:346–352.

Nyirjesy P, Peyton C, Weitz MV, et al. Causes of chronic vaginitis: analysis of a prospective database of affected women. *Obstet Gynecol.* 2006;108:1185–1191.

Nyirjesy P. Postmenopausal vaginitis. *Curr Infect Dis Rep.* 2007;9: 480–484.

Perry D, Lynch PJ, Fazel N. Pseudoepitheliomatous, keratotic, and micaceous balanitis: case report and review of the literature. *Dermatol Nurs.* 2008;20:117–120.

Suckling J, Lethaby A, Kennedy R. Local oestrogen for vaginal atrophy in postmenopausal women. *Cochrane Database Syst Rev.* 2006;(4):CD001500.

Wakatsuki A. Clinical experience of streptococcal balanoposthitis in 47 healthy adult males. *Hinyokika Kiyo.* 2005;51:737–740.

CHAPTER 16

Special Issues in Genital Dermatology: Psychosexual Matters, Concerns of Immunosuppression, and Aging

PETER LYNCH AND LIBBY EDWARDS

PSYCHOLOGICAL ISSUES

Although the situation is improving slowly, discussion about genital disorders and their role in the patient's psychological, social, and sexual function has historically been indirect, played down, or even avoided completely. In order to maximize the quality of care offered, these aspects need to be explored with virtually every patient presenting with a genital problem. There are two ways of doing so. One is to offer patients a chance to express these concerns indirectly by way of a computerized questionnaire filled out privately by the patient prior to a face-to-face interaction with the clinician. The other is for the clinician to take the initiative in bringing up this discussion at the time of the examination. Rarely, with individuals, who by culture or temperament are very shy, it may be appropriate to defer this discussion until the second or third visit. Because of space limitations only a few aspects or psychosocial and sexual function related to genital disease can be covered in this chapter.

Psychological factors obviously can play some role in the pathophysiology of all diseases and the degree to which they do so probably exists on a spectrum. Unfortunately, for most diseases, there is no consensus as to what these factors are and how important a role they play in the etiology, extent, severity, and duration of the problem. In addition, there is always controversy over the degree to which psychological factors cause the disease versus the degree to which the disease causes the psychological factors. Essentially this presents a "chicken and egg" situation that, while it can be discussed, can never be resolved to the satisfaction of all participants. With this in mind, I have divided this chapter into three segments: (1) psychosocial and sexual dysfunction may cause the disease, (2) psychosocial and sexual dysfunction may influence the course of the disease, and (3) psychosocial and sexual dysfunction may occur as a result of the disease.

PSYCHOSOCIAL DYSFUNCTION MAY CAUSE DISEASE

The major genital disorders for which I believe psychosocial and sexual dysfunction plays a significant etiologic role are (1) chronic idiopathic genital pain, (2) chronic itching in the absence of a recognizable disease, (3) chronic scratching or gouging occurring in the absence of a recognizable disease, (4) fixed ideation that some aspect of the genitalia, although normal on clinical examination, is in fact abnormal (body dysmorphic disorder), and (5) intentional or unintentional self-mutilation (dermatitis artefacta).

Chronic Idiopathic Genital Pain

Mucocutaneous pain can arise secondary to an underlying cutaneous or neurologic disorder or occur as an idiopathic problem. The main idiopathic mucocutaneus pain disorders include unexplained pain involving the head (tongue, lips, face, and scalp) and the anogenital area (vulva, penis, scrotum, and anus). Idiopathic pain that occurs at these latter four sites is generally termed vulvodynia, penodynia, scrotodynia, and anodynia. Of these, only vulvodynia has been studied sufficiently to warrant discussion here. Nevertheless, one of us (PJL) believes that the information regarding vulvodynia, as cited below, can be generalized to pain occurring at the three other sites of involvement.

Nearly all patients with vulvodynia have psychological, social, and sexual dysfunction, although the degree to which this occurs is quite variable (1–4). The major question, of course, is whether the presence of pain causes this dysfunction or whether the dysfunction causes the pain. While the majority of clinicians currently favors the former explanation, the minority including one of us (PJL) favors the latter. Support for this latter point of view is perhaps best established by examination of the data suggesting that psychosocial and/or sexual dysfunction precedes the development of the pain. In that regard, there is arguably acceptable evidence that significant depression, anxiety, somatization, relationship dysfunction, and painful physical, sexual, or psychological trauma precede the development of vulvar pain (4). Depending on the degree to which these data are correct and acceptable, vulvodynia might then be considered as a somatoform disorder (4).

Regardless of whether psychosocial and sexual dysfunction either causes the pain or arises from it, all agree that vulvodynia is a very debilitating condition and that it has a dramatic adverse effect on quality of life (QOL) (5). In fact, it appears that women with this condition have significantly poorer QOL than do women with most other general dermatologic diseases and also worse than women with other vulvar disorders (6). Finally, while both medical and procedural therapy can lead to good results for most patients with vulvodynia, it is clear that these individuals can also benefit from a variety of psychological approaches to therapy (7).

Chronic Itching in the Absence of Recognizable Disease

As is true for cutaneous pain, pruritus can arise either as an idiopathic process or develop secondary to an underlying systemic, cutaneous, or neurologic (neuropathic) disorder. Idiopathic pruritus, often termed psychogenic pruritus or pruritus sine materia, is associated with a variety of psychogenic problems, notably anxiety and depression (8,9). It, also, like chronic idiopathic pain, can be classified as a somatoform disorder (10). The fact that psychogenic pruritus responds very well to psychotropic medications such as the tricyclics, benzodiazepines, SSRIs (selective serotonin reuptake inhibitors), and antipsychotic agents supports the supposition that this form of itching is primarily caused by psychological dysfunction (11).

Chronic Scratching and Gouging in the Absence of Recognizable Disease

Psychogenic excoriation ("neurotic excoriation") is the term used for those patients who chronically scratch, gouge or pick at skin that is otherwise visibly normal. This condition differs from the scratching and rubbing that occurs in pruritic skin disorders such as atopic dermatitis and lichen simplex chronicus in several ways. First, there is no atopy or other recognizable underlying disorder. Second, the excoriations are appreciably deeper and thus usually appear as ulcers rather than erosions. Third, individual gouge marks are separated one from another by areas of intervening normal skin. And, fourth, the scratching and picking is often not preceded by a sensation of itching but rather by the perception that there is something in the skin and that its presence requires removal by the patient.

Essentially all patients with the milder forms of psychogenic excoriation have underlying psychological dysfunction, primarily related to depression or bipolar disorder (12). In addition, most of these patients meet the criteria for impulse-control disorder or obsessive–compulsive disorder (12). This type of psychogenic excoriation is one of the commonest forms of psychocutaneous disorders (13) and often involves the genitalia. These patients can be considered to have a somatoform disorder.

On the other hand, patients with the more severe form of psychogenic excoriation, those who believe that their skin contains "bugs" ("delusions of parasitosis") or fibers ("Morgellons disease") are almost always delusional (14,15). These latter two conditions (which are essentially identical from a psychological viewpoint) only occur on the genitalia when other parts of the body are also involved.

All forms of psychogenic excoriation may be associated with the use of recreational drugs, and evidence for this possibility should be sought before ascribing the problems solely to a psychiatric etiology (12). Psychotropic agents, to include the SSRIs and antipsychotics, are useful for the milder forms and are required for the more severe forms of psychogenic excoriation (14–16). Additional information on this subject can be found in the section on self-induced ulcers in Chapter 10.

Body Dysmorphic Disorder

Body dysmorphic disorder (BDD) is defined as preoccupation with some slight, or nonexistent, defect in appearance that causes significant distress resulting in psychosocial or sexual dysfunction. BDD is quite common with an overall prevalence of 1% to 2% of the general population and about 5% of the patients seen in dermatology practices (17). BDD is classified with the somatoform disorders, but in those instances where no defect whatsoever is present, patients may be delusional. The severity of preoccupation with the perceived defect is generally at the level of that found in patients with obsessive–compulsive disorder and, in fact, these two conditions frequently coexist (18).

Not surprisingly, preoccupation with minor or imagined defects most often involves the face, head, and hair but it can also involve the genitalia (17). The level of preoccupation may be relatively mild and only obsessive in nature or it may be more severe, representing fully developed BDD. Preoccupation regarding the genitalia most often revolves around size or color.

In terms of preoccupation with size, men not surprisingly, most often focus on the penis perceiving that their normal size penis is too small ("small penis syndrome") (19,20). On the other hand, in women it is usually the misperception that their labia minora are too large or too asymmetric (21,22). Penile concerns in men have resulted in a huge industry involving the use of nonprescription medications advertised as "guaranteed" to result in penile enlargement. Similarly, misperception about labia size or asymmetry has resulted in a booming business for female genital cosmetic surgery (23).

There is very little published about preoccupation with genital color. However, a search of the Internet reveals a considerable level of concern on the part of women regarding the perception that their external genitalia (primarily the labia majora) or anal area are too darkly pigmented. Because of this concern, many products and services are offered for genital and anal bleaching. In addition, many women who develop vestibular pain examine the vulvar vestibule and perceive that the color is abnormally red. This perception may be reinforced by clinicians who on examination confirm the presence of "excessive" redness. This "excessive" redness is then perceived as an inflammatory process responsible for the occurrence of vestibular pain. This led to use of the term "vulvar vestibulitis." However, several studies have demonstrated that normal, asymptomatic women, with entirely normal biopsies, frequently have a similar degree of vestibular redness. This suggests that the red color is a normal finding unrelated to inflammation and the development of pain (24). In recognition of this information, the ISSVD has recommended that the term "vestibulodynia" replace the term "vestibulitis" (24).

A similar situation also occurs in men. A small number of men develop idiopathic scrotal skin pain and on self-examination, they perceive that excessive redness is present. They then believe that the redness is abnormal and that it is directly related to the development of their pain. This association may be supported by clinicians who are unfamiliar with genital skin color. The severity of preoccupation with this redness often reaches the level of BDD. However, invariably examination by experienced clinicians reveals that the redness is within the normal variability of scrotal wall color and that there is no local pathology present. Very little has been written about this "red scrotum syndrome" (25), but we have seen at least 20 such patients suggesting that it is appreciably more common than the medical literature would suggest.

Self-mutilation (Dermatitis Artefacta, Factitial Dermatitis)

Self-mutilation involving the skin is an uncommon condition in which individuals knowingly and repeatedly damage the skin through burning, cutting, abrasion, chemical application, or other similar behaviors (13,26,27). We exclude those conditions that occur on a one-time basis such as tattooing and skin piercing. Self-mutilation can occur at any age, but some forms, especially cutting, occur most often in adolescents and young adults (27,28). Characteristically, patients strenuously deny that they are doing anything injurious to the skin. Surprisingly often these patients have a background of work in health care (26).

Self-mutilation occurs in two major settings: with malingering, where secondary gain is the driving factor, and in those individuals with moderate to severe psychological impairment, where the behavior is carried out to satisfy an internal, unknown, and unrecognized emotional need. The underlying psychiatric abnormalities present in these individuals are variable but include anxiety, depressive, bipolar, and personality disorders (13).

These traumatically self-induced lesions are fairly easy to recognize although it is extremely difficult to prove that they occur directly as a result of self-induction. A major clue is the observation that they develop only where the patient can reach. The most common sites are the face, arms, and legs, but the genitalia may be involved in a small percentage of cases (27). There are very few publications in the medical literature about genital self-mutilation, but a short search on the Internet suggests that the problem is much more common than physicians believe. Based mostly on anecdotal information, one of us (PJL) has concluded that major forms of mutilation (such as penile self-amputation) are more common in men, whereas less damaging behaviors such as genital cutting are more likely to occur in young women. A dramatic and disturbing example of this latter problem figured prominently in a recent movie, *The Piano Teacher*.

PSYCHOSOCIAL DYSFUNCTION INFLUENCES THE COURSE OF DISEASE

Psychosocial problems play an important, but not causative, role for many genital disorders. Since this is true of numerous genital diseases, this section will focus on only two examples, atopic dermatitis and psoriasis, wherein psychological factors may play an important role regarding the time of onset, extent, severity, and duration of the disease. The published literature on these two disorders relates almost entirely to generalized forms of the disease, but it is reasonable to expect that when the genital area is involved, there will be even greater psychosocial dysfunction than is described for generalized involvement (29).

Atopic Dermatitis and Lichen Simplex Chronicus

As indicated in Chapter 4, we believe that lichen simplex chronicus represents the localized form of atopic dermatitis, and these two conditions will be treated as a single entity in this section. Atopic dermatitis develops in only a portion of patients who are biologically predisposed to develop the disease through defects (such as filaggrin mutations) in the differentiation of epithelial keratinocytes. Psychological dysfunction appears to be one of the major factors influencing which of these predisposed individuals develop the disease. Often these psychological aspects are present very early in life and frequently occur as a result of a dysfunctional mother–child relationship (30). Other sorts of psychosocial dysfunction associated with atopic dermatitis may develop in childhood and young adult life (31).

For adults, several studies of patients with atopic dermatitis reveal increased levels of both state and trait anxiety (32,33). This heightened anxiety leads to increased itching that in turn leads to incessant scratching. This then is responsible for the development of the "itch–scratch cycle," which characterizes the disorder. In addition, there is evidence that patients with atopic dermatitis have increased levels of depression, somatization, obsession–compulsion, interpersonal sensitivity problems, anger–hostility, and dissociation (29,34). In more psychoanalytic terms, atopic dermatitis patients are often described as irritable, resentful, guilt-ridden, and hostile (31). In what might be called a "proof of concept" observation, the significant improvement in lesional severity, itch intensity, and scratch activity that can be obtained by way of psychological intervention demonstrates the high level of importance that psychological factors play in the development of atopic dermatitis and lichen simplex chronicus (35).

Psoriasis

It is clear that there is a genetic, biologic predisposition for the development of psoriasis. But, as for atopic dermatitis, psychological factors appear to influence the time of lesion development, severity of disease, and response to therapy. There is some consensus that high stress levels frequently precede the development and exacerbation of psoriasis (31,36,37). Patients with psoriasis have significantly higher levels of anxiety and depression than control populations (36,38,39), and it is reasonable to believe that heightened stress plays a role in the development of the abnormal levels of anxiety and depression that are so regularly found in patients with psoriasis (38). Moreover, men with psoriasis consume more alcohol, and patients of both genders are more likely to smoke than do controls (40–42). These behavioral events are also likely to be associated with the noted anxiety and depression (43).

Patients with psoriasis are also appreciably more likely to exhibit alexithymia (an inability to understand, process, or describe emotions), and it is possible that this personality trait plays a role in the development of their disease (36,44). Lastly, psoriatic patients are found to have higher than normal levels of stigmatization and social avoidance/attachment and tend to perceive that social support is lacking (36,37). These findings however probably occur as a result, rather than as a cause, for their disease.

PSYCHOSOCIAL DYSFUNCTION OCCURS AS A RESULT OF DISEASE

Poor health always has a detrimental effect on patients' QOL. The magnitude of this detrimental effect has been primarily determined through the use of questionnaire surveys. These have been carried out for a very large number of dermatologic diseases (45,46). Four aspects regarding the results of these QOL studies are worth exploring.

First, dermatologic disorders, compared to significant systemic medical disease, appear to have a disproportionably large detrimental effect on overall QOL. Two studies suggest that the impact of psoriasis on QOL is greater than that for patients with arthritis, cancer, diabetes hypertension, and heart disease (47). For patients with severe psoriasis, more than 7% reported suicidal ideation; this rate was higher than the approximately 3% of general medical patients (47).

Second, skin disease, again when compared with significant medical disease, has a disproportionably large effect on the sexual function aspect of QOL. This is probably self-evident based on the realization that visible, palpable clearly abnormal, skin problems (when compared to "invisible problems such as diabetes and hypertension") will likely have a very detrimental effect on the patient's self-image and on the partner's response in intimate situations. In a recent study, 35% to 70% of patients with psoriasis were reported to have experienced sexual problems because of their psoriasis (48,49). This problem is probably accentuated in patients who have lesions in the genital area (30). Similarly, more than 50% of patients with atopic dermatitis and 30% of their partners indicated that the disease had an adverse effect on their sex lives (48,50).

Third, dermatologic problems occurring on face and in the anogenital area have more impact on QOL than that same disease occurring at other body sites (29,30). As regards disease at a genital site, some of this effect on QOL is directly due to symptoms of pain such as that occuring with genital lichen sclerosus and erosive lichen planus. But, in other instances it is due to high levels of concern by patients and partners about intimacy and sexual function. And, in still other situations, there will be concern about potential contagiousness. This may, of course, be entirely appropriate when conditions like genital warts are present or may be related to ignorance about what is transmissible and what is not. For instance in one study, 15% of the sexual partners of patients with atopic dermatitis, a clearly noncontagious disease, thought that the disease was potentially contagious (50).

Fourth, the assessment of disease severity and its impact on QOL is quite different between patients and clinicians (51). Clinicians very frequently believe that the decrement in QOL due to a given disease is much less than that perceived by patients. This is largely related to the fact that clinicians base their estimate of disease effect on QOL almost entirely on their observation of the extent and severity of the disease without taking into account what even trivial disease may mean to individual patients. The use of patient-completed QOL questionnaires would alleviate this discrepancy between the viewpoint of the patient and the clinician, but, unfortunately, such surveys have almost only been used in a clinical research setting rather than for individual patient encounters. This needs to change as such underestimation of a patient's perception of disease effect on QOL is demeaning to the patient and will inevitably have an adverse effect on the clinician–patient relationship and possibly also on the patient's response to therapy.

IMMUNOSUPPRESSION

Patients who are immunosuppressed are more likely not only to develop infections but also to exhibit atypical morphology, more severe disease, and unusual infections. Some malignancies are more common, and malignant tumors invade and metastasize more quickly than in immunocompetent patients. In addition, patients who are immunosuppressed by virtue of infection with the human immunodeficiency virus (HIV) are at risk of developing several inflammatory but noninfectious diseases, most notably psoriasis, Reiter disease, and aphthae.

INFECTIONS

Herpes Simplex Virus Infection (see also Chapter 9)

Genital ulcers in an immunosuppressed patient are most often the result of chronic herpes simplex virus (HSV) infection.

Clinical Manifestations

Chronic HSV can occur in any immunosuppressed patient who has been exposed to this virus. However, this occurs more often in those who are immunosuppressed due to HIV. This is because HSV is more common in individuals with a history of intravenous drug use and with multiple sexual partners, which are also risk factors for HIV. With the availability of highly active antiretroviral therapy, the frequency of chronic HSV ulcerations has decreased remarkably.

Like immunocompetent patients, individuals with chronic HSV describe pain, and careful questioning usually reveals prior, more typical recurrent HSV infection outbreaks. HSV infections in these patients begin as the typical grouped vesicles on an erythematous base, disintegrating almost immediately into well-demarcated, discrete erosions. Unlike immunocompetent patients, immunosuppressed patients often experience nonhealing erosions that coalesce and deepen to form large, well-demarcated, painful, chronic ulcers (Figs. 16-1 through 16-4). The ulcers may be superficial initially but may become deeper and more poorly demarcated if untreated or secondarily infected. Coinfection with *Candida* or human papillomavirus (HPV) is common and can change the clinical appearance (Fig. 16-5).

Men most often experience chronic HSV ulcers in a perianal and gluteal cleft distribution as well as on the penis, scrotum, or groin. In the female patient, ulcers may involve the mucous membrane portion of the vulva and may extend to the labia majora, lateral labia minora and even to the crural creases or inner thighs. As in the male patient, HSV infection also often extends

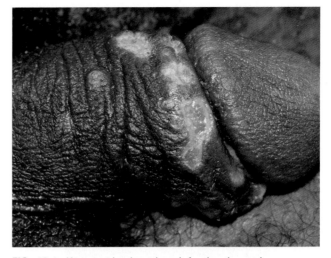

FIG. 16-1. Herpes simplex virus infection in an immunosuppressed patient, with both small superficial macerated new vesicles and early, small, coalescing ulcerations.

to a perianal location and gluteal cleft. Any chronic nonhealing ulcer located on or near a mucocutaneous surface in an immunosuppressed patient is statistically an HSV infection until proven otherwise. Herpes simplex ulcers occasionally are exophytic rather than ulcerative, with prominent elevation above the skin because of prominent fibrin debris and exudate on the surface, and sometimes due to thickened tissue producing a pseudotumor (Fig. 16-6) (52).

Diagnosis

A high index of suspicion should be present for HSV in any chronic nonhealing ulcer in the immunosuppressed person. Although a viral culture can usually confirm a diagnosis of HSV infection type 1 or 2 within 1 to 2 weeks, a biopsy is the fastest means to confirm the

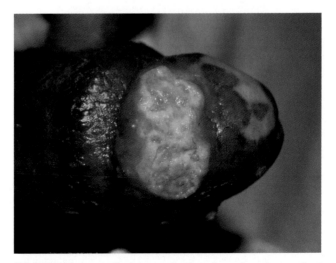

FIG. 16-2. These penile herpes simplex ulcerations in a patient with HIV have enlarged and become firm from inflammation.

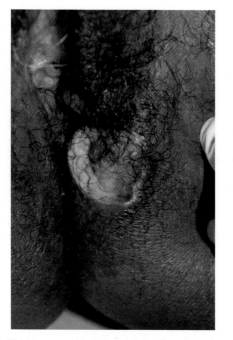

FIG. 16-3. This large perianal herpes simplex ulcer in a woman with chronic lymphocytic leukemia has a yellow adherent fibrin base characteristic of ulcerations of any cause.

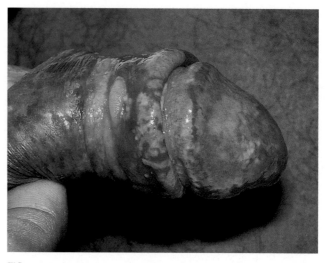

FIG. 16-5. Immunosuppressed patients are likely to develop mixed infections. A microscopic fungal preparation revealed *Candida albicans* infection, but the concomitant herpes virus infection must be suspected, diagnosed, and treated for the patient to improve significantly.

suspicion of a herpes infection in most circumstances, and it may also rule out other concomitant infections such as cytomegalovirus (CMV). However, a biopsy does not distinguish HSV from varicella-zoster infection (herpes zoster and varicella). Direct immunofluorescent antibody testing gives immediate results, and polymerase chain reaction technique for the identification of HSV infection is exquisitely sensitive and is now available commercially for reasonable prices. These require several days at most laboratories.

A biopsy from the edge of a chronic herpes ulcer shows the same histologic features as that of herpes in an immunocompetent person.

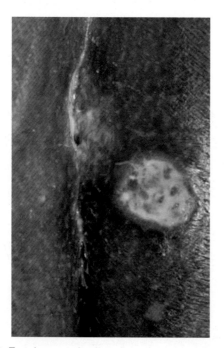

FIG. 16-4. Two herpes simplex ulcerations in an immunosuppressed patient, with a deep, burrowing lesion in the crural crease.

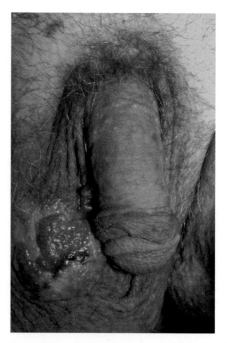

FIG. 16-6. This patient with HIV and chronic scrotal herpes exhibits an unusual morphology of exophytic lesions that resembles human papillomavirus infection; a biopsy, however, distinguishes the two.

The differential diagnosis of genital ulcers in an immunosuppressed host is extensive, although the presence of multiple well-demarcated, painful, chronic ulcers is highly suggestive of HSV infection. Each of these causes generally does not need to be ruled out, unless testing for HSV is negative or the patient does not respond to therapy.

Syphilis and CMV should be seriously considered in many with the acquired immunodeficiency syndrome (AIDS) because they are at higher risk than most for these unusual infections. Biopsy confirmation or polymerase chain reaction testing is often needed, because HSV infection can be a concomitant infection with CMV and may overgrow CMV in viral culture. In patients with negative studies for herpes and poor response to antiviral medications, the uncommon diseases of chancroid, lymphogranuloma venereum, granuloma inguinale, tuberculosis, atypical mycobacterial infections, and deep fungal infection (blastomycosis, coccidioidomycosis, and sporotrichosis), should be considered, although these are very uncommon and do not generally deserve extensive evaluation. These fungal infections do not, in general, show a disposition for the genitalia and, in addition the clinical presentation is that of infiltrated, ulcerated nodules or plaques, unlike HSV ulcers. Rarely, amebiasis may produce serpiginous ulcers with violaceous heaped-up borders, representing an extension of abdominal wall or perineal abscesses to the skin.

Patients with poorly controlled HIV occasionally exhibit unusually large aphthae, or "canker sores," which are indistinguishable morphologically from chronic HSV ulcers. These aphthae can occur in the mouth, but may be extensive and produce impressively large and destructive genital ulcers as well.

Pathophysiology

HSV ulcers in immunosuppressed patients most often arise from reactivation of preexisting recurrent disease, rather than from a primary outbreak. Patients who have altered cellular immunity, such as HIV infection, or patients receiving immunosuppressive agents are at increased risk of more severe herpes infections. HSV infection, usually type 2, becomes chronic and ulcerative rather than recurrent, because it is unchecked by the host's incompetent immune system. In addition, some HSV ulcerations are coinfected with CMV.

Management

Herpes simplex ulcers should be treated with oral acyclovir, famciclovir, or valacyclovir, except in ill patients who require hospitalization and intravenous acyclovir or those with malabsorption. Oral doses include acyclovir 200 mg five times a day, but if clinical improvement does not occur promptly, 400 mg five times a day may be more effective. Famciclovir 125 mg twice daily and valacyclovir 500 mg twice daily are equally effective.

Once healing occurs, long-term suppressive oral antiviral therapy is generally required because recurrence rates are high, and chronic ulceration increases the risk of transmission of both HSV and other infections—including HIV—to others. Also, HSV and HIV appear to be synergic (53). Antiviral agents for HSV used in men with both HIV and HSV decrease the amount of HIV found in semen (54). Suggested doses for suppression, rather than treatment, of HSV infection include acyclovir 400 mg twice daily, famciclovir 250 mg twice daily, or valacyclovir 1 g once daily. Immunosuppressed patients are more likely to experience recurrences at these standard doses, so higher doses can be instituted if this occurs.

Viral resistance occasionally develops in immunosuppressed patients, a much more common and serious event before the development of highly active antiretroviral therapy, although this is still much more likely in immunosuppressed individuals (55). A viral culture with sensitivities should be performed in a patient with known HSV infection not responding to therapy. A primary therapy for HSV resistant to standard therapies is intravenous foscarnet, and a topical formulation has been shown effective as well. Cidofovir, both intravenously and as a topical preparation, has been found beneficial in many patients with acyclovir-resistant cutaneous HSV infections. Topical trifluorothymidine has also been used in acyclovir-resistant HSV infection with some success. Finally, there is evidence of a role for topical imiquimod in the treatment of resistant HSV in immunosuppressed patients.

Genital Warts (see also Chapter 12)

Genital warts are sometimes extremely large, producing local irritation and obstruction in immunosuppressed patients. There is also an increased risk for high-risk HPV types to eventuate into squamous cell carcinoma (SCC).

Clinical Manifestations

In the immunosuppressed host, wart infections on all skin surfaces are more severe. Warts are more numerous, larger, and recalcitrant to treatment (Figs. 16-7 and 16-8). Occasionally, they can be unusually hyperkeratotic (Fig. 16-9).

Genital warts are also markedly increased in the immunosuppressed host. Warts of all morphologies are seen: lobular, papular, flat, and filiform. The warts are larger, may coalesce to form plaques, and are highly recalcitrant to therapy. The warts may become so large that they obstruct an orifice. Genital warts often extend into the anal canal and may cause difficulty with defecation. When the warts enlarge to form plaques, they may become secondarily infected with bacteria, especially *Staphylococcus aureus* or *Streptococcus* sp., or with yeast.

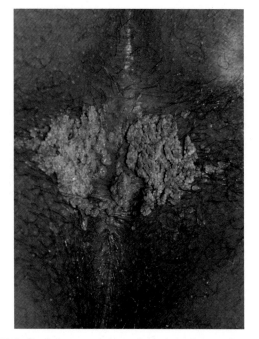

FIG. 16-7. Genital warts grow quickly in patients who are immunosuppressed and produce confluent and resistant plaques.

There is also an increased proportion of potentially oncogenic HPV serotypes found in warts in the immunosuppressed patient (HPV 16, 18, 31, 33) (6). This finding, as well as the ineffective immune system, explains the increased incidence of anogenital SCC in immunosuppressed patients, especially those with AIDS (56).

Diagnosis

The diagnosis of genital HPV infection usually can be made by clinical impression. However, a biopsy of the lesion can be easily performed for confirmation. The

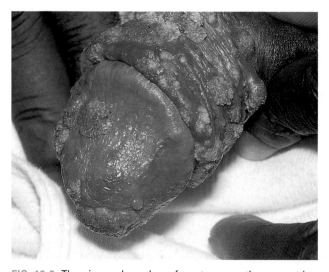

FIG. 16-8. The size and number of warts correctly suggest immunosuppresion in this man with acquired immunodeficiency syndrome.

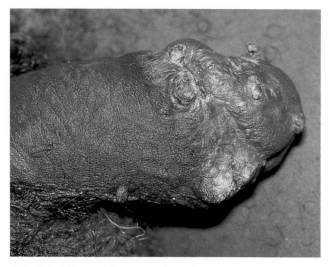

FIG. 16-9. Although dry, keratotic, and verrucous warts generally do not occur in the genital area, this atypical morphology is more likely in immunosuppressed patients.

biopsy is performed by shaving the lesion near its base. A biopsy is suggested if warts are flat, very bulky, or hyperpigmented (except in patients with a naturally dark complexion), because these signs are sometimes associated with dysplasia.

The histopathology of genital warts in immunosuppressed patients is identical to warts in immunocompetent hosts, with epithelial cells that show perinuclear vacuolization. These koilocytes also have large hyperchromatic nuclei with adjacent vacuolization.

Seborrheic keratoses may appear clinically similar to warts as may molluscum contagiosum or pigmented nevi. Intradermal nevi, skin tags, pearly penile papules, vulvar papillae, and condylomata lata can also mimic genital warts. Large lesions, especially if ulcerated, should be examined by biopsy to rule out SCC or an additional, unexpected infection.

Pathophysiology

HPV infection that is uncontrolled by a compromised immune system results in infection that is more recalcitrant and often more florid than the usual HPV infection.

Management

Anogenital warts do not clear spontaneously in the immunosuppressed patients. Many modalities have been employed for the treatment of genital warts, in both immunologically normal and immunosuppressed hosts, but existing therapies do not eradicate the virus, even in the normal host. The lack of adequately functioning immunity translates into a condition that can be somewhat controlled only, requiring ongoing therapy. One alternative for therapy is the removal of the largest lesions, particularly plaques that are obstructing orifices or are becoming secondarily infected. Ulcerated, indurated lesions should be surgically removed and examined by biopsy to rule out SCC. The higher risk of malignant transformation on the transitional epithelium of the cervix and within the anal canal as compared with squamous epithelium should be remembered so that these areas can be reevaluated frequently in high-risk patients.

Traditional therapies used for immunocompetent patients are also the standard of care for immunocompromised patients. Liquid nitrogen treatment, podophyllin resin, home application of podofilox, cantharidin, cold steel surgery, and laser surgery can all be used, either singly or in combination. The home use of imiquimod, a topical immune enhancer, although less effective in patients with an incompetent immune system, can be somewhat helpful in some patients (57). Topical cidofovir has also been shown to be beneficial.

Molluscum Contagiosum (see also Chapters 8 and 12)

Clinical Manifestations

Molluscum contagiosum infection in the adult, when it is severe or extragenital, is now recognized as a cutaneous marker for possible immunodeficiency. It has been seen in many clinical settings, including HIV infection, mycosis fungoides, sarcoidosis, lymphoma, and leukemia. In the immunosuppressed host, molluscum contagiosum is characterized by numerous lesions that are often recalcitrant to therapy, similar to wart infections (Fig. 16-10). The lesions are not self-limited, as in the immunologically

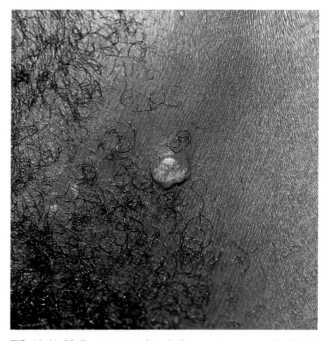

FIG. 16-11. Mollusca contagiosa in immunosuppressed patients are sometimes extremely large and atypical.

normal host, and occur not only on the face, beard area, abdomen, and genitalia, but also over the entire body. Genital molluscum lesions in patients with AIDS are quite common.

Although lesions may present as classic, pink, white, or skin-colored, waxy, umbilicated papules, they are more numerous and may be morphologically atypical in immunosuppressed patients. Lesions in these patients often coalesce to form plaques, and they may individually be much larger than 2 to 3 mm (Fig. 16-11). Lesions are found on the shaft of the penis, scrotum, and inner thighs and in a perianal distribution in men. In women, lesions are found on the labia and inner thighs and also in a perianal location.

Diagnosis

Biopsy of an individual lesion is the test of choice in confirmation of molluscum contagiosum when required. Epidermal cells contain characteristic large, intracytoplasmic eosinophilic inclusion bodies caused by the virus, as occurs in biopsy specimens of immunocompetent patients. A biopsy may be needed in the immunosuppressed host to differentiate molluscum from a deep fungal infection. If the biopsy does not show the pathognomonic intracytoplasmic eosinophilic inclusion bodies or if a different infectious origin is strongly suspected, tissue should also be sent for culture because the organism may not always be seen on routine staining. Mollusca contagiosa in the immunosuppressed host can mimic a number of different infections. Disseminated cryptococcosis, histoplasmosis, coccidioidomycosis, and *Penicillium marneffei* have all been

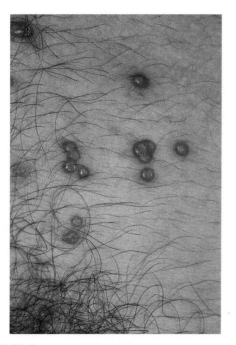

FIG. 16-10. Mollusca contagiosa are more numerous, larger, and resistant to treatment in immunosuppressed patients.

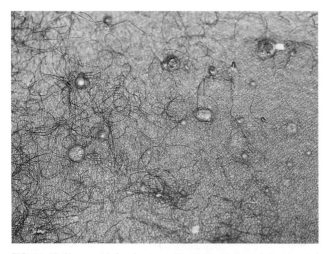

FIG. 16-12. Unusual infections such as histoplasmosis or cryptococcosis, as seen here, can mimic molluscum or herpes simplex virus infection. Any atypical lesions in an immunosuppressed patient should be assessed by culture or biopsy.

described as clinically resembling mollusca (Fig. 16-12). Mollusca also may have a shiny, umbilicated appearance resembling vesicles, so HSV infections also should be considered at times in the differential diagnosis. Occasionally, warts, nevi, and basal cell carcinomas can resemble mollusca contagiosa.

Pathophysiology

Mollusca contagiosa occurring on the adult genitalia are sexually transmitted nodules produced by a poxvirus. As occurs with genital warts, large, atypical, recalcitrant lesions often develop as a result of this infection in the setting of an ineffective immune system.

Management

Molluscum contagiosum in immunosuppressed patients can be very resistant to therapy. Although immunocompetent hosts eventually clear the virus irrespective of therapy, the lesions do not clear spontaneously in those without normal immune function. Treating the largest, most bothersome lesions is more practical than the widespread destruction of affected skin. Many therapies have been tried, but liquid nitrogen treatment is a mainstay of therapy. Curettage is effective but painful and bloody. Large mollusca are best treated by surgical removal. Cantharidin can also be used, but in the USA this may have to be compounded because it is not commercially available. Occasionally, cantharidin can cause marked blistering, particularly in the genital region, so care should be used to apply this sparingly until tolerance is ascertained. Topical tretinoin has been used to decrease the occurrence of new lesions, but it is extremely irritating when used in the genital region. Imiquimod cream 5% has been reported to be somewhat useful in immunocompetent patients with mollusca contagiosa and may be helpful in

immunosuppressed patients. Topical cidofovir has been beneficial in some immunosuppressed patients with mollusca contagiosa. Mollusca exhibit no malignant potential and generally do not obstruct orifices.

Tinea Cruris (see also Chapter 6)

Clinical Manifestations

Dermatophyte infections are more common in the immunosuppressed host and may be atypical in presentation. Although tinea cruris may show typical inflamed plaques with central clearing and a scaly "ringworm" border, usually the infection is more extensive (Fig. 16-13). The penis and scrotum are sometimes affected; this is extraordinarily uncommon in the immunocompetent patient (Fig. 16-14). Tinea cruris may involve the buttocks and occasionally extends to the abdomen in immunosuppressed patients. Although tinea cruris occurs much less often in women, it can extend to involve the hair-bearing portion of the vulva. In addition, follicular involvement is common and is manifested by papules or pustules within the plaques.

Tinea cruris sometimes presents as hyperkeratotic, scaly plaques, often without the typical annular scaly border and central clearing. In black patients, hyperpigmentation rather than erythema is often present in association with scaly patches and plaques. This is often accompanied by onychomycosis.

Diagnosis

Dermatophyte infections involving the skin usually are easily diagnosed by microscopic examination of scale

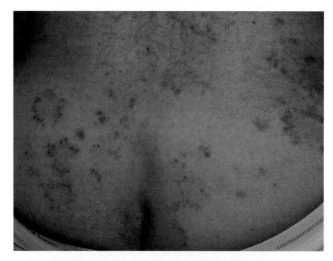

FIG. 16-13. Dermatophytosis in an immunosuppressed patient, or in a patient using topical corticosteroids, is more likely to present with extensive disease, and fungal folliculitis; there are annular plaques composed of red papules that represent extention of the fungal infection into hair follicles in this immunosuppressed man.

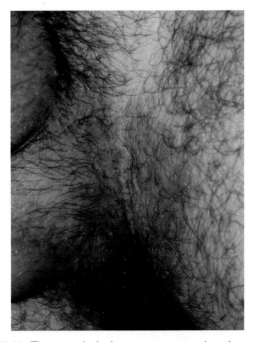

FIG. 16-14. Tinea cruris in immunosuppressed patients often does not show the classic central clearing and peripheral scale, but is more likely to show uniform scale throughout the plaque; also, scrotal involvement is more common in immunosuppressed individuals.

from the periphery of the patch or plaque in a potassium hydroxide preparation. A biopsy also shows the organism.

Erythematous scaly eruptions involving inguinal creases elicit a differential diagnosis, including tinea cruris, *Candida albicans* infection, erythrasma, and intertrigo. Because HIV-infected patients are more likely than other patients to have psoriasis, this disease should be remembered in the differential diagnosis of tinea cruris. Seborrheic dermatitis has also been increased in incidence in the HIV-infected patient, and it occurs as yellow scale along the inguinal creases.

Pathophysiology

Dermatophyte infections are superficial fungal infections that may affect hair, nails, and the skin. These can be atypical, more extensive, and recalcitrant in immunosuppressed patients.

Management

Tinea cruris in immunosuppressed patients is treated in the same manner as in immunocompetent patients, discussed in Chapter 6. However, immunosuppressed hosts have more extensive disease or have follicular involvement that often requires oral therapy.

Topical antifungal therapy is helpful for immunosuppressed patients to use early when the eruption recurs. There are many effective topical antifungal medications, which include any of the azoles, such as clotrimazole, econazole, and ketoconazole, or the non-azole, terbinefine.

Norwegian Scabies (Crusted Scabies)

Clinical Manifestations

Normally, scabies is characterized by intense pruritus and excoriations, with occasional linear, edematous papules called "burrows" concentrated in finger web spaces and skin fold areas. Usually, there is no involvement above the neck, except in infants and very ill people.

Norwegian scabies, however, is manifested by thick, yellow, hyperkeratotic papules and plaques, rather than discrete excoriated and crusted papules (Fig. 16-15). The hyperkeratotic plaques commonly occur on hands, feet, scalp, ears, buttocks, and genitalia, but they can occur on any skin surface. The nails may be thickened with subungual and periungual crusting, which contain numerous mites. In the immunosuppressed host, hyperkeratotic, yellow, scaling plaques involving the scrotum, glans, or shaft of the penis may occur.

Diagnosis

A suspected diagnosis may be confirmed by microscopic examination of material scraped from a scaling plaque. In Norwegian scabies, mites, eggs, and feces are abundant and easily visualized because of the immunosuppressed state of the patient. When needed, however, a biopsy reveals epidermal spongiosis and a mixed perivascular inflammatory infiltrate, prominent with eosinophils, often with a mite, ova, eggshells, or fecal deposits seen. Persistent nodules of scabies show a dense, inflammatory infiltrate in which eosinophils are prominent.

Because scabies presents with marked secondary eczematous changes and occasional vesicles, the differential diagnosis of genital Norwegian scabies includes eczema or atopic dermatitis and allergic contact

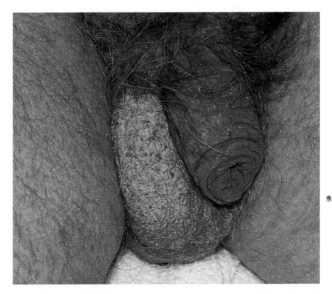

FIG. 16-15. Norwegian, or crusted, scabies, which is scabies in an immunocompromised host, presents as very characteristic hyperkeratotic, yellowish plaques.

dermatitis. Nondescript excoriated papules also suggest a differential diagnosis of any bite reaction. Intense itching, worse at night, and abrupt onset of an eruption in a patient with no history of eczema should make scabies high in the differential diagnosis.

Because Norwegian scabies presents with hyperkeratotic plaques, rather than discrete excoriated papules, it may elicit a differential diagnosis that includes unusual psoriasis, tinea cruris, and even seborrheic dermatitis, when it occurs on the genitalia or scalp. Impetiginized eczema may also appear similar to scabies.

Pathophysiology

Sarcoptes scabiei var. *hominis* is a mite responsible for the infestation known as scabies. Because the mite is poorly contained by the immunosuppressed host, a severe form of scabies, Norwegian scabies, is sometimes seen. The severity of the infestation is entirely the result of the host's poor immunity, not a more virulent mite.

Management

Although the mainstay of therapy for scabies is 5% permethrin cream, the severity of Norwegian scabies, together with its crusted, relatively impenetrable skin indicates that it is usually best treated orally with ivermectin 200 µg. Resistent disease occasionally requires both topical and oral therapy, or a repeat dose of ivermectin (58). Permethrin is applied from the neck to the toes, is left on for 8 to 10 hours, and then is washed off. Those immunosuppressed patients with head and scalp involvement should treat these areas also, and care should be taken to treat under the fingernails as well as possible. All other household members and close contacts are also treated. Recently worn clothing and bed linens should be washed in hot water.

NONINFECTIOUS INFLAMMATORY DISEASES ASSOCIATED WITH HIV

Psoriasis (see also Chapters 6 and 8)

Psoriasis can be triggered by sunburn, a streptococcal infection, and HIV disease. It is not more common in other types of immunosupression.

Clinical Manifestations

Psoriasis is well known to be increased in incidence in patients with HIV infection. Those patients with preexisting psoriasis may worsen, and patients sometimes present with new-onset psoriasis when they develop HIV. This occurs in patients with advanced HIV.

Psoriasis occurring in these patients is typical in appearance, showing well-demarcated, erythematous papules or plaques covered with silvery scale. Psoriasis preferentially occurs on the knees, elbows, scalp, umbilicus, lumbosacral region, hands, and feet. However, AIDS-associated psoriasis is much more extensive and recalcitrant to treatment than in the immunologically normal host.

Psoriasis may occur as the common plaque type, but, in HIV, there is an increased incidence of "inverse" psoriasis, which preferentially affects the anogenital skin. Well-demarcated plaques may involve the inguinal creases, suprapubic region, intergluteal cleft, axillae, inframammary skin, and umbilicus. Scale is less dense than the silvery scale that is classic for psoriasis on drier skin surfaces (Figs. 16-16 and 16-17). Psoriasis may affect the labia majora and occasionally occurs on the scrotum and the shaft of the penis (Figs. 16-17 and 16-18).

Severe psoriasis can become generalized. This generalized erythema and scale, called exfoliative erythroderma, are seen more commonly in the HIV-affected patient than in others, and they involve the genitalia incidentally. However, exfoliative erythroderma can also result from other severe dermatoses such as atopic dermatitis and from medication reactions, both more common in HIV-infected patients than noninfected individuals.

Diagnosis

A high index of suspicion is needed on clinical grounds, based on the morphology of the lesions and knowledge of the preferential "inverse" distribution of psoriasis in the immunosuppressed host. A biopsy is helpful if typical of psoriasis, but if it is not diagnostic, this should not deter one from the diagnosis. Evaluating the patient for other typical psoriatic lesions is sometimes

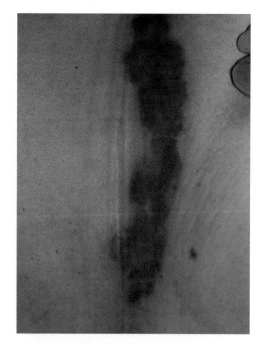

FIG. 16-16. Although a microscopic examination of skin scale showed yeast, this red, moist crural crease plaque did not clear with antifungal therapy, and the new onset of psoriasis as a concomitant condition was missed for several months.

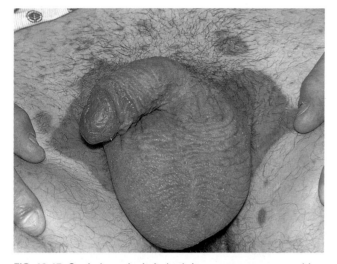

FIG. 16-17. Genital psoriasis in both immunocompetent and immunosuppressed patients often does not show the classic, silvery scale.

helpful (nails, elbows, knees, and scalp). Ruling out other diagnostic possibilities with a potassium hydroxide preparation and Wood's lamp examination is also important.

A biopsy shows the same abnormalities as found in psoriasis occurring in immunocompetent patients. Histologically, well-developed psoriasis is characterized by regular elongation of the epidermal rete ridges, the absence of granular cells, and confluent parakeratosis (cornified cells near the top of the epidermis that have retained their nuclei). Munro microabscesses and spongiform pustules of Kogoj are also characteristic. These findings are nearly pathognomonic for psoriasis. Psoriasis in the HIV-affected patient clinically may be

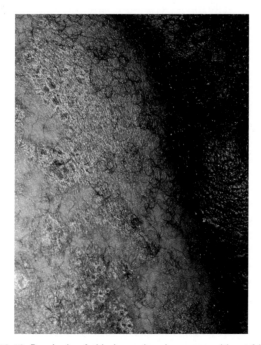

FIG. 16-18. Psoriasis of skin in cooler, dry areas without friction is more likely to exhibit the typical, silvery scale.

classic morphologically, but often does not show classic histopathologic changes of psoriasis, showing instead a nondiagnostic picture of psoriasiform dermatitis.

Psoriasis occurring in the inguinal creases and intergluteal cleft may mimic or coexist with tinea cruris, candidiasis, erythrasma, seborrheic dermatitis, or even eczema. Although psoriasis classically presents with well-demarcated erythematous plaques with silver scale, scale may not be prominent when psoriasis occurs on the genitalia. As long as infection is ruled out, topical corticosteroids are the mainstay in therapy for psoriasis, eczema, and seborrhea so that absolute differentiation is not always crucial.

Pathophysiology

The predisposition of individuals with HIV to develop psoriasis is not intuitive. HIV suppresses T-cells, whereas psoriasis is a T-cell driven disease. Also, type 2 cytokines predominate in HIV, whereas type 1 cytokines are operative in psoriasis. However, gamma interferon produced by memory CD8 T and other cells may be important in psoriasis both associated and unassociated with HIV (59).

Management

Most important for the improvement of psoriasis in these patients is antiviral therapy for HIV, which usually results in substantial improvement in their psoriasis. Otherwise, usual first-line therapy for genital psoriasis occurring in the immunosuppressed host is the same as for that occurring in immuncompetent individuals (Chapter 6). Aggressive therapy including systemic retinoids and immunosuppressive agents such as methotrexate, cyclosporine, and tumor necrosis-alpha blockers such as adalimumab and etanercept can be used with care (60). Supportive care, including treatment of secondary infection with *S. aureus, Streptococcus* sp., or *C. albicans,* is often needed and crucial to comfort.

Reiter Syndrome (see also Chapter 8)

Etiology

Reiter syndrome is a reactive skin condition related to psoriasis and defined by the presence of arthritis, urethritis, and conjunctivitis for greater than 3 months. Various organisms have been thought to act as triggering agents including *Chlamydia, Salmonella, Shigella, Yersinia,* and *Ureaplasma.* Many patients with Reiter syndrome are found to have a human leukocyte antigen (HLA)-B27 genotype or closely related genotypes.

Clinical Manifestations

Reiter syndrome occurs predominantly in young male patients, and the incidence is increased in male patients with HIV disease. The clinical presentation is similar to that in the immunologically normal host. About two

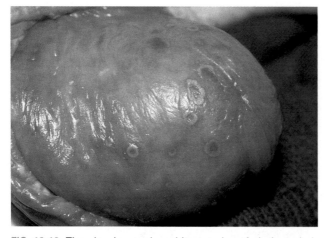

FIG. 16-19. The classic annular white papules of circinate balanitis on the uncircumcised glans of a patient with Reiter syndrome can be mistaken for a yeast infection.

thirds of patients exhibit cutaneous lesions, primarily on the genitalia, palms of the hands, and soles of the feet. Genital lesions occur primarily on the penis, especially on the glans or the prepuce, and much less often on the vulva, particularly on the hair-bearing portion. The lesions closely resemble those of pustular psoriasis. In uncircumcised men, lesions are white, annular, "circinate" papules or plaques usually occurring on the glans (balanitis circinata) (Fig. 16-19). These lesions may also be seen on the mucous membrane and modified mucous membrane portion of the vulva, vagina, or cervix. In circumcised men and on the hair-bearing portion of the vulva, the plaques are

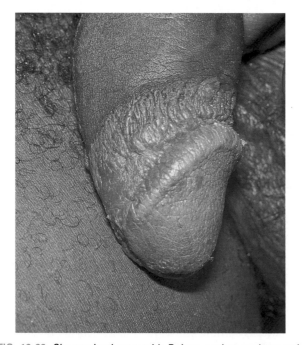

FIG. 16-20. Circumcised men with Reiter syndrome show redness and scale indistinguishable from psoriasis of the glans, rather than circinate, white papules.

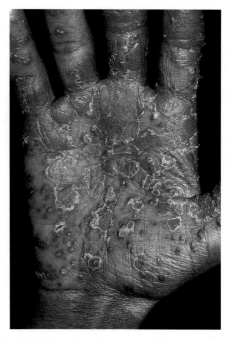

FIG. 16-21. The diagnosis of Reiter syndrome can sometimes be made when genital lesions are accompanied by typical, well-demarcated, crusted, pustular, keratotic plaques on the palms or soles of a patient.

erythematous and scaly, often with crust (Fig. 16-20). These skin findings are indistinguishable from those of psoriasis. Lesions on the palms and soles exhibit pustules that evolve into thick, hyperkeratotic plaques, a condition termed *keratoderma blenorrhagica* (Fig. 16-21). Occasionally, there are pustular or crusted hyperkeratotic lesions elsewhere on the skin. Conjunctivitis and urethritis also occur in most patients. Arthritis affecting the large joints in an asymmetric distribution is common.

Diagnosis

The diagnosis of Reiter syndrome is made by a combination of clinical findings. Urethritis often precedes skin findings, and evaluation for gonorrhea or *Chlamydia* infection is often performed. Asymmetric arthritis, conjunctivitis, and dermatitis may occur. Circinate balanitis and keratoderma blenorrhagica are classic, as described earlier. Reiter syndrome and psoriasis with arthritis exist on a spectrum, and therefore the differentiation sometimes cannot be made with certainty. Unlike Reiter syndrome, psoriasis associated with arthritis usually lacks conjunctivitis and urethritis.

A skin biopsy is identical to that of pustular psoriasis. Early lesions of Reiter syndrome show a spongiform pustule in the epidermis, called a spongiform pustule of Kogoj. More developed lesions exhibit thickening of the stratum corneum with associated intermingled pyknotic nuclei of neutrophils.

Reiter syndrome should be distinguished from pustular psoriasis, secondary syphilis, and unusual impetiginized

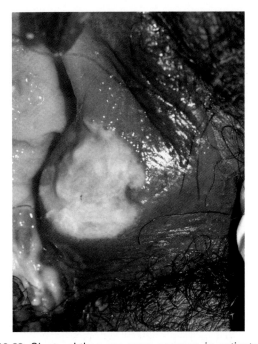

FIG. 16-22. Giant aphthae are more common in patients with human immunodeficiency virus disease, and they are generally indistinguishable from ulcerative herpes simplex virus infection.

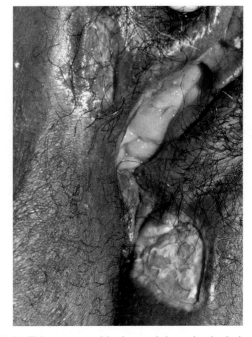

FIG. 16-23. This woman with giant aphthae also had ulcerative herpes simplex virus infection, producing difficulty in diagnosis and a delay in treatment.

eczema. Cutaneous candidiasis or HSV infection should be ruled out in the patient with prominent erosions. Disseminated gonococcemia can mimic the noncutaneous aspects of Reiter syndrome, but the skin lesions are very different, consisting of occasional hemorrhagic pustules over joints.

Management

Topical steroids are somewhat useful for the skin disease of Reiter syndrome. Systemic therapy for Reiter syndrome is immunosuppressive and should be used with caution. Patients with arthritis often benefit from nonsteroidal anti-inflammatory agents, analgesics, and/or rest. As for psoriasis, patients with either severe skin disease or arthritis require methotrexate or anittumor necrosis factor medications with careful monitoring. The skin disease is sometimes improved remarkably by oral retinoids such as acitretin or isotretinoin, but these medications often aggravate joint disease. The conjunctivitis is self-limited.

Aphthae (see also Chapter 10)

Patients with HIV are more likely than other people to develop unusually large, deep, and recalcitrant aphthae. These painful lesions are probably immune complex mediated.

Although typical, small aphthae are round, 1- to 3-mm erosions with a white fibrin base and a surrounding white flare, aphthae associated with HIV are deep and large. These are sometimes several centimeters in diameter and

can deeply ulcerate with, usually, well-demarcated, clean, irregular borders (Figs. 16-22 and 16-23). There is often significant scarring following healing.

Ulcerative HSV infection is the primary disease in the differential diagnosis, although any cause of infectious or neoplastic ulcers should be considered and ruled out with a biopsy. Topical and intralesional therapies are generally inadequate for these ulcers, and systemic corticosteroids maybe required to initiate healing. Dapsone and colchicine can be tried, but thalidomide is the treatment of choice in these patients; however, the neurotoxicity can be limiting (61).

NEOPLASTIC DISEASES

Malignancy is more common in chronically immunosuppressed patients in general, as the routine occurrence of atypical cells is not checked by the surveillance of a normal immune system. Skin lymphoreticular cancers are the most common of these malignancies. However, HIV is associated with Kaposi sarcoma, lymphomas, and SCC. With the advent of highly active antiretroviral therapy, the longer life span of individuals with HIV may allow these patients to develop and die of their cancers.

Squamous Cell Carcinoma
(discussed primarily in Chapter 12)

All chronically immunosuppressed patients are at higher risk than other for the development of this common

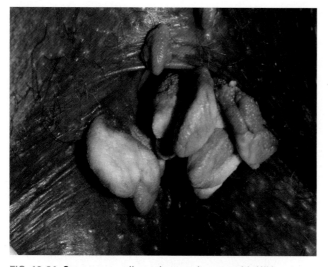

FIG. 16-24. Squamous cell carcinomas in men with HIV are usually associated with HPV infection, and are most likely to be anal; unusually large warts should be removed and submitted for histologic evaluation.

malignancy. Most often, anogenital SCCs are associated with HPV infection, although patients with other at-risk diseases such as lichen sclerosus should be followed especially carefully as well. Immunosuppressed patients also have a higher risk of ultraviolet light-induced skin cancers, but not in the anogenital area. Anogenital SCC and intraepithelial neoplasia grade 3 are also discussed in Chapters 6, 7, 10, and 11–13.

Clinical Manifestations

Anogenital SCC is more common in the immunosuppressed host, and tumors often are larger and more keratotic than in other patients. The earliest clinical presentation usually is that of a genital wart, with lesions often multifocal or coalescent. These classically are either flat warts or are exuberant lobular warts (Bushke–Lowenstein wart). Growth is often more rapid, and response to wart therapy is poor. The plaques or nodules often become hyperkeratotic or impressively large (Fig. 16-24). Penile SCC occurs on the prepuce, glans, or coronal sulcus, but it may occur elsewhere.

Anorectal SCC is seen in HIV-infected men who engage in receptive anal intercourse. It is found also in the setting of multiple genital warts. These lesions present as an indurated ulcerated plaque or occasionally a large, hyperkeratotic, verrucous nodule or plaque.

Diagnosis

The diagnosis is by biopsy, which shows the same features as in immunocompetent patients. In contradistinction, verrucous, hyperkeratotic anogenital SCCs can be indistinguishable from large genital warts, with no evidence of malignancy on biopsy. This does not rule out SCC. Any remarkably large wart (in both immunouppressed and immunocompetent patients) that yields a biopsy showing

no signs of malignancy on biopsy should be re-evaluated in toto and sectioned for foci of malignancy.

The primary condition in the differential diagnosis of anogenital SCC is that of HPV infection. Ulcerated plaques or nodules of SCC evoke a differential diagnosis of many malignant neoplasms, including malignant melanoma or unusual basal cell carcinoma. In the immunosuppressed patient, this form of SCC can also mimic infectious processes, such as deep fungal infections, unusual atypical mycobacterial infection including tuberculosis, viral infections such as those produced by HSV or CMV, ecthyma, and even parasitic infections, including cutaneous *Acanthamoeba* infection.

Pathophysiology

This topic is discussed in Chapter 12. However, infectious agents play a role in most immunosuppressed patients. HPV DNA is often found in invasive SCC. HPV types 16, 18, and 33 are strongly associated with anogenital SCC and are found more commonly in the immunosuppressed host, especially those with HIV (62). In all likelihood, immunosuppression and increased incidence of oncogenic HPV types are responsible for the increase in anogenital SCC in HIV-infected patients.

Management

Therapy for anogenital SCC is by surgical excision. Local radiation may or may not be used in conjunction with surgery, depending on the staging of the SCC.

AIDS-Associated Kaposi Sarcoma

Kaposi sarcoma is an unusual tumor strongly associated with HIV and herpesvirus 8, although classically found in older men from the Mediterranian gene pool. This lesion is seen most commonly in the male homosexual patient with AIDS. Kaposi sarcoma occurring in the HIV-affected patient usually begins as a pink or red papule, which becomes violaceous. Lesions often enlarge to form plaques, and older lesions are red brown, as hemosiderin is deposited in the skin (Fig. 16-25). Occasionally, early lesions may be flat and resemble a bruise. Kaposi sarcoma in patients of African background often is nearly black.

The initial lesions of AIDS-associated Kaposi sarcoma frequently occur on the face and ears, and 10% to 15% of patients experience oral mucosal lesions as the first site of involvement. Kaposi sarcoma occurs in all areas, and extracutaneous disease affecting the lymph nodes, gastrointestinal tract, and lungs is not uncommon.

Genital lesions occasionally occur and, when present, are most common on the shaft of the penis, but they may also be found in the suprapubic region. When plaques evolve, there is often associated lymphedema of the penis. As the plaques enlarge, they may ulcerate, becoming a source of recurrent infection, particularly with *S. aureus*, *Streptococcus* sp., or *C. albicans*. Because Kaposi sarcoma

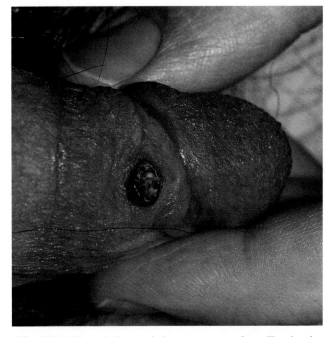

FIG. 16-25. Although the penis is not an area of predilection for Kaposi sarcoma, this tumor can appear in the genital area.

occurs almost exclusively in homosexual or bisexual men, few reports exist of female genital involvement.

The diagnosis is made on biopsy, which is always indicated, because bacillary angiomatosis may be indistinguishable clinically. A biopsy may also rule out concomitant infection, such as deep fungal (histoplasmosis, cryptococcosis) or viral (CMV) infections, which have been reported to occur in Kaposi lesions.

Kaposi sarcoma associated with HIV is due to herpesvirus 8, which has been shown by polymerase chain reaction technique to be present in Kaposi sarcoma lesions. CMV, HPV, and even hepatitis B virus have also been described as associated with Kaposi sarcoma.

The therapy of Kaposi sarcoma depends on the clinical stage and location of the lesion. Small lesions do not require therapy other than for psychological or cosmetic reasons, but these can be treated successfully with liquid nitrogen or surgical removal. Larger patches or plaques may be treated with radiation therapy. Therapies currently approved by the Food and Drug Administration include alitretinoin gel for topical administration and liposomal daunorubicin, liposomal doxorubicin, paclitaxel, and interferon-α for systemic administration (63).

GERIATRIC ISSUES

Older people have difficulties that differ from and compound those of younger patients, especially in the arena of genital dermatology. There are multiple interrelated issues that produce problems when individuals age, and attention

to these factors is important for maximal alleviation of the patient's genital symptoms.

Normal Genital Aging

The Aging Female Genitalia

Primarily due to low estrogen, the postmenopausal vulva and vagina typically exhibit differences from the well-estrogenized external genitalia. However, overweight women experience peripheral conversion of estrogen, and women who remain sexually active generally exhibit fewer signs of genital atrophy.

One of the most obvious changes seen in the postmenopausal vulva is the loss of hair. As body hair disappears, hair on the mons diminishes as well. Often, this is most obvious in the center of the mons. The very elderly may lose almost all genital hair.

The modified mucous membranes of the vulva become pale, thin, and smooth compared to the fuller, more erythematous epithelium of premenopausal women, which generally exhibits Fordyce spots and vulvar papillomatosis (Fig. 16-26). The labia minora shrink, occasionally disappearing altogether, so that differentiation from resorption due to lichen sclerosus and lichen planus can be difficult. The vaginal epithelium is smooth, with loss of the estrogenized rugae. The vagina is also dry, and with more advanced atrophy, the mucosa becomes pale. Pelvic floor muscles lose tone, and cystoceles and rectoceles sometimes occur (Fig. 16-27). Vaginal secretions are scant. Microscopically, epithelial cells are small and round (parabasal cells) rather than large, flat,

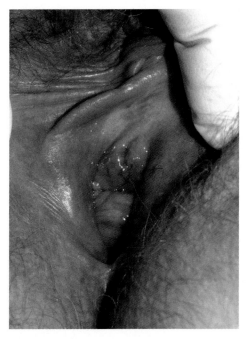

FIG. 16-26. The postmenopausal vulva exhibits smooth, dry, pale modified mucous membrane, with shrinkage of the labia minora.

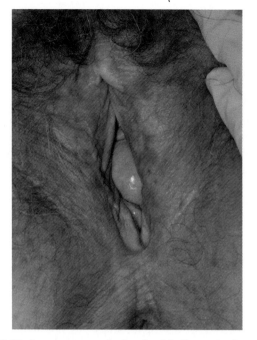

FIG. 16-27. As women age, laxity of pelvic floor muscles sometimes result in a rectocele or cystocele, as seen here with the smooth protuberance of a cystocele at the introitus.

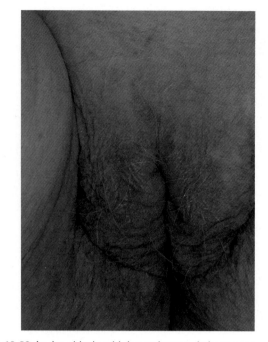

FIG. 16-28. In the elderly with incontinence, irritant contact dermatitis is common.

and folded. Lactobacilli are absent. With longstanding loss of estrogen, vaginal secretions are nearly acellular microscopically.

The Aging Male Genitalia

The normal changes of the male genitalia with age are less obvious. Like women, men experience a decrease in genital hair. The skin of the penis and scrotum becomes more lax.

Factors that Exacerbate Genital Symptoms in the Elderly

Incontinence

As patients age, incontinence becomes a factor in chronic anogenital irritation. Most elderly women experience urinary incontinence as a natural sequela of childbirth, waning estrogen levels, and loss of muscle tone from aging. Men with prostate disease also experience urinary incontinence as a result of surgery. Neurologic disease interferes with normal bowel and bladder function in both genders (Fig. 16-28).

Constant moisture produces maceration of skin, promotes the growth of yeast, and increases friction between skin folds (Fig. 16-29). This results in intertriginous dermatitis, either as a primary disease or as a factor in other skin conditions (see Chapter 4). The management of intertriginous dermatitis consists of keeping the areas as dry as possible, using adult diapers, soft cloths placed between skin folds and changed frequently, and, when skin

is only slightly wet, powders. Barrier pastes applied heavily to irritated skin helps to protect from feces and urine.

Obesity

Overweight, common in older individuals, complicates genital symptoms in several manners. Obesity compounds the irritation of incontinence by trapping both urine and sweat in skin folds, and increasing friction between skin surfaces.

When genital symptoms occur, treatment is more difficult for the obese patient. Application of medication is

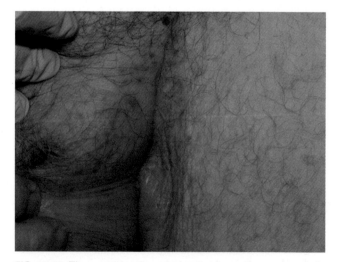

FIG. 16-29. The combination of obesity, incontinence, and diabetes has resulted in an intertriginous dermatitis due to candidiasis.

difficult, in part because the areas to be treated are difficult to visualize. Skin folds can be difficult to both separate and treat with only two hands. This sometimes best is achieved by application of medications when the patient is sitting on the toilet, where skin folds can be separated by positioning on the seat. Also, excess weight interferes with adequate removal of feces, sweat, and smegma/desquamated epithelial cells from skin folds.

Obesity interferes with sexual function in many people; positioning can be difficult and body image can suffer. This is especially difficult for individuals who already experience compromised sexual functioning due to chronic genital pain or itching, and for older individuals who may have loss of libido and natural lubrication.

Arthritis

Joint pain and stiffness, like obesity, interferes with hygiene, application of medications, and sexual functioning.

Psychological Factors

Depression from declining health, loss of friends and family (by death or dementia), pain of arthritis, waning strength, diminished intellectual capacity, decreased body image, and fear of incapacity and malignancy are common emotional stresses for the elderly. These all affect the patient's ability to treat and tolerate genital disease, and depression and anxiety escalate pain and itching.

Declining Sexual Capability

Sexual function diminishes as people age. Falling hormone levels; effects of diabetes mellitus, cardiovascular disease, and neurologic disease; adverse effects to medication; depression; loss of a partner; pain; declining muscle strength and endurance; prostate surgery; and decreasing self-confidence in one's appearance and sexual ability are factors that interfere with sexual ability and pleasure. For many patients with these issues, genital itching and pain can be the final factors that end sexual activity. Emotional support, referral for counseling, and understanding of the patient and her/his partner's wishes and expectations for future sexual functioning can minimize the impact of chronic genital disease while conveying a realistic outlook. Simply helping the patient to acknowledge his/her desires and expectations for future sexual function can be a significant help for planning therapy. For example, the elderly woman with scarring associated with lichen sclerosus may be unable to engage in sexual intercourse. A frank discussion of her and her partner's wishes help to make the decision of whether to lyse her adhesions.

Anogenital Diseases Most Common in the Elderly

Specific genital diseases associated with aging occur primarily in women. The only skin diseases that occur more commonly in older men are malignancies, particularly SCC. Extramammary Paget disease, basal cell carcinoma, and malignant melanoma occur more often in older men as well, but are quite uncommon.

Atrophic Vaginitis (see also Chapter 15)

Until the results of the Women's Health Initiative were widely publicized, postmenopausal women regularly received estrogen replacement. Symptoms of an atrophic vagina or atrophic vaginitis were uncommon for many years, and the index of suspicion for this diagnosis has decreased. Now, an atrophic vagina is a common cause of dyspareunia and vulvovaginal irritation, rawness, and burning.

Nearly all women experience an atrophic vagina when the ovaries cease estrogen production. The vagina becomes dry, and the epithelium is thin. Women who are not sexually active are usually comfortable and unaware of these changes. However, women who are sexually active often experience irritation and pain with intercourse because of the lack of lubrication. The fragility of skin and mucosa may result in erosions from friction between vaginal walls pressed together by a cystocele or rectocele, or with sexual activity. The presence of erosions causes secondary inflammation, and the patient develops atrophic vaginitis. The vaginal secretions become clinically and microscopically purulent, with the wet mount characterized by an increase in white blood cells, parabasal cells, and a lack of lactobacilli.

The diagnosis of atrophic vaginitis is made by the setting of low estrogen, the wet mount, and response to estrogen replacement. The management of atrophic vaginitis is primarily estrogen replacement. This can be achieved with topical estrogen or systemic estrogen replacement. Topical therapies include estradiol or conjugated equine estrogen cream, 1 g inserted three times a week, estradiol vaginal tablets inserted thrice weekly, or sustained release estradiol formulated into a ring that is inserted into the vagina and changed every three months. Or, estrogen replacement can be achieved by estrogens administered orally or by patch, with concomitant progesterone provided to women who have not undergone a hysterectomy. Some clinicians believe that estrogen replacement substantially increases the risk of candidiasis during the first month of therapy; fluconazole weekly can prevent this uncomfortable complication.

Treatment is easy for most women, and improvement is prompt. Women who are not sexually active often can stop or decrease estrogen after vaginal secretions normalize. Patients who want to be sexually active generally require ongoing estrogen replacement.

Lichen Sclerosus (see also Chapter 11)

Lichen sclerosus is a disease primarily diagnosed on the vulva of postmenopausal women. This condition has been found in up to 3% of incontinent women in a nursing home environment (64). Lichen sclerosus is characterized by pruritus, the presence of white crinkled plaques, resorption of the labia minora, and entrapment of the clitoris by the clitoral hood. The etiology is multifactorial and includes autoimmune issues, genetic factors, and local environmental aspects. Usually, lichen sclerosus responds to ultrapotent topical steroids and care of accompanying factors such as secondary infection, estrogen deficiency, and maceration from incontinence. Poorly controlled disease eventuates into SCC in about 3% to 5% of women, usually the elderly with thickened lesions.

Erosive Mucosal Lichen Planus

(see also Chapters 6 and 9)

Once felt to be rare, erosive genital lichen planus now is recognized as a frequent cause of vulvovaginal itching, burning, and scarring. By far most often seen in postmenopausal women, the commonest lesion is the vestibular erosion. Dyspareunia and resorption of the labia minora and clitoral hood are prominent. Erosive vulvovaginal lichen planus is usually accompanied by oral lichen planus. Gingival and posterior buccal mucosal erosions and white striae and white hyperkeratosis of the tongue are typical lesions. Vulvar lichen planus is generally associated with erosive vaginal lichen planus. Vaginal lichen planus can result in synechiae that scar the vagina closed. Also, the inflammation of vaginal lichen planus results in vaginal secretions that irritate the vulva, compounding the discomfort of the vulvar lichen planus itself.

Like lichen sclerosus, lichen planus is treated primarily with ultrapotent topical corticosteroids and local supportive care. Except for mild lichen planus, however, improvement is usually partial, and additional therapies such as tacrolimus or pimecrolimus, methotrexate, hydroxychloroquine, etc. are often required to improve efficacy. Also like lichen sclerosus, there is an increased risk of SCC in poorly controlled diseases.

Elderly individuals experience remarkable life and health changes. Specific issues such as incontinence and genital diseases that occur most often in older patients should be investigated and treated, and the issues of depression and loss of body image addressed with compassion.

REFERENCES

1. Sutton KS, Pukall CF, Chamberlin S. Pain ratings, sensory thresholds, and psychosocial functioning in women with provoked vestibulodynia. *J Sex Marital Ther*. 2009;35:262–281.
2. Plante AF, Kamm MA. Life events in patients with vulvodynia. *BJOG*. 2008;115:509–514.
3. Desrochers G, Bergeron S, Khalifé S, et al. Fear avoidance and self-efficacy in relation to pain and sexual impairment in women with provoked vestibulodynia. *Clin J Pain*. 2009;25:520–527.
4. Lynch PJ. Vulvodynia as a somatoform disorder. *J Reprod Med*. 2008;53:390–396.
5. Sargeant HA, O'Callaghan F. Predictors of psychological well-being in a sample of women with vulval pain. *J Reprod Med*. 2009;54:109–116.
6. Ponte M, Klemperer E, Sahay A, et al. Effects of vulvodynia on quality of life. *J Am Acad Dermatol*. 2009;60:70–76.
7. Masheb RM, Kerns RD, Lozano C, et al. A randomized clinical trial for women with vulvodynia: cognitive-behavioral therapy vs. supportive psychotherapy. *Pain*. 2009;141:31–40.
8. Tuerk MJ, Koo J. A practical review and update on the management of pruritus sine materia. *Cutis*. 2008;82:187–194.
9. Yosipovitch G, Samuel LS. Neuropathic and psychogenic itch. *Dermatol Ther*. 2008;21:32–41.
10. Gupta MA. Somatization disorders in dermatology. *Int Rev Psychiatry*. 2006;18:41–47.
11. Shaw RJ, Dayal S, Good J, et al. Psychiatric medications for the treatment of pruritus. *Psychosomatic Med*. 2007;69:970–978.
12. Mutasim DF, Adams BB. The psychiatric profile of patients with psychogenic excoriation. *J Am Acad Dermatol*. 2009;61: 611–613.
13. Ehsani AH, Toosi S, Shahshahani MM, et al. Pscho-cutaneous disorders: an epidemiologic study. *J Eur Acad Dermatol Venereol*. 2009;23:945–947.
14. Lee CS. Delusions of parasitosis. *Dermatol Ther*. 2008;21:2–7.
15. Accordino RE, Engler D, Ginsburg IH, et al. Morgellons disease? *Dermatol Ther*. 2008;21:8–12.
16. Ravindran AV, da Silva TL, Richter MA, et al. Obsessive-compulsive spectrum disorders: a review of the evidence-based treatments. *Can J Psychiatry*. 2009;54:331–343.
17. Robles DT, Romm S, Combs H, et al. Delusional disorders in dermatology: a brief review. *Dermatol Online J*. 2008;14:2.
18. Chosak A, Marques L, Greenberg JL, et al. Body dysmorphic disorder and obsessive compulsive disorder: similarities, differences and the classification debate. *Expert Rev Neurother*. 2008;8:1209–1218.
19. Wylie KR, Eardley I. Penile size and the 'small penis syndrome'. *BJU Int*. 2007;99:1449–1455.
20. Tiggeman M, Martin Y, Churchett L. Beyond muscles: unexplored parts of men's body image. *J Health Psychol*. 2008;13:1163–1172.
21. Miklos JR, Moore RD. Labiaplasty of the labia minora: patients' indications for pursuing surgery. *J Sex Med*. 2008;5:1492–1495.
22. Pardo J, Solà V, Ricci P, et al. Laser labioplasty of the labia minora. *Int J Gynaecol Obstet*. 2006;93:38–43.
23. Goodman MP. Female cosmetic genital surgery. *Obstet Gynecol*. 2009;113:154–159.
24. Moyal-Barracco M, Lynch PJ. 2003 ISSVD terminology and classification of vulvodynia. A historical perspective. *J Reprod Med*. 2004;49:772–777.
25. Prevost N, English JC III. Case reports: red scrotal syndrome: a localized phenotypical expression of erythromelalgia. *J Drugs Dermatol*. 2007;6:935–936.
26. Koblenzer CS. Dermatitis artifacta. Clinical features and approaches to treatment. *Am J Clin Dermatol*. 2000;1:47–55.
27. Nielsen K, Jeppesen M, Simmelsgaard L, et al. Self-inflicted skin disease. A retrospective analysis of 57 patients with dermatitis artefacta seen in a dermatology department. *Acta Derm Venereol*. 2005;85:512–515.

28. Laukkanen E, Rissanen M-J, Honkalampi K, et al. The prevalence of self-cutting and other self-harm among 13- to 18-year-old Finnish adolescents. *Soc Psychiatry Psychiatr Epidemiol.* 2009;44:23–28.

29. Lotti T, Buggiani G, Prignano F. Prurigo nodularis and lichen simplex chronicus. *Dermatol Ther.* 2008;21:42–46.

30. Koblenzer CS. The emotional impact of chronic and disabling skin disease: a psychoanalytic perspective. *Dermatol Clin.* 2005;23:619–627.

31. Panconesi E, Hautmann G. Stress and emotions in skin disease. In: Koo J, Lee CS, eds. *Psychocutaneous Medicine.* New York: Marcel Decker, Inc; 2003:41–63.

32. Annesi-Maesano I, Beyer A, Marmouz P, et al. Do patients with skin allergies have higher levels of anxiety than patients with allergic respiratory diseases? Results of a large-scale cross-sectional study in a French population. *Br J Dermatol.* 2006;154:1128–1136.

33. Buske-Kirschbaum A, Ebrecht M, Kern S, et al. Personality characteristics in chronic and non-chronic allergic conditions. *Brain Behav Immun.* 2008;22:762–768.

34. Konuk N, Koca R, Atik L, et al. Psychopathology, depression and dissociative experiences in patients with lichen simplex chronicus. *Gen Hosp Psychiatry.* 2007;29:232–235.

35. Chida Y, Steptoe A, Hirakawa N, et al. The effects of psychological interventions on atopic dermatitis. A systematic review and meta-analysis. *Int Arch Allergy Immunol.* 2007;144:1–9.

36. Fortune DG, Richards HL, Griffiths CEM. Psychologic factors in psoriasis: consequences, mechanisms, and interventions. *Dermatol Clin.* 2005;23:681–694.

37. Janović S, Raznatović M, Marinković J, et al. Relevance of psychosomatic factors in psoriasis: a case control study. *Acta Derm Venereol.* 2009;89:364–368.

38. Karanikas E, Harsoulis F, Giouzepas I, et al. Neuroendocrine stimulatory test of hypothalamus-pituitary-adrenal axis in psoriasis and correlative implications with psychopathological and immune parameters. *J Dermatol.* 2009;36:35–44.

39. Nasreen S, Ahmed I, Effendi S. Frequency and magnitude of anxiety and depression in patients with psoriasis vulgaris. *J Coll Physicians Surg Pak.* 2008;18:397–400.

40. Behnam SM, Behnam SE, Koo JY. Smoking and psoriasis. *Skinmed.* 2005;4:174–176.

41. Bijan D, Laufer D, Filaković P, et al. Psoriasis, mental disorders and stress. *Coll Antropol.* 2009;33:889–892.

42. Janović S, Raznatović M, Marinković J, et al. Risk factors for psoriasis: a case-control study. *J Dermatol.* 2009;36:328–334.

43. Kirby B, Richards HL, Mason DL, et al. Alcohol consumption and psychological distress in patients with psoriasis. *Br J Dermatol.* 2008;158:138–140.

44. Masmoudi J, Maale I, Masmoudi A, et al. Alexithymia and psoriasis: a case-control study of 53 patients. *Encephale.* 2009;35:10–17.

45. Both H, Essink-Bot M-L, Busschbach J, et al. Critical review of generic and dermatology-specific health-related quality of life instruments. *J Invest Dermatol.* 2007;127:2726–2739.

46. Basra MK, Fenech R, Gatt RM, et al. The dermatology life quality index; a comprehensive review of validation data and clinical results. *Br J Dermatol.* 2008;159:997–1035.

47. Hong J, Koo B, Koo J. The psychosocial and occupational impact of chronic skin disease. *Dermatol Ther.* 2008;21:54–59.

48. Lynch PJ. Dermatologic disorders resulting in sexual dysfunction. In: Goldstein I, Meston CM, Davis SR, Traish AM, eds. *Women's Sexual Function and Dysfunction. Study, Diagnosis and Treatment.* London: Taylor & Francis; 2006:627–635.

49. Sampogna F, Gisondi P, Tabolli S, et al. Impairment of sexual life in patients with psoriasis. *Dermatology.* 2007;214:144–150.

50. Misery L, Finlay AY, Martin N, et al. Atopic dermatitis: Impact on quality of life of patients and their partners. *Dermatology.* 2007;215:123–129.

51. Grob JJ. Why are quality of life instruments not recognized as reference measures in therapeutic trials of chronic skin disorders? *J Invest Dermatol.* 2007;127:2299–2301.

52. Cury K, Valin N, Gozlan J, et al. Bipolar hypertrophic herpes: an unusual presentation of acyclovir-resistant herpes simplex type 2 in a HIV-infected patient. *Sex Transm Dis.* 2010;37(2):126–128. [Epub 2009, October 23.]

53. Van de Perre P, Segondy M, Foulongne V, et al. Herpes simplex virus and HIV-1: deciphering viral synergy. *Lancet Infect Dis.* 2008;8:490–497.

54. Zuckerman RA, Lucchetti A, Whittington WL, et al. HSV suppression reduces seminal HIV-1 levels in HIV-1/HSV-2 co-infected men who have sex with men. *AIDS.* 2009;23:479–483.

55. Lolis MS, González L, Cohen PJ, et al. Drug-resistant herpes simplex virus in HIV infected patients. *Acta Dermatovenerol Croat.* 2008;16:204–208.

56. Chaturvedi AK, Madeleine MM, Biggar RJ, et al. Risk of human papillomavirus-associated cancers among persons with AIDS. *J Natl Cancer Inst.* 2009;101:1120–1130.

57. Saiag P, Bauhofer A, Bouscarat F, et al. Imiquimod 5% cream for external genital or perianal warts in human immunodeficiency virus-positive patients treated with highly active antiretroviral therapy: an open-label, noncomparative study. *Br J Dermatol.* 2009;161:904–909.

58. Perna AG, Bell K, Rosen T. Localised genital Norwegian scabies in an AIDS patient. *Sex Transm Infect.* 2004;80:72–73.

59. Fife DJ, Waller JM, Jeffes EW, et al. Unraveling the paradoxes of HIV-associated psoriasis: a review of T-cell subsets and cytokine profiles. *Dermatol Online J.* 2007;1(13):4.

60. Menon K, Van Voorhees AS, Bebo BF Jr, et al. For the National Psoriasis Foundation. Psoriasis in patients with HIV infection: From the Medical Board of the National Psoriasis Foundation. *J Am Acad Dermatol.* 2010;62(2):291–299. [Epub 2009, July 29.]

61. Shetty K. Current role of thalidomide in HIV-positive patients with recurrent aphthous ulcerations. *Gen Dent.* 2007;55:537–542.

62. McCloskey JC, Metcalf C, French MA, et al. The frequency of high-grade intraepithelial neoplasia in anal/perianal warts is higher than previously recognized. *Int J STD AIDS.* 2007;18:538–542.

63. Potthoff A, Brockmeyer NH. HIV-associated Kaposi sarcoma: pathogenesis and therapy. *J Dtsch Dermatol Ges.* 2007;5:1091–1094.

64. Myers WA, Gottlieb AB, Mease P. Psoriasis and psoriatic arthritis: clinical features in disease mechanisms. *Clin Dermatol.* 2006;24:438–447.

SUGGESTED READINGS

Chaturvedi AK, Madeleine MM, Biggar RJ, et al. Risk of human papillomavirus-associated cancers among persons with AIDS. *J Natl Cancer Inst.* 2009;101:1120–1130.

Gormley RH, Kovarik CL. Dermatologic manifestations of HPV in HIV-infected individuals. *Curr HIV/AIDS Rep.* 2009;6: 130–138.

Guldbakke KK, Khachemoune A. Crusted scabies: a clinical review. *J Drugs Dermatol.* 2006;5:221–227.

Menon K, Van Voorhees AS, Bebo BF Jr, et al. For the National Psoriasis Foundation. Psoriasis in patients with HIV infection: from the Medical Board of the National Psoriasis Foundation. *J Am Acad Dermatol.* 2010;62(2):291–299. [Epub 2009, July 29.]

Patel RV, Weinberg JM. Psoriasis in the patient with human immunodeficiency virus, part 1: review of pathogenesis. *Cutis.* 2008;82:117–122.

Patel RV, Weinberg JM. Psoriasis in the patient with human immunodeficiency virus, part 2: review of treatment. *Cutis.* 2008;82:202–210.

Potthoff A, Brockmeyer NH. HIV-associated Kaposi sarcoma: pathogenesis and therapy. *J Dtsch Dermatol Ges.* 2007;5: 1091–1094.

A

Classification of Genital Disorders

PETER J. LYNCH

Two components are necessary in order to organize information regarding medical disorders: "nomenclature" (or "terminology") that encompasses the names and definitions of individual diseases and "classification" that represents the orderly arrangement of these diseases into specific groups, categories, or classes. Our preferred *terminology* for disorders of the genitalia has been provided for each disease in the main body of this book. The purpose of this Appendix is to provide information regarding *classification*. This information consists of four parts: the rationale for classification, approaches used for classification, our preferred classification, and alternative classifications.

THE RATIONALE FOR CLASSIFICATION

A random list of genital disorders would be of little use for clinicians involved in the care of patients with these problems. Even if one could identify the disease as, say, "atopic dermatitis," it would be cumbersome to locate additional information such as therapy or prognosis. You could start with the index, but would you start your search by looking under "atopic" or "dermatitis"? And knowing that "dermatitis" is a synonym for "eczema," would you also have to look under "eczema"? At the very least, this would be an inefficient approach. More importantly, what if you didn't recognize the condition and therefore could not put a name on it? In that rather common situation, there would be no way to find the disease in a textbook short of turning each page in an attempt to match a picture with the appearance of the patient's problem. Clearly this would be even more inefficient. Simply speaking, in a clinical setting, the goal of classification should be to assist in diagnosis and to make the retrieval of disease information easier and quicker.

APPROACHES USED FOR CLASSIFICATION

Many systems are available for classification. For instance, diseases could be listed alphabetically, but this would leave you with the same inefficiencies noted above. Alternatively, diseases could be organized and grouped by etiology or pathogenesis into categories such as "infections," "malignancies," or "endocrinopathies." But, what if you didn't know whether the disease was an infection, or a malignancy, or an endocrinopathy? And, what if the etiology was controversial or even unknown? This approach may be intellectually satisfying for the author, and it is certainly used in many textbooks but is much less satisfactory for the clinician. A better approach for the clinician would be to classify the disorders by the region of the skin involved. You would then find categories such as clitoral, scrotal, and penile diseases. This would help you to identify an unknown disorder, but it would lead to long lists of diseases within each category and to considerable redundancy since lichen planus, for instance, would have to be listed under almost every region.

OUR PREFERRED APPROACH FOR CLASSIFICATION

We believe that it is most sensible to classify genital disorders (actually, all dermatologic conditions) on the basis of clinical morphology. This approach groups the diseases on the basis of shared similarities in appearance. So, once you have described the disease using standard dermatologic nomenclature, you can go directly to a single group containing a small number of conditions. The number of diseases contained within each group would be determined by the frequency with which they are encountered and by their relative importance. The conditions listed in a given group would then constitute one's list of differential diagnoses. Then, from that list, you could quickly pick the top two or three candidates. After a few moments of additional reading on those most likely diagnoses, you would likely find a final candidate that would represent your most probable single diagnosis. In addition to offering usefulness and efficiency, this approach to classification would even allow one to make a diagnosis of a disease that had never previously been encountered. A classification based on this principle and modified for genital diseases is used for the diagnostic algorithm found in Chapter 2. Additional information regarding the rationale and application of this morphologic approach to classification can be found in two general dermatology textbooks (1,2).

ALTERNATIVE CLASSIFICATIONS

The International Society for the Study of Vulvovaginal Disease (ISSVD) is an organization that has purposefully recruited members from various medical specialties and from various countries. While English is the official language of the ISSVD, many of the members have been educated using medical terminology and classifications that are parochial to a specific specialty and/or their own native language. The founding members of the ISSVD recognized that these disparate systems of nomenclature and classification would cause significant problems in communication. Thus, a major goal of the society was to develop and promulgate an international standardized nomenclature and classification system for vulvar disease. The guiding principles that were used to achieve this goal included: (1) acceptability to members from all specialties; (2) acceptability to members from all countries regardless of the language used therein; (3) sufficient simplicity and conciseness for daily clinical use; and (4) sufficient inclusiveness and flexibility in structure so as not to require frequent revision.

The ISSVD began their efforts by looking at the two single problems of vulvodynia and squamous intraepithelial neoplasia. More recently, the society has tackled the larger and more complex problem of classifying the vulvar dermatoses. In our view, the ISSVD has been remarkably successful in their venture. We are, of course, aware that the three classifications currently approved and used by the ISSVD were meant to apply only to vulvar disease, but we believe that they work equally well for male genital disorders. These classifications, with minor editorial revision, are presented in the three sections that follow.

ISSVD CLASSIFICATION OF VULVODYNIA (2003)

Pain involving the vulva occurs in two major settings: pain related to a specific, identifiable disease and pain that is ostensibly idiopathic. The ISSVD elected not to deal with pain falling into the first category and, instead, focused on the very controversial subject of idiopathic vulvar pain. Historically, this type of pain was termed "the burning vulva syndrome" and subsequently, "vulvar dysesthesia." The term "vulvodynia," as popularized by the ISSVD has now become the standard terminology for idiopathic vulvar pain. Initially "vestibulitis" was identified as a subset of vulvodynia and was used for women who appeared to have an abnormal degree of vestibular redness, histologic inflammation, and accompanying entrance dyspareunia. It has since been determined that, for patients with this diagnosis, the degree of redness falls within the normal spectrum of vestibular color and that there is no abnormal inflammation present. Accordingly,

TABLE A.1 ISSVD classification of vulvar pain (2003)

Vulvar pain related to a specific disorder
    Infections (candidiasis, herpes, etc.)
    Inflammatory disorders (lichen planus, immunobullous diseases)
    Neoplasms (Paget disease, squamous cell carcinoma, etc.)
    Neuropathies (postherpetic neuralgia, pudendal nerve neuralgia, etc.)
Vulvodynia
    Generalized idiopathic vulvar pain
        Provoked (sexual, nonsexual, or both)
        Unprovoked
        Mixed (provoked and unprovoked)
    Localized idiopathic vulvar pain (vestibulodynia, clitorodynia, etc.)
        Provoked (sexual, nonsexual, or both)
        Unprovoked
        Mixed (provoked and unprovoked)

the term "vestibulitis" has been replaced by "vestibulodynia" and this condition is now subsumed into the general category of vulvodynia (Table A.1). Note that this table has been very slightly edited and that it does not contain the definitions and notes that were found in the original publication (3).

ISSVD CLASSIFICATION OF SQUAMOUS CELL VULVAR INTRAEPITHELIAL NEOPLASIA (2004)

In 1986, based on analogy with cervical intraepithelial neoplasia (CIN), the ISSVD classified vulvar intraepithelial neoplasia (VIN) into the three categories of VIN 1, VIN 2, and VIN 3. Over the next 15 years, it became apparent that there were several major differences between CIN and VIN. First, it was found that VIN 1, unlike CIN 1, was not an obligate precursor to the development of invasive squamous cell carcinoma. Second, it was determined that VIN has two categories of etiology (viral and nonviral) compared to CIN that has only one (viral). Third, the course of CIN 1 through CIN 3 is known to be steadily progressive, whereas the course of VIN is variable depending on whether the pathogenesis is viral or nonviral. With these observations in mind, the ISSVD approved a new classification that (1) deleted VIN 1 (indicating that this histologic appearance was really only HPV viral effect); (2) combined VIN 2 and VIN 3 into a single category (because of poor ability to dependably

TABLE A.2 ISSVD classification of vulvar squamous cell intraepithelial neoplasia (2004)

VIN, usual (HPV viral) type
 VIN, warty type
 VIN, basaloid type
 VIN, mixed (warty/basaloid) type
VIN, differentiated (nonviral) type

TABLE A.3 ISSVD classification of the vulvar dermatoses: pathologic subsets and their clinical correlates

Spongiotic pattern
 Atopic dermatitis
 Allergic contact dermatitis
 Irritant contact dermatitis
Acanthotic pattern (formerly, squamous cell hyperplasia, and psoriasiform dermatitis)
 Psoriasis
 Lichen simplex chronicus
  Primary (idiopathic)
  Secondary (superimposed on lichen sclerosus, lichen planus, or other vulvar disease)
Lichenoid pattern
 Lichen sclerosus
 Lichen planus
Dermal homogenization/sclerosis pattern
 Lichen sclerosus
Vesiculobullous pattern
 Pemphigoid, cicatricial type
 Linear immunoglobulin A disease
Acantholytic pattern
 Hailey–Hailey disease
 Darier disease
 Papular genitocrural acantholysis
Granulomatous pattern
 Crohn disease
 Melkersson–Rosenthal syndrome
Vasculopathic pattern
 Aphthous ulcers
 Behçet disease
 Plasma cell vulvitis

identify these two grades of dysplasia separately); and (3) identified and named the two kinds of VIN based on their different pathogenesis and prognosis (Table A.2). Note that this table has been very slightly edited and that it lacks the notes that were included in the original publication (4).

ISSVD CLASSIFICATION OF VULVAR DERMATOSES (2006)

The ISSVD previously classified the conditions now called vulvar dermatoses as "nonneoplastic epithelial disorders." However, the society eventually concluded that not all of the disorders found in this classification were "epithelial" in nature and that at some time in the future, it might be desirable to include one or more neoplastic conditions. With this in mind, a new classification committee was appointed. The first action of the committee was to change the title to the much more inclusive "vulvar dermatoses." However, beyond that step there was great controversy over the manner in which diseases within the vulvar dermatoses would be classified. Some simply wanted to list all of the dermatologic diseases that involve the vulva, whereas others wanted a classification based on clinical morphology. Unfortunately, consensus could not be reached for either approach.

Consideration of three points led to an alternative methodology of classification. First, if the clinician could correctly identify the disease, there would be no need for a new classification because the disease could be looked up in any standard dermatology textbook. Second, if the clinician could not identify the disease, a biopsy would be undertaken and the pathologist would then provide the correct diagnosis. And again, the disease could be easily looked up. Third, if the pathologist could not provide a specific diagnosis, a descriptive report of a general histologic pattern would be rendered. In that situation, the clinician would have to use clinicopathologic correlation to come up with the single most likely diagnosis.

The committee concluded that any new classification should be designed to assist the clinician in making this clinicopathologic correlation. Accordingly, the committee identified the eight most common general histologic patterns and then listed within each pattern the two or three most common and important diseases for which that histology would be found on biopsy. Then, when a clinician received a biopsy report that contained only a histologic description rather than a specific diagnosis, it would be easy to go to the classification, find the histologic pattern and see which diseases make up the differential diagnoses for that pattern. A minimal amount of textbook reading should then allow clinicopathologic correlation and establishment of the single most likely diagnosis. Note that the classification as found in Table A.3 has been very slightly modified for simplicity and does not contain the notes that were included in the original publication (5).

REFERENCES

1. Lynch PJ. *Dermatology.* 3rd ed. Baltimore: Williams & Wilkins; 1994:89–105.

2. Lynch PJ. Problem oriented diagnosis. In: Sams WM Jr, Lynch PJ, eds. *Principles and Practice of Dermatology.* 2nd ed. New York: Churchill Livingstone; 1996:33–44.

3. Moyal-Barracco M, Lynch PJ. 2003 ISSVD terminology and classification of vulvodynia: a historical perspective. *J Reprod Med.* 2004;49:772–777.

4. Sideri M, Jones RW, Wilkinson EJ, et al. Squamous vulvar intraepithelial neoplasia. 2004 modified terminology, ISSVD Vulvar Oncology Subcommittee. *J Reprod Med.* 2005;50:807–810.

5. Lynch PJ, Moyal-Barracco M, Bogliatto F, et al. 2006 ISSVD classification of vulvar dermatoses: pathological subsets and their clinical correlates. *J Reprod Med.* 2007;52:3–9.

Patient Education Handouts

LIBBY EDWARDS

ATROPHIC VAGINA AND ATROPHIC VAGINITIS

Estrogen is a hormone that maintains the elastic, moist, and supple skin of the vulva and vagina. The ovaries produce estrogen, so after woman goes through menopause or her ovaries are surgically removed, estrogen levels decline, and the vaginal skin becomes thin, dry, and fragile. This is called vaginal atrophy (meaning thin). Some women remain comfortable although often they need to use a lubricant, but others experience dryness, irritation, rawness, painful sexual activity, and burning of the opening to the vagina. This is a common and normal—but uncomfortable—experience for women as they age. Overweight women and women who are sexually active are often less troubled by thinning from low estrogen.

Fortunately, the treatment of an atrophic vagina and atrophic vaginitis is easy and extremely effective. Estrogen can be used in the vagina, with minimal effects to the body as a whole, or estrogen can be taken orally or by patch, if other symptoms of low estrogen are a problem, such as hot flashes, bone loss, or psychologic symptoms. When estrogen is given by pill or patch, care must be taken to monitor for the increased risk of breast cancer, heart attack, and stroke. This risk usually depends upon the individual woman and her family history for these problems.

Estrogen cream is a treatment that has been used for many years. Either conjugated equine estrogen cream (Premarin) can be inserted three times a week with an applicator or estradiol (Estrace) cream can be used in the same way, which is slightly less irritating. For minor symptoms, these creams can be applied inside the vagina with a finger, so that even less estrogen cream is used. Although estrogen cream inserted in the vagina is absorbed into the blood stream to a small degree, when used as directed, this exposes the body to far, far less hormone than pills by mouth or patch. Even most cancer doctors allow their breast cancer patients to use this. Alternatives include a small estradiol tablet (Vagifem) inserted into the vagina about three nights a week. Finally, a flexible ring containing estradiol (ESTring) can be inserted into the vagina, where the hormone is released gradually over 3 months, when it is replaced. Almost no estrogen from the ring is absorbed into the rest of the body. The tablet and ring are less messy, but conjugated equine estrogen cream is the least expensive alternative.

After only a week or two of estrogen, most women notice a significant increase in vaginal moisture, which can be mistaken for a discharge from infection, rather than a return of normal vaginal secretions. The frequency of use of the local estrogen can be adjusted to that needed to remain comfortable. Sometimes, the estrogen can be stopped altogether when the patient is comfortable. Most of the time, however, without this added estrogen, the vaginal skin again thins, dries, and becomes uncomfortable.

CANDIDA (YEAST) VAGINITIS

Yeast infections are extremely common occurrences. These arise almost entirely between the ages of puberty and menopause, but postmenopausal women who use vaginal or systemic estrogen also have vaginal yeast infections. Babies and elderly incontinent adults sometimes experience yeast of the vulva, but generally do not have vaginal yeast. Factors that increase the chance of developing a yeast infection include diabetes, sexual activity, and the use of antibiotics, birth control pills, and cortisones or other medications that lower the immune system. Diet is not important in causing or curing a yeast infection, except for women with diabetes that is poorly controlled.

Yeast usually is not a sexually transmitted disease. Yeast lives normally in the intestines and, often, in the vagina. So any irritation or factor such as antibiotic or cortisone use can allow the yeast to become an infection.

Most yeast infections are caused by a yeast called *Candida albicans*. The overwhelming symptom of a *C. albicans* infection is itching. Sometimes, the scratching and rubbing can cause irritation, burning, and pain with intercourse. Less often, yeast infections are caused by different but related yeasts, especially *Candida glabrata*, or, *Candida parapsilosis*, *Candida krusei*, and *Saccharomyces cerevisae*. Most of the time, a non-*albicans Candida* infection causes no symptoms or injury to the body, so treatment is unnecessary. However, when these yeasts do cause symptoms, the symptoms are more often irritation and burning rather than itching.

In the past, some health care providers believed that *C. albicans* caused depression, bloating, constipation, fatigue, and headaches. Now we know that this is not true.

Vaginal yeast infections caused by *Candida albicans* are easily treated with any of several types of medication. Fluconazole tablets by mouth are effective, generally requiring only one tablet to cure an infection. Any prescription or over-the-counter "azole" cream or vaginal suppository is equally beneficial; these include miconazole, clotrimazole, terconazole, tioconazole, and butconazole. Any of these medications regularly cure a yeast infection, but some women experience frequent recurrences. Frequent recurrences are extremely annoying, but not dangerous, and they are not generally a sign of significant, silent underlying illness such as diabetes or an immune problem. Most often, using regular doses of a yeast medication, such as a fluconazole tablet once a week, or an "azole" cream or vaginal suppository two to three times a week prevents the return of yeast. Often, after several months, the medication can be stopped successfully. There is no good scientific evidence that acidophilus, yogurt, probiotics, lactobacilli, or diet are useful in preventing or curing a yeast infection.

Chronic pain with sexual activity, as well as burning, irritation, and rawness are common complaints of many women. Many women are mistakenly diagnosed with yeast as the cause of these symptoms, and, not surprisingly, yeast treatment either is unhelpful, or only partly and briefly improves the symptoms. These women should undergo a formal culture rather than only an examination of vaginal secretions under the microscope. Long-standing pain with sexual activity is not usually due to yeast infections, but more often caused by a skin condition, or vulvodynia. Vulvodynia consists of burning and rawness because of pelvic floor muscle abnormalities and neuropathic pain/neuralgia/neuritis. Or, in postmenpausal women, low estrogen causes these symptoms. Women with itching that does not clear with yeast medications are more likely to have eczema than a yeast infection.

Infections caused by non-*albicans Candida* often are much more difficult to clear, so it is fortunate that most of these infections are unimportant and do not require therapy. Fluconazle and "azole" creams and suppositories very often do not cure these infections. Rather, boric acid capsules inserted into the vagina, nystatin ointment or vaginal tablets, or flucytosine cream are used more successfully.

Yeast can be annoying and uncomfortable, but it is a common infection in women that should not be a cause of concern for overall health.

DESQUAMATIVE INFLAMMATORY VAGINITIS

Desquamative inflammatory vaginitis (DIV) is a cause of vulvovaginal irritation and discharge. This is a relatively common problem, but there is little information on the causes of DIV. It is not dangerous in any way, and it is not contagious.

DIV sometimes only causes a yellow discharge, but at other times causes redness and irritation of the opening of the vagina. Pain with sexual activity can be another symptom. This happens to both young and older women.

Although DIV can feel like a vaginal infection, this is not an infection. The redness and discharge result from irritation of the vaginal walls. The reason for this irritation is not known, but many people believe this irritation is caused by an overactive immune system. The immune system, the part of the body that fights off infection, becomes overactive and mistakenly attacks the vaginal skin or normal bacterial in the vagina.

This diagnosis is made by the presence of a discharge that, under the microscope, shows inflammation (increased white blood cells), when there is no infection on vaginal cultures. Occasionally, a culture shows bacteria called group B streptococcus, but group B strep is normal in many women, and it is unrelated to a strep throat or "flesh-eating strep."

The treatment is either cortisone or clindamycin cream or suppository inserted into the vagina at bedtime. Cortisone is very effective for inflammation, and although clindamycin cream is an antibiotic, it also is useful for inflammation even in the absence of infection. For example, clindamycin is used for acne, another inflammatory skin problem that is not caused by an infection.

While occasionally, this treatment cures DIV, more often, a cortisone or clindamycin has to be used either off and on or once or twice a week to control the symptoms of DIV.

HIDRADENITIS SUPPURATIVA

Hidradenitis suppuratuva (HS) is a skin condition that consists of tender nodules, which sometimes drain, and are located mostly in the underarm area and groin. Although these appear to be infectious boils, this is not an infection, but actually is acne of the underarm and genital area.

Like acne, HS most often begins after puberty. It occurs in men and women and is often more severe in men. It is more common in people of African descent as well. People with HS experience painful, deep, firm areas that come to the surface as red nodules. These usually open and drain. They sometimes heal, or, at other times, they continue to drain, or recur in the same spot. Scarring is common.

HS does not spread outside the underarm area or the genital area. However, the genital area occasionally includes not only the vulva and scrotum, but also the buttocks, upper thighs, and lower abdomen, so that the occasional patient experiences rather widespread genital nodules.

The first-line treatment of HS is the same as that for cystic acne. Some antibiotics by mouth improve inflammation, even though HS is not an infection. Doxycycline, minocycline, clindamycin, and trimthoprim-sulfamethoxyzole are the most often used. Because this is not a curable infection, the antibiotics must be used continuously, and requires a month for any improvement, and about three months for maximal improvement. Topical medications normally used for acne are too irritating to use in the sensitive underarm and groin areas.

For people who have an occasional painful nodule, a few drops of cortisone injected into the nodule in the office can shrink it very quickly without a worry of exposing the whole body to a cortisone. Unfortunately, cortisone creams and ointments are not significantly useful and may worsen the overall HS.

For patients who are not controlled with long-term antibiotics and local injections, either individual nonhealing nodules or a whole affected area can be surgically removed. Underarm skin is loose and the area is small, so underarm HS is usually cured by surgery. But, in the genital area, the areas of involvement can be too large to entirely take out although, the worst areas can be removed.

Most recently, several medications developed for rheumatoid arthritis and psoriasis have been found effective for HS. These are etanercept (Enbrel), adalimumab (Humira), and infliximab (Remicaid). These are extraordinarily expensive and sometimes denied for this condition by insurance companies.

Although HS is a chronic skin problem, careful therapies often improve symptoms enormously.

LICHEN PLANUS

Lichen planus is a common skin condition that sometimes affects the genital skin. This is especially common on the vulva and in the vagina of older women who have gone through menopause. However, this occasionally affects men, most often the head of the penis of uncircumcised men. Lichen planus can affect rectal skin of both men and women. This skin problem does not affect the genital area of children. Patients with lichen planus of genital skin usually have lichen planus of the mouth also, especially the insides of the cheeks, or sometimes on the gums, but other areas of the skin are generally not affected.

Lichen planus usually looks like red patches, but sometimes there is white skin, or white streaks. The skin can be itchy, but usually there is soreness and burning as well. Sexual activity is often painful or may be impossible. Untreated lichen planus eventually can cause scarring, and, occasionally, narrowing of the opening to the vagina in women. In men, the foreskin can scar to the head of the penis.

Lichen planus is caused by an overactive immune system. The immune system, the part of the body that fights off infection, becomes overactive and attacks the skin by mistake. Why this happens is not known.

Lichen planus improves with treatment. For men, circumcision is the best treatment. For those who do not clear with circumcision, or who are already circumcised, remaining lichen planus is treated by a very strong topical corticosteroid, also called a cortisone, or a steroid (but not the same kind of steroid as used illegally by some athletes).

Women require not only a very strong corticosteroid, but also attention to any vaginal infection; avoidance of irritating products such as creams, panty-liners, and soaps; and local replacement of estrogen when low estrogen has thinned the vaginal skin.

The corticosteroid (most often used is clobetasol ointment) is applied very, very sparingly once or twice a day. If the skin feels greasy after medication is applied, too much is being used. This is very safe medication when used in the correct amount and for the correct length of time. When too much medication is used, or when medication is used for too long, the skin can thin and become irritated and red. Therefore, a health care provider should examine the area monthly initially. The itching and irritation usually improve within a few days. Mild lichen planus sometimes clears altogether, whereas severe lichen planus may only improve a moderate amount.

Although lichen planus usually improves with a corticosteroid, it is not cured. Therefore, if the medication is stopped, itching and irritation reappear. Scarring continues, sometimes even before itching or irritation returns. At times, the corticosteroid ointment does not improve the skin enough, so some patients need additional medications by mouth or injection to become comfortable. These medications include methotrexate, mycophenylate mofetil, azathioprine, cyclosporine, griseofulvin, hydroxychloroquine, cyclophosphamide, etanercept, and adalimumab. There is no good research for any treatments of genital lichen planus, but experience has shown that these are sometimes very useful.

Because lichen planus often affects the inside of the vagina, most women need to use a corticosteroid inside the vagina. Corticosteroids can be used in the vagina by inserting a rectal hydrocortisone suppository into the vagina at bedtime (there are no corticosteroids designed for the vagina.) Because women with lichen planus are usually postmenopausal, they have thinning of the vagina due to low estrogen as well as lichen planus. Therefore, postmenopausal women with lichen planus of the vulva and vagina should use an estrogen cream, tablet, or ring inserted into the vagina. Or, estrogen replacement by oral medication or patch are other alternatives.

Lichen planus is not cured with treatment. However, it improves. Most patients become comfortable, although some require time and trying several medications before the best combination of therapy is discovered. Patients should be followed carefully to evaluate for scarring and side effects to medications. Lichen planus of genital skin increases the risk of skin cancer of this area. Although skin cancers are uncommon, this is another reason that the area should be evaluated at least twice a year, even when doing well.

LICHEN SCLEROSUS

Lichen sclerosus (sometimes called lichen sclerosus et atrophicus or LS&A) is a skin condition that is most common on the vulva of older women who have gone through menopause. However, lichen sclerosus sometimes affects girls before puberty as well as young adult women, and the penis of uncircumcised males. In females, lichen sclerosus can affect rectal skin also. Only rarely does lichen sclerosus affect skin outside the genitalia, and this is usually the back, chest, or abdomen. Lichen sclerosus almost never appears on the face or hands.

The causes of lichen sclerosus are not completely understood, but a main cause is an overactive immune system. The immune system, that part of the body that fights off infection, becomes overactive and attacks the skin by mistake. Why this happens is not known.

Lichen sclerosus typically appears as white skin that is very itchy. The skin is also fragile, so that rubbing and scratching can cause breaks, cracks, and bruises, which then hurt. Sexual activity is often painful or may be impossible. Untreated lichen sclerosus eventually can cause scarring, and, occasionally, narrowing of the opening of the vagina in women. In boys and men, the foreskin can scar to the head of the penis. Also, untreated lichen sclerosus is associated with skin cancer of the vulva in about 1 out of 30 women, and there is an increased risk of skin cancer of the penis with untreated lichen sclerosus as well. Well-controlled lichen sclerosus is at much less risk.

Lichen sclerosus usually improves very quickly with treatment. For boys and men, circumcision usually cures this disease. Women require not only a very strong corticosteroid, but also attention to any vaginal infection, low estrogen, or things that irritate the area.

Irritating creams, unnecessary medications, soaps, and overwashing should be avoided. Washing should be limited to once a day with clear water only. Some irritants, such as sweat in overweight people and urine in incontinent people, can be hard to avoid. Otherwise, the most common irritant is rubbing and scratching. Many people can keep from scratching during the day, but much rubbing and scratching occur during normal sleeping hours, when people do not realize they are scratching. Although there are no effective anti-itch pills, a medication that produces a very deep sleep can stop nighttime scratching and allow the skin to heal.

Then, for all girls and women, and for men either awaiting circumcision or who have not cleared adequately, the best treatment is a very strong topical corticosteroid ointment, also called cortisone, or steroid (but not the same kind of steroid as used illegally by some athletes). The corticosteroid (most often used is clobetasol ointment) is applied very, very sparingly once or twice a day to start. If the skin feels greasy after medication is applied, too much is being used. This is very safe medication when used in the correct amounts and for the correct length of time. When too much medication is used, or when medication is used for too long, the skin can thin and become irritated and red. Therefore, a health care provider should examine the area monthly while medication is being used daily. The itching and irritation usually improve within a few days. With ongoing use of the corticosteroid, the color and strength of the skin gradually return to normal.

Lichen sclerosus usually is well controlled with a corticosteroid, but it is not cured. Therefore, if the medication is stopped, itching and irritation reappear. Scarring continues, sometimes even before itching or irritation return. Daily use of the corticosteroid usually is needed for 2 to 4 months for the normal color and strength to return. When the skin is controlled, either application of the strong corticosteroid ointment is decreased to about once a day, three days a week, or a milder corticosteroid ointment is used daily.

Occasionally, patients do not improve enough with the corticosteroid ointment. These patients can be treated with the application of tacrolimus (Protopic) or pimecrolimus (Elidel) twice a day. These medications do not cause thinning of the skin, but they are often irritating. Also, there are concerns about long-term use possibly increasing the risk of skin cancer in this skin.

Occasionally, lichen sclerosus is well controlled with treatment, but symptoms of irritation continue. This can result from irritation from medications or overwashing, an infection that is unrecognized, low estrogen, or scarring. Also, infrequently, women experience a pain or irritation syndrome (called vulvodynia) triggered by the lichen sclerosus, but different and good therapies in the event of this uncommon occurrence are available.

Nearly all patients do extremely well following treatment for lichen sclerosus. Even when lichen sclerosus is completely controlled, however, patients should be followed every 6 months to be sure the disease remains controlled, to detect side effects of the medication, and to examine for very early skin cancers.

GENITAL LICHEN SIMPLEX CHRONICUS
(ECZEMA, NEURODERMATITIS, AND DERMATITIS)

Lichen simplex chronicus (LSC), or eczema, is a common skin condition that is very itchy. Although not dangerous in any way, the itching, and sometimes the pain from rubbing and scratching, can be miserable. Eczema/LSC of the genital area most often affects the scrotum of men, the vulva of women, or the rectal skin of both. Many people with eczema/LSC have had sensitive skin or eczema/LSC on other areas of the skin at some point, and many have a tendency toward allergies, especially hay fever or asthma.

The skin usually appears red or dark, and thick from rubbing and scratching, sometimes with sores from scratching.

The cause of eczema/LSC is not entirely clear. However, eczema/LSC starts with irritation that triggers itching. Often, at the office visit with the health care provider, the original infection or other initial cause of irritation is no longer present. Common triggers include a yeast or fungus infection, an irritating medication, moisturizer or lubricant, a wet bathing suit, anxiety or depression, overwashing, panty liners, sweat, heat, urine, contraceptive jelly, irritating condom, or any other activity or substance that can irritate the skin and start the itching.

Although rubbing and scratching often feel good at first, rubbing irritates the skin and ultimately makes itching even worse, so that there is more scratching, then more itching, then more scratching. This is called the "itch–scratch cycle."

Treatment is very effective and requires clearing infection and avoiding irritants as well as using medication. In addition to the elimination of creams, unnecessary medications, soaps, overwashing, etc., the irritation of rubbing and scratching must be stopped. Many people can keep from scratching during the day, but much rubbing and scratching occur during normal sleeping hours, when people do not realize they are scratching. Although there are no effective anti-itch pills, a medication that produces a very deep sleep can stop nighttime scratching and help to break the itch–scratch cycle. Besides scratching, the most common things that irritate are overwashing, soaps, and creams. Therefore, soap should be avoided, and washing should be limited to once a day with clear water only. Some irritants, such as sweat in overweight people and urine in incontinent people, can be hard to avoid.

Then, eczema/LSC usually improves very quickly with a very strong or ultrapotent topical corticosteroid ointment, also called cortisone, or steroid (but not the same kind of steroid as those illegally used by some athletes). The corticosteroid is applied very sparingly once or twice a day to start. This is very safe medication when used in the correct amounts and for the correct length of time. A small pea-sized amount usually covers the entire genital area. The use of too much medication or for too long can cause overthinning of the skin, so that a check of the skin by a health care provider after a month of treatment is generally required.

Stopping the medication as soon itching and irritation improve is a common mistake, because eczema/LSC recurs quickly if the skin has not yet returned to normal. Once itching is controlled and the skin has lost its redness and thickness, the corticosteroid should be gradually used less and less before being stopped. Otherwise, when the corticosteroid is stopped abruptly and too soon, the itching and itch–scratch cycle return.

After the corticosteroid has been discontinued, a patient with LSC/eczema remains at risk for recurrence of itching, because the genital skin is an area with ongoing irritation from normal sweat, friction, sexual activity, etc. A patient with eczema/LSC should not be surprised when itching returns, but immediate treatment can prevent the return of the itch–scratch cycle and LSC/eczema.

PHYSIOLOGIC VAGINAL SECRETIONS (PHYSIOLOGIC VAGINAL DISCHARGE)

Vaginal secretions, or discharge, are a normal part of vaginal health. A physiologic discharge is a normal discharge, except that it is uncomfortably heavy. Normal vaginal secretions are made mainly of mucous, old skin cells from the lining of the vagina, and many kinds of normal bacteria. The amount of vaginal secretions changes with hormone levels and with factors that are not well understood. The amount, color, and odor can suddenly change, even when there is no infection or disease causing these changes. Abundant normal vaginal secretions can be either caused by infection or disease, or they can be a sign of a healthy vagina. To make a diagnosis of physiologic discharge, the health care provider must find no abnormalities in vaginal secretions examined under a microscope, as well as no infection on a culture sent to the laboratory. Treatment for infection either does not clear the discharge or there is partial or temporary improvement only.

However, large amounts of vaginal secretions are a common complaint by women who do not like the messy, uncomfortable, constant wetness, and this explains the large number of panty liners in stores. Although panty liners are sometimes irritating, most women find this a partially acceptable answer for controlling the effects of a vaginal discharge. Some women, once they are diagnosed with a physiologic discharge rather than an infection, are less bothered because they know that this is not a medical problem.

Although douching is never needed for vaginal health, an occasional patient may find a weak vinegar and water douche flushes excess discharge and allows for a period of discharge-free time. A half-teaspoon vinegar in a pint of warm water is an acceptable fragrance- and preservative-free as well as inexpensive mixture.

As mysteriously as a heavy physiologic discharge can appear, it can just as mysteriously disappear. Unfortunately, there are no medications, creams, or pills that eliminate a physiologic discharge.

VULVAR CARE

Despite all of the products available for vulvar care, the vulva needs no special cleaning or medications. Many women believe that scrupulous washing prevents infections and skin disease, but, actually, overwashing with soap produces more irritation than poor hygiene. Panty liners help to prevent the wet feeling from vaginal secretions, but many have fragrances, deodorants, or additives that cause irritation or allergy. Similarly, some wipes have irritating preservatives and fragrances, yet have no health benefit over toilet paper. Douching is not needed for vaginal health, and commercial douches contain scents, preservatives, deodorants, etc., which sometimes irritate the skin. Although these products are not needed, most women do not experience problems with their use. But when vulvovaginal itching, irritation, or pain occurs, these should be avoided.

Many health care providers believe that only white cotton underwear should be worn. However, there is no evidence that colored fabric or synthetic fabric cause skin problems or infection. Fabric softeners and detergents are not the cause of vulvovaginal problems unless other areas of skin covered by clothing is affected as well.

Diet does not play a role in the development of infection, to include yeast, so avoidance of yeast breads or sugars is not useful, and there is no convincing evidence that yogurt or acidophilus helps to prevent yeast.

Guidelines for vulvar care to reduce irritation include:

Wash only once a day, with clear water. Avoid soap when irritated. Pat dry, do not use a hairdryer

Avoid panty liners, especially Always brand

Use tampons if tolerated rather than pads

Douching is not needed and does not promote vaginal health; if necessary for psychologic reasons, avoid commercial douches with additives, and use a homemade recipe of a half teaspoon of vinegar per cup of water

Avoid KY products as lubricants; instead, use vegetable oil, olive oil, almond oil, or commercial products such as SlipperyStuff (slipperystuff.com) or Astroglide

Wear loose fitting clothing if irritated

VULVODYNIA/VESTIBULODYNIA/VESTIBULITIS

Vulvodynia is defined as vulvovaginal irritation, burning, painful sex, stinging, soreness, or pain that has been present for at least 6 months, when there is no infection or skin disease causing the discomfort. Vestibulodynia, previously called vulvar vestibulitis, refers to vulvodynia that is located only at the opening of the vagina. Vulvodynia is a very common problem with up to one woman in six experiencing unexplained irritation at some point in her life.

Vulvodynia is a symptom most often caused by several problems occurring at the same time. First is abnormalities of the pelvic floor muscles, those muscles a person uses to stop urinating mid-stream. These muscles are supposed to be very relaxed, but strong. However, some women have tenseness and irritability of these muscles, although the muscles are overall weak. An abnormal pelvic floor often leads to symptoms of constipation, diarrhea, cramping, frequent urination, burning with urination, or urine leakage with coughing or sneezing.

Second is nerve pain (also called neuropathic pain, neuritis, or neuralgia). People with pelvic floor abnormalities are at risk for the development of neuropathic pain, which is often set off by any irritation or injury, such as a vaginal infection, delivery of a baby, etc. How pelvic floor abnormalities cause neuropathic pain is not understood.

Thirdly anxiety and depression are always factors in vulvar and vaginal pain, as is the understandable fear of painful sexual activity in women who want to be sexually active. Depression regularly worsens pain of any kind, and anxiety increases the tenseness of the pelvic floor muscles and intensifies pain.

Vulvodynia is never associated with dangerous illness. Vulvodynia is not caused by sexually transmitted diseases, cancer, diabetes, or other dangerous conditions. Vulvodynia is not associated with infertility. However, the effects of the pain of vulvodynia seriously interfere with normal activities of daily life, and disrupt enjoyment of life and relationships.

There is no cure for vulvodynia, but there are treatments that make the discomfort much better. The goal for the treatment of vulvodynia is to relieve discomfort so that daily activities, including sexual activity, exercise, and sitting, are comfortable.

Treatment begins with the avoidance of irritation. These include irritating medications, moisturizers and some lubricants, overwashing, panty liners, contraceptive jelly, irritating condom, or any other activity or substance that can irritate the skin. Women with low estrogen due to menopause, breastfeeding, or some hormonal contraceptives should be given estrogen replacement or causes of low estrogen corrected.

A first-line therapy for vulvodynia targets pelvic floor muscle abnormalities with a pelvic floor evaluation and physical therapy. This strengthens the pelvic floor muscles while retraining them to relax.

Also important are medications for neuropathic pain. These include tricyclic medications (amitriptyline, desipramine, and imipramine), gabapentin (Neurontin), pregabalin (Lyrica), venlafaxine (Effexor), and duloxetine (Cymbalta). These are medications that were originally developed for depression or seizures, but have been discovered to alleviate neuropathic pain. These are not pain medications that immediately produce short-term relief, bur rather help to regulate the nerve pain long-term. Normally, the medications are begun at very low doses and gradually increased, especially since women with vulvodynia are often very sensitive to medications.

Some health care providers use topical medications as well, including topical estrogen, lidocaine, gabapentin, or amitriptyline/baclofen combination. There is much less experience with these as a means of clearing vulvodynia.

There are two main patterns of vulvodynia. Most common is vestibulodynia, or vestibulitis, where burning, stinging, or stabbing pain occurs only at the opening or just inside the vagina, mostly with sexual activity, tampons, tight clothing—anything that touches or rubs the area. Some women experience pain occurring in a larger area; this type is called generalized vulvodynia. The treatment for these types of vulvodynia is the same for the most part. However, women with the very localized pain of vestibulodynia have the option of an additional therapy, surgical removal of the painful area. This surgery, called a vestibulectomy, is extremely beneficial, especially when the pelvic floor muscle abnormalities have been corrected before the procedure.

Many women find that, after a long period of pain with sexual activity, reestablishing comfortable and fun sexual activity is difficult. Fear and the psychologic effects of this chronic genital pain very often require counseling, to include couple counseling.

With proper therapy, the discomfort of vulvodynia usually is controlled and women are able to lead a normal life.

INDEX

Page numbers ending in "*f*" refer to figures. Page numbers ending in "*t*" refer to tables.